X-ray Department
Royal United Hospital
Bath

Computed Body Tomography

COMPUTED BODY TOMOGRAPHY

Editors

Joseph K. T. Lee, M.D.

.

Stuart S. Sagel, M.D.

.

Robert J. Stanley, M.D.

The Edward Mallinckrodt Institute of Radiology
Washington University School of Medicine
St. Louis, Missouri

Raven Press ▪ New York

Raven Press, 1140 Avenue of the Americas, New York, New York 10036

Made in the United States of America

Great care has been taken to maintain the accuracy of the information contained in the volume. However, Raven Press cannot be held responsible for errors or for any consequences arising from the use of the information contained herein.

Library of Congress Cataloging in Publication Data
Main entry under title:

Computed body tomography.

Includes bibliographical references and index.
1. Tomography.   I. Lee, Joseph K. T.   II. Sagel,
Stuart S.   III. Stanley, Robert J.
RC78.7.T6C6415   1983   616'.07'572   81-40546
ISBN 0-89004-703-0

First printing, November 1982
Second printing, February 1983
Third printing, September 1983

This work is dedicated to our wives,
Christina, Beverlee, and Sally,
and to our children,
Alexander, Betsy, and Catherine
Scott, Darryl, and Brett
Ann, Robert, Cathy, and Sara

Preface

Computed tomography was first developed for intracranial imaging in the late 1960s by Godfrey Hounsfield at the Central Research Laboratories of EMI Limited. Since that time, major technical advances have resulted in substantial improvements in image quality concomitant with a marked reduction in scanning time. In the past seven years, CT has become gradually accepted as an accurate and practical diagnostic technique, with its clinical applications broadened to include virtually every part of the body. This has occurred despite the initial skepticism of many regarding the value of extracranial CT in comparison to its cost. We have been fortunate to personally witness the germination and development of computed body tomography from its inception, to a technique that now has an enormous impact upon our practice of radiology. This radiological method has fulfilled the expectations of its early users and has proven to be an important and efficacious procedure for the evaluation of a myriad of pathologic problems.

In many cases, the information obtained by CT is unique. On occasion, data derived from CT have enabled reevaluation of traditional concepts of various disease processes. Body CT has supplanted or encroached upon other radiological procedures. Laryngography has been replaced. Lymphangiography for staging lymphoma and other neoplasms has declined drastically. Rapid, sequential, contrast-enhanced CT scans have been successfully substituted for angiography in many patients to diagnose or exclude suspected vascular lesions (e.g., aneurysm, dissection) or to assess the extent of a neoplastic process.

This volume has been prepared to present a comprehensive text on the application of CT to the extracranial regions of the body. It is intended primarily for use by the radiologist either in clinical practice or in training. The internist, pediatrician, and surgeon also will derive beneficial information about the relative value and indications for CT of the body, with their patients as the ultimate beneficiaries. Anatomy in each area is stressed initially, since such knowledge is basic to proper interpretation. Regions often are presented serially to portray the caudad progression of structures. The CT findings in a variety of pathologic conditions are described and illustrated. Instruction is provided to optimize the conduct, analysis, and interpretation of CT scans. Both technical and interpretative errors can occur in CT examinations, and hopefully the reader will benefit from our previous innumerable mistakes.

Comprehensive discussions of how CT is compatible with other clinical and radiological procedures for a variety of problems have been attempted. Both radiologist and referring clinician often are faced with the dilemma of determining the best radiologic approach toward documenting a specific diagnosis given a set of clinical findings. With the burgeoning availability of a wide variety of new radiologic techniques, there is often a tendency to perform a large number of examinations before drawing a conclusion. Such an approach, however, is extremely expensive and puts undue constraints on the total resources available for health care, besides being unfair to the individual patient who is subjected to unnecessary discomfort and risk.

The uses of CT we suggest have been developed through the cooperative efforts of the diagnostic radiology staff at the Mallinckrodt Institute. Each member has established an interest and expertise in a specific area. The proper sequencing of radiologic tests for a variety of clinical indications has been discussed in countless, joint consultations and conferences during the past several years. From this ongoing dialogue, our current ideas have evolved. We are well aware that equally valid alternative radiologic approaches to certain clinical problems are possible. It is obvious that available equipment and personal experience could modify the evaluation of any particular problem. Clearly our recommendations on the optimal use of CT are not final, and the enlightened physician continually will need to update his ideas about how CT fits in with other modalities as clinical research and technology continue to develop.

J.K.T.L.
S.S.S.
R.J.S.

Acknowledgments

Providing recognition to everyone involved in the production of this volume is extremely difficult because of the large number of individuals who aided immeasurably in forming the final product. We graciously thank the various contributors who kindly provided chapters in their areas of expertise in order to bring depth and completeness to the book.

A special note of gratitude goes to our secretaries, Sue Day, Lynn Losse, Carol Keller, and Karen Abdelhamid, who spent endless hours in typing the manuscripts and checking the references. Our appreciation is also extended to Patty Haring for her continuous assistance in organizing the CT files and locating CT cases for photography. Cramer Lewis and his staff in the Department of Medical Illustration at Washington University Medical School and Thomas Murry in our Photography Laboratory were extremely helpful in preparing the illustrative material.

Our thanks go to our residents and the many radiologic technologists who performed and monitored the CT studies. Their dedication is reflected in the high quality of scans used throughout this book.

We also would like to express our appreciation to the publisher, Raven Press, for the professional and sympathetic way they have handled the myriad problems encountered in publication. Most particularly, we would like to thank Anne Patterson and Mary Rogers for their timeless dedication and advice during each stage in the production of this book.

Finally, and most importantly, we would like to acknowledge the immeasurable debt of gratitude the authors owe to Dr. Ronald G. Evens, Chairman of our department, who, through the years, has provided us with the proper academic atmosphere conducive to such an endeavor. Without his constant encouragement, understanding, and support, this book could not have been written.

J.K.T.L.
S.S.S.
R.J.S.

Contents

Foreword xv
Ronald G. Evens

1. Physical Principles and Instrumentation 1
Michel M. Ter-Pogossian

2. Techniques 9
Dixie J. Aronberg

3. Larynx 37
Stuart S. Sagel

4. Thoracic Anatomy and Mediastinum 55
Stuart S. Sagel and Dixie J. Aronberg

5. Lung, Pleura, Pericardium, and Chest Wall 99
Stuart S. Sagel

6. Normal Abdominal Anatomy 131
Dennis M. Balfe, Roy R. Peterson, and Joseph K. T. Lee

7. Liver and Biliary Tract 167
Robert J. Stanley

8. Pancreas 213
Matthew A. Mauro and Robert J. Stanley

9. Spleen 243
Robert E. Koehler

10. Retroperitoneum 257
Joseph K. T. Lee

11. Abdominal Wall and Peritoneal Cavity 287
Robert G. Levitt

12. Alimentary Tract 307
Matthew A. Mauro and Robert E. Koehler

13. Kidneys 341
Bruce L. McClennan and Joseph K. T. Lee

14. Adrenals 379
Philip J. Weyman and Harvey S. Glazer

15. Pelvis 393
   Joseph K. T. Lee and Dennis M. Balfe

16. Spine 415
   Mohktar H. Gado, Fred J. Hodges III, and Jash I. Patel

17. Musculoskeletal System 453
   William A. Murphy, Louis A. Gilula, Judy M. Destouet, Barbara S. Monsees, Chandrakant C. Tailor, and William G. Totty

18. Pediatric Applications 517
   Marilyn J. Siegel

19. Comparative Imaging 535
   G. Leland Melson, Daniel R. Biello, and Joseph K. T. Lee

20. Radiation Oncology 547
   Miljenko V. Pilepich, Satish C. Prasad, and Todd H. Wasserman

21. The Economics and Politics of Computed Tomography 559
   Ronald G. Evens and R. Gilbert Jost

Subject Index 565

Contributors

The Edward Mallinckrodt Institute of Radiology
Washington University School of Medicine
St. Louis, Missouri 63110

Dixie J. Aronberg, M.D.
Assistant Professor of Radiology

Dennis M. Balfe, M.D.
Assistant Professor of Radiology

Daniel R. Biello, M.D.
Associate Professor of Radiology

Judy M. Destouet, M.D.
Assistant Professor of Radiology

Ronald G. Evens, M.D.
Elizabeth Mallinckrodt Professor of Radiology
Director, Mallinckrodt Institute of Radiology

Mokhtar H. Gado, M.D.
Professor of Radiology
Director, Neuroradiology Section

Louis A. Gilula, M.D.
Professor of Radiology
Co-Director, Musculoskeletal Section

Harvey S. Glazer, M.D.
Assistant Professor of Radiology

Fred J. Hodges III, M.D.
Professor of Radiology

R. Gilbert Jost, M.D.
Associate Professor of Radiology

Robert E. Koehler, M.D.
Currently, Professor and Vice Chairman
Department of Radiology
University of Alabama School of Medicine
Birmingham, Alabama

Joseph K. T. Lee, M.D.
Associate Professor of Radiology
Co-Director, Computed Body
Tomography Section

Robert G. Levitt, M.D.
Associate Professor of Radiology

Matthew A. Mauro, M.D.
Currently, Assistant Professor of Radiology
Director, Section of Gastrointestinal Radiology
University of North Carolina School of Medicine
Chapel Hill, North Carolina

Bruce L. McClennan, M.D.
Professor of Radiology
Director, Abdominal Radiology Section

G. Leland Melson, M.D.
Associate Professor of Radiology
Director, Diagnostic Ultrasound

Barbara S. Monsees, M.D.
Instructor in Radiology

William A. Murphy, M.D.
Associate Professor of Radiology
Co-Director, Musculoskeletal Section

Jash I. Patel, M.D.
Instructor in Radiology

Roy R. Peterson, Ph.D.
Professor of Anatomy
Department of Anatomy

Miljenko V. Pilepich, M.D.
Associate Professor of Radiology
Division of Radiation Oncology

Satish C. Prasad, M.D.
Currently, Assistant Professor of Radiology
Division of Radiological Sciences
Upstate Medical Center
Syracuse, New York

Stuart S. Sagel, M.D.
Professor of Radiology
Director, Chest Radiology Section
Co-Director, Computed Body
Tomography Section

Marilyn J. Siegel, M.D.
Assistant Professor of Radiology

Robert J. Stanley, M.D.
Currently, Professor and Chairman
Department of Radiology
University of Alabama School of Medicine
Birmingham, Alabama

Chandrakant C. Tailor, M.D.
Currently, Staff Radiologist
Christian Hospitals
St. Louis, Missouri

Michel M. Ter-Pogossian, Ph.D.
Professor of Radiology
Director, Division of Radiation Sciences

William G. Totty, M.D.
Assistant Professor of Radiology

Todd H. Wasserman, M.D.
Associate Professor of Radiology
Division of Radiation Oncology

Philip J. Weyman, M.D.
Assistant Professor of Radiology

Foreword

Ronald G. Evens

It is my privilege to introduce a book dedicated to many aspects of computed tomography (CT) and its role in modern medical care. It seems appropriate to begin with a history of CT, which in its early stages has many similarities to the early history of radiology. Both radiology and CT are relatively new to the practice of medicine; the X-ray was discovered in 1895 and CT was introduced in 1972. Both are identified with scientists, Wilhelm Conrad Roentgen and Godfrey Hounsfield (Fig. 1), respectively, who had little if any medical or biological background. Both radiology and CT were declared to be "revolutionary" in less than two years and were established as important and significant scientific contributions leading to Nobel prizes in less than ten years. Both were highly controversial due to economic and social issues in their early development.

EARLY INVESTIGATIONS

Exercises in reconstruction of images from individual data points have been of interest in mathematics or physics for many years. Investigators include Radon (1917), Bracewell (1956), Oldendorf (1961), Kuhl (1963), and Cormack (1963) (2).

Allan M. Cormack, who shared the Nobel Prize in Medicine with Godfrey Hounsfield in 1979, was relatively unknown to many radiologists and scientists who were closely involved with CT. Dr. Cormack was serving as a lecturer in physics to the University of Capetown, South Africa, in 1955 when he was assigned as the hospital physicist to the Groote Schuur Hospital Department of Radiation Therapy for 1½ days per week, because the full-time physicist had resigned. He quickly noted the problems, still apparent today, of inhomogeneities of normal body tissue that create difficulties in radiation therapy treatment planning. He developed a mathematical approach to this problem and intermittently performed experimental work over the next six years (3). Publications of his work appeared during 1963 and 1964 with "virtually no response."

Although the work of Cormack and others was fundamental, serious medical or commercial interest was not stimulated. It remained for Godfrey Hounsfield at EMI to develop independently a practical system for clinical radiological studies.

In 1968, Mr. Hounsfield was completing a major project using large-scale computers for the EMI Corporation and the government of the United Kingdom. He was at a transition time in his personal responsibilities and was asked by the Central Research Laboratory (CRL), the basic research organization of EMI, for his opinion about his next project. He suggested that computers and mathematics could be used to reconstruct an image from sets of accurate X-ray measurements through the body from multiple angles. CRL and the management of EMI agreed to set aside resources to pursue this idea.

During the next several months, Mr. Hounsfield pursued this project in a laboratory located in Hayes, England (a short distance from Heathrow Airport). The early laboratory experiments were performed on relatively primitive equipment that included a standard metal working lathe and an americium isotopic source of gamma rays. Early images were produced from simple phantoms and an anatomical specimen of human brain. The initial results were highly encouraging, showing a computer reconstructed image that was similar to the anatomical specimen, although it required 9 days to scan the object and 2½ hours to process a single image (5).

Further investigations and the major decision to utilize an X-ray tube as a source of photons to replace the gamma source reduced the mechanical scanning time from 9 days to 9 hours. As is typical for research and development, many triumphs and catastrophes occurred during the early months of research. For example, the first experiments were performed with formalin-preserved cadaver specimens, and early apparent "anatomical observations" that confused the researchers were due to the formalin treatment. Research experiments then were performed on fresh tissue of cows and other animals from the butcher shop that were more "anatomical," but difficulties arose because the specimens aged during the long scan times and small gas bubbles were produced. Finally, a prototype unit was prepared for clinical studies of the brain and placed in the Atkinson Morley Hospital near Wimbledon in 1972.

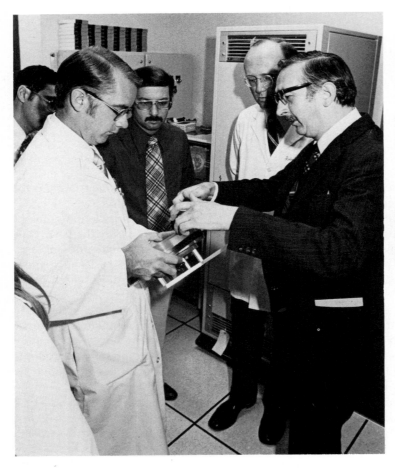

FIG. 1. Godfrey N. Hounsfield (right) describing CT phantom correlation with the EMI 5000 (prototype-body) scanner in 1976 with Dr. Ronald Evens (left). In background (left to right) Drs. Gilbert Jost (partially hidden), Stuart Sagel, and Robert Stanley.

CLINICAL DEVELOPMENT OF CT

The early clinical results were reported at the April 1972 Annual Congress of the British Institute of Radiology, and were quickly recognized as a major improvement in neuroradiology (1). Essentially all early clinical research was performed in the United Kingdom and the United States with equipment from EMI. The clinical importance of this new radiologic technique was not recognized initially by the manufacturer, and the EMI Corporation projected the need for the production of only 25 units. The first production model, called the Mark I, was limited to use on the head because of the slow scanning time (4½ min) and the need for a bag of water to be in close contact with the part of the anatomy scanned to eliminate any air gap. The first three production CT head units were installed at the Mayo Clinic, Massachusetts General Hospital, and the Presbyterian–St. Luke's Hospital in Chicago. The Mallinckrodt Institute of Radiology installed the 9th and 16th units built during 1973 and was the first institution to have two CT scanners.

The impact on neuroradiology was spectacular. Quickly, it was obvious to many observers that CT was a major advance. It was amazing to visualize the ventricles of the brain without having to instill air or contrast material. In a very few months, by the spring of 1974, CT was recognized as a major improvement by radiologists throughout the world and had become a term that was known to politicians, government regulators, and the general public. In the early years it was described as computerized axial tomography or "CAT" scanner and the word "CAT" became both famous and infamous.

The years of 1974 and 1975 were dynamic and controversial. The growth of the CT industry and the incorporation of CT into neuroradiologic practice were dynamic. Concern over the uncontrolled expansion of this highly expensive new technology led to national controversy. Computed tomography became essential to modern neuroradiologic evaluation; many commercial corporations developed or announced plans to develop some form of a CT unit (in 1976 at least 22 separate companies were advertising products); and serious concerns were voiced by politicians, health planners, and government regulators on the "dangers" (primarily economical) of this new technology.

Commercial competition was at a high level and generally was useful to the development of this new technology. An early commercial development from

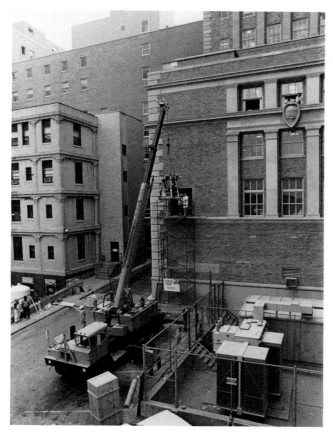

FIG. 2. Prototype EMI body scanner being brought by derrick through an opening made in the outer wall of the Mallinckrodt Institute in August 1975.

several manufacturers (1974) was a body scanner with scanning times of 2½ minutes or longer that eliminated the water bag and had a larger gantry aperture so that the thorax or abdomen could be studied. Unfortunately, the contrast and spatial resolution were poor. Respiratory and other physiological motions caused severe degradation of the reconstructed images. Accordingly, diagnostic body CT was not initially viewed as providing clinically valuable information.

In the summer of 1975, EMI announced a CT unit (the 5000 series) with an 18-second scanning time and no requirement for a water bag. It produced the first images of the chest and abdomen with reproducible and satisfactory resolution. The era of clinically useful body CT had finally arrived. The prototype EMI 5000 was initially located in London at Northwick Park and two other units were soon installed at the Mallinckrodt Institute of Radiology and the Mayo Clinic in the United States. A series of important clinical evaluations, at these and other medical centers, demonstrated the importance of CT as a diagnostic method for use throughout the body (4,6–8).

Although CT development was very important for

patients, it came at a time when considerations of cost for medical care were rapidly becoming a national concern. Questions of "cost control" and "efficacy" were especially prominent not only in the United States, but also throughout the world in the early 1970s. Computed tomography became the focus of questions about technology in medicine by politicians, regulators, and economists. Radiologists and clinicians had to evaluate critically the appropriate role of CT both in a medical and cost-controlling environment; thorough discussion of the economic considerations will be presented in a later chapter of this book.

Computed tomography has now become a major factor in most radiologic facilities throughout the world. It is available to most patients in the developed countries and in general is of high quality. Dedicated head units have, for the most part, been replaced by general purpose scanners with rapid scanning time (1–5 sec), rapid reconstruction (1–35 sec), and narrow collimation (2–10 mm), capable of producing high resolution images. With sufficient clinical experience, CT has become a major part of diagnostic and therapeutic radiology.

PERSONAL EXPERIENCE AND REFLECTIONS

When I first saw the early images of the Atkinson Morley-EMI unit in 1972, it was clear that a major revolution was about to occur. The ability to see the ventricles of the brain without air was very important. Anyone who had participated in a pneumoencephalogram (especially the patient) recognized a major improvement.

The staff of the Mallinckrodt Institute of Radiology recognized the importance of CT soon after the early presentations of clinical work from the United Kingdom. We contacted EMI and two head CT units were in place and operational by the fall of 1973. It was immediately obvious that the specialties of neurology and neurosurgery would be altered dramatically. By current standards, the CT images were crude. The images required more than 3 minutes of scanning time and any movement of the head produced significant degradation. The matrix size was 80 × 80, producing a very coarse, checkerboard image. The equipment itself was not very reliable, resulting in frequent downtime, and, of course, we were quite inexperienced. Despite these early problems, diagnostic evaluation and resultant treatment of patients were improved dramatically.

In early 1974, I met with the senior members of the scientific and corporate management of EMI, including Godfrey Hounsfield, Bill Ingham (Director of CRL-EMI), and Bob Froggatt (Chief Scientist, EMI). The outcome of this meeting was that this group subsequently requested that the MIR be an evaluation site of their prototype body scanner (the EMI 5000).

On arrival of the prototype unit in St. Louis in August 1975, it was discovered that it was too large to fit onto an elevator. Our quick solution was literally to knock a hole in the outer wall of the building and bring the instrument to the second floor by derrick (Figure 2). The unit was made operational within a week and clinical trials were begun.

As I view the history of radiology before CT, it was generally believed that contributions to improved diagnosis would be correlated with improvement in spatial resolution. Computed tomography is a technique that certainly improved diagnostic methods, even with comparatively poor spatial resolution in comparison to conventional radiography. I have always found it interesting that the combination of an inventive scientist and a non-radiologic corporation was able to develop this new technique.

Finally, I would like to record my personal appreciation for Godfrey Hounsfield. We have developed a close relationship that began in 1974. It was my pleasure to invite him as an early Wendell Scott Lecturer at the Mallinckrodt Institute in 1976. This was his third visit to St. Louis but the first of a personal nature. Godfrey has many interesting and unique talents and patterns. At that time, he insisted on staying on London time even with visits to the United States. Accordingly, it was difficult for him to visit my home (6:00 p.m. in St. Louis is 12:00 midnight in London), but we arranged an appropriate schedule. In 1976 I had a selfish interest—I wanted my wife, Hanna, and my children to meet and dine with a gentleman whom I predicted would be a Nobel laureate of the future. The scheduling worked and my prediction came true.

REFERENCES

1. Ambrose J, Hounsfield G: Computerized transverse axial tomography. *Br J Radiol* 46:148, 1973
2. Cormack AM: Representation of a function by its line integrals, with some radiological application. *J Appl Physiol* 34: 2722–2727, 1963
3. Cormack AM: Early two-dimensional reconstruction (CT scanning) and recent topic stemming from it. *J Comput Assist Tomogr* 4:658–664, 1980
4. Evens RG: New frontier for radiology: Computed tomography. *Am J Roentgenol* 126:1116–1129, 1976
5. Hounsfield GN: Computed medical imaging. *Science* 210:22–28, 1980
6. Sagel SS, Stanley RJ, Evens RG: Early clinical experience with motionless wholebody computed tomography. *Radiology* 119:321–330, 1976
7. Sheedy PF, Stephens DH, Hattery RR, Muhm JR, Hartman GW: Computed tomography of the body: Initial clinical trial with the EMI prototype. *Am J Roentgenol* 127:23–51, 1976
8. Stanley RJ, Sagel SS, Levitt RG: Computed tomography of the body: Early trends in application and accuracy of the method. *Am J Roentgenol* 127:56–67, 1976

Computed Body Tomography

Chapter 1

Physical Principles and Instrumentation

Michel M. Ter-Pogossian

The development in the early 1970s of computerized axial tomography, now more commonly called computed tomography (CT), led to the award of the Nobel Prize in 1979 to Godfrey Hounsfield of EMI, Ltd. and to Allen Cormack of Tufts University. This technique not only provided radiologic imaging with a well proven and broadly utilized clinical tool but also led to an extensive reevaluation of radiologic imaging stimulated by the understanding of the physical principles pertaining to CT.

Tomography (from the Greek *tomos*–meaning section) has been used extensively in diagnostic radiology, well before the advent of CT, to provide transverse as well as longitudinal sections of the human body. In these forms of "conventional" tomography the image forming variable is the spatial distribution of X-ray attenuation coefficients in the imaged sections. The tomographic effect is achieved by moving the roentgenographic film and the source of X-rays in synchrony about the patient (Fig. 1) in such a fashion that the structures in the tomographic plane remain in focus while those in planes above and below are blurred out. For this reason conventional tomography is sometimes referred to as "in-focus" or blurring tomography.

Computed tomography became an important component of our radiologic armamentarium at a time when conventional tomography was widely recognized as a highly useful clinical procedure. The most striking difference between the two tomographic radiographic imaging methods lies in the ability of CT to depict considerably more subtle differences in the absorption or attenuation of X-rays than is possible with the conventional roentgenographic techniques including tomography. This is, however, at the cost of spatial resolution, which is appreciably inferior in CT examinations than that which can be achieved with standard roentgenograms. This primary virtue of computed tomography, the ability to detect very minor differences in radiographic contrast, thus expands the ability of radiology to portray boundaries between different tissues that are normally indistinguishable on conven-

tional radiographic examinations. For example, in the brain, tumors and edematous areas that were invisible on standard skull radiographs and required an invasive angiographic procedure for their depiction, became apparent in many instances on CT images.

THE PHYSICAL BASIS OF CT

The ability of CT to detect minute differences in the X-ray attenuation properties of the tissues to be visualized stems from three factors: (a) the signal to noise ratio of the data acquisition in CT is more favorable than in conventional diagnostic radiology; (b) scattered radiation, which depresses contrast resolution substantially in most conventional diagnostic examinations, is considerably reduced in CT; (c) the method of image reconstruction with CT is unique and different from that of conventional tomography.

How these three factors operate can be explained with the help of a schematic representation of the simplest CT system (Fig. 2). A narrow beam of X-rays scans across the structure to be imaged in a linear fashion. While traversing the object (patient), the nonabsorbed X-rays are detected by some form of radiation detector that scans synchronously with the beam. This linear scan sequence is repeated at different angles around the object. The data thus acquired consist of a series of "profiles" that reflect simply the attenuation properties of the object scanned at different angles. From these profiles, through the application of a complex mathematical algorithm, a transverse tomographic image (section) of the object examined can be reconstructed.

The data acquired from CT for the reconstruction of the image exhibit a better signal-to-noise ratio than that achieved in conventional radiography because the number of X-ray photons used per resolution element in the examination is considerably greater than in conventional diagnostic radiology, and the detector utilized in CT exhibits less noise than radiographic film.

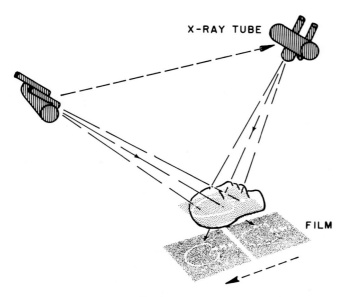

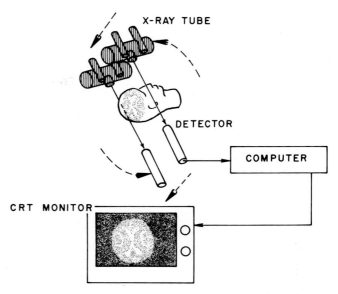

FIG. 1. Diagram illustrating the principle of longitudinal radiographic tomography (reproduced from *Semin Roentgenol* 12: 13–25, 1977).

FIG. 2. Diagram illustrating the principle of CT (reproduced from *Semin Roentgenol* 12:13–25, 1977).

In CT the beam of radiation is narrowly collimated, both before entering and after emerging from the patient; under these circumstances only a minimal fraction of the scattered radiation reaches the detector. Consequently, the tissue contrast differentiation capability of CT is considerably superior to that which can be achieved with conventional radiography, even when grids are used to decrease the unwanted contribution of scattered radiation.

Finally, the filtered back-projection method of image reconstruction used in CT provides images that are unencumbered by superimposed underlying and overlying structures, which, although blurred, are recorded in conventional tomography.

THE CT APPARATUS

The different components of the CT apparatus are shown in Fig. 3. Generation of the CT image is accomplished in several steps.

The data, in the form of profiles from which the image is reconstructed, are acquired by measurement of the attenuation of the X-radiation passing through the part to be imaged. The ability of a CT device to faithfully reproduce the morphology of the assessed structures in the reconstructed image depends on the number of physical measurements taken per unit image area. Consequently, if an anatomical structure is to be imaged with a resolution of several lines per millimeter, the detector used in the imaging process must "sample" the structure with a precision much finer than expected in the image—in this particular case, several samples per millimeter. In fact, analytical de-

terminations have established that the sampling "frequency" in reproducing a structure must be at least two to three times as "fine" as the expected resolution in the image. Thus, if a structure is to be reproduced with a resolution of 4 lines per mm, the number of measurements that must be sampled by the detector system should be no less than 8 to 12 per mm. In CT this requires suitable linear and angular sampling of the object to be imaged by the X-ray beam. Data acquisition in the projection of the image of the structure along a line perpendicular to the direction of the beam of X-rays (often called the CT profile) is reflected in the linear sampling frequency. The number of measurements taken at different angles around the object is the angular sampling frequency.

A large number of different motions have been incorporated into CT gantries to achieve the proper linear and angular sampling. At this time, two configurations are used in the majority of commercially available CT devices (Fig. 4). In the first configuration (rotate–rotate) the X-ray tube and the array of detectors rotate synchronously about the patient to be imaged. In the other (rotate–stationary detector array) the detectors are arranged in a stationary ring encircling the patient and the X-ray tube rotates around the patient usually within the detector array. Both of these configurations exhibit some specific physical and technological advantages and concomitant disadvantages, with no clear superiority for either.

These data, often after some preliminary mathematical preprocessing, are converted by a computer applied algorithm into an "image," which is stored in a digital form in the computer's memory. The stored "image" can be displayed either in an analog form as

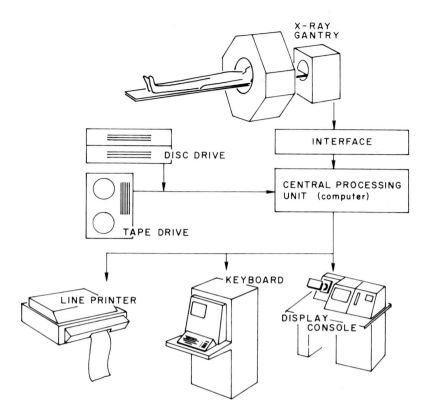

FIG. 3. Diagram illustrating the components of a CT system (reproduced from *Semin Roentgenol* 12:13–25, 1977).

an optical image on a cathode ray oscilloscope (television monitor) or as a digital matrix produced by a line printer.

The faithful display of the CT image on the cathode ray oscilloscope screen requires that the display matrix be sufficiently fine to reproduce without, or with, minimal distortion, the image-forming data provided by the CT reconstruction algorithm. Typically, image matrices used in CT displays vary from 256×256 to 512×512 pixels. Computed tomographic devices also incorporate the ability to magnify a portion of the image (zooming). For example, a quarter of the original image may be displayed over the whole screen. In its simplest form, this process is accomplished after image reconstruction by assigning several display pixels (e.g., four) to every original pixel and by interpolation of data between adjacent display pixels to achieve a smooth image. Such a magnification process does not improve the inherent resolution of the CT image, but it may render some details more perceptible. In some of the newer CT systems, recalculation of the raw data from a region of interest prior to image reconstruction is possible; this approach potentially can improve the image quality in a given area. The same raw data can be used to produce different transaxial reconstructions depending on the user's needs. High resolution small area scans (e.g., 5 cm in diameter with a voxel size of 0.2 mm $\times$ 0.2 mm $\times$ 1 cm) can be

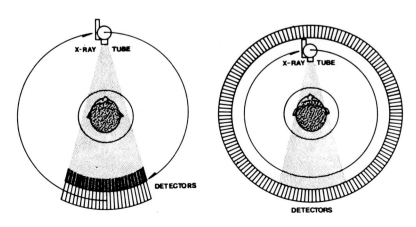

FIG. 4. Two configurations commonly used for data acquisition in current CT devices. **Left:** Rotate-moving detector array (3rd generation) configuration. **Right:** Rotate-stationary detector array (4th generation) configuration (reproduced from *Semin Roentgenol* 12:13–25, 1977).

produced in addition to or instead of the usual large area scans (e.g., 32 cm in diameter with a voxel size of 1 mm × 1 mm × 1 cm).

Reducing as much as possible the range of attenuation values of the tissues traversed by the X-ray beam and thus measured by the detectors is advantageous for the algorithmic reconstruction process. It is desirable to eliminate air surrounding the body part examined to make the region as close to a sphere as practicable for optimal imaging. In the early CT devices, this was accomplished by placing the upper portion of the patient's head in a box filled with water. Obviously, such an approach is not very practical for body imaging, nor was it for the cranium. Modern CT devices minimize the range of absorptions by the use of wedge-shaped filters, which tend to equalize the attenuation of X-radiation throughout the part examined. The shape and size of the wedges vary with the size of the reconstruction field selected for the study.

The image displayed on the oscilloscope can be permanently recorded by various photographic methods, including Polaroid film or a conventional photographic emulsion. The majority of hard copy imaging is now performed using multiformat cameras that are capable of recording simultaneously a number of images on an X-ray film that can be conveniently developed in the radiology department. The numerical data that provide the CT image can be stored on video tape or magnetic disks; relatively inexpensive "floppy" disks are now commonly used for archival storage.

The earliest CT devices utilized scintillation detectors as radiation sensors. These consist of a crystal that fluoresces when struck by ionizing radiation; it is optically coupled to a photomultiplier tube that converts the fluorescence into an electronic signal. A number of different crystals has been used, including sodium iodide initially and then bismuth germanate. Later, gas detectors, such as xenon, were introduced. These consist of a gas, usually at high pressure, surrounded by two electrodes; the radiation is detected by collecting the ions generated in the gas. Large arrays of such gas detectors can be effectively packed in various configurations. Most recently, detectors made of a fluorescent crystal optically coupled to a photo diode that generates an electric current when struck by light have been utilized and are proving increasingly popular.

The computers employed in CT devices basically are systems that have been developed for other purposes and that usually incorporate large buffer memories needed for the large amounts of data contained in the CT images. Most modern CT devices incorporate array processors that carry out a portion of the image reconstruction process without the use of the computer per se. The image display systems utilized in CT also have been adapted from systems developed for

other purposes. They consist of a high quality television monitor (oscilloscope) interfaced to the computer memory.

THE CT IMAGE

The CT image generated represents a slice of selected thickness. This selection is achieved by collimating the beam of X-rays produced; the thickness usually is between 2 mm and 1 cm and varies depending on the requirements of each clinical study. Thus, although the CT image consists of a two-dimensional series or matrix of resolution elements, called pixels for picture elements, each pixel actually is a representation of a three-dimensional slice of tissue or voxel for volume element (Fig. 5). Each pixel in the tomographic image is proportional to the linear attenuation of X-rays within the actual voxel represented. The unit most widely used in expressing the attenuation of X-rays in a CT image is the "Hounsfield unit" (HU), in honor of the inventor of CT. This unit is defined as $\mu - \mu_\omega / \mu_\omega \times 1{,}000$ where μ is the attenuation coefficient of X-rays of tissue imaged and μ_ω is the attenuation coefficient for water. Thus an attenuation value given in HU is a relative expression referenced to the attenua-

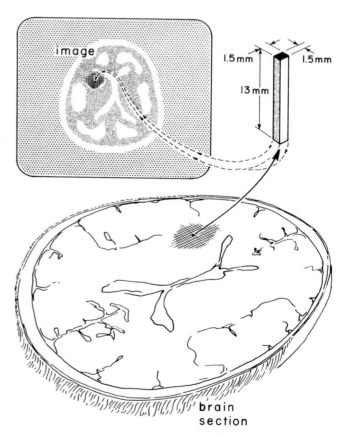

FIG. 5. Illustration of the relationship between the CT pixel displayed on the image and the voxel of tissue which it represents (reproduced from *Semin Roentgenol* 12:13–25, 1977).

tion of radiation in water. Positive values represent tissues with attenuation values higher than that of water and negative values lower. The purpose of incorporating the number 1,000, sometimes called the magnifying value, into the above equation is simply to expand the scale sufficiently to provide whole number attenuation values.

It is imperative to recognize that *Hounsfield values yielded by a specific CT system are not absolute.* The Hounsfield value represents the attenuation of a polychromatic beam of X-rays generated at energies (kVp) that may vary from examination to examination and/or for different CT devices. Furthermore, the spectral distribution of the initial X-radiation is modified by its passage through higher atomic number Z materials, such as bone and contrast media; the final CT values may vary appreciably depending on the amount of high Z materials encompassing the region where the Hounsfield number is determined. Furthermore, the Hounsfield number may be affected by the reconstruction algorithm used, detector efficiency, and electronic noise. It is really not possible to convert with accuracy CT numbers on any given scanner by establishing a comparative calibration. If CT values are to be compared, even within the same unit for different examinations, it is prudent to calibrate the unit at frequent intervals, which can be accomplished by means of suitably designed phantom.

Because the CT image is recorded in a digital form, it is relatively easy to apply to it a number of manipulations designed to improve the perceptibility of potentially diagnostic information encoded in the reconstructed data. Various interactive devices have been incorporated to alter the image displayed on the monitor and hopefully enhance recognition of diagnostic findings. These include adjustment of the window width and level, magnifying a region of interest, or producing reformatted sagittal or coronal images. A most important manipulation called "windowing" consists of selecting an upper and lower contrast level, between which the tissues are displayed. This endows the radiologist with the ability to either expand or decrease the dynamic range of contrast densities displayed. A narrow window width, which is particularly valuable, increases perceptibility of objects with little difference in inherent contrast. The window level can also be adjusted to make it optimal for the structure being assessed (e.g., approximately −600 HU for viewing the lungs and approximately +200 HU for assessing bone). It should be emphasized that none of these image manipulations in any way really increases information content, but they simply permit the display of the data in a manner that, hopefully, facilitates diagnosis.

The alteration of the spectral distribution of the beam of X-rays as it traverses the tissues to be imaged by filtration (beam hardening) limits the accuracy possible with the reconstruction process. The method of image acquisition and reconstruction in CT renders these images particularly susceptible to artifact formation because any measurement affects the whole image, and noise is easily propagated. In many instances very small differences in X-ray attenuation form the CT image; therefore the physical measurements must be carried out with high accuracy and precision, often under conditions of relatively low signal-to-noise ratio. A condition required for the faithful reproduction of the object in the image is that the attenuation of X-rays in any given voxel be the same no matter what the incidence of the radiation is. This condition would be fulfilled for monochromatic X-rays, but the X-radiation used in CT is polychromatic (or polyenergetic) and it undergoes filtration as it traverses the tissues. This results in an unequal removal of lower energy photons from the X-ray spectrum. As long as the tissues traversed contain only low Z elements, as is the case for soft tissues, the beam hardening is minuscule. But if higher Z materials are included in the traversed tissues, such as bone, iodinated contrast media, or metallic objects, then the spectral distribution of X-rays may change radically for measurements taken at different angles, thus providing the CT reconstruction algorithm with incompatible information. Under this situation not only are unreliable Hounsfield values generated, but at worst annoying artifacts may be created. Most CT devices incorporate physical and mathematical means to compensate at least partially for bone and iodinated contrast media, but metallic objects, such as surgical clips, are often less well tolerated and result in artifacts.

An additional important factor that greatly influences the Hounsfield value determination is the partial volume effect. The pixel depicted in the CT image may include within its true volume (voxel) structures with different X-ray attenuation properties. Under this circumstance, the Hounsfield number will represent a weighted average of the tissues included. Interpretation of the value represented by the pixel must include the understanding that sometimes this value refers to an inhomogeneous sample. The partial volume effect on CT number may be particularly important when the voxel incorporates structures of widely different X-ray absorption properties (e.g., pulmonary nodule and lung parenchyma).

Another source of artifact is motion of the patient during data acquisition. Such a situation provides the reconstruction algorithm with incompatible pieces of information that result in artifacts. This effect is particularly noticeable for high-absorption structures. Drift in the sensitivity of detectors also creates artifacts that may assume different appearances depending on the design of the CT device used.

THE PERFORMANCE OF CT DEVICES

Three criteria of performance can be applied to most imaging systems, particularly CT devices. They are *spatial resolution, contrast resolution,* and *temporal resolution.*

Spatial resolution is a measure of the system to discriminate images of objects separated by a small distance. An accepted method for this determination consists of measuring the point spread function of the system and calculating its modulation transfer function. Often a test object consisting of a series of radioopaque lines embedded in a plate transparent to X-rays is used. Contrast resolution in a radiologic image is usually expressed as the percentage of the X-radiation transmitted in one area of the image with respect to the radiation transmitted by the surrounding or adjacent area. This can be mathematically expressed as $C_{ab} = B_a - B_b/B_a \times 100$, where C_{ab} is the contrast of area *a* with respect to area *b;* B_a is the number of photons per unit area in area *a* and B_b is the recorded number of photons per unit area in area *b.* Temporal resolution is the length of time required by the system to yield an image of predetermined quality. A similar conceptual determination is the ability of a system to repeat examinations at frequent time intervals.

As with most imaging systems, these three variables in CT are not independent. Measurement of spatial resolution carried out with a test object exhibiting 100% contrast difference will yield a value disparate from the one obtained with an object with lower inherent contrast. Contrast resolution determinations depend strongly on the size of the area in which the contrast is measured. The temporal resolution of the system generally will vary depending on the quality of the image desired by the radiologist. These comments emphasize that any measure of the performance of a CT device is valid only for certain circumscribed conditions. Most modern CT devices exhibit a spatial resolution of somewhat better than 1 line per mm, a contrast resolution of better than 0.5%, and a temporal resolution of approximately 1 to 4 sec. Such precision presumes that there is no significant statistical variation in the number of X-ray photons yielding the image. But under normal conditions of utilization of CT systems, these performances are seldom achieved simultaneously. This is particularly true when examining a markedly obese patient; it is seldom possible to fulfill this requirement without exposing the patient to an unduly high dose of radiation. In some CT devices the radiologist is provided with the ability to alter the reconstruction algorithm or filter function. In general, this ability means trading spatial resolution for contrast resolution. Thus, a "smoother" filter function provides an image that contains a lower spatial frequency range (resolution) but with improved contrast resolution.

Most CT devices are operated with heavily filtered X-rays generated with an energy somewhere between 120 and 140 kVp. This energy range was selected as a compromise because practical considerations had to be interfaced with basic physical principles. Much lower X-radiation energy cannot be used in CT since at lower energies the production of X-rays by the tube is inefficient and a sufficiently large enough number of photons could not be generated in a tolerably short period of time. In addition, many of the lower energy X-rays produced would be attenuated in the tissues traversed and the beam hardening effect would be much more troublesome than with the higher energy photons. Although higher energy radiation than used for CT could be created with a higher efficiency in the target of the X-ray tube, it would be more difficult to produce and less desirable because of lower contrast resolution.

One of the limiting factors in temporal resolution is imposed by the X-ray tube. In most current CT de-

TABLE 1. *Single slice maximum doses for various body CT scanners[a]*

Device	kV	mA	Time (sec)	Maximum skin dose (rad)	Ref.
Ohio-Nuclear 50FS	140	35	20/36	2.4/4.8	(1)
Ohio-Nuclear 2020P	130	40/200	2	1.5/6.5	(1)
Siemens Somatom	125	230	4	1.6	(1)
EMI-5005	140	—	20	2.3/2.8	(2)
GE CT/T-8800	120	75/1200	4.8/9.6	0.4/6.5	(3)
EMI 7070	120	96	3	2.3	(4)

(1) McCullough EC, Payne JT: *Radiology* 129:457–463, 1978
(2) Hobday P, Parker RP: *Brit J Radiol* 51:926–927, 1978
(3) Cohen J: *J Comput Assist Tomogr* 3:197–203, 1979
(4) Eichling JO: Personal communication
[a] It should be noted that through better equipment design, the radiation doses are being lowered and these values, as well as those in Table 2, are probably high. Radiation doses resulting from CT examination can vary widely depending upon the size of the patient and on the radiologist's decision concerning the exposure factors used. Thus, these figures should be regarded only as approximations.

TABLE 2. *Comparison of maximum skin absorbed doses for torso studies*[a]

Study	Max absorbed dose (rad/exam)
CT multiple-scan study	8
Chest film	0.030−0.050
Barium enema	15−20
Cardiac angiography	75

[a] Courtesy of J. O. Eichling.

TABLE 3. *Comparison of intergral absorbed doses for selected situations*[a]

Situation	Integral dose (grams-rad)
Tc-99m pertechnetate brain scan (20 mCi IV)	17,500
Chest radiography	300−500/film
Image-intensified abdominal fluoroscopy	40,000/min
Background radiation (St. Louis)	8,400/yr
Upper-limit recommended for radiation workers	350,000/yr
CT multi-scan torso study	20,000

[a] Courtesy J. O. Eichling.

vices the X-ray tube is subjected to much higher loading compared to conventional X-ray examinations. Limitations on obtaining fast repetitive scans are frequently imposed by the X-ray tube. And even with prudent operation, costly X-ray tubes often must be replaced.

Computed tomographic devices, in spite of extensive engineering improvements, remain relatively complex devices that operate properly only if they are regularly subjected to tight quality control. Such quality control involves usually at least two operations. The first one is a measure of the standard deviation of the Hounsfield values for a uniform object. Deviations from an optimal value indicate potentially serious irregularities in the performance of the system. Another important quality control test consists of obtaining CT images of a well-designed phantom. Phantoms are commercially available and can provide a convenient measure of field uniformity, spatial resolution, and calibration of the Hounsfield scale. Both of these tests ideally should be carried out daily.

RADIATION EXPOSURE

It is difficult to compare meaningfully the patient's radiation exposure in CT examinations to radiation exposures with the more conventional diagnostic radiologic procedures. In a conventional radiologic study, the patient's skin facing the X-ray tube receives the highest dose of radiation as it is exposed to the unattenuated beam; the skin at the exit side receives the lowest dose and the structures encompassed between receive doses that crudely decrease exponentially from the maximum to the minimum value. In CT the skin receives the highest dose of radiation, but

there is no difference between the entrance and exit sides because the source of radiation rotates about the patient. Also, the dose of radiation measured in the midbody is generally higher than that observed in the more conventional radiological procedures. This effect is enhanced because the energy of the radiation used for CT (heavily filtered radiation generated at 120 to 140 kVp) is somewhat higher than in conventional radiology.

An alternative expression of the radiation dose received by the patient is the integral dose, which varies considerably with the field size exposed. The integral dose in CT usually is lower than with comparable roentgenographic procedures because the total volume of tissue irradiated is smaller.

Tables 1 through 3 give some values of radiation exposures in conventional diagnostic procedures and in CT. It is probably fair to state that CT examinations in general do not deliver more radiation to the patient than conventional roentgenographic procedures, particularly if the radiation dose is assessed as integral dose.

BACKGROUND READING

Gordon R, Herman GT, Johnson SA: Image reconstruction from projections. *Sci Am* 233:56−68, 1975

Robb RA: X-ray computed tomography: An engineering synthesis of multiscientific principles. In: *Critical Reviews in Biomedical Engineering,* ed. by JR Bourne, Boca Raton, CRC Press, 1982, pp 265−333

Ter-Pogossian MM: Computerized cranial tomography: Equipment and physics. *Semin Roentgenol* 12:13−25, 1977

Chapter 2

Techniques

Dixie J. Aronberg

In the practice of medicine and radiology there should be a constant endeavor to maximize diagnostic information while minimizing risks and cost. Computed tomography seems to have an added responsibility to be efficient, having been thrust into the spotlight as a classic example of expensive technology. In this context, determining the most appropriate method of conducting the CT examination becomes an important consideration. The complexity of a CT unit need not dissuade one from becoming familiar with both the fine points of technique and the general concepts of CT. As with any other procedure, to understand the limitations of CT is to be able to use it more effectively. Based on the experience of others, as well as our own, this chapter attempts to answer the following questions: What makes a CT scan unique? What technical variables can we control and which ones make a significant difference? How does one conduct specific problem-oriented CT examinations for diagnostic or therapeutic purposes? How can oral and intravenous contrast media be used most effectively?

The physical principles of CT are detailed in Chapter 1. A review of the unique qualities of CT, however, is in order as a basis for discussing technique variables. Computed tomography requires roughly the same photon density as conventional radiography (approximately 10^7 photons/cm^2) but is designed to focus X-rays on a limited cross-sectional tissue plane and to utilize those X-rays more efficiently. The strong point of this imaging method is contrast sensitivity. The capability of resolving attenuation differences on the order of 0.5% is much superior to conventional radiography, which requires approximately a 10-fold difference in density for detection. The reasons for the improved contrast sensitivity include: (a) reduction in scatter, (b) removal of superimposed information, (c) sophisticated detection systems, and (d) sensitive display techniques (13). Scatter reduction is accomplished by use of a narrowly collimated X-ray beam. Overlapping information is successfully removed in the image display through the combination of transverse scanning and computer reconstruction techniques. The detecting systems employ a high signal-to-noise ratio with a wide dynamic range and are coupled with image processing that makes use of virtually all the available data.

The spatial resolution of CT is intimately related to quantum mottle and subject contrast. With high subject contrast and good precision, spatial resolution is approximately 1.5 times the pixel size, or, using standard CT systems, about 0.5 to 1 mm. This compares poorly to mammography studies (with resolution of approximately 0.1 mm) or to conventional film/screen imaging (0.2–0.4 mm). It is important to remember that spatial resolution does not represent the smallest size object that is detectable on a CT scan, since the contrast of the object is more important than size in determining whether a specific lesion will be distinguishable. A lesion relatively small as compared to pixel size may be seen if it is sufficiently different in attenuation value from the surrounding tissue.

Finally, the ability to display a detailed cross-sectional image adds a valuable dimension to radiology.

MACHINE VARIABLES AND OPTIONS

Multiple machine variables are controlled by the operator. These include kilovoltage (kV), milliamperage (mA), scan speed, collimation, scan interval, field of view, pixel size, and gantry tilt. There may be some minor variation among CT body scanners but, for the most part, these comments apply equally well to all scanning units.

The kilovoltage is maintained at a set level except in unusual circumstances. At our institution, 140 kVp is used for virtually all body CT exams. Variation of the kilovoltage will affect attenuation values (89). In fact, dual energy scanning (2,68) has the theoretical advantage of extending the sensitivity of CT for establishing more precise attenuation values. Some reasonably simple methods of applying the technique have been described (65,69). This may have implications for contrast enhanced CT, pulmonary nodule evaluation, and many other CT studies.

The milliamperage is adjusted for the size and composition of the part of the body being examined. This may vary from very low values (20 mA) for an

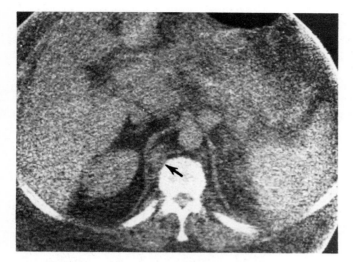

FIG. 1. Photopenia artifact. Coarse mottling caused by a paucity of X-rays reaching the detectors in this obese patient partially obscures an enlarged retrocrural node (arrow).

examination of the larynx to maximal output for an examination of the pelvis in a large patient. Photon deficiency (Fig. 1) may be noted when scanning an unusually obese person or it may result from an inappropriately low milliamperage; unnecessary radiation exposure is delivered to the patient if the milliamperage is too high.

Optimal scan speed is, in general, the fastest speed available within the limitation of achieving adequate photon flux. Faster scan speeds qualitatively improve images, especially where physiological motion is a problem, such as in the upper abdomen. This improvement has been shown to be diagnostically significant (66); however, most patients can be satisfactorily imaged by an 18-sec scanner. Fast scanning (2–5 sec) virtually eliminates motion artifact due to peristalsis

and dramatically decreases respiratory motion artifact (Fig. 2). Short scan times also allow "dynamic" scanning (rapid sequential scans), important in the CT evaluation of blood vessels and organ or lesion perfusion.

The collimation used is dependent on the purpose of the examination. If the intent is to demonstrate 1-cm or larger nodes in the retroperitoneum, then 1-cm collimation suffices. If, however, one is concerned with imaging the larynx, the disc spaces, or small adrenal masses, then thin slices from 2 to 5 mm may be needed. For most examinations, 1-cm collimation is used; 2- to 5-mm slice widths are reserved for detailed examinations, sometimes as a supplement to the initial study in which a small lesion is identified or suspected. Thick scans may result in incorrect attenuation values due to partial volume averaging of small structures. Contrariwise, a CT examination with very narrow collimation requires more slices to cover the same longitudinal area, thereby increasing time and radiation dose per study. In addition, in larger individuals, reduced slice thickness may lead to photon deficiency.

The scan interval, or the spacing distance between adjacent scans, is closely related to scan collimation as well as to the clinical problem. Contiguous scans or nearly contiguous scans are most frequently used. In certain instances, it is more practical to use 2-cm spacing, e.g., in retroperitoneal surveys, 2-cm intervals have been shown to be very nearly as accurate as contiguous scans (28).

The five variables discussed above are the determining factors of radiation dose. Repeating scans or obtaining overlapping slices will increase radiation dose, in an essentially additive fashion. Increased scan time will increase the dose linearly if the kilovoltage and milliamperage are kept the same, as they usually are; therefore, going from a scan time of 3 sec to a scan

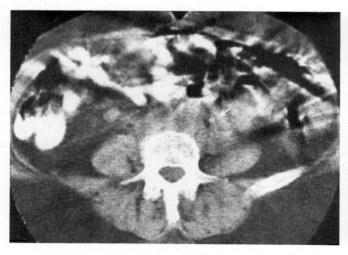 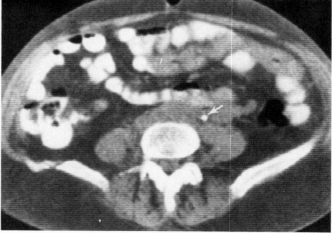

FIG. 2. Effect of scanning time on peristaltic motion artifact. **Left:** Streak artifacts from bowel peristalsis, despite prior glucagon administration, are noted on this 18-sec scan of the lower abdomen. **Right:** Repeat examination at a comparable level on a 3-sec CT scanner shows no motion artifact. Arrow identifies a ureteral stent.

time of 6 sec will double the radiation dose. In addition, decreased slice width (collimation) usually will increase the dose. The exposure due to primary radiation stays the same, but to cover the same longitudinal distance, more thin cuts will be required, thus increasing the scatter component.

The field of view, which determines the pixel size, is selected to match the cross-sectional size of the part to be examined. Selecting an inappropriately large field of view will tend to compromise spatial resolution, which is partially related to pixel size. Even more importantly, an inordinately large field of view introduces uncertainties in the attenuation values since the computer algorithm is designed for and based on examining a volume of tissue density without the extreme variations of attenuation introduced by including a large volume of surrounding air. A field of view smaller than the cross-section being examined, sometimes called a target scan, is appropriate in selected instances to improve spatial resolution (1). Although this may exclude important findings in the periphery, reprocessing the raw data at the larger field size can demonstrate the entire image.

Gantry tilt provides some flexibility in designing CT examinations to accommodate special situations. Gantry angulation has proved most helpful in evaluation of the spine (see Chapter 16) and has not been used extensively in other body CT applications.

Other technical variables, usually available as options or computer programs, include the computed radiograph (Scanogram, Scout view, Pilot scan), dynamic scanning, and multiplanar reconstruction.

A computed radiograph, similar in appearance to a conventional radiograph, is a feature present on most CT scanners. The image is obtained by moving the patient through the gantry as the now-stationary X-ray tube is rapidly pulsed, producing many contiguous narrow image bands. These are "stacked" together to form the complete digital image. This radiograph (Fig. 3) does not have the spatial resolution of a quality conventional radiograph, but it may be used to localize appropriate scan levels (e.g., disc space or the level of the diaphragm), which then may be marked on the viewing console by a line cursor and entered into the computer to initiate scanning at precisely defined levels.

Most CT units provide automatic incrementation of the patient couch and sequential numbering of images. This does not solve the problem of accurately choosing the level for the initial scan, however, nor does it eliminate the practical problems of precise patient repositioning or possible faulty table indexing. The computed radiograph described above circumvents some of these problems. In the absence of that capability, several techniques have been described. One of the first was based on the use of regularly spaced radio-

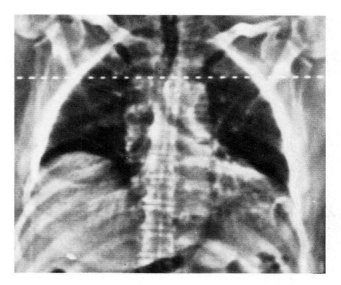

FIG. 3. Computed radiograph. A scan at the level of the aortic arch has been selected (dotted line) from this preliminary radiologic image of the thorax.

paque catheters of incrementally varying lengths taped to the patient during scanning such that the number of catheters visualized indicates the level of the scan (71). The reconstruction artifacts and image degradation associated with the catheters make the use of this otherwise practical system suboptimal. Other methods (16,34,49,59,67,85) have been described, but none seem to have broad application or particular merit.

Dynamic scanning is the ability to scan consecutively with variable interscan delay. A zero time delay between scans combined with postponed processing allows continuous scanning. Wide differences in technical capabilities exist among CT scanners ranging from as few as 2 scans per minute to as many as 16 scans in a minute. In CT angiography (87), where dynamic scanning has been used most widely, obtaining 4 consecutive scans during a minute is usually sufficient. For other examinations, such as the examination of pulmonary nodules or the larynx, it is often convenient to do a series of scans during a single suspended respiration (i.e., 3 or 4 scans in a 15-sec period).

Multiplanar reconstruction, as a software program, will reorient the CT data in other planes, typically sagittal or coronal (Fig. 4). These reformatted images are optimized by contiguous or even overlapping, narrowly collimated scans. Commonly, contiguous 2.0- to 5-mm slices are utilized. When compared to the directly imaged cross-sectional views, such reconstructed images are of inferior quality partly due to inconsistencies in breath holding (50). Multiplanar reconstructions are most valuable in selected areas, such as the spine and the peridiaphragmatic area. Presently,

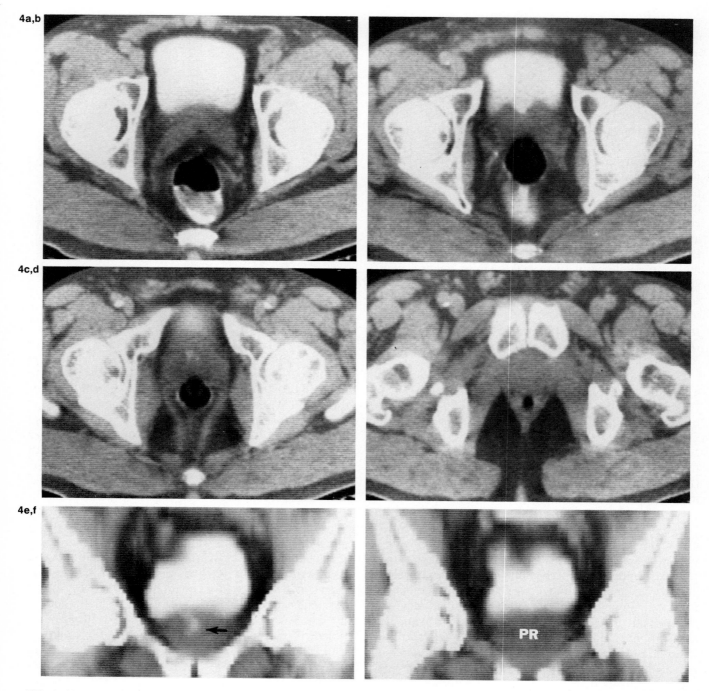

FIG. 4. Multiplanar reconstruction. **a–d:** Contiguous CT scans at 1-cm intervals caudad through the pelvis demonstrate an enlarged prostate. **e and f:** Reconstructed coronal images define the bladder-prostate interface more clearly. A portion of the prostatic urethra is indicated by the arrow. PR, prostate.

the utility of reformatted images is limited by (a) the quality of these studies, (b) increased radiation dose required for multiple thin contiguous or overlapping slices, (c) the necessity to anticipate the need for multiplanar views, and (d) the prolonged scanning and processing times required for obtaining the initial scans.

Various approaches have been tried to obtain direct images in multiple planes to achieve high resolution and avoid the above problems. Special support devices are available to obtain direct coronal and saggital views by allowing the patient to intersect the scanning gantry in some nonaxial orientation. A bicycle-type apparatus has been designed at Utrecht (80) and modified at Mallinckrodt (Fig. 5), which affords direct coronal views of the pelvis of excellent quality. This type

5a,b

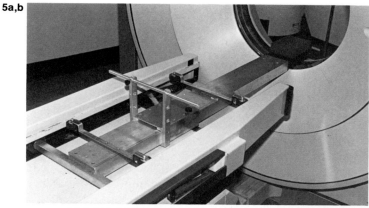

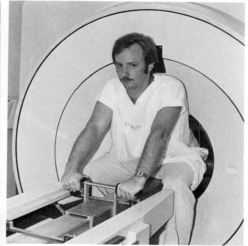

5c

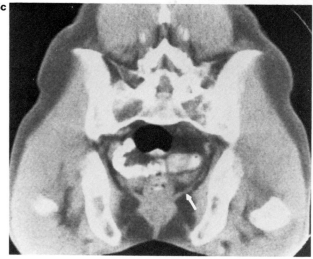

FIG. 5. a: Direct coronal pelvic CT may be accomplished with the patient seated on an attachment to the CT couch. b: Patient position for direct coronal views of the pelvis. c: Direct coronal image of the pelvis. Arrow denotes levator ani muscle.

of special bicycle (51) is coupled to the indexing table after removing the original patient couch. The patient then sits on the seat with his back to the gantry. The angle of the patient may be controlled by adjusting the variable screw set position of the "handle bar." Technique factors are the same as those used for transaxial scanning of the pelvis. The entire examination, including the time to attach the accessory seat, requires about 20 min and is applicable to the majority of patients.

Another attachment that allows direct sagittal and coronal CT of the pelvis is a special accessory table adapted for wide-aperture body scanners (61). This device allows the patient to lie almost parallel to the scanning gantry, either supine for sagittal views or in a decubitus position for coronal scans of the pelvis.

IMAGE MANIPULATION

Attenuation Values

Initially, major emphasis was placed on determining the specific CT attenuation value of lesions. However, as experience has accumulated, it has become clear that CT numbers cannot be considered absolute values (8). The reasons for inaccurate or inconsistent density values include beam hardening, eccentric or peripheral location within the scanning ring, size of the field of view, calibration drift, poor quality control, and various scanning artifacts. Therefore, it is much more appropriate to observe CT numbers in a relative fashion, e.g., compare the attenuation value of a renal mass with the density of a paraspinal muscle in the same patient. An excellent application of this concept is the proven validity of comparing liver and spleen CT numbers to predict the presence of diffuse fatty infiltration of the liver (63). If one finds liver values significantly lower than the spleen in a given patient, then fatty infiltration can be diagnosed with confidence.

Window Width and Level

Computed tomography images on the digital image processor screen may be viewed at any of a range of window levels and window widths. The window level is the CT number at the midpoint of the gray-scale display and, at least theoretically, should be at or near the attenuation value one is most interested in defining.

The window width, usually varying from 0 to 1,000, will determine the range of attenuation values included in the gray scale. For example, a window width of 100 at a window level of 0 would assign white to any individual voxel with a CT number greater than 50 and black to any CT number less than −50. The shades of grey would be applied to the values in between. Optimal CT images for photographic reproduction may require individual experimentation. A wide window width is appropriate whenever wide differences in CT attenuation values need to be displayed, e.g., pelvic bone and surrounding soft tissues, whereas narrow window widths maximize small differences among CT numbers, e.g., metastases in liver parenchyma.

Optimal window settings must be developed for particular regions of the body. In the chest it is virtually mandatory to obtain at least two separate images at any given level due to the wide variation in attenuation between the mediastinum and the pulmonary parenchyma. One image is obtained at an optimum "lung" window, usually the widest setting available (i.e., window width of 800 for EMI 7070) and a very negative window level (i.e., window level of −700 for EMI 7070). The other "mediastinal" or soft tissue image utilizes a narrower window width and a window level of zero (Fig. 6). These guidelines need to be individualized to particular CT units and even to individual cases when specific details, e.g., bronchial anatomy, require optimization. Bone structure detail also demands particular attention. Use of negative CT image displayed with a wide window width may be valuable in evaluating some bone lesions (72).

Size Determinations

The CT image may be used to obtain accurate size determinations of organs or lesions. However, substantial errors may occur unless one is aware of the

6a,b

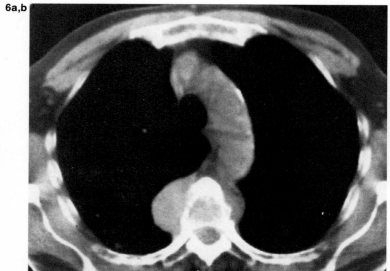
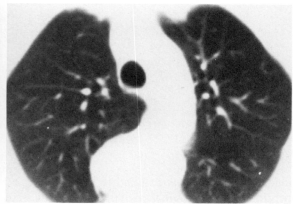

6c

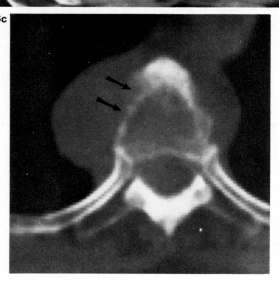

FIG. 6. Three different window settings of the same scan allow specific evaluation of **(a)** soft tissue of the mediastinum and chest wall, **(b)** the lungs, and **(c)** bone in this patient with a plasmacytoma originating from and eroding a thoracic vertebral body (arrows).

various factors that affect the CT image display. Partial volume effect, inappropriate or noncomparable CT window settings, limited spatial resolution in the axial plane, and CT calibration errors in the reconstruction algorithm all may contribute to the problem of accurate CT depiction of a lesion (46). Of these factors, the first two may be controlled or influenced by the CT operator. Partial volume averaging (discussed in Chapter 1) may be minimized by keeping the slice width at least half of the lesion diameter. The CT window settings are critical for the evaluation of the size of a lesion. The greater the difference in attenuation values between the object to be measured and the background or adjacent tissue, the more variation there will be in the size of that object on the CT display. Similarly, the smaller the lesion, the greater the variation. It has been determined, using phantoms, that for accurate measurement of size the CT window level should be set halfway between the lesion density and the density of the background (6). The window width is not so important. In almost all cases this "measure" window level will be different from the usual window settings used for routine photography of CT scans.

PATIENT VARIABLES

Detailing the machine controls tends to overshadow or diminish the importance of relating to the person being examined. It is essential that someone, usually the technologist, communicates with the patient both before and during the CT study. Usually a brief description of the examination and a review of any commands will assure patient cooperation and a diagnostic quality examination. Other patient-oriented concerns are the respiratory phase of scanning and patient positioning on the scanning couch.

The optimal phase of respiration varies by region and is included in the examination protocols later in this chapter. Asking the patient to practice these commands prior to scanning is effective in achieving patient cooperation. Variations in scan appearance due to respiratory phase differences are not trivial, especially in the lower chest and upper abdomen. In this region, it may be critical to have complete patient cooperation.

Although most CT examinations are performed with the patient supine, other positions are helpful at times. For example, a prominent gastroesophageal junction may be differentiated from a mass by left lateral decubitus or prone views (Fig. 7). Certain anatomical structures change their relative location according to the scanning position (4). The descending aorta and the kidneys show dramatic caudal and ventral displacement on prone views as compared to supine. The heart, pulmonary nodules, pulmonary hila, liver, spleen, stomach, and transverse colon also move caudally and ventrally in the prone position. Other structures such as the gastroesophageal junction, duodenum, and pelvic structures show minimal or no change.

Radiation treatment planning scans should be performed in the position that will be used to deliver the radiation therapy, noting the position of the arms as well as the patient's treatment position. A change in the position of the arms, for example, will change some organ relationships (64). Also the difference between the usual curved couch of the CT scanner and the flat surface of the radiation treatment table is sufficient to cause some discrepancies that are significant in therapy planning. Simple insertion of a flat wooden table top overcomes this problem.

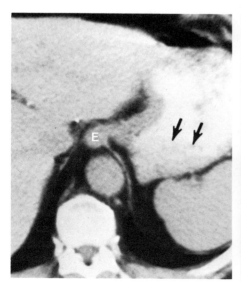 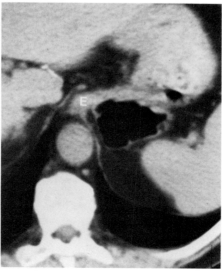

FIG. 7. Patient position. **Left:** With the patient supine, the posterior gastric fundus is incompletely opacified even after additional contrast material administration, suggesting a possible gastric wall mass (arrows). **Right:** A scan after prone positioning demonstrates a normal posterior gastric fundus. (A left lateral decubitus position is helpful when the medial aspect of the posterior fundus is considered possibly pathologic.)

CONTRAST ENHANCEMENT

Computed tomography is a sensitive detector of differences in tissue contrast density as compared to conventional radiography, an advantage that can be maximized by introducing exogenous contrast materials. Lumen opacification of hollow viscera has been used, for example, to demonstrate the bladder wall, as well as to identify bowel loops and other segments of the gastrointestinal tract. The other major category of contrast enhancement methods is intravenous administration of contrast material. Although the usual urographic agents are neither organ nor lesion specific, they frequently provide additional information.

Oral Contrast Material

Oral contrast media have proved invaluable in performing CT of the abdomen since unopacified bowel may simulate abdominal masses (42). Indeed, one of the most common interpretive problems in abdominal CT is distinguishing unopacified fluid filled bowel loops from an abdominal or pelvic mass (Fig. 8). For this reason, virtually every abdominal CT examination is done with oral contrast material administration.

The optimal bowel enhancement agent for CT would be an easily administered, inert substance that would render the bowel distinctly identifiable by an exclusive and specific attenuation value without causing ar-

tifacts. The high density of conventional barium suspensions causes computer-generated artifacts (Fig. 9). Flavored low density barium preparations have been developed specifically for CT, and are commercially available (35). E-Z CAT® (1.5% weight per volume barium suspension) (E-Z EM Company, Inc., Westbury, NY), the primary oral contrast agent used at our institution, has proved to be effective and well tolerated. The relatively slow transit time, although not optimal, is only a minor disadvantage.

The other available alternative to barium is a water-soluble agent such as a diatrizoate preparation—diatrizoate meglumine-diatrizoate sodium (Gastrografin®). Used in dilute solution (e.g., 10 cc Gastrografin® to 300 cc water), the diatrizoate mixtures usually provide adequate bowel opacification, a fast transit time, and are not significantly absorbed from the intestinal tract. However, the peristaltic stimulation may cause artifacts, sometimes necessitating use of an antiperistaltic agent (0.50−1.0 mg intravenous glucagon), especially when scan times of about 10 sec or more are employed. Other disadvantages of the diatrizoates are the side effect of diarrhea in a few patients, the inconsistent bowel coating, and the objectionable taste (even when "flavored" with a powdered lemonade mix). We generally use the low density barium preparation, reserving the dilute diatrizoate solution for situations when water-soluble

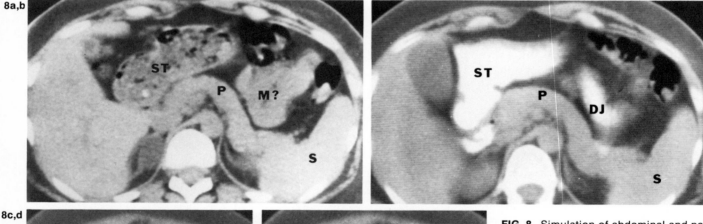

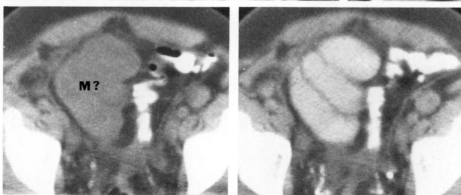

FIG. 8. Simulation of abdominal and pelvic masses by unopacified bowel. **a:** A scan through the upper abdomen shows a questionable soft tissue mass (M?). P, pancreas; S, spleen; ST, stomach. **b:** A subsequent scan after the administration of oral contrast agent demonstrates opacification as well as a change in the configuration consistent with a small bowel loop at the duodenal-jejunal junction (DJ). **c:** A scan of the pelvis in another patient shows a questionable large mass (M?). **d:** Rescanning after additional administration of low density barium and a suitable delay shows the suspected mass to be some mildly dilated ileal loops.

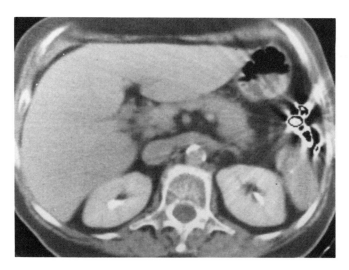

FIG. 9. Computer generated artifacts. Previously administered conventional barium retained in the splenic flexure of the colon compromises this scan quality only slightly. However, more extensive collections can seriously degrade the image, and preclude or delay CT examination.

agents seem prudent (e.g., question of perforated bowel) or when a faster transit time is desirable.

Once an oral agent is selected, the details of administration are dependent on the type of examination being performed. Excellent opacification of the proximal bowel is provided by giving 300 cc of contrast material 15 min prior to scanning the upper abdomen. Earlier administration of a larger volume is required to opacify bowel in the mid-abdomen or pelvis. Our usual method is to give 600 cc approximately 1 hr prior to scanning and another 300 cc about 15 min prior to scanning. Giving contrast material the night before the CT exam will opacify the colon and is sometimes helpful in examining the pelvis or the pediatric abdomen.

Specific oral contrast-related problems are commonly encountered but can be easily solved. When it is uncertain whether a mass represents a fluid-filled loop of bowel due to incomplete intestinal opacification, repeat scanning after additional oral contrast material administration and a suitable delay is necessary (Fig. 8). Esophageal enhancement, e.g., to confirm a hiatal hernia that may be simulating a retrocrural mass, is easily achieved by scanning while the patient is sipping barium. The region of the pancreatic tail is best visualized by maximally distending the stomach to displace adjacent small bowel loops (75). In the pelvis, an

enema of 300 cc of contrast material is occasionally necessary to define the rectosigmoid colon.

Intravenous Contrast Material

Indications

Iodinated intravenous contrast agents, first introduced for urography in 1929, are now used widely in CT. The specific indications are enumerated in Table 1. In general, the indications include determining the vascular characteristics of a mass, differentiating a vascular anomaly or abnormality from a neoplastic mass, and maximizing lesion detectability. Iodinated intravenous contrast agents aid in the search for subtle findings or occult lesions. Often the attenuation value difference between normal parenchyma and abnormal mass lesions will increase after contrast media administration. This is particularly true in the liver where mildly dilated intra- or extrahepatic bile ducts sometimes are recognized confidently only on postcontrast scans and metastases frequently are more obvious after intravenous contrast material is given.

Techniques of Administration Based on Tissue Dynamics

A variety of techniques of administration of contrast media have been used, reflecting the inadequacies of any one method. However, the two major approaches have been bolus and infusion, both of which involve injecting contrast media into a large peripheral vein. Bolus refers to a quick injection of 10 to 20 g of iodine; this method is preferred at our institution. An infusion refers to a large volume (150–300 cc) of a 30 to 60% iodine solution administered usually at a flow rate around 20 to 30 cc/min.

By observing the arteriovenous iodine difference as measured on CT scans, three phases can be differentiated: a bolus effect phase, a nonequilibrium phase, and an equilibrium phase (9). Maximum vascular enhancement, the bolus effect, occurs only with the rapid injection of contrast medium (60) (Fig. 10). This phase is very transient, lasting only about 40 to 60 sec. The second or nonequilibrium phase occurs about 1 min after bolus administration or during rapid infusion of a relatively large volume of contrast material. The final phase, or equilibrium, occurs when there is a negligible arteriovenous iodine difference. This phase corre-

TABLE 1. *Indications for intravenous contrast material*

Distinguish normal or anomalous vascular structure(s) and define pathologic vessel(s), e.g., question aneurysm.
Characterize the relative vascularity of a mass.
Improve anatomic definition, e.g., imaging the common bile duct.
Increase the detectability of a lesion(s), e.g., focal hepatic mass(es).
Opacify the urinary tract.

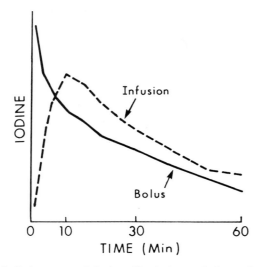

FIG. 10. Bolus versus infusion. The bolus technique of administering intravenous iodinated contrast media results in a higher concentration of intravascular iodine than infusion methods can achieve when equal amounts of contrast material are injected. A bolus of contrast material combined with sequential or dynamic scanning is the optimal method for administering intravenous contrast material when high intravascular levels are desired. (Modified from Ono et al., ref. 60.)

sponds to approximately 2-min postbolus adminstration or to the end of infusion. Based on these types of observations (9,88), it is apparent that a bolus of contrast material produces the best quality vascular enhancement (Fig. 11) and, in general, it is during the bolus effect and nonequilibrium phase that clinically useful information is provided.

Small-volume (25–50 cc) bolus technique at one or few scan levels is used to obtain vessel opacification and to determine the vascular characteristics of a specific lesion. The injection of contrast material, performed quickly to ensure a well-defined bolus, should be delivered into a large vein through an 18- or 19-gauge needle. A medially directed antecubital vein that enters the basilic system should be chosen if possible since it has a more direct route to the superior vena cava and will not be obstructed by the over-the-head arm position usually adopted during CT. This method is often coupled with dynamic scanning, i.e., serial images at a predetermined level. Although bolus administration is the most effective method of achieving excellent vascular enhancement, it is usually difficult or impossible to obtain a sufficient number of scans after a single injection to assess more than one plane of interest since the effect lasts less than a minute. Due to limitations on the amount of urographic contrast media that may be safely administered (a total dose less than or equal to 1 g iodine/kg has been recommended) (3), repeating multiple large volume injections is not clinically feasible. This dilemma has led many radiologists to use an infusion of contrast material since it allows more flexibility in terms of scanning time. Infusion

flow rates of 20 to 50 ml/min will achieve good vascular enhancement (48) and are clinically effective in many instances such as when evaluating both kidneys or the entire liver and extrahepatic biliary tree. There are other ways of achieving optimal studies while limiting contrast media administration. One method is to repeat the small volume bolus technique at selected levels. Another practical approach is a modification combining a small bolus injection with a drip infusion. Initially a small volume (25–50 cc) bolus is given, followed by prompt infusion of a 300-cc volume of a 30% iodine solution through an 18- or 19-gauge needle. This usually allows 12 to 18 scans to be obtained while infusing contrast media. If reconstruction times are relatively long, delayed processing may be appropriate. These methods combine the desirable bolus effect with the convenience of obtaining several scans, at different levels if necessary.

Enhancement of the soft tissues, which corresponds to phases two and three, is dependent on diffusion and is more variable than vascular opacification. Diffusion of the contrast media from vessels begins almost immediately following injection, so that after one pass through the body, 50 to 75% of the material has diffused from the vascular space and at about 45 min after injection CT numbers return to baseline (88). Pragmatically, soft tissue enhancement has some value in improving lesion detectability, e.g., in kidney and liver, and in separating normal organs from pathologic processes. For example, a questionably enlarged head of the pancreas that enhances to the same degree as the rest of the gland becomes less suspicious and more likely to be a normal pancreas.

When prolonged arterial or venous phase enhancement to evaluate various levels is necessary, administering 100 to 150 cc of contrast media through an 18- or 19-gauge needle is a useful alternative technique (45). This "large volume bolus" requires someone in the examination room to inject the contrast agent continuously while the examination is in progress. Different levels are selected by moving the couch between the scans.

The appearance of a lesion after contrast material injection can be crucial in making a specific diagnosis. For example, a cavernous hemangioma of the liver or an arteriovenous malformation has unique enhancement characteristics (5,39). The dose and type of injection and the timing of the study are critical in obtaining maximum information from contrast material administration for this purpose. The optimal volume of contrast agent depends somewhat on the size of the lesion relative to the anticipated vascular supply, with larger lesions requiring larger doses. In general, however, 25 to 50 cc of contrast media will suffice, administered as a bolus injection followed by immediate serial scanning with a minimum of three scans obtained

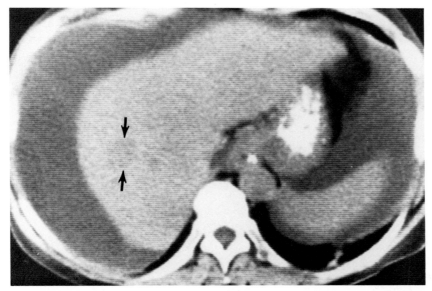

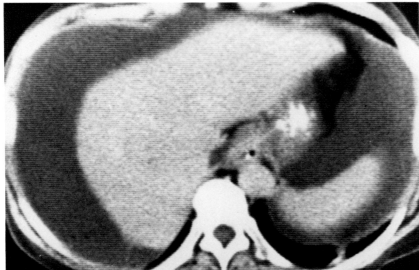

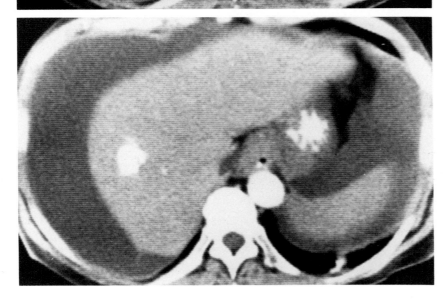

FIG. 11. Bolus versus infusion techniques of contrast material administration. **Top:** A low-density hepatic lesion (arrows) is present on the precontrast image in this patient with cirrhosis and ascites. **Middle:** After administration of contrast medium by a rapid drip infusion, there is subtle enhancement of the lesion as compared to surrounding normal liver parenchyma. **Bottom:** A subsequent CT after a bolus injection of contrast media clearly demonstrates marked enhancement of the lesion consistent with an arteriovenous malformation.

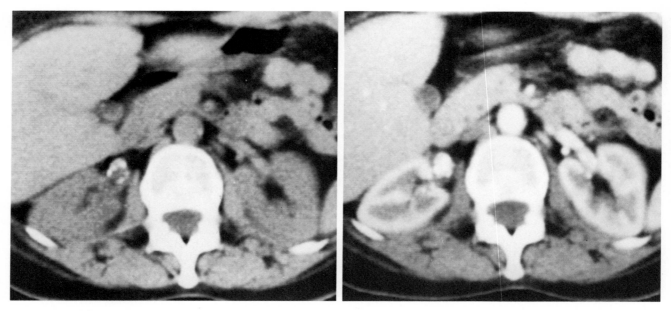

FIG. 12. CT angiography. **Left:** A curvilinear calcification in the region of the right renal hilum is seen. **Right:** This is shown to be a renal artery aneurysm after bolus administration of intravenous contrast media.

in the first minute. If a hepatic cavernous hemangioma, which typically demonstrates delayed central contrast enhancement, is suspected, larger doses, e.g., 100 cc, are often required combined with delayed scanning at 1- to 3-min intervals up to 10 min.

In many cases the kinetics of contrast enhancement are such that dynamic scanning capabilities are required to make intravascular contrast material administration rewarding (43). To delineate specific vessels,

e.g., suspected aortic dissection or renal vein thrombosis, a bolus technique as described above combined with dynamic scanning, so-called CT angiography, is required for optimal evaluation. Computed tomographic angiography (45,87) involves scanning a single plane sequentially after bolus administration of contrast material (Figs. 12 and 13). These serial images may better define a confusing finding, e.g., demonstrate tortuous or anomalous vessels that were sim-

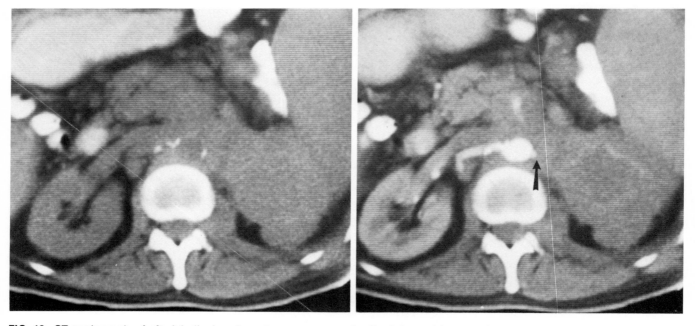

FIG. 13. CT angiography. **Left:** A bulky lymphomatous mass occupies the left renal fossa and merges with paraaortic lymph nodes surrounding the aorta on a precontrast scan. **Right:** A scan after a bolus injection of contrast media shows an opacified normal right renal artery but the left renal artery is totally obstructed near its origin (arrow).

TABLE 2. *Intravenous contrast agent variables*

Agent	Iodine content (mg/ml)	Viscosity (in CPS) at 37°C
Conray 400®	400	4.1–5.0
Renografin 76®	370	9.0
Conray 60®	282	4.0
Renografin 60®	288	3.9
Hypaque 50®	300	2.3
Hypaque 76®	370	9.0

ulating a mass (54). Time-density curves have been obtained using this technique; however, they have limited practical value.

Intravenous Contrast Agents

Among the distinctions of the many available iodinated contrast agents, two characteristics, the iodine content and viscosity, are important for use in CT since they affect the ability (a) to inject a maximum amount of iodine in a small volume and (b) to deliver that volume quickly. These features of the commonly used contrast media are listed in Table 2. The pharmacology of these urographic contrast agents is otherwise similar; there are no significant differences in tissue dynamics or distribution. Based on this information, we have preferred to use iothalamate meglumine (Conray® 400) in the majority of CT studies and have used it almost exclusively for bolus injection.

One of the attributes of these agents is the low risk of reaction or serious complication. The technique of contrast material administration does not affect the incidence of adverse reaction (33). Diabetics, elderly patients, individuals with compromised renal function on any basis, and those with cardiovascular disease are more likely to develop contrast-related complications. Contrast media should be used judiciously and closely monitored, therefore, if elected at all in these patients.

Although water-soluble contrast media are readily available, widely accepted, and relatively risk free, the tissue dynamics of these agents are far from ideal (23). The iodinated compounds, extensively studied long before the advent of CT (10,11), are not specifically metabolized or concentrated except in the kidney and, even more importantly, as has been described, are

quickly equilibrated with the extravascular space (47,58). These characteristics limit the specificity of today's intravenous contrast agents. Research has been directed toward developing organ- or lesion-targeted compounds (15,36,70,86). Contrast agents specifically designed for CT are evolving. One such agent, a liposoluble organ-specific contrast agent (EOE 13) (82), is an ethiodized oil emulsion injected intravenously. Selective uptake by the reticuloendothelial system results in contrast enhancement of the liver and spleen. Associated with some minor side effects and currently available on an experimental basis only, this agent has improved the capability to detect small hepatic and splenic lesions (81,84). EOE 13 also allows greater specificity in evaluating upper quadrant masses (83) when normal splenic tissue is a consideration.

Preliminary studies with non-ionic iodinated contrast media indicate two advantages over the ionic iodine compounds: (a) even lower incidence of side effects and (b) a transiently higher level of intravascular iodine after bolus injection. These contrast agents are potentially well suited for use in dynamic CT.

TECHNIQUES UNIQUE TO SPECIFIC REGIONS

Tables 3 to 15 summarize our general approach to the conduct of CT examinations by region of interest. (The conduct of CT examinations of the spine and other musculoskeletal regions, as well as pediatric CT, is addressed in their respective sections.) Kept in the CT examination room, these protocols serve as an immediate reference and as a teaching tool for technologists and radiologists being introduced to CT. These guidelines are not designed to avoid all thought processes, but rather to provide a basic approach that may be further tailored according to the clinical question to be answered and the initial scan findings. There may be a relatively large number of cases that cannot be neatly categorized according to the following tables. Also, some examinations will overlap two or more regions of interest. Modification will be required in each instance.

TABLE 3. *Region of interest: Abdominal survey (retroperitoneum and pelvis)*

Oral contrast agent	300–600 cc oral contrast agent 1 hr before scanning; plus 300 cc oral contrast agent 15 min before scan begins
Phase of respiration	Suspended expiration
Slice thickness	10 mm
Slice interval	20 mm
Superior extent	Xiphoid (to include all of retrocrural area)
Inferior extent	Symphysis (or lower if inferior inguinal nodes need to be studied)
IV contrast agent	To evaluate vascularity of a mass or to define suspected lesions or suspected anomalies of retroperitoneal vascular structures.

TABLE 4. *Region of interest: Pancreas*

Oral contrast agent	300 cc oral contrast agent 15 min before scanning
Phase of respiration	Suspended expiration
Slice thickness	10 mm (occasionally 5 mm in areas of special interest)
Slice interval	10 mm
Superior extent	Approximately 20 mm below xiphoid
Inferior extent	Through third duodenum
IV contrast agent	Enhancement of pancreatic parenchyma and surrounding vessels is exceedingly helpful in defining an observed or suspected abnormality.
Comments	IV contrast agent is administered to visualize the pancreas and distinguish tortuous splenic vessels that may simulate a pancreatic mass. Aneurysms or pseudoaneurysms about the pancreas or dilated pancreatic duct may be documented as well. In thin patients, study of the entire pancreatic area may be optimized by scanning during an infusion of contrast media. The suspicious area in or near the pancreas is first localized, then rescanned using bolus technique. Maximum distention of the stomach by administering additional contrast agent may be indicated when pancreatic tail images are equivocal.

TABLE 5. *Region of interest: Liver–spleen*

Oral contrast agent	300 cc oral contrast agent 15 min before scanning
Phase of respiration	Suspended expiration
Slice thickness	10 mm
Slice interval	10 mm
Superior extent	Dome of liver (approximately 20 mm above xiphoid)
Inferior extent	Through the inferior tip of right lobe
IV contrast agent	Both pre- and post-IV contrast scans may be necessary if searching for focal lesions (hepatoma or liver metastases).
Comments	In characterizing a focal mass, 3–4 scans during the first 60 sec after a bolus injection of contrast agent, followed by a scan at 2 min, is required. To differentiate a cavernous hemangioma from other hepatic masses, additional scans through the lesion should be obtained at 4, 6, 10, and 15 min, if necessary.

TABLE 6. *Region of interest: Liver–pancreas in jaundiced patient*

Oral contrast agent	300 cc oral contrast agent 15 min before scanning, unless a common bile duct stone is strongly suspected
Patient position	Supine
Phase of respiration	Suspended expiration
Slice thickness	10 mm; 5 mm collimation for improved spatial resolution should be considered especially when (a) a point of transition from a dilated biliary system to a more normal biliary duct is seen and (b) common bile duct stones are suspected.
Slice interval	2 cm down to the junction of right and left hepatic ducts, then 1 cm inferiorly; 5 mm intervals should be used if 5 mm collimation is selected.
Superior extent	Dome of liver
Inferior extent	Through third duodenum
IV contrast agent	Infusion of contrast medium should be begun once the appropriate level through the superior aspect of the liver parenchyma is established. Bolus injections (25–50 cc) may be used to clarify selected scans.

TABLE 7. *Region of interest: Kidney*

Oral contrast agent	300 cc oral contrast agent 30–60 min before scanning
Phase of respiration	Suspended expiration
Slice thickness	10 mm
Slice interval	10 mm
Superior extent	Just above upper poles
Inferior extent	Through lower poles
IV contrast agent	To define the vascular character of a mass, an injection of 50 cc of contrast media will suffice in most instances.
Comments	Precontrast scans are usually of minimal value unless renal calculi, perinephric hematoma, or calcified masses are suspected (18). When the need for dynamic scanning is anticipated, precontrast scans are obtained to select the appropriate level(s) for evaluation. Otherwise, the precontrast scans may be bypassed completely.

TABLE 8. *Region of interest: Adrenal*

Oral contrast agent	300 cc oral contrast agent 30 min before scanning
Phase of respiration	Suspended expiration
Slice thickness	10 mm collimation
Slice interval	10 mm (5 mm intervals to be used when collimation is reduced to 5 mm)
Superior extent	Dome of diaphragm
Inferior extent	To lower poles of kidneys
IV contrast agent	Occasionally helpful, e.g., to differentiate tortuous splenic artery from left adrenal mass or to accentuate the difference between a small non-enhancing mass from surrounding structures.
Comments	10 mm collimation is usually adequate if screening for pheochromocytoma or adenoma in Cushing's syndrome. In Conn's syndrome, however, 5 mm collimation is essential to exclude a small adenoma. If screening for pheochromocytoma in an adult, and the adrenal area is normal, scans to a level just below aortic bifurcation are done to search for possible extra adrenal pheochromocytoma (organ of Zuckerlandl).

TABLE 9. *Region of interest: Pelvic survey*

Oral contrast agent	500 cc oral contrast agent at least 1 hr before scanning; if possible, 300 cc dilute barium suspension the evening before scanning to identify the colon
Phase of respiration	Suspended expiration or normal respiration
Slice thickness	10 mm[a]
Slice interval	10–20 mm
Superior extent	Iliac crest
Inferior extent	Symphysis pubis
IV contrast agent	To define the bladder and ureters or to define vascular characteristics of pelvic tumors.
Comments	In females, a vaginal tampon is inserted prior to the exam (14). If oral contrast agent has not progressed to the colon, a contrast material enema or rectal catheter is helpful in defining the rectosigmoid colon. Direct coronal scans or reformatted images should be considered if suspicious densities are seen about the pelvic floor on the transaxial views.

[a] 5 mm collimation is helpful when trying to depict clearly the extent of gross disease, such as in primary prostate, cervix, or bladder carcinoma.

TABLE 10. *Region of interest: Pelvis—search for undescended testicle*

Oral contrast agent	500 cc oral contrast agent at least 1 hr before scanning; if possible, 300 cc dilute barium suspension the evening before scanning to identify the colon
Phase of respiration	Suspended expiration or normal respiration
Slice thickness	10 mm
Slice interval	10 mm
Inferior extent	Begin at level of inferior pubic symphysis and proceed superiorly.
Superior extent	If testis or mass is defined in the inguinal ring or true pelvis, the abdomen need not be scanned.
Comments	In pediatric patients, contiguous scans using 5-mm slice thickness are required.

TABLE 11. *Region of interest: Mediastinum survey*

Oral contrast agent	None
Phase of respiration	Suspended inspiration
Slice thickness	5–10 mm
Slice interval	10–20 mm
Superior extent	Sternal notch
Inferior extent	Ventricular level
IV contrast agent	Bolus or rapid infusion if needed to evaluate mediastinal or hilar anatomy.
Comments	If IV contrast agent is administered to define the superior mediastinum, it is advantageous to use the left arm since this approach is most apt to opacify the left brachiocephalic vein, a vessel that is seen longitudinally and is frequently poorly defined.

TABLE 12. *Region of interest: Whole lung survey*

Oral contrast agent	None
Phase of respiration	End tidal volume (breathe in, breathe out, relax, hold your breath).
Slice thickness	10 mm
Slice interval	10 mm
Superior extent	Pulmonary apices
Inferior extent	Diaphragm
IV contrast agent	None
Comments	Differentiating pulmonary nodules from peripheral vessels seen on the cross-sectional images may be difficult. In general, a CT-defined nodule must be larger than the pulmonary vessels seen in cross-section in that region. In addition, it is sometimes useful to obtain additional scans in the prone position to help interpret confusing scans (74). Vessels will change; lung nodules will stay the same.

TABLE 13. *Region of interest: Pulmonary mass*

Oral contrast agent	None
Patient position	Supine
Phase of respiration	End tidal volume (breathe in, breathe out, relax, hold your breath).
Slice thickness	See comments
Slice interval	2–10 mm relative to size of lesion
Superior extent	Relative to site of lesion
Inferior extent	Relative to site of lesion
IV contrast agent	Usually not necessary unless a vascular malformation is suspected.
Comments	10 mm collimation is used to localize the nodule, then if the nodule is greater than or equal to 1 cm in diameter, 5 mm collimation at 2 mm increments. For lung nodules less than 1 cm, scan through the nodule using 2 mm collimation at 2 mm increments. Using the circular cursor, the attenuation value of the nodule on the scan showing the greatest diameter is measured. The very negative attenuation values of normal lung parenchyma make partial volume averaging a major problem in determining accurate CT values; therefore, the collimator width should always be less than half the diameter of the lesion in question (73). Furthermore, the scan used for CT number determination should be through the middle of the nodule, which pragmatically is the scan that shows the nodule to be the largest. Inconsistent respiratory motion makes localization of small nodules difficult. Multiple serial fast scans during a single breath holding helps circumvent this problem.

TABLE 14. *Region of interest: Oncologic survey of lung and mediastinum*

Oral contrast agent	None
Phase of respiration	Suspended inspiration
Slice thickness	10 mm; 5 mm collimation may improve spatial resolution and should be considered when scans demonstrate questionable findings.
Slice interval	10 mm; 5 mm intervals if 5 mm collimation is used.
Superior extent	Superior margin of clavicles
Inferior extent	Through adrenals
IV contrast agent	May be used to define the mediastinum and/or determine the relationship of a mass to mediastinal vessels; it is not routinely administered.

TABLE 15. *Region of interest: Larynx survey*

Oral contrast agent	None
Phase of respiration	During slow inspiration[a]
Slice thickness	5 mm
Slice interval	5 mm
Superior extent	Base of tongue[b]
Inferior extent	Proximal trachea
IV contrast agent	Occasionally to determine relation of tumor mass to vessels or differentiate small nodes from vessels.
Comments	The neck should be hyperextended. A small field of view (120–250 cm) affords the best resolution.

[a] Various laryngography maneuvers may be used to define problem areas (Fig. 14): *phonation* ("e") for definition of cord mobility; used for distending the pyriform sinuses and is valuable at times in evaluating the extent of supraglottic tumors around the sinuses and aryepiglottic folds; and *reverse "e"* for laryngeal ventricles (very difficult for most patients to accomplish in supine position).

[b] Since the inferior landmarks are easier to identify, it is often more practical to start from below and proceed superiorly.

CT-GUIDED INTERVENTIONAL PROCEDURES

Needle Biopsy

Percutaneous biopsy using radiological guidance has become common over the past few years and has become increasingly accepted as a method of establishing a tissue diagnosis without surgery; frequently the procedure can be performed on an outpatient basis. Certainly, when thin aspirating needles are used, a key factor in establishing this as an effective diagnostic procedure is the availability of an experienced cytopathologist. Also important to the success of needle biopsy is the availability of cross-sectional imaging capable of producing exquisitely detailed images. Radiographically guided biopsy may totally obviate surgery and dictate appropriate palliative therapy in a patient with incurable malignancy; in others it will allow more precise preoperative planning.

Aspiration Versus Cutting Needles

One of the first considerations is which needle to use. Aspirating needles are simple beveled needles of narrow gauge that obtain only a cytological specimen. Cutting needles are larger bore with various configurations of the needle tip capable of producing cores or chunks of tissue. There is a significant difference in risk between aspirating needle biopsy and cutting needle biopsy. In an intermediate category are the modified aspirating needles, which are very versatile and often provide a specimen suitable for histologic processing. Technically, some needles, e.g., the Rotex® and Franseen® needles, have a cutting action but are probably more appropriately thought of with the group of modified aspirating needles since indications and risks are generally considered equivalent. The structural differences among some of the commercially available needles are illustrated in Fig. 15. Table 16 describes a selection of biopsy needles with some of the more commonly used gauges listed. In addition to these needle variations, several "handled syringes" have been designed to facilitate biopsy procedures (90).

The standard Chiba or "spinal" needle, also referred to as a thin or skinny needle, is adequate for many needle biopsies. However, a modified aspirating needle, such as the Turner (52), or the Greene (38), appears to combine the safety of a "skinny" needle with the ability to obtain a tissue core that may provide a histologic diagnosis often useful in patient management. Among abdominal masses percutaneously sampled with one of these two core needles, more than 80% were successfully biopsied, often with sufficient biopsy material for histological as well as cytological analysis (38,52).

Large bore and cutting needles are reserved for large, easily accessible lesions. For example, the Menghini needle capable of extracting small chunks of tissue with CT guidance has been used for focal liver lesions (32). Computed tomography with bolus administration of contrast material to determine the vascularity of the lesion and the adjacent vascular structures is considered mandatory when such biopsies are undertaken in the abdomen (30). Because of the potential bleeding risk, blood typing and cross-matching are recommended prior to large bore needle biopsy. Cutting needle biopsies probably should be reserved for hospitalized patients. Large bore needle puncture of bowel, gallbladder, and hypervascular lesions as well as major vessels is considered dangerous and should be avoided. Therefore, when considering large bore or cutting needle biopsies, one must weigh the advantage of larger tissue specimens against the risk of bleeding and other complications from puncture of various organs.

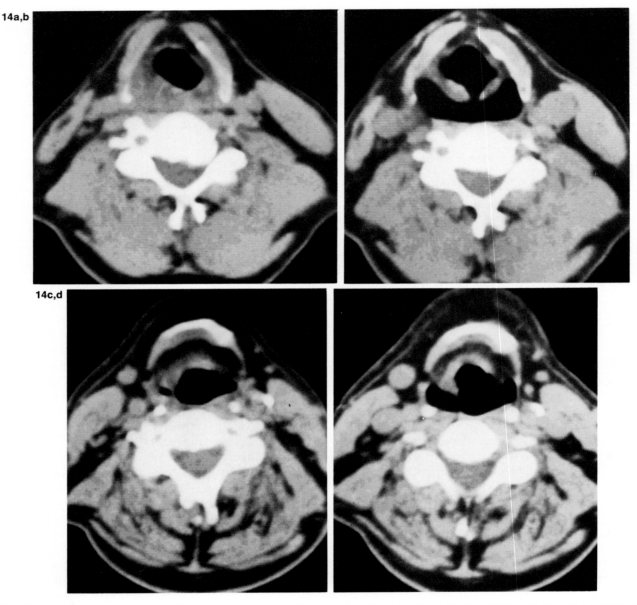

FIG. 14. Laryngeal maneuvers. **a:** The pyriform sinus is often not visualized during quiet inspiration. **b:** Repeat scanning during phonation ("e") distends the pyriform sinuses allowing more precise evaluation of the soft tissues in this region. **c:** In another patient with carcinoma of the epiglottis, the right pyriform sinus is not well distended. **d:** Scan during phonation shows a normally distended uninvolved right pyriform sinus, but neoplasm is seen to extend into the right aryepiglottic fold.

Indications and Results

Virtually all organs and abdominal compartments are considered amenable to percutaneous biopsy (40,44,57). As with any invasive procedure one should be sure that the potential benefits outweigh the possible risks and that it will provide clinically valuable information. The rate of recovery of positive tissue samples of aspiration biopsies has been high (60–90%) (22,29,44). The overall diagnostic yield for aspiration biopsy of abdominal masses is about 80% with few complications. Biopsy of lymphomatous masses and

lymph nodes has a significantly lower yield, but has also been shown to be efficacious (17,22). Aspiration biopsy of chest lesions has a yield of about 90%, with the only substantial risk being that of a pneumothorax.

Cytological analysis of aspiration biopsies is quite sensitive. Although it may be only possible to differentiate benign from malignant cells by cytological examination, a specific histological diagnosis can be rendered on occasion. Cutting needles and needles capable of obtaining larger specimens often increase the specificity, albeit with the acceptance of some increased risk.

TABLE 16. *Needles*

	Gauge	Comments
Aspiration		
Chiba (Cook)	22,23	Very flexible; hard to control
(Cook)	22	Slightly larger internal diameter than Chiba; very flexible; harder to control; may obtain slightly more tissue than Chiba
(Cook)	21	Less flexible than the Chiba and easier to control; suitable for obese patients
Modified aspiration		
Turner (Cook)	16,18,20,22	Potential for obtaining tissue fragments or core
Greene (Cook)	18–22	Potential for obtaining tissue core
Madayag (Waters Instruments)	22	Potential for obtaining tissue core
Rotex (Surgimed)	21	Potential for obtaining tissue fragments
Franseen (Cook)	16,18,20,22	Potential for obtaining tissue core
Johannah (Med. Serv. Inc.)	22,23	Potential for obtaining tissue core
Cutting		
Trucut (Cook)	14,16	
Lee (Cook)	20	Excellent for node biopsies
Westcott (Becton-Dickinson)	20	

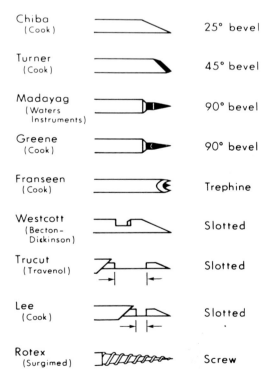

FIG. 15. Biopsy needles. Structural differences among the common biopsy needles presented in diagrammatic form; the stylet tips are shown in black.

Imaging Guidance

The radiologic guidance system employed for percutaneous biopsy largely depends on the size and location of the target lesion. The simplest imaging method that allows adequate definition of the mass with minimal risk to the patient should be selected. Most thoracic and bony lesions, as well as large superficial masses, can be biopsied under fluoroscopic guidance. Opacified lymph nodes are also amenable to biopsy under fluoroscopy (29). Large cystic collections, 4 cm or more in diameter, are ideal for ultrasound guidance, whereas deep and/or small lesions usually are best biopsied under CT control. Computed tomography offers precise three-dimensional localization of lesions (Fig. 16). Accurate depiction of relationships to vital structures is also a major advantage, but the greatest impact of CT as a guide for biopsy procedures is its ability to define exactly the location of the needle tip within a lesion (Fig. 17). Computed tomography is also extremely versatile, i.e., biopsy can be performed in a variety of positions with a variety of needles.

Although CT provides excellent images, disadvantages of CT-controlled biopsies include the encumbrance of the bulky CT gantry and competition with completing a usually quite busy CT schedule. We and others feel that CT should be reserved for those cases

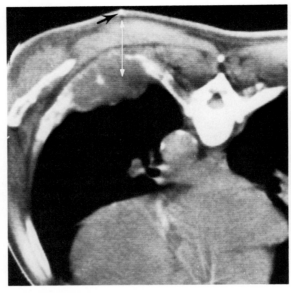 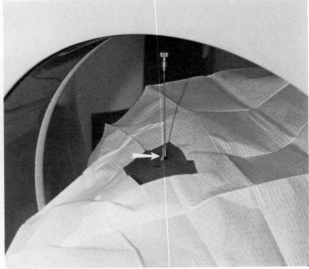

FIG. 16. CT-guided biopsy. CT guidance was selected for this posterior rib lesion since the mass was difficult to appreciate fluoroscopically. Computed tomography safely permitted placement of the tip of an 18-g Franseen needle directly in the tumoral mass. **Left:** Pre-biopsy planning scan was obtained with a 25-g needle (black arrow) in the anesthetized skin marking the entry site. The precise distance from the skin to the center of the mass (double white arrow) was measured directly on the CT monitor. **Right:** A photograph of the patient positioned in the scanning gantry with a biopsy needle inserted to a predetermined depth marked by a needle stop (arrow). Histologic analysis of the biopsy specimen disclosed metastatic prostatic carcinoma.

in which the lesion cannot be localized or the needle path cannot be guided safely by any other method (62).

Computed tomographic guidance should be strongly considered for biopsy of the following lesions: (a) non-opacified lymph nodes in the abdomen or pelvis, (b) small pancreatic masses, (c) any deeply seated lesion less than 5 cm in diameter, (d) lesions in the pelvis, and (e) lesions high in the abdomen that may require an angled approach to avoid the pleural space. No series of unselected patients is available to compare CT-guided biopsies with biopsies controlled under fluoroscopy or ultrasound. However, in one study (20), CT-guided biopsy was successful in 100% of cases versus 78% yield with fluoroscopic or ultrasound guidance.

Technique

Successful biopsies require planning and cooperation between and among technologists and radiologists. The details of couch position, gantry size, needle length, and availability of various paraphernalia become very important. A list of the basic equipment required for biopsy or drainage procedures is shown in Table 17. These items should be available as a unit at the time of the examination. An alternate needle or drainage tube may be added to the basic tray for a particular problem.

In general, the technique of aspiration biopsy is relatively simple to learn. This assertion is supported by the report that 10 different radiologists of all levels of experience contributed to a series of CT-controlled needle biopsy with 100% yield (20). They attributed their success to the CT depiction of the exact location of the needle tip.

The actual technique of CT-guided biopsy is straightforward, usually requiring no particular patient preparation other than discussing the procedure with the patient, obtaining the standard operative permit, and requiring the patient to fast for 3 hr prior to the biopsy. From the preliminary scans, taken in the same position and phase of respiration optimal for the biopsy, the one best level for biopsy is selected (Fig. 17). It is important to remember that biopsying the periphery of a suspected neoplastic lesion is more likely to yield diagnostic material, especially with a large mass. When the lesion to be biopsied is near a hemidiaphragm, either above or below, the phase of respiration may be crucial. End tidal volume ("breathe in, breathe out, relax, and stop breathing") seems to be the most reproducible respiratory pattern and best tolerated by the patient. A metallic marker (buckshot is adequate) is taped to the skin at the same level as the proposed entry site. In a sterile field, sterile buckshot or a 25-gauge needle tip placed into the anesthetized skin can be used. The scan is then repeated to confirm the marker location as ideal for needle entry. The approach is planned using the line cursor to simulate the needle path. Ideally, the shortest vertical line from skin to target volume is chosen, although a longer angled needle path may be selected to avoid critical structures.

The needle is advanced to the previously determined precise depth marked on the biopsy needle either with a needle stop, sterile tape, or the protective plastic needle sheath cut to the correct length (12). With the needle in place, a scan is obtained to confirm the needle tip location (Fig. 17). Several CT scans may be required to document the exact location of the needle tip, especially if the needle becomes angled. Although usually unnecessary, it is possible with this technique to inject a small amount of contrast material via the localizer needle if there is difficulty locating the needle tip. Once the needle tip is documented to be in the lesion, material is sampled by the appropriate technique. Negative pressure on the attached syringe is sufficient to obtain material through an aspirating needle; a twisting motion combined with suction is necessary for modified aspirating and cutting needles.

Because it is difficult to predict the adequacy of an aspirate by the gross appearance, most radiologists empirically obtain from two to six samples, especially when using an aspirating needle (22).

The sample can be smeared on glass slides with immediate fixation in 95% alcohol or the aspirate may be drawn into a syringe containing a balanced electrolyte solution to be delivered to the pathology lab for microbiology or cytopathology evaluation the same day. The latter technique allows centrifugation, which theoretically results in a more efficient cell harvest.

Post-biopsy monitoring is usually continued for about 4 hr, and should include an expiration chest radiograph if upper abdomen or chest lesions have been biopsied.

To eliminate repetition of the time-consuming localization process for each pass, two different methods have been developed. The first is a "double needle"

17a,b

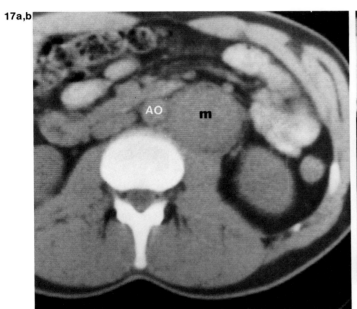
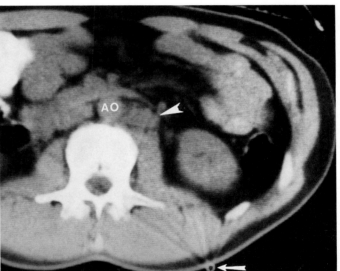

17c

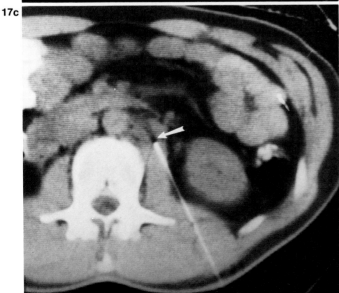

FIG. 17. CT-guided biopsy. **a:** CT scan demonstrates a large mass (m) due to metastatic seminoma lateral to the aorta (AO) and medial to the lower pole of the left kidney. Scans obtained after 6 months of chemotherapy demonstrated that the paraaortic mass had markedly diminished in size. **b:** To determine whether this mass represented residual tumor or fibrotic tissue, a percutaneous biopsy under CT control was elected. On a scan performed in the prone position, a metallic marker (arrow) is placed on the skin surface at a likely entry site for needle biopsy of the paraaortic mass (arrowhead). **c:** After advancing the biopsy needle, a CT scan confirms that the tip is in the paraaortic mass. "Shadowing" (arrow) of the needle distally confirms that the needle tip is within the scan plane.

TABLE 17. *Biopsy or drainage procedure*

Scalpel blade
"BB" for skin marker
Tape
Transparent centimeter ruler
Marking pen
Betadine
1% Lidocaine
Polysol or fixative/preservative
Sterile 4 × 4's
Sterile drape
Sterile needles: 23, 21, 18 gauge
Sterile syringes
Tubes
Sterile paper tape (or needle stop)
Needles:
   Greene 19, 21 gauge
   Spinal needles 18, 20, 22 gauge; 10, 15 cm lengths
   Chiba 22 gauge; 10, 15 cm lengths
   Trucut and Lee 18, 16, 14 gauge
   Franseen 20, 18 gauge
Clot tubes for chemistries
Pigtail catheter 8.3 F
Sump tube
Guide wires 0.025, 0.035, 0.038
Aerobic and anaerobic culture tubes
Gloves
(Albuminized glass slides)

technique. A large gauge needle (18 or 19 gauge) acts as a sleeve for the thin needle or an "introducing" needle. The first needle may be a short (3.8 cm) needle used to cross the abdominal musculature or a needle of sufficient length to approach the lesion (17,31). The 22-gauge needle is then passed through the large bore "introducer" to obtain samples. The introducing needle, although it may be helpful in crossing the anterior abdominal musculature, takes away one big advantage of the thin needle, i.e., its flexibility. The safety of thin needles is attributed to the flexibility of the needle as well as the size so that, for example, respiratory motion with the needle in place does not cause significant damage to internal organs.

The second method, which has largely replaced the double needle technique, is the "tandem needle" approach. A thin needle is advanced to the margin of the lesion and is left in place to act as a guide for the actual biopsy needle. Subsequent needle passes with fluoroscopic or CT confirmation of needle location are made immediately adjacent to the guide needle. The first needle is not withdrawn until the final sample is obtained. Thus, reproducibility of the needle path, angle, and depth is assured (20). Careful placement of an initial localization needle with CT documentation of the location of the needle tip makes it possible to carry out the actual biopsy under fluoroscopic control. This kind of compromise may make more efficient use of CT equipment.

An angled approach to avoid violating the pleura, vital organs, or peritoneum when performing large bore needle biopsy or a drainage procedure is some-

times required. Localization aids such as triangulation methods (20,24,78) and a grid marker system (34) have helped develop precise, angled biopsy routes when such meticulous needle placement is required. Triangulation applies the fundamentals of geometry to calculate the length and angulation of the needle path required to get to the lesion X from a proposed safe skin entry Y (Fig. 18). The calculation begins with determining the straight vertical distance from the skin surface to the lesion. The point on the skin overlying the lesion is marked Z and the lesion is designated X. The distance from Z to X is measured by CT and can be labeled *B*. Thus far the method is no different from the usual vertical approach. But now a safe entry point in the same parasagittal plane as Z is marked Y for the actual needle insertion. The distance from Z to Y is labeled *A*. A right triangle can be constructed. Since two sides, *A* and *B*, are known, the third side, representing the path of the needle, can be calculated by the Pythagorean theorem from $A^2 + B^2 = C^2$. In addition the angle, *a*, can be calculated since the tangent of *a* is equal to the ratio of the opposite side, *B*, over the adjacent side, *A*. The angle of the needle to the horizontal, 0, will be equal to angle *a*. Once the needle path length and the angle are calculated, the biopsy procedure is performed as any other. It is mandatory that the needle stay in the intended parasagittal plane and that a goniometer be available to allow the operator to obtain the proper needle angle.

A simpler application of the triangulation approach (24) has been to transfer the full scale distances *A* (measured directly from the patient) and *B* (measured by CT) onto two edges and the enclosed corner of a large index card. Connecting X and Y, the triangle can be completed with *C* representing the length of the desired needle path. The angle of the approach can also be measured directly from the index card by measuring angle *a* using a goniometer. This method

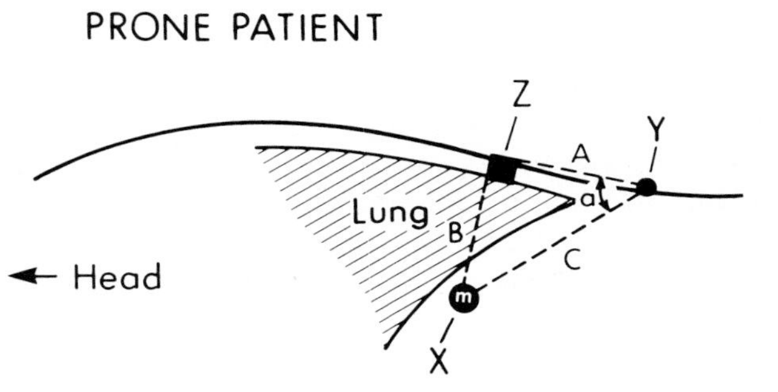

PRONE PATIENT

FIG. 18. Triangulation method. Construction of a right triangle (X,Y,Z) with "Z" at a point directly above the mass ("X") to be biopsied and "Y" the prospective needle entry site will allow the needle path length (C) to be determined according to the Pythagorean theorem and the angle "a" calculated from the ratio of B to A. This triangle can be constructed full scale directly on a large index card enabling one to obtain length C and angle "a" by direct measurement (24).

circumvents the need to use mathematics tables and is less likely to lead to mistakes.

Complications

Based on a vast collective experience, thin needle biopsies within the abdomen can be performed without undue concern for vascular structures, ducts, and bowel loops (7,29,37,53). Inadvertent puncture of the bowel, urinary bladder, gallbladder, ureter, and even large vessels (40) is almost always without clinical sequelae. Potentially, percutaneous abdominal biopsies are associated with risks of bleeding, bacterial contamination, peritoneal leakage, and pancreatitis; these events, however, are rare (19,21). The overall incidence of complications is quite low, about 5% (20), including transient hypotension and pneumothorax. Theoretically the risk of needle biopsy increases as the bore or diameter of the needle increases. In addition there is a significant increment in risk when a cutting needle is employed. Still, complications of large bore and cutting needles are minimal when adequate precautions are taken and CT guidance is available (30).

An adverse effect of needle biopsy on patient survival has not been documented (7) despite the theoretical possibility of inducing intravascular dissemination of malignant cells. Contraindications to percutaneous biopsy are few. One absolute contraindication due to the risk of peritoneal contamination might be that an abdominal lesion represents an echinococcal cyst. A relative contraindication is a bleeding disorder, which frequently can be remedied by administering appropriate blood products. Highly vascularized lesions impose an increased risk for percutaneous biopsy; however, again, thin needle biopsies performed in the routine manner with post-biopsy monitoring are almost always well tolerated.

Drainage Procedures

Percutaneous abscess drainage (PAD), an increasingly common procedure, is a logical extension and application of the biopsy technique. The basic principles of surgical management of abscess can be applied without the insult of general anesthesia and major surgery (26,27,55,76). In many centers, PAD has become the method of choice for the initial treatment of intraabdominal abscess.

Imaging Guidance

There are three distinct functions required of the imaging study directing percutaneous drainage. The first is to diagnose an abdominal abscess; conventional radiography, ultrasound, radionuclide gallium imaging, and CT all may be used to diagnose an abscess.

When the overwhelmingly likely clinical diagnosis is abscess, CT is certainly the diagnostic method of choice (26) as it will allow precise definition of the collection and relationship to surrounding structures. Even if CT cannot specifically differentiate an abscess from a hematoma, seroma, or necrotic neoplasm, the detailed cross-sectional view will localize the collection precisely. The second function of imaging is to plan a safe catheter route. This requires visualization of both bowel loops and the abscess and usually is best accomplished with CT, although the combination of ultrasound and fluoroscopy may suffice. The third function is to guide the actual placement of the drainage catheter. Ultrasound, with its scan-plane flexibility and instantaneous imaging capability, is sometimes favored for this purpose.

All things considered and given equal availability, CT would be the number one choice of guidance techniques for abscess drainage (25).

Indications

In general, four criteria are used (26,55,76) to define patients who are amenable to percutaneous drainage: (a) a well-defined unilocular abscess cavity, (b) a safe percutaneous drainage route, (c) concurring evaluation by surgical and radiologic services, and (d) immediate operative capability in case of failure or complication. These criteria include a large proportion, probably near 90% (26), of intraabdominal abscesses. Abscesses that have a higher likelihood of requiring surgical intervention (26,31) are (a) multiloculated, (b) situated between bowel loops or deep in pelvis, (c) filled with thick, viscid material, or (d) pancreatic abscesses.

Catheter Systems

Adequate drainage requires a large bore catheter with multiple side holes to minimize occlusion. The many catheters that satisfy these prerequisites (25, 31,56,76) can be divided into three basic types: (a) a pigtail angiocatheter, (b) a trocar catheter, and (c) a sump tube (Fig. 19).

The curled distal configuration of the pigtail catheter is atraumatic to cavity walls and provides stability within a lesion. It has been used primarily for parenchymal and deep abscesses. This catheter is available in a variety of sizes. The major disadvantage is the relatively small side holes.

Trocar-catheter units have been used to drain large, superficial lesions by direct puncture (27). The major merit of this system is that the side holes are larger than the pigtail angiocatheter. The unit illustrated has a small inflatable balloon that can be used to secure the catheter further, although this is not of much practical value. Depending on the unit, the catheter may not be

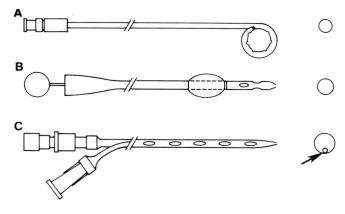

FIG. 19. Drainage catheters. Pigtail (A), trocar (B), and sump-type (C) catheters are shown diagrammatically. The cross-sectional view to the right of each catheter demonstrates the single lumen of both the pigtail and trocar catheters and the double lumen of the sump catheter. The air vent lumen of the sump tube is indicated by the arrow.

as flexible as either the pigtail or the sump catheters and the straight configuration of a trocar system is a disadvantage. Because of the weight and size of this system, direct control of catheter placement by cross-sectional radiologic imaging is not possible; however, the previous confirmatory needle aspiration provides important guidance.

The system that is probably most effective and most widely applicable is the sump catheter. The van Sonnenberg sump catheter (Medi-Tech, Inc.) is a flexible, double lumen tube with large oval side holes (41,55,77). This catheter may be used for either deep focal collections or the larger, more accessible abscesses since it is prepared for placement using either the guide wire exchange method or the trocar method. The dual lumen design allows for concomitant irrigation and drainage, but, perhaps even more importantly, it allows for active withdrawal of fluid. Suction applied to pigtail or trocar units tends to cause cavity walls to collapse around the catheter, occluding drain holes.

These systems, therefore, are usually left to dependent drainage. The sump catheter, however, prevents tissue encroachment by allowing air ingress through the smaller lumen while suction is being applied to the major lumen.

Technique

The technique of abscess drainage begins with radiologic imaging of a mass. Often with clinical information a relatively specific diagnosis of abscess can be made, however, a preliminary diagnostic aspiration is always performed. The needle biopsy technique described previously is followed with three exceptions. First, the initial incision is slightly more generous, usually about 4 mm, and is widened with blunt dissection using a hemostat. Second, a 16- to 20-gauge needle may be used since it is theoretically more difficult to aspirate pus through a 22-gauge needle. Third, the needle path takes on added importance since it is usually the route used for catheter placement. The path of a needle biopsy is not so critical; however, the route for placing an indwelling catheter must be planned to avoid bowel loops, intervening organs and vascular structures, and the posterior pulmonary sulcus. Abdominal abscesses typically displace surrounding viscera providing a "window" for a percutaneous approach. Aspiration of a significant amount of the lesion's contents may change the relationship of the collection to neighboring structures such that placement of a drainage catheter is made more difficult; therefore, only a few cc's of aspirate are obtained with the thin needle in place. Although an extraperitoneal approach is preferred, both transperitoneal and extraperitoneal approaches have been shown to be safe (26). The remainder of the procedure of actual catheter placement varies somewhat depending on the catheter system selected. The details specific for each catheter type are described separately.

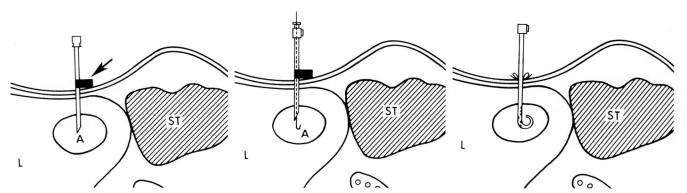

FIG. 20. Percutaneous abscess drainage using pigtail catheter. **Left:** The angiocatheter technique of this diagrammatic representation of a liver abscess (A) begins with placing a needle into the collection. Arrow indicates a strip of sterile tape used as a needle stop. L, liver; ST, stomach. **Center:** A guide wire is passed through the needle into the collection. The needle is then removed leaving the guide in place. **Right:** A pigtail catheter is threaded over the guide wire and the guide wire removed. The catheter is secured in place with suture material. (Modified from Gerzof et al., ref. 27.)

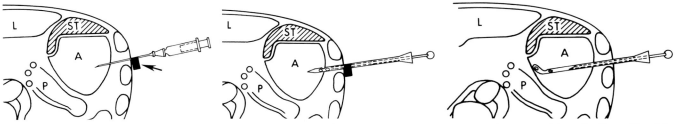

FIG. 21. Percutaneous abscess drainage using trocar catheter. **Left:** Aspiration of this diagrammatic retrogastric collection with a thin needle is done as an initial confirmatory procedure. The needle stop is indicated by the arrow. L, liver; P, pancreas; ST, stomach; A, abscess. **Center:** The trocar unit is advanced to a previously determined distance with a needle stop in place to prevent puncture of the back wall of the abscess. **Right:** Keeping the stylet in place, the catheter is advanced over the stylet until the drainage tube is well seated in the cavity. The trocar is removed and dependent drainage begun. (Modified from Gerzof et al., ref. 27.)

Pigtail catheter placement.

A pigtail catheter is placed using a modified Seldinger technique (27) (Fig. 20). Specifically, a .038-inch 80-cm floppy or J-tip guide wire is passed through an 18-gauge needle. The needle is removed, and an 8-F angio dilator is passed over the guide and removed while the position of the guide is carefully maintained. Finally, the catheter is threaded over the guide wire and into the lesion. The guide wire is removed and the position of the pigtail confirmed with repeat scanning. Contrast media injection may be of value to ensure proper location of the catheter.

Trocar catheter placement.

After confirmation of the abscess by needle aspiration and removal of the needle (Fig. 21), a 12- to 16-F trocar catheter with a cutting edge stylet is passed through the front wall of the abscess. The catheter is advanced over the stylet to the back wall. The stylet is then removed. After securing the catheter, pus is manually aspirated from the lesion with a syringe.

Sump catheter placement.

The van Sonnenberg sump can be introduced by either the angiocatheter or the trocar catheter technique. With successful drainage, the patient usually becomes afebrile after 48 hr (26). The catheter is left to gravity drainage or suction as long as fluid continues to drain. Follow-up imaging studies, as well as clinical parameters, frequently provide objective measures of the endpoint of the procedure (Fig. 22). To avoid recurrence, the catheter is generally left in place for 2 to 4 days after cessation of drainage (26). The mean duration of treatment has been 7 to 10 days. It has been noted that abscesses with enteric communication require longer periods of drainage but don't necessarily require surgical intervention.

Although seldom absolutely required, it has been suggested (76) that catheter irrigation hastens debridement of the cavity, maintains catheter patency, improves abscess drainage, and prevents loculation. Irrigation should be gentle to avoid bacteremia. Sinograms, performed gently to avoid spillage, are occa-

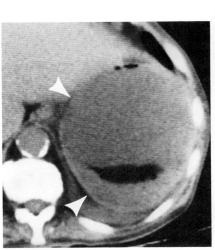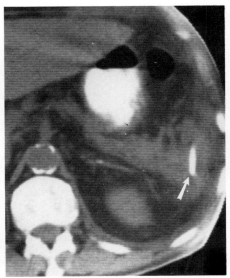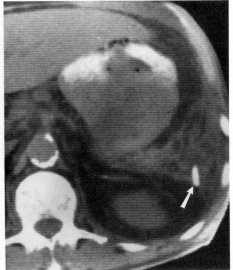

FIG. 22. Drainage procedures. **Left:** A splenic bed collection (arrowheads) was defined in this man who had undergone a splenectomy one month earlier. **Center:** Scan post-insertion of a catheter confirms that the abscess is decreasing in size. **Right:** Scan 2 weeks later confirms that successful drainage has been accomplished. Arrows indicate a portion of the drainage catheter.

sionally helpful to evaluate the abscess cavity when contemplating catheter withdrawal or possible re-treatment. Intravenous antibiotic coverage is used in all instances of percutaneous drainage.

Although the experience is limited, acetyl cysteine (Mucomyst®) (Mead Johnson Pharmaceutical), a mucolytic agent, has been reported to be useful in maintaining patency of drainage catheters by liquefying thick pus (79). Small quantities (2–5 cc) of a 10 to 20% acetyl cysteine solution are used to flush the catheter. A sump tube facilitates such flushing maneuvers.

Results and Complications

Percutaneous drainage of abscess compares favorably to operative treatment in terms of complication rate, adequacy of drainage, duration of drainage, and recurrence rate. It has been stated that these improved results may in part be related to the diagnostic accuracy of CT, which facilitates earlier diagnosis and therapy (26). Although the sump catheter has been advocated as a slightly better approach, the success rate of PAD does not seem to be dependent on the catheter system used.

Complication rates of 10 to 15% have included peritoneal spill, empyema, diaphragmatic perforation, enteric fistula, and laceration of a mesenteric vessel (26,76). The incidence of recurrence of an abscess collection after successful PAD is approximately 5%. These figures compare favorably to surgical management of abscess, which is associated with a mortality rate of about 10% and a recurrence rate of about 14%.

Summary

Percutaneous drainage of abdominal abscesses is a technique that minimizes manipulation of the abscess and, theoretically, in comparison to surgery, would be less likely to cause spillage, hematogenous spread, or sepsis. In addition it has the specific advantages of (a) avoiding the risks of surgery and anesthesia, (b) saving considerable time and expense, (c) making nursing care easier, and (d) lowering recurrence rate. Surgical treatment of abdominal abscesses perhaps should be reserved for those collections that have evidence of loculation or have no safe drainage route or in which a percutaneous drainage has failed. Even when surgery is ultimately required, the benefits of percutaneous drainage, as the initial approach to abscesses, far outweigh the potential risks and do not appear to complicate surgical drainage. It is clear that optimal management of abscesses requires the cooperative effort of the primary physician, surgeon, and radiologist.

REFERENCES

1. Albrechtsson U, Stahl E, Tylen U: Evaluation of coronary artery bypass graft patency with computed tomography. *J Comput Assist Tomogr* 5:822–826, 1981
2. Alvarez RE, Marcovski A: Energy-selective reconstructions in x-ray computerized tomography. *Phys Med Biol* 21:733–744, 1976
3. Baert AL: *CT Angiographic Techniques.* Fifth Annual Course in Computed Body Tomography, Tarpon Springs, Florida, 1982
4. Ball WS, Wicks JD, Mettler FA Jr: Prone-supine change in organ position: CT demonstration. *AJR* 135:815–820, 1980
5. Barnett PH, Zerhouni EA, White RI, Siegelman SS: Computed tomography in the diagnosis of cavernous hemangioma. *AJR* 134:439–447, 1980
6. Baxter BS, Sorenson JA: Factors affecting the measurement of size and CT number in computed tomography. *Invest Radiol* 16:337–341, 1981
7. Berg JW, Robbins GF: A late look at the safety of aspiration biopsy. *Cancer* 15:826–827, 1962
8. Brooks RA, Keller MR, O'Connor CM, Sheridan WT: Progress toward quantitative computed tomography. *IEEE Trans Nucl Sci* 27:1121–1127, 1980
9. Burgener FA, Hamlin DJ: Contrast enhancement in abdominal CT: Bolus vs. infusion. *AJR* 137:351–358, 1981
10. Cattell WR: Excretory pathways for contrast media. *Invest Radiol* 5:473–497, 1970
11. Cattell WR, Fry IK, Spencer AG, Purkiss P: Excretion Urography 1. Factors determining the excretion of hypaque. *Br J Radiol* 40:561–580, 1967
12. Chen SM: A simple method of limiting needle depth during percutaneous biopsy. *Radiology* 143:269, 1982
13. Cohen G, DiBianca FA: Information content and dose efficiency of computed tomographic scanners. In: *The Physics of Medical Imaging,* ed. by AG Haus, New York, American Institute of Physics, 1979, pp 356–357
14. Cohen WN, Seidelmann FE, Bryan PF: The use of a tampon to enhance vaginal localization in computed tomography of the female pelvis. *AJR* 128:1064–1065, 1977
15. Cohen Z, Seltzer SE, Davis MA, Hanson RN: Iodinated starch particles: New contrast material for computed tomography of the liver. *J Comput Assist Tomogr* 5:843–846, 1981
16. Dossetor RS, Veiga-Pires JA, Kaiser M: Localization of scanning level in computed tomography of the spine. *J Comput Assist Tomogr* 3:284–285, 1979
17. Dunnick NR, Fisher RI, Chu EW, Young RC: Percutaneous aspiration of retroperitoneal lymph nodes in ovarian cancer. *AJR* 135:109–113, 1980
18. Engelstad BL, McClennan BL, Levitt RG, Stanley RJ, Sagel SS: The role of pre-contrast images in computed tomography of the kidney. *Radiology* 136:153–155, 1980
19. Evans WK, Ho C, McLoughlin MJ, Tao L: Fatal necrotizing pancreatitis following fine-needle aspiration biopsy of the pancreas. *Radiology* 141:61–62, 1981
20. Ferrucci JT Jr., Wittenberg J: CT biopsy of abdominal tumors: Aids for lesion localization. *Radiology* 129:739–744, 1978
21. Ferrucci JT, Wittenberg J, Margolies MN, Carey, RW: Malignant seeding of the tract after thin-needle aspiration biopsy. *Radiology* 130:345–346, 1979
22. Ferrucci JT Jr, Wittenberg J, Mueller PR, Simeone JF, Kirkpatrick RH, Taft PD: Diagnosis of abdominal malignancy by radiologic fine-needle biopsy. *AJR* 134:323–330, 1980
23. Gardeur D, Lautrau J, Millard JC, Berger N, Metzger J: Pharmacokinetics of contrast media: Experimental results in dog and man with CT implications. *J Comput Assist Tomogr* 4:178–185, 1980
24. Gerzof SG: Triangulation: Indirect CT guidance for abscess drainage. *AJR* 137:1080–1081, 1981
25. Gerzof SG, Robbins AH, Birkett DH, Johnson WC, Pugatch RD, Vincent ME: Percutaneous catheter drainage of abdominal abscesses guided by ultrasound and computed tomography. *AJR* 133:1–8, 1979
26. Gerzof SG, Robbins AH, Johnson WC, Birkett DH, Nabseth

DC: Percutaneous catheter drainage of abdominal abscesses. *N Engl J Med* 305:653–657, 1981

27. Gerzof SG, Spira R, Robbins AH: Percutaneous abscess drainage. *Semin Roentgenol* 16:62–71, 1981

28. Glazer GM, Goldberg HI, Moss AA, Axel L: Computed tomographic detection of retroperitoneal adenopathy. *Radiology* 143:147–149, 1982

29. Gothlin JH: Post lymphographic percutaneous fine needle biopsy of lymph nodes guided by fluoroscopy. *Radiology* 120:205–207, 1976

30. Haaga JR: New techniques for CT-guided biopsies. *AJR* 133:633–641, 1979

31. Haaga JR, Reich NE, Havrilla TR, Alfidi RJ: Interventional CT scanning. *Radiol Clin North Am* 15:449–456, 1977

32. Haaga JR, Vanek J: Computed tomographic guided liver biopsy using the Menghini needle. *Radiology* 133:405–408, 1979

33. Hagman LA, Evans RA, Fahr LM, Hinick VA: Renal consequences of rapid high dose contrast CT. *AJR* 134:553, 1980

34. Hammerschlag SB, Wolpert SM, Carter BL: Computed tomography of the spinal canal. *Radiology* 121:361–367, 1976

35. Hatfield KD, Segal SD, Tait K: Barium sulfate for abdominal computer assisted tomography. *J Comput Assist Tomogr* 4:570, 1980

36. Havron A, Seltzer SE, Davis MA, Shulkin P: Radiopaque liposomes: A promising new contrast material for computed tomography of the spleen. *Radiology* 140:507–511, 1981

37. Holm HH, Als O, Gammelgaard J: Percutaneous aspiration biopsy procedures under ultrasonic visualization. In: *Clinics in Diagnostic Ultrasound. Vol. I. Diagnostic Ultrasound in Gastrointestinal Disease,* ed. by KJW Taylor, New York, Churchill Livingstone, 1978, pp 137–149

38. Isler RJ, Ferrucci JT Jr, Wittenberg J, Mueller PR, Simeone JF, van Sonnenberg E, Hall DA: Tissue core biopsy of abdominal tumors with a 22 gauge cutting needle. *AJR* 136:725–728, 1981

39. Itai Y, Furui S, Araki T, Tasaka A: Computed tomography of cavernous hemangioma of the liver. *Radiology* 137:149–155, 1980

40. Jacques PF, Staab EV, Richey W, Photopoulos G, Swanton M: CT-assisted pelvic and abdominal aspiration biopsies in gynecological malignancy. *Radiology* 128:651, 1978

41. Karlson KB, Martin EC, Fankuchen EI, Mattern RF, Schultz RW, Casarella WJ: Percutaneous drainage of pancreatic pseudocysts and abscesses. *Radiology* 142:619–624, 1982

42. Kaye MD, Young SW, Hayward R, Castellino RA: Gastric pseudotumor on CT scanning. *AJR* 135:190–193, 1980

43. Kivisaari L, Kormano M, Rantakokko V: Contrast enhancement of the pancreas in computed tomography. *J Comput Assist Tomogr* 3:722–726, 1979

44. Kline TS, Neal HS: Needle aspiration biopsy: A critical appraisal eight years and 3,267 specimens later. *JAMA* 239:36–39, 1978

45. Koehler PR, Anderson RE: Computed angiotomography. *Radiology* 137:843–845, 1980

46. Koehler PR, Anderson RE, Baxter B: The effect of computed tomography viewer controls on anatomical measurements. *Radiology* 130:189–194, 1979

47. Kormano M, Dean PB: Extravascular contrast material: The major component of contrast enhancement. *Radiology* 121:379–382, 1976

48. Kormano M, Dean PB, Hamlin DJ: Upper extremity contrast medium infusion in computed tomography of upper mediastinal masses. *J Comput Assist Tomogr* 4:619–620, 1980

49. Kuhns LR, Seigel R, Borlaza GS: A simple method of localizing the level of computed tomography cross-sectioning. *J Comput Assist Tomogr* 2:233–234, 1978

50. Kuhns LR, Thornbury J, Siegel R: Variation of position of the kidneys and diaphragm in patients undergoing repeated suspension of respiration. *J Comput Assist Tomogr* 3:620–621, 1979

51. Lee JKT, Barbier JY, McClennan BL, Stanley RJ: A support device for direct coronal CT imaging of the pelvis. *Radiology (in press)*

52. Lieberman RP, Hafez GR, Crummy AB: Histology from aspiration biopsy: Turner needle experience. *AJR* 138:561–564, 1982

53. McLouglin MJ, Ho CS, Langar B, McHattie J, Tao LC: Fine needle aspiration biopsy of malignant lesions in and around the pancreas. *Cancer* 41:2413–2419, 1978

54. Marchal GJ, Baert AL, Wilms G: Intravenous pancreaticography in computed tomography. *J Comput Assist Tomogr* 3:727–732, 1979

55. Martin EC, Karison KB, Fankuchen EI, Cooperman A, Casarella WJ: Percutaneous drainage of postoperative intraabdominal abscesses. *AJR* 138:13–15, 1982

56. Mauro MA, Jacques PF: Modified trocar-cannula system for percutaneous pancreatic abscess drainage. *Radiology* 139:227–228, 1981

57. Mueller PR, Wittenberg J, Ferrucci JT Jr: Fine needle aspiration biopsy of abdominal masses. *Semin Roentgenol* 16:52–61, 1981

58. Newhouse JH, Murphy RX: Tissue distribution of soluble contrast: Effect of dose variation and changes with time. *AJR* 136:463–467, 1981

59. Nikesch W: Using a radiation therapy simulator to localize the anatomical level of computed tomography slices. *J Comput Assist Tomogr* 5:593–595, 1981

60. Ono N, Martinez CR, Fara JW, Hodges FJ III: Diatrizoate distribution in dogs as a function of administration rate and time following intravenous injection. *J Comput Assist Tomogr* 4:174–177, 1980

61. Osborn AG, Koehler PR, Gibbs FA, Leavitt DD, Anderson RE, Lee TG, Ferris DT: Direct sagittal computed tomographic scans in the radiographic evaluation of the pelvis. *Radiology* 134:255–257, 1980

62. Pereiras RV, Meiers W, Kunhardt B, Troner M, Hutson D, Barkin JS, Viamonte M: Fluoroscopically guided thin needle aspiration biopsy of the abdomen and retroperitoneum. *AJR* 131:197–202, 1978

63. Piekarski J, Goldberg HI, Royal SA, Axel L, Moss AA: Difference between liver and spleen CT numbers in the normal adult: Its usefulness in predicting the presence of diffuse liver disease. *Radiology* 137:727–729, 1980

64. Purdy JA, Prasad SC: Computed tomography applied to radiation therapy treatment planning. Medical physics of CT and ultrasound: Tissue imaging and characteristics. *Med Phys,* Monograph No. 6:224, 1980

65. Ritchings RT, Pullan BR: A technique for simulating dual energy scanning. *J Comput Assist Tomogr* 3:842–846, 1979

66. Robbins AH, Pugatch RD, Gerzof SG, Spira R, Rankin SC, Gale DR: An assessment of the role of scan speed in perceived image quality of body computed tomography. *Radiology* 139:139–146, 1981

67. Russell WJ, Murakami J, Kimura S, Hayabuchi N: Computed tomography localizer. *Comput Tomogr* 5:215–220, 1981

68. Rutherford RA, Pullan BR, Isherwood I: Measurement of effective atomic number and electron density using an EMI scanner. *Neuroradiology* 11:15–21, 1976

69. Rutt B, Fenster A: Split-filter computed tomography: A simple technique for dual energy scanning. *J Comput Assist Tomogr* 4:501–509, 1980

70. Seltzer SE, Adams DF, Davis MA, Hessel SJ, Havron A, Judy PF, Paskins-Hurlburt AJ, Hollenberg N: Hepatic contrast agents for computed tomography: High atomic number particulate material. *J Comput Assist Tomogr* 5:370–374, 1981

71. Sheldon JJ, Sersland T, Leborgne J: Computed tomography of the lower lumbar vertebral column. *Radiology* 124:113–118, 1977

72. Shirkhoda A, Johnston RE, Staab EV, McCartney WH: Optimal computed tomography technique for bone evaluation. *J Comput Assist Tomogr* 3:134–139, 1979

73. Siegelman SS, Zerhouni EA, Leo FP, Khouri NF, Stitik FP: CT of the solitary pulmonary nodule. *AJR* 135:1–14, 1980

74. Spirt BA: Value of the prone position in detecting pulmonary nodules by computed tomography. *J Comput Assist Tomogr* 4:871–873, 1980

75. Stuck KJ, Kuhns LR: Improved visualization of the pancreatic tail after maximum distension of the stomach. *J Comput Assist Tomogr* 5:509–512, 1981

76. van Sonnenberg E, Ferrucci JT Jr, Mueller PR, Wittenberg J, Simeone JF: Percutaneous drainage of abscesses and fluid col-

lections: Technique, results, and applications. *Radiology* 142:1–10, 1982

77. van Sonnenberg E, Mueller PR, Ferrucci JT Jr, Neft C, Simeone J, Wittenberg J: A specially designed catheter for abscess and fluid drainage: A double lumen sump catheter with large side holes and options for insertion by direct trocar puncture or guidewire technique. *Radiology (in press)*

78. van Sonnenberg E, Wittenberg J, Ferrucci JT Jr, Mueller PR, Simeone JF: Triangulation method for percutaneous needle guidance: The angled approach to upper abdominal masses. *AJR* 137:757–761, 1981

79. van Waes PFGM: *Management of Loculated Abscesses Containing Hardly Drainable Pus: A New Approach.* Presented at the Annual Meeting of the Society of Uroradiology, March 22–25, 1982

80. van Waes PFGM, Zonneveld FW: Direct coronal body computed tomography. *J Comput Assist Tomogr* 6:58–66, 1982

81. Vermess M, Bernardino ME, Doppman JL, Fisher RI, Thomas JL, Velasquez ES, Fuller LM, Russo A: Use of intravenous liposoluble contrast material for the examination of the liver and spleen in lymphoma. *J Comput Assist Tomogr* 5:709–713, 1981

82. Vermess M, Chatterji DC, Doppman JL, Grimes G, Adamson RH: Development and experimental evaluation of a contrast medium for computed tomographic examination of the liver and spleen. *J Comput Assist Tomogr* 3:25–31, 1979

83. Vermess M, Inscoe S, Sugarbaker P: Use of liposoluble contrast material to separate left renal and splenic parenchyma on computed tomography. *J Comput Assist Tomogr* 4:540–542, 1980

84. Vermess M, Javadpour N, Blayney DW: Post-splenectomy demonstration of splenic tissue by computed tomography with liposoluble contrast material. *J Comput Assist Tomogr* 5:106–108, 1981

85. Villafana T, Lee SH, Lapayowker MS: A device to indicate anatomical level in computed tomography. *J Comput Assist Tomogr* 2:368–371, 1978

86. Young SW, Muller HH, Marincek B: Contrast enhancement of malignant tumors after intravenous polyvinylpyrrolidone with metallic salts as determined by computed tomography. *Radiology* 138:97–106, 1981

87. Young SW, Noon MA, Nassi M, Castellino RA: Dynamic computed tomography body scanning. *J Comput Assist Tomogr* 4:168–173, 1980

88. Young SW, Turner RJ, Castellino RA: A strategy for contrast enhancement of malignant tumor using dynamic CT and intravascular pharmacokinetics. *Radiology* 137:137–147, 1980

89. Zatz LM: The effect of the kVp level on EMI values. *Radiology* 119:683–688, 1976

90. Zornoza J: Abdomen. In: *Percutaneous Needle Biopsy*, ed. by J Zornoza, Baltimore, William & Wilkins, 1981, pp. 103–105

Chapter 3

Larynx

Stuart S. Sagel

Computed tomography of the larynx, using thin collimation (5 mm) combined with a rapid scan time (less than 5 sec), is a clinically valuable tool in assessing carcinoma of and trauma to the larynx (1–3,10–13,16,17). The entire larynx, including the cartilage and surrounding soft tissues, can be evaluated. Computed tomography is the radiologic procedure of choice to supplement the findings at laryngoscopy when additional diagnostic information is required to determine the feasibility of conservation surgery. Following trauma, CT is the best radiologic technique to assess possible cartilaginous injury and any concomitant airway encroachment.

Laryngeal carcinomas are detected by indirect and direct laryngoscopy, but the limitations of clinical methods to determine the exact anatomic location, size, and extent of such tumors are well recognized. Only the mucosal surfaces are seen, and deep (submucosal) spread must be inferred from increased bulk or altered physiology. Frequently, the surface extension of a laryngeal carcinoma represents only the "tip of the iceberg." Neoplastic invasion of the paralaryngeal and pre-epiglottic space or adjacent supporting cartilaginous structures may be difficult or impossible to ascertain, even with deep biopsy, and the base of the epiglottis and subglottic space often are poorly seen. In the past, when the only treatment alternatives for carcinoma of the larynx were total laryngectomy or radiation therapy delivered through relatively large ports, correct delineation of the extent of tumor was less important. With the development of conservation surgery designed to preserve a useful voice and food swallowing function, precise delineation of tumor has become imperative for proper surgical planning (9,15). The usefulness of radiologic examination, especially laryngography (7), to provide supplemental information to the clinical examination, has been known for many years. Nevertheless, certain areas—such as the paralaryngeal soft tissues and supporting cartilages—may still be difficult to assess. Computed tomography provides a noninvasive imaging technique capable of a unique three-dimensional

anatomic display of these areas of the larynx (Figs. 1 and 2).

TECHNIQUE

Since significant anatomical relationships change within millimeters, and because respiratory motion may cause the entire larynx to move 1 cm or more, *thinly collimated sections* obtained with *rapid scanning times* are necessary for optimal portrayal of laryngeal anatomy and tumor extent. Almost all of the latest commercially available CT scanners provide such technical capabilities. A rotary motion, stationary detector array CT scanner (EMI 7070) is used in our medical center. The scanner is operated at 120 kVp, between 20 and 60 mA, with a 3-sec scan time and small field of view (125 to 250 mm). With the patient supine, the neck is extended (with the orbitomeatal line approximately 25 to 30° from the vertical) to make the larynx as parallel and the vocal cords as perpendicular to the table top as possible. Contiguous 5 mm thick sections are obtained over the entire laryngeal area (from the base of the tongue above the hyoid down to the upper trachea). Approximately 14 slices are required to cover the area of interest. Most scans are performed during a slow inspiratory effort. The patient is cautioned against swallowing, moving, or talking. Scanning is occasionally performed during phonation ("e") or during a modified Valsalva maneuver (to fill out the pyriform sinuses and better delineate the aryepiglottic folds) (6) or a reverse "e" maneuver (to fill out the ventricles and aid separation of the true from false vocal cords) whenever clarification is required. Iodinated intravenous contrast medium administration is used in only selected cases to document that a structure is vascular in origin or to determine the relationship of neoplasm to major vessels.

NORMAL ANATOMY (FIGS. 3–9)

Accurate interpretation of CT scans of the larynx requires high quality images and rigid control of tech-

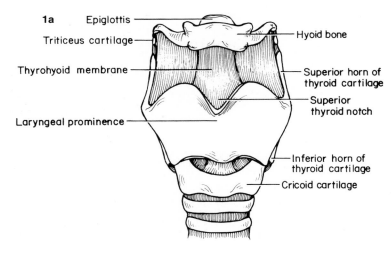

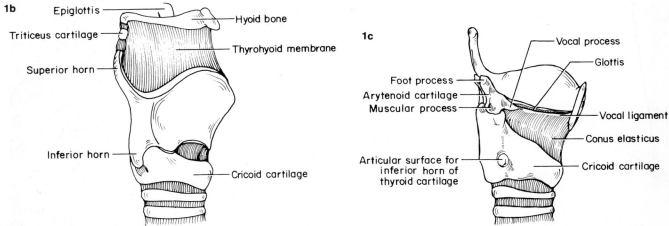

FIG. 1. Schematic drawings of laryngeal skeleton. **a:** Frontal view. **b:** Lateral view. **c:** Lateral view after removal of the right lamina of the thyroid cartilage.

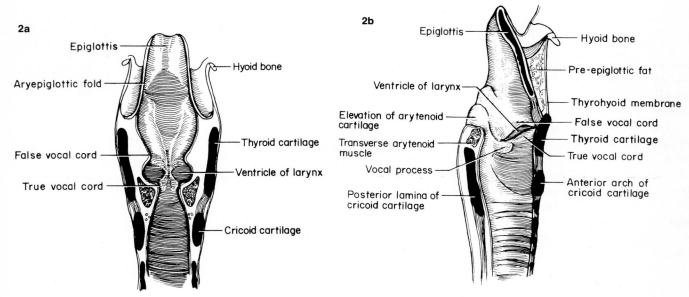

FIG. 2. Sections through larynx and surrounding tissues. **a:** Coronal view. **b:** Sagittal view.

3a,b

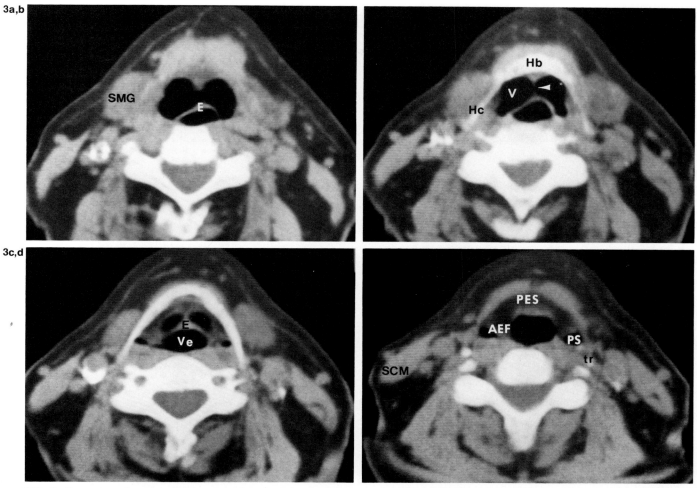

3c,d

FIG. 3. Normal anatomy: hyoid bone region (serial scans at 5 mm intervals in caudad direction).

a: Above the level of the hyoid bone, the thin epiglottis (E) is seen posterior to the valleculae. The free edge of the epiglottis abuts but does not attach to the posterior pharyngeal wall. A portion of the right submandibular gland (SMG) is present; this structure often appears somewhat asymmetric and should not be confused with enlarged lymph nodes.

b: At the next inferior level, the body of the hyoid bone (Hb) is visible, as well as the upper portion of the major cornua of the hyoid bone (Hc). The paired, air-filled valleculae (V) are seen, anterior to the epiglottis, separated by the median glossoepiglottic fold (arrowhead).

c: More inferiorly, the valleculae have become smaller and slightly asymmetric, a normal variation. The top of the pyriform sinuses can be seen lateral to the laryngeal vestibule (Ve), which lies posterior to the epiglottis (E).

d: The fat-containing pre-epiglottic space (PES) is seen anterior to the soft tissue density epiglottis. The fat in this space extends posterolateral into the aryepiglottic folds (AEF), which separate the air-containing pyriform sinuses (PS) and laryngeal vestibule. The calcified triticeus cartilages (tr) are seen in the area just caudad to the posterior cornua of the hyoid bone. The sternocleidomastoid muscle (SCM) lies lateral to the major neck vessels.

nical details. Symmetry of most of the laryngeal structures assists in the diagnosis of abnormalities. The degree of normal asymmetry, however, must be appreciated to avoid misinterpretation.

The larynx is a fibromuscular organ supported by a group of cartilaginous structures (5). Certain features of the normal cross-sectional anatomy of the larynx as displayed on CT could cause confusion in interpretation. Patterns of mineralization of the laryngeal cartilaginous skeleton vary greatly, tending to increase with age and be more extensive in men (4). Generally, the amount of calcium is sufficient in adults to distin-

guish the cartilages from the surrounding soft tissues on CT.

Hyoid Bone

Surrounding the upper end of the epiglottis, the hyoid bone is always calcified and visible (Fig. 3); a tripartite origin frequently can be appreciated with posteriorly projecting cornua arising from a central anterior body. Immediately posterior are the two air-containing valleculae, divided by the median glossoepiglottic fold. The valleculae frequently appear asymmetric.

Epiglottis

Forming the anterior border of the supraglottic laryngeal airway, the epiglottis is a thin band-like structure whose superior margin extends above the hyoid bone and whose apex or inferior margin, the petiole, ends immediately superior to the anterior attachment of the true vocal cords to the thyroid cartilage (Figs. 3, 4, and 7). It is attached superiorly to the base of the tongue by the glossepiglottic ligament (fold). The cartilage is visible immediately anterior to the mucosa of the airway as a condensation of soft tissue density, which rarely may calcify in part (Fig. 6a).

Aryepiglottic Fold and Pyriform Sinus

The bilateral folds, which demarcate the lateral aspect of the laryngeal vestibule, form the medial wall of the pyriform sinus on each side (Fig. 4). They extend from the tip of the epiglottis superiorly to the arytenoid cartilages inferiorly. These obliquely oriented folds are about 2.5 mm thick superiorly and broaden to about 5 mm inferiorly. They may be moderately asymmetric during inspiration, but become appreciably thinner and more symmetric during phonation or a modified Valsalva maneuver when the pyriform sinuses are distended maximally (Fig. 5). The folds are continuous with the pre-epiglottic space anteriorly, and the fibrofatty tissue of this space frequently extends directly into the folds. The pyriform sinuses are bilateral air-containing structures that bulge into the paralaryngeal space (Fig. 4). As mentioned, they are separated from the air in the laryngeal vestibule by the aryepiglottic folds; the lateral wall is closely applied to the inner margin of the thyroid ala. Asymmetry in the size and caudal extent of the sinuses is common, especially during inspiration. During phonation, their inferior portions distend to within 5 mm of the true vocal cords. While the pyriform sinuses are not truly part of the larynx, management of tumors arising in or extending into these structures is similar to primary supraglottic laryngeal lesions.

Thyroid Cartilage

Composed of paired laminae, which extend vertically for approximately 3 cm, the thyroid cartilages are fused anteriorly to form the laryngeal prominence (Fig.

4a,b

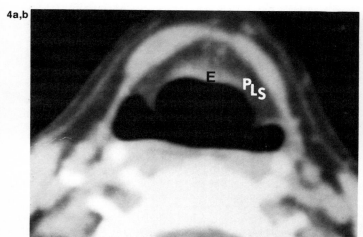
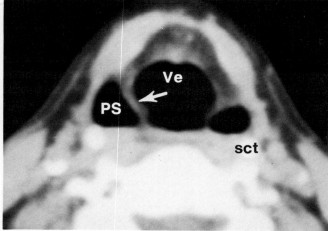

4c

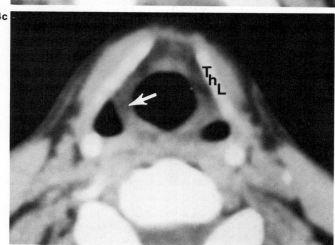

FIG. 4. Normal anatomy: aryepiglottic folds and pyriform sinuses (serial scans at 5 mm intervals in caudad direction).

  a: The soft tissue density epiglottis (E) is well demarcated by the fibrofatty tissue in the pre-epiglottic space anteriorly and the air in the laryngeal vestibule posteriorly. The fat in the pre-epiglottic space extends laterally on both sides into the paralaryngeal spaces (PLS) and then into the upper portion of the aryepiglottic folds, which begin to separate the laterally positioned pyriform sinuses from the vestibule.

  b: The pyriform sinuses (PS) are well demarcated from the vestibule (Ve) by the obliquely oriented aryepiglottic folds (arrow), which now broaden. The superior cornua of the thyroid cartilage (sct) are seen posterolateral to the sinuses. The anterior wall of the vestibule is wider than the posterior portion.

  c: The pyriform sinuses are smaller and slightly asymmetric (such asymmetry in their size and caudal extent is a common variation). The lateral walls of the sinuses are in close apposition with the inner margin of the lamina (or ala) of the thyroid cartilage (ThL). The aryepiglottic folds (arrow) are thicker than on more cephalad scans.

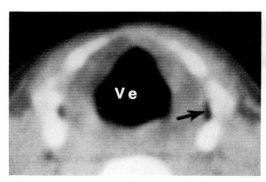
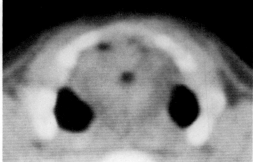

FIG. 5. Left: During slow inspiration, the laryngeal vestibule (Ve) is filled with air, but the caudad portions of the pyriform sinuses (arrow) appear quite small. **Right:** During modified Valsalva maneuver, pyriform sinuses become maximally distended, while the vestibule is almost completely obliterated.

7). Above the prominence is the superior thyroid notch, where the laminae do not meet in the midline; this normal defect should not be mistaken for cartilaginous destruction. The shape of the laminae tends to be similar on both sides, but there is no consistency in their density or contour, which may be variably composed of calcified or noncalcified hyaline cartilage or bone (with even a marrow cavity). The process of calcification and ossification often is irregular, resulting in short segmental interruptions along both the outer and inner margins of the laminae that may simulate neoplastic invasion. Localized tubercles may form along the margins. The superior and inferior cornua (horns) are extensions of the posterior border of the laminae. The triteceus cartilages are located between the superior cornua of the thyroid cartilage and the posterior portion of the cornua of the hyoid. The inferior cornua of the thyroid cartilage, which appear as dense homogeneous circles or peripherally calcified rings, articulate with the posterolateral margins of the cricoid cartilage.

Cricoid Cartilage

The most inferior of the supporting laryngeal cartilages, the cricoid cartilage is a signet-ring shaped structure with a broad posterior quadrate lamina, measuring 2 to 3 cm in vertical height, and a much narrower anterior arch (Figs. 7–9). Like the thyroid laminae, the posterior ring often has a mixed composition of cartilage and bone. A dense cortical bony rim with a relatively low density center due to a medullary space is the most common occurrence. The lateral aspect of the cricoid cartilage is in close contact bilaterally, usually within 1.5 mm, with the inner aspect of the thyroid cartilage at the cricothyroid articulation. In the area of the cricoid ring, which demarcates the subglottic space, the mucosa normally is closely adherent to the surface of the cartilage. No appreciable intraluminal soft tissue density should be seen on CT scans taken at the level of the cricoid ring or below. The complete ring usually is seen about 15 mm below the true vocal cords.

6a,b
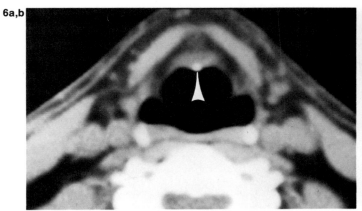
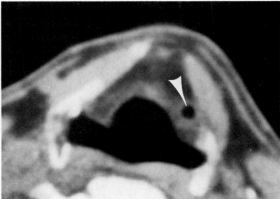

FIG. 6. Anatomic variations. **a:** Calcification (arrowhead) noted in portion of epiglottic cartilage. **b:** Air in a vestigial appendix of the laryngeal ventricle (arrowhead) in the left paralaryngeal space. (This occurrence most frequently is a normal variation. A pathologic lesion about the laryngeal ventricle causing obstruction has been present in less than 50% of our patients with this CT finding.)

7a,b

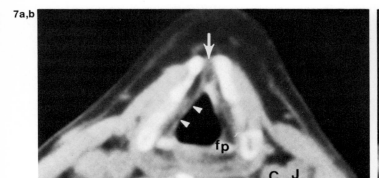

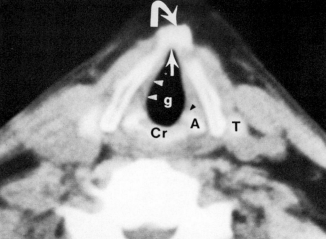

FIG. 7. Normal anatomy: false and true vocal cord levels.

a: The false vocal cords (arrowheads), medial to the paralaryngeal space, are seen at a level where the foot processes (fp) of the arytenoid cartilage are present. A space is noted anteriorly, the superior thyroid notch (arrow), between the paired thyroid laminae (note the incomplete calcification of the left ala). The air in the vestibule at the level of the false vocal cords is separated from the thyroid notch region by the fibrofatty tissue in the pre-epiglottic space. Posterolateral to the larynx, and deep to the sternocleidomastoid muscle, lie the common carotid artery (C) and the internal jugular vein (J).

b: The anteromedially projecting vocal processes (black arrowhead) of the arytenoid cartilages (A), which lie superolateral to the upper border of the posterior cricoid lamina (Cr), demar-

cate the plane of the true vocal cords (white arrowheads). Each cord (and laterally positioned vocalis muscle) is thickest posteriorly and tapers anteriorly where it meets the contralateral cord at the anterior commissure (straight arrow). In front of this, the thyroid laminae fuse to form the thyroid angle or laryngeal prominence (curved arrow). The airway or glottis (g) is elliptical with a long anteroposterior axis. The soft tissue space of the anterior commissure behind the thyroid cartilage should be less than 2 mm in thickness. Likewise, the glottic airway closely abuts the cricoid cartilage at the posterior commissure between the arytenoid cartilages. Sufficient iodine is present in this patient's thyroid (T) to demarcate the upper portion of the glands lateral to the thyroid laminae. Note the incomplete calcification and/or ossification of the ala just posterior to the midline.

Arytenoid Cartilages

Paired structures lying superior and slightly lateral to the middle of the upper border of the posterior cricoid lamina, the arytenoid cartilages are roughly pyramidal in shape (Figs. 7 and 8). The sharp anteriorly projecting vocal process, seen clearly in about 50% of patients, extends from the base of the arytenoid and attaches to and defines the plane of the true vocal cord, while the superiorly projecting foot process spans a height from the base to the level of the false cord. The laterally projecting muscular process is separated from the inner surface of the thyroid cartilage by 2 mm or less. The arytenoid cartilages usually are homogeneously dense and symmetric, although apparent inequality in size may occur due to some differences in bony or cartilaginous composition.

True Vocal Cords

These bilateral soft tissue density structures are normally seen in an abducted position during slow inspiration (Figs. 7b and 8). They should be similar in density and configuration on both sides. Roughly triangular in shape, at their widest horizontal portion posteriorly, the true vocal cord measures about 9 mm in thickness. In this region between the anteriorly projecting vocal processes of the arytenoids lies the posterior commissure; only a minimal mucosal soft tissue density should be seen in this area when the cords are abducted. The true cord tapers to a thickness of about 2 mm anteriorly, where it meets the contralateral cord to form the anterior commissure just behind the thyroid cartilage attachment. Again only a very small amount of mucosal tissue should be seen behind the

8a,b

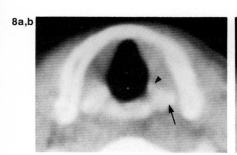

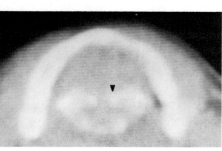

FIG. 8. a: During a slow inspiratory effort, the vocal processes (arrowhead) of the arytenoid cartilages are abducted and the glottis is distended with air. The muscular processes (arrow) of the arytenoid are directed posterolaterally. **b:** During expiration, the vocal processes (arrowhead) are adducted and point medially; the glottis is closed.

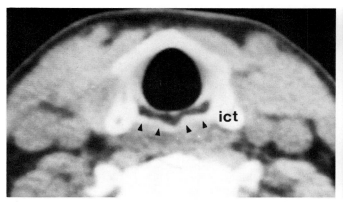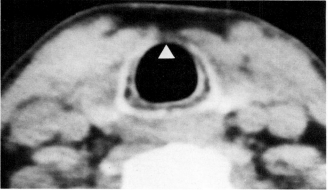

FIG. 9. Normal anatomy: subglottic region. **Left:** The superior portion of the posterior cricoid lamina (arrowheads), composed of a dense cortical rim and low density medullary center, is seen. Note the close contact of its lateral portion with the lamina and inferior cornu (ict) of the thyroid cartilage. **Right:** One centimeter inferiorly, the cricoid ring is now virtually complete, except anteriorly at the cricothyroid membrane (arrowhead). The circular airway is in apposition to the internal surface of the cricoid cartilage.

midline thyroid cartilage at the level of the true vocal cords. In contradistinction, the false cords are seen as a thicker band of density crossing the midline anteriorly (Fig. 7a). Only in approximately 10% of patients can the laryngeal ventricle be seen on the cross-sectional images separating the true and false cords.

Paralaryngeal Space

These bilateral spaces consist of a mixture of fibrous and fatty tissue deep to the endolarynx, bounded laterally by the thyroid laminae (Figs. 3, 4, and 7). At the level of the true cords, it is a very thin space, but it markedly widens superiorly. Anterolaterally, the paralaryngeal space is contiguous with the pre-epiglottic space, which extends superiorly to the valleculae. The normal fat content in this space, present in virtually every adult patient, causes a definite decreased density on CT in comparison to the paralaryngeal musculature or neoplastic tissue.

Laryngeal Airway

The vestibule, or portion of the laryngeal airway above the false cords, assumes an elliptical shape with a long lateral axis (Fig. 4). It is widest superiorly and narrower in its lower portion, with the anterior wall wider than the posterior. The airway at the level of the true cord also is elliptical, but with a long antero-posterior axis (Fig. 7b). The subglottic area is circular (Fig. 9), while the tracheal air column is either circular or horseshoe shaped with a flat posterior aspect.

Vascular Structures

The major vascular bundle lies posterolateral to the thyroid cartilages; the jugular veins, which typically

are larger and usually asymmetric, lie posterolateral to the carotid arteries (Figs. 6a and 7a). Identification of the major arteries and veins may be improved by intravenous contrast medium administration.

PATHOLOGY
Carcinoma
CT Appearance

Neoplasm is identifiable on CT because it contains tissue of greater density than the normal laryngeal soft tissues or because it distorts, displaces, or destroys normal anatomic structures (Figs. 10 and 11). Computed tomography is especially valuable in assessing the paralaryngeal and pre-epiglottic spaces, areas that should be considered a continuum and that serve as a pathway for the superior, anterior, and inferior spread of supraglottic neoplasm. Deeply infiltrating tumor usually obliterates the normal low density fat content of these spaces (Fig. 12). Such early extension of epiglottic carcinoma to the pre-epiglottic space is difficult to assess clinically or by laryngography. Lack of approximation of the hyoid bone to the thyroid cartilage during a Valsalva maneuver on laryngography has been described as a sign of infiltration of tumor into the pre-epiglottic space (7), but this sign is relatively insensitive. Computed tomography also can demonstrate deep spread of epiglottic tumor to encircle the hyoid bone with infiltration of its attached muscles, necessitating more extensive surgery. The presence of mobile vocal cords is not adequate evidence for the absence of deep invasion of neoplasm (Fig. 13).

Computed tomography presents accurate estimation of the posteroinferior spread of tumor (Figs. 14 and 15). Spread between thyroid and arytenoid cartilages, with or without insinuation of tumor between the inferior cornu of the thyroid cartilage and the cricoid

10a

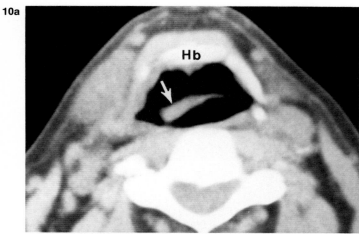

10b,c

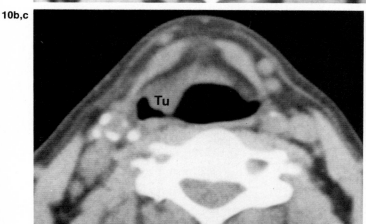

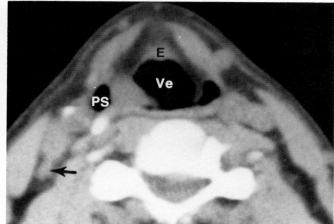

FIG. 10. Epiglottic carcinoma. **a:** Neoplasm producing moderate thickening of the right side of the tip of the epiglottis (arrow), at the level of the hyoid bone (Hb). **b:** The tumor (Tu) extends into the right aryepiglottic fold 1.5 cm inferiorly. **c:** One centimeter caudad, the neoplasm markedly widens the right aryepiglottic fold, causing some compression of the medial aspect of the right pyriform sinus (PS) and the right lateral wall of the laryngeal vestibule (Ve). The epiglottis (E) and pre-epiglottic space at this level are normal. A mildly enlarged lymph node (arrow) is seen posterior to the right jugular vein. No gross tumor was visible at the level of the false cords or below. *Supraglottic laryngectomy and right radical lymph node dissection performed.*

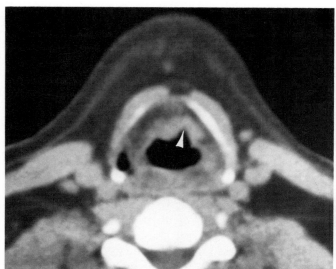

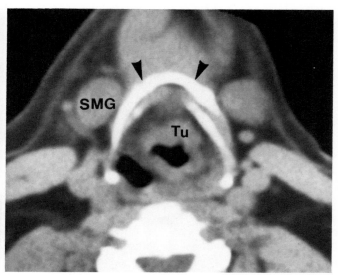

FIG. 11. Supraglottic carcinoma. **Left:** Scan during slow inspiration shows an ulcerating (arrowhead) neoplasm of the epiglottis extending toward the left aryepiglottic fold. There is no air seen within the left pyriform sinus. **Right:** Scan during phonation demonstrates distension of the right pyriform sinus but continued lack of filling of the left side. The tumor (Tu) of the epi- glottis and left aryepiglottic fold is again seen. Note that the patient has flexed his neck somewhat, causing the hyoid bone (arrowheads) to overlap the cephalad portion of the thyroid cartilage. The inferior portions of the submandibular glands (SMG) and the base of the tongue also are visible. *Supraglottic laryngeopharyngectomy performed.*

12a,b

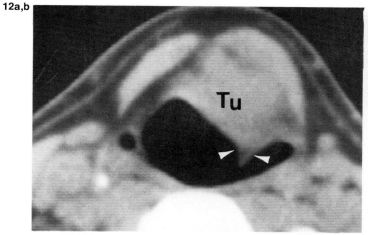
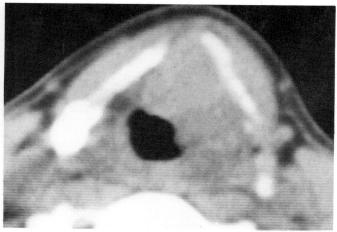

12c

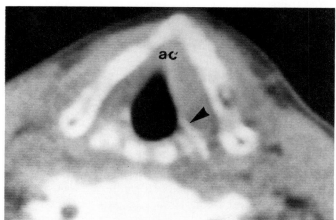

FIG. 12. Transglottic carcinoma. **a:** A bulky supraglottic tumor (Tu), probably originating in the epiglottis, infiltrates the left pre-epiglottic space and extends into the aryepiglottic fold (arrowheads). **b:** 1.5 cm inferiorly the tumor involves the entire pre-epiglottic and the left paralaryngeal space; the vestibule is displaced toward the right. **c:** At the level of the vocal process of the arytenoid (arrowhead), the left true vocal cord and the anterior commissure (ac) are thickened by tumor invasion. *Total laryngectomy performed.*

cartilage, a virtually pathognomic finding of pyriform sinus lesions (Figs. 16 and 17), is well demonstrated (8).

The arytenoid cartilages are mobile and most frequently are displaced by neoplasm rather than invaded. Spread across the midline deep to the anterior or posterior commisure is reliably detected on CT (Fig.

18). The extent of this spread across the midline may decide the feasibility of conservative hemi-laryngectomy operation. Such determination can be very difficult on laryngography with bulky tumors.

Computed tomography can corroborate that the true vocal cord is fixed in the midline, but it may be impos-

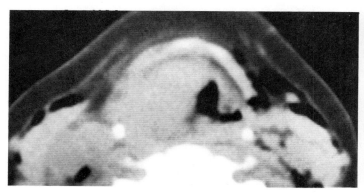
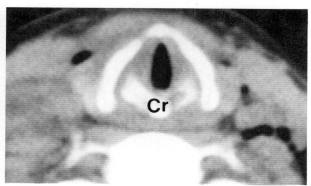

FIG. 13. Supraglottic carcinoma. **Left:** An extensive carcinoma, which necessitated a tracheostomy (accounting for the air seen in the soft tissues), involves the epiglottis, pre-epiglottic space, right aryepiglottic fold, and pyriform sinus, and compromises the vestibule. Tumor extended around the hyoid bone and into the vallecula on more cephalad scans. **Right:** At the level of the cricoid cartilage (Cr), the true vocal cords are abducted. *Total laryngectomy considered necessary for management of this large neoplasm despite the presence of mobile cords.*

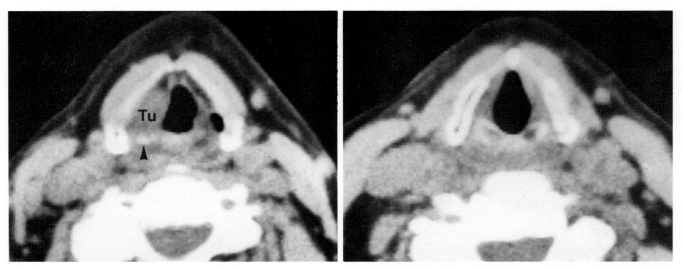

FIG. 14. Localized false vocal cord carcinoma. **Left:** At level of foot process of arytenoid (arrowhead), tumor (Tu) involves the right false vocal cord with bulging into the vestibular airway. **Right:** Right true vocal cord area is normal. *Supraglottic laryngectomy performed.*

sible to determine whether the cord is paramedian due to paresis or involvement with tumor. If neoplasm is seen separating the cricoid and thyroid cartilages, then infiltration of the paralaryngeal space can be presumed. A paramedian cord with an otherwise normal larynx on clinical examination is most likely the result of recurrent laryngeal nerve disruption (often in the mediastinum). In this circumstance, CT study of the larynx would add little to the clinical evaluation. However, if there is any laryngoscopic finding that suggests a neoplasm or prior trauma, CT can provide useful diagnostic information. In the presence of a laryngeal mass without a mucosal lesion on laryngoscopy, CT may demonstrate distortion of the laryngeal skeleton compatible with an old healed, often "occult" fracture (Fig. 19).

The relationship between any subglottic tumor and the cricoid cartilage, well demonstrated on CT (Figs. 18b, 20–22), is critical information for the surgeon to know and is more important than some arbitrary measurement (e.g., 6 mm posteriorly or 10 mm anteriorly) of the extent of tumor downward from the inferior margin of the true vocal cords. The cricoid cartilage provides major support for the larynx, and only a minimal portion of the superior margin can be sacrificed in conservation surgery if the patient is to retain a viable airway, voice, and "sphincter" to prevent aspiration.

Computed tomography is an excellent method for detecting cartilaginous invasion, although definite pitfalls and limitations exist. Especially in the thyroid cartilage, because of the normally irregular and non-

15a,b

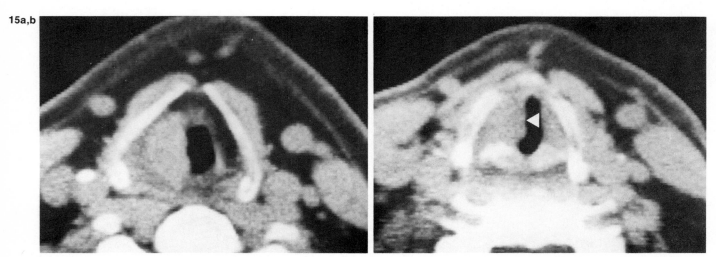

FIG. 15. False vocal cord carcinoma with extension. **a:** Large right supraglottic tumor involving the false vocal cord and paralaryngeal space. **b:** Lesion extends transglottic to produce paralysis of right true vocal cord (arrowhead), which is seen in the midline. *Total laryngectomy performed.*

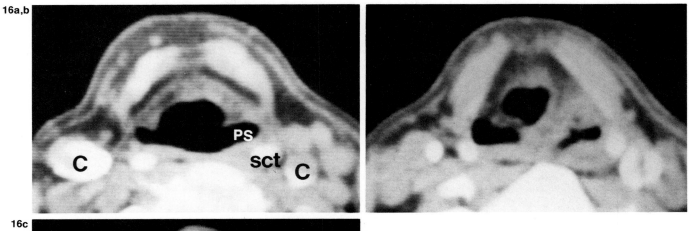

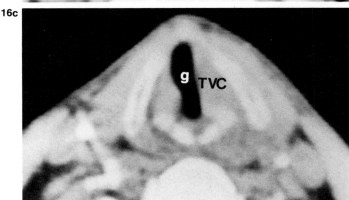

FIG. 16. Pyriform sinus carcinoma. **a:** Some increase in density in left pre-epiglottic and paralaryngeal spaces about upper portion of pyriform sinus (PS), due to tumor extension, at level of superior cornu of the thyroid cartilage (sct). Extensive calcification of carotid arteries (C) is present. **b:** The bulk of the tumor involves the midportion of the left pyriform sinus, extending into the left aryepiglottic fold. **c:** At the level of the glottis (g), a paralyzed left true vocal cord (TVC) caused by tumor infiltration is seen in the midline. *Radical laryngopharyngectomy performed.*

uniform patterns of calcification and ossification, only moderate to far advanced involvement can be confidently identified (Fig. 22). Disruption of the thyroid cartilage may be gross, with fragments displaced away from the normal contour of the cartilage or tumor seen extending lateral to the margin of the cartilage (Fig.

23). Care must be exercised in diagnosing neoplastic invasion of the cartilaginous structures. Irregularity due to foci of noncalcified cartilage should not be mistaken for tumor extension, since conservative surgery would be contraindicated. Even the proximity of tumor to the cartilage can be misleading, and it is best

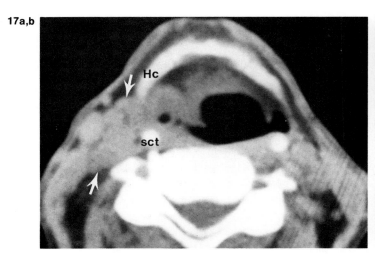

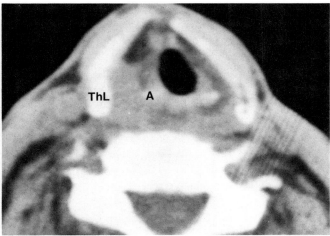

FIG. 17. Pyriform sinus carcinoma. **a:** Tumor originating in right pyriform sinus extends directly through the thyrohyoid ligament, between the cornu of the hyoid bone (Hc) and the superior cornu of the thyroid cartilage (sct), to involve the soft tissues of the neck (arrows) surrounding the carotid and jugular vessels. *Clinically, lymph node metastases were felt responsible for the palpable right neck mass.* **b:** Tumor extends inferiorly in the paralaryngeal space at the false vocal cord level to widen the distance between the right lamina of the thyroid cartilage (ThL) and the foot process of the arytenoid cartilage (A).

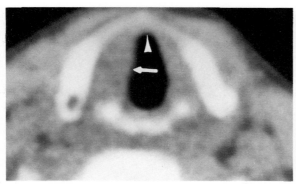

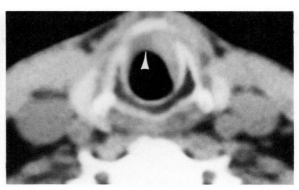

FIG. 18. True vocal cord carcinomas. **Left:** A right true vocal cord tumor (arrow) produces thickening of this structure. The neoplasm extends to the anterior commissure (arrowhead) but does not cross the midline. *Right hemilaryngectomy performed.* **Right:** In another patient, at a level 1 cm below the center of the true cords, a lesion arising from the left true vocal cord is seen to extend across the midline (arrowhead) behind the thyroid cartilage. In addition, the tumor spreads from the undersurface of the cord and widens the space between the subglottic airway and the left anterior cricoid ring. *Total laryngectomy performed.*

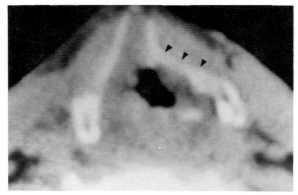

FIG. 19. An apparently old, "occult" fracture of the left thyroid lamina (arrowheads) explains a bulge seen at laryngoscopy in the left false vocal cord area; no mucosal lesion was present.

with suspected early involvement to tell the surgeon that the findings are equivocal and that inspection and possible biopsy of the cartilages should precede commitment to radical surgery. Despite the problems encountered, CT is the best radiologic technique, superior to soft tissue radiography (including xeroradiography) (14), in determining cartilaginous invasion (18). Clinical appreciation of such involvement comes only very late when fixation is present.

The cross-sectional area of the airway lumen, especially when it is irregular, can be very difficult to estimate on conventional radiography. Computed tomography accurately depicts the airway size.

Only rarely are enlarged lymph nodes identified on CT that cannot be palpated clinically (Fig. 24). Com-

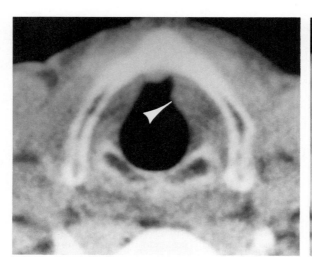

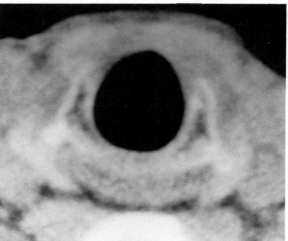

FIG. 20. Localized true vocal cord carcinoma. **Left:** Tumor seen on undersurface of anterior portion of left true vocal cord (arrowhead). **Right:** No subglottic extension; the airway is in close apposition to the cricoid cartilage. *Left hemilaryngectomy performed.*

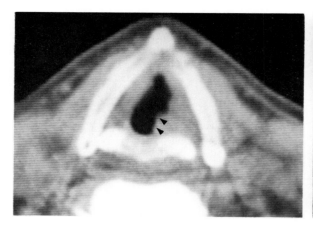

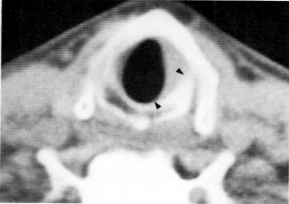

FIG. 21. True vocal cord carcinoma with extension. **Left:** Tumor of the left true vocal cord spreads posteromedially over arytenoid cartilage (arrowheads) toward posterior commissure. **Right:** In-

ferior extension of tumor in the subglottic area is manifested as soft tissue thickening (arrowheads) separating the airway from the left side of the cricoid arch. *Total laryngectomy performed.*

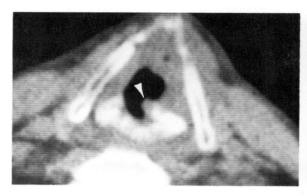

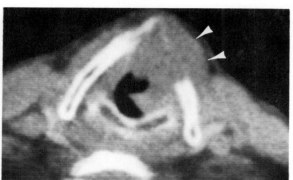

FIG. 22. True vocal cord carcinoma with thyroid cartilage destruction. **Left:** Tumor of left true vocal cord spreads both posteromedially over vocal process of arytenoid (arrowhead) and across the midline at the anterior commissure. **Right:** Tumor extends subglottically adjacent to the cricoid cartilage posterior

and through the left thyroid ala. Not only is there destruction of the left thyroid lamina, but neoplasm can be seen to infiltrate into the subcutaneous tissues (arrowheads), a finding not appreciated on clinical examination. *Total laryngectomy performed.*

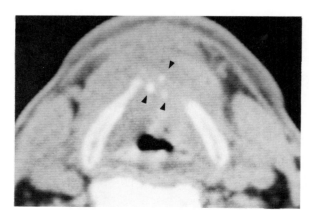

FIG. 23. A bulky carcinoma involving the anterior commissure extends into the thyroid cartilage, producing destruction and fragmentation (arrowheads).

puted tomography may be useful in identifying the relationship of tumor extension or metastatic lymphadenopathy to the carotid artery and jugular vein (Figs. 25 and 26); if neoplasm totally surrounds or invades these structures, surgical salvage becomes unlikely. On occasion, CT may demonstrate that a neck mass thought to be due to enlarged lymph nodes is due to direct extension from a supraglottic carcinoma (Fig. 17a).

Limitations of CT

A weakness of CT is its inability to define consistently a transition zone from the false to the true vocal cords. The ventricle is seen in only about 10% of patients. Spread of tumors from the false to the true

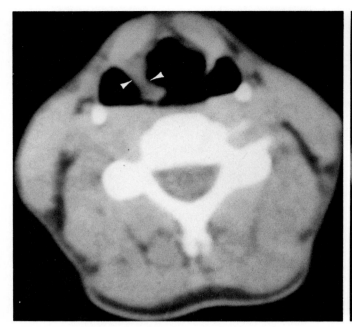

FIG. 24. Supraglottic carcinoma, no neck masses initially palpated. **Left:** Tumor involving right aryepiglottic fold (arrowheads). **Right:** Enlarged lymph node mass (arrows) seen on most cephalad scan in suprahyoid region. With knowledge of scan finding, repeat clinical examination disclosed a palpable posterior cervical mass; at surgery, metastatic involvement of lymph node was confirmed.

cords, or vice versa, may be difficult to ascertain on CT. Invasion of the ventricle is presumed when tumor is seen involving both the false and true cords. The use of coronal and sagittal reconstruction may diminish this problem somewhat, but in most instances reconstructed views provide no more clinical information than is well depicted on the cross-sectional transverse scans. While theoretically those additional views might supply a different perspective of the relationship of neoplasm to normal structures, in reality, once the cross-sectional anatomy is understood fully, no new diagnostic understanding is gained. This should be ex-

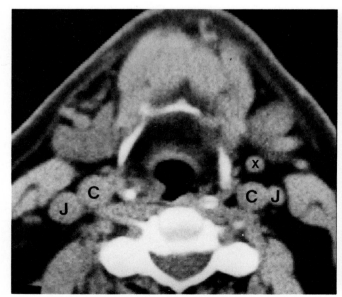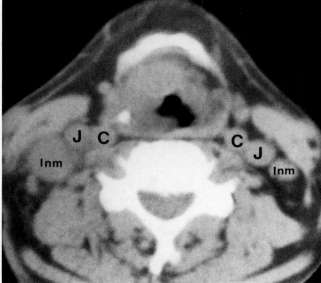

FIG. 25. Left: Small carcinoma of right aryepiglottic fold, no cervical lymph node metastases. Note normal internal (C) and external (X) carotid arteries and internal jugular vein (J). The carotid arteries are usually bilaterally symmetric, whereas the internal jugular veins are frequently asymmetric (with the right usually larger than the left). **Right:** Bulky supraglottic carcinoma involving epiglottis and right aryepiglottic fold in patient with palpable neck masses bilaterally. Note cervical lymph node metastases (lnm) lateral to carotid artery (C) and internal jugular vein (J).

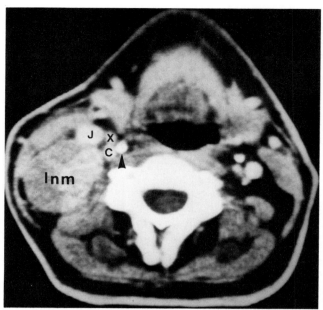

FIG. 26. Supraglottic carcinoma with palpable large right neck mass. CT scan (narrow window width setting to accentuate contrast differences) following intravenous contrast medium injection. Large lymph node metastases (lnm) seen posterolateral and separate from internal jugular vein (J) and external (X) and internal (C) carotid arteries, at level of cornua of hyoid bone (arrowhead).

pected, since only data present on the transaxial images are used by the computer to generate the sagittal and coronal views (18).

Minor mucosal abnormalities will not be imaged with CT, but this is generally of no clinical importance since such irregularities can be delineated well by endoscopy. Motion, also, is evaluated more easily by clinical examination, since CT is essentially an anatomic study.

Computed tomography only identifies changes in tissue density and fascial planes and does not permit a histologic diagnosis. Consequently, fibrosis or edema in adjacent tissues can simulate malignant extension on CT. Because of this, a CT study should be performed prior to any biopsy or at least 48 hours after such a procedure.

Accuracy and Comparison to Laryngography

Computed tomography is cost-competitive (actually slightly less expensive at our hospital) with laryngography. It can be performed with no appreciable discomfort or morbidity to the patient. Laryngography is an invasive procedure carrying some risk, albeit small, particularly in massive tumors. Premedication and substantial cooperation are required for that examination. Most important, equal or superior clinically relevant information is provided by CT in over 90% of cases studied by both modalities (2,11). In most cases, CT demonstrates more extensive disease than is appreciated by laryngography. Computed tomography is clearly superior in assessing the laryngeal cartilages and deep extension and should be the initial radiologic procedure, and usually the only one, when a radiologic examination is required. Computed tomography displays the larynx in a three-dimensional format allowing direct demonstration of tumor in both the larynx and paralaryngeal soft tissues, as well as the cartilages. In contradistinction, laryngography (and laryngoscopy) suggests extension of tumor involvement more by inference than by direct determination.

An accuracy of greater than 90% in the staging of laryngeal carcinomas can be achieved with CT. With experience, most false positive interpretations can be eliminated (e.g., overcalling cartilaginous destruction). Still there will be cases of microscopic extensions of neoplasm into the surrounding tissues that are undetectable with CT.

Clinical Applications

The classic division of laryngeal carcinoma into supraglottic, glottic, subglottic, and transglottic lesions provides the rationale for selecting either conservation surgery or radical total laryngectomy. Conservative surgery (supraglottic or vertical partial laryngectomy) may successfully manage tumors restricted to either the supraglottic or glottic compartments; once the neoplasm extends beyond these boundaries (transglottic) or deeply into the paralaryngeal tissues, to involve, for example, the laryngeal cartilages or the apex of the pyriform sinus, total laryngectomy usually is indicated.

Computed tomography is a quick (usually requiring less than 20 min to complete) and noninvasive (no discomfort or risk to the patient) method of examining the larynx. It provides information that supplements or reinforces the clinical examination. Deep extension of neoplasm into the paralaryngeal and pre-epiglottic spaces is well depicted, and the supporting cartilages and subglottic area can be assessed. Cartilage involvement indicates that the lesion cannot be cured by conservation surgery or radiation therapy. Computed tomography is complementary to, rather than a substitute for, laryngoscopy. Laryngoscopy should precede the CT examination and is the best study to assess the mucosal surface of the larynx and motion of the intrinsic structures. The clinical indications for the use of CT are similar to those established previously for laryngography: when additional data are required to decide whether conservative surgery as opposed to a more radical operation or irradiation is the therapy of choice. Patients with early mucosal or very far advanced lesions usually do not require the procedure.

Computed tomography plays an important role in the management of the patient with carcinoma of the larynx at our medical center. Recent technological improvements (thin collimation, rapid scan time) permit detailed studies during suspended respiration or during physiological maneuvers on a routine basis. The study can be accomplished in virtually every cooperative adult. Not only can the structures deep to the mucosal surface and the laryngeal cartilages be accurately evaluated, but subglottic extension of tumor and the cross-sectional size of the airway can be depicted.

When the CT findings are discrepant with the laryngoscopic results, CT always shows the carcinoma to be further advanced than clinically suspected, with deep extension into the paralaryngeal and pre-epiglottic space or inferiorly to the subglottic region, with or without cartilage destruction. Some valuable information about the soft tissues of the neck also may be provided. The combination of CT with laryngoscopy and biopsy almost always supplies all the structural and functional information necessary for appropriate therapy planning. Laryngography can be obviated in almost all patients with carcinoma of the larynx. If conservation surgery is being contemplated, a CT study of the larynx is essential.

Trauma

Injury to the larynx may be associated with substantial problems related to glottic function and airway maintenance. Even in severe injury, the larynx can be examined easily and conveniently by CT. The ability of CT to show minor degrees of mineralization makes it ideal for demonstration of the cartilaginous supporting structures. The unique cross-sectional display can show the extent of cartilaginous injury and dis-

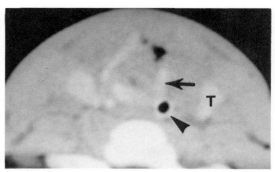

FIG. 28. Multiple laryngeal fractures. *Emergency tracheostomy required for airway compromise sustained in automobile accident.* CT scan demonstrates extensive disruption of the laryngeal cartilages. The posterior cricoid lamina is fractured, with dislocation of the left sided fragment anteromedially (arrow). Subcutaneous air is seen in the expected position of the left thyroid lamina, which has been fractured and displaced more cephalad. Hemorrhage and edema obliterate the glottic airway and displace the left lobe of the thyroid gland (T) laterally. A nasogastric tube (arrowhead) is present. *The patient requires a permanent tracheostomy as a result of the severe laryngeal injury.*

placement, related soft tissue changes, and the degree of resulting airway encroachment. The cricoarytenoid joint and the other supporting cartilages can be depicted, permitting differentiation of dysfunction due to soft tissue changes from fracture or dislocation. In the acute phase, supraglottic swelling may prevent complete examination of the airway during laryngoscopy, making CT especially valuable.

In blunt trauma to the larynx, the force is almost invariably directed anteroposteriorly, compressing the larynx against the cervical spine. Laryngeal injuries may include transverse and/or vertical fractures of the thyroid cartilage (Figs. 19 and 27). The fragments may become widely dispersed, resulting in lack of support

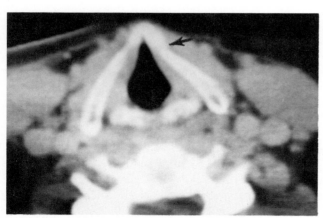

FIG. 27. Minimally depressed fracture of left thyroid lamina (arrow). Some enlargement of the left thyrohyoid muscle (due to hemorrhage and/or edema) can be seen surrounding the injured ala, but the vocal cords and cricoid cartilage are normal. *No therapy considered necessary.*

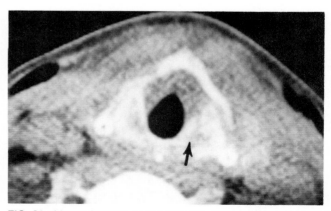

FIG. 29. Linear fracture of the left side of the posterior cricoid lamina (arrow), with swelling of the soft tissues beneath the anterior portion of the subglottic airway. Air within the subcutaneous tissues suggest an associated laceration of the endolaryngeal mucosa. *Fractures of the cricoid generally presage an unfavorable prognosis; despite several operations this patient has persistent subglottic stenosis.*

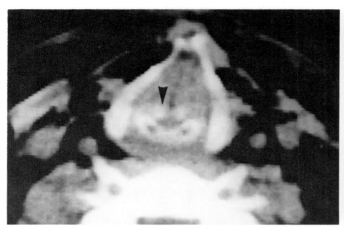 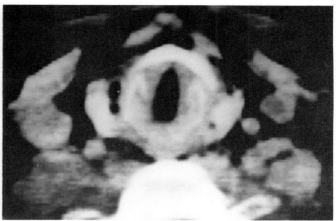

FIG. 30. Soft tissue injury of larynx with intact cartilage. *Direct trauma to anterior neck during automobile accident caused airway compromise necessitating emergency tracheostomy.* **Left:** Marked hemorrhage and edema thicken the vocal cords with obliteration of the glottic airway. The thyroid alae and top of the posterior cricoid laminae are intact; the arytenoid cartilages (arrowhead) are adducted. Extensive air is present in the tissues surrounding the larynx; a mucosal tear may have resulted directly from the accident or the tracheostomy. **Right:** One centimeter inferiorly, the remainder of the cricoid ring is intact, and the subglottic airway is normal. *Complete recovery followed conservative therapy with a temporary tracheostomy.*

for the true and false cords (Fig. 28). The arytenoid cartilages usually do not fracture, but often dislocate, especially upward and anteriorly, at the cricoarytenoid joint. The epiglottis may be avulsed just above the anterior commissure, with its base displaced posteriorly. Because the cricoid cartilage is a ring, fractures occur in two places. Springing apart of the posterior cricoid ring is common (Fig. 29) and may actually serve to widen the airway. Disruption of the cricothyroid joint may cause dysfunction of the true vocal cords.

Hematoma and edema secondary to trauma may spread throughout the same deep planes of the larynx that serve as pathways for neoplasm. Spreading hematomas and edema in the aryepiglottic folds and the pre-epiglottic and paralaryngeal spaces surrounding the vocal cords can encroach on the airway to varying degrees (Fig. 30).

REFERENCES

1. Archer CR, Friedman WH, Yeager VL, Katsantonis GP: Evaluation of laryngeal cancer by computed tomography. *J Comput Assist Tomogr* 2:618–624, 1978
2. Archer CR, Sagel SS, Yeager VL, Martin S, Friedman WH: Staging of carcinoma of the larynx: Comparative accuracy of computed tomography and laryngography. *Am J Roentgenol* 136:571–575, 1981
3. Archer CR, Yeager VL, Friedman WH, Katsantonis GP: Computed tomography of the larynx. *J Comput Assist Tomogr* 2:404–411, 1978
4. Archer CR, Yeager VL: Evaluation of laryngeal cartilages by computed tomography. *J Comput Assist Tomogr* 3:604–611, 1979
5. *Cunningham's Manual of Practical Anatomy* (revised by GJ Romanes), *Vol 3, Head and Neck,* London, Oxford University Press, 1967, pp 168–178
6. Gamsu G, Mark AS, Webb WR: Computed tomography of the normal larynx during quiet breathing and phonation. *J Comput Assist Tomogr* 5:353–360, 1981
7. Holtz S, Powers WE, McGavran MH, Ogura JH: Contrast examination of the larynx and pharynx: Glottic, infraglottic and transglottic tumors. *Am J Roentgenol Radium Ther Nucl Med* 89:10–28, 1963
8. Larrson S, Mancuso A, Hoover L, Hanafee W: Differentiation of pyriform sinus cancer from supraglottic laryngeal cancer by computed tomography. *Radiology* 141:427–432, 1981
9. Lesinski SG, Bauer WC, Ogura JH: Hemilaryngectomy for T$_3$ (fixed cord) epidermoid carcinoma of the larynx. *Laryngoscope* 10:1563–1571, 1976
10. Mancuso AA, Calcaterra TC, Hanafee WN: Computed tomography of the larynx. *Radiol Clin North Am* 16:195–208, 1978
11. Mancuso AA, Hanafee WN: A comparative evaluation of computed tomography and laryngography. *Radiology* 133:131–138, 1979
12. Mancuso AA, Hanafee WN: Computed tomography of the injured larynx. *Radiology* 133:139–144, 1979
13. Mancuso AA, Tamakawa Y, Hanafee WN: CT of the fixed vocal cord. *Am J Roentgenol* 135:529–534, 1980
14. Nathan MD, Sagel SS, Gall AM, Griffith RC, Ogura JH: Diagnostic accuracy of xeroradiographic assessment of extent of carcinoma of the larynx. *Trans Ophthalmol Otolaryngol* 84:609–621, 1977
15. Ogura JH, Heeneman H: Conservation surgery of the larynx and hypopharynx—Selection of patients and results. *Can J Otolaryngol* 2:11–16, 1973
16. Parsons CA, Chapman P, Counter RT, Grundy A: The role of computed tomography in tumors of the larynx. *Clin Radiol* 31:529–533, 1980
17. Sagel SS, Aufderheide JF, Aronberg DJ, Stanley RJ, Archer CR: High resolution computed tomography in the staging of carcinoma of the larynx. *Laryngoscope* 91:292–300, 1981
18. Scott M, Forsted DH, Rominger CJ, Brennan M: Computed tomographic evaluation of laryngeal neoplasms. *Radiology* 140:141–144, 1981

Chapter 4

Thoracic Anatomy and Mediastinum

Stuart S. Sagel and Dixie J. Aronberg

It is generally acknowledged that the greatest value of computed tomography of the thorax is in the evaluation of the mediastinum. The cross-sectional CT images display the fine anatomic detail of this area with great precision, and often yield unique and useful diagnostic information directly affecting the management or prognosis of the patient (11,18,21,27,38).

Compared with conventional radiographic techniques, the transverse anatomic plane CT sections provide an unparalleled view of the superimposed structures of the mediastinum. For recognition of a mediastinal lesion by conventional roentgenographic studies, sufficient expansion to deform the mediastinal contour and displace the pleuropulmonary interface laterally is required. Using CT, enlargement of an individual mediastinal component or replacement of the normal mediastinal fat by a denser soft tissue mass is detectable at an earlier stage. The size, contour, tissue density, and homogeneity of a mediastinal lesion can be defined as well as its relation to other mediastinal structures. Computed tomography is more valuable than any other radiologic technique to determine the exact extent and localization of a mediastinal mass. The improved density discrimination of CT aids distinction between the vascular, solid, lipomatous, or cystic nature of various mediastinal lesions. Such tissue characterization may be crucial in differentiating benign from malignant disease, and, in some patients, removes the necessity for further invasive diagnostic evaluation (1,4,35).

NORMAL ANATOMY

To emphasize the cross-sectional relationships in various regions of the thorax, nine basic mediastinal levels have been selected to provide an orderly demonstration of the major structural associations. These levels, in caudad order, are illustrated both in diagrammatic form and with comparable CT scans (Figs. 1–10). Common deviations from these most typical CT patterns also will be described.

Fat, with its characteristic CT number, always can be recognized and distinguished from other mediastinal structures. In most adult patients sufficient fat is present to sharply outline and allow identification of structures that cannot be separated out by conventional radiographic techniques. Generally the aorta and great vessels, superior vena cava and major venous channels, and the central pulmonary vessels all can be seen with regularity and confidence even without intravenous contrast administration. The diameter of the ascending aorta, which is larger than the descending aorta by a factor of approximately 1.5, is approximately 3.5 cm in the adult; measurements more than 4.5 cm should be considered abnormal. The pulmonary artery, which lies to the left and slightly anterior to the ascending aorta, has a diameter of approximately 3 cm. The normal pulmonary artery is smaller than the ascending aorta. The intrapericardial portions of the great vessels can be evaluated for possible displacement by masses, to demonstrate their relationship to one another as in suspected transposition, and to assess their size as in possible pulmonary artery hypertension. Whereas lung normally is seen lateral to the aortic arch and aortopulmonary window, scans may demonstrate the cephalad portion of the main and left pulmonary arteries in this location. Such an appearance is common if scanning is not done during full inspiration or if a high variant position of the pulmonary artery is present. Generally, study of sequential images can establish that a structure partially imaged on a particular scan merges with and represents part of a major vessel. If doubt persists that something in the mediastinum represents a vascular structure, scans after the intravenous injection of iodinated contrast medium should be performed since the CT numbers of the major arteries and veins can be increased well beyond the range of the other mediastinal components (Fig. 11). With proper contrast administration, enhancement of the major vessels is always grossly obvious, and there is no need to carefully measure attenuation values.

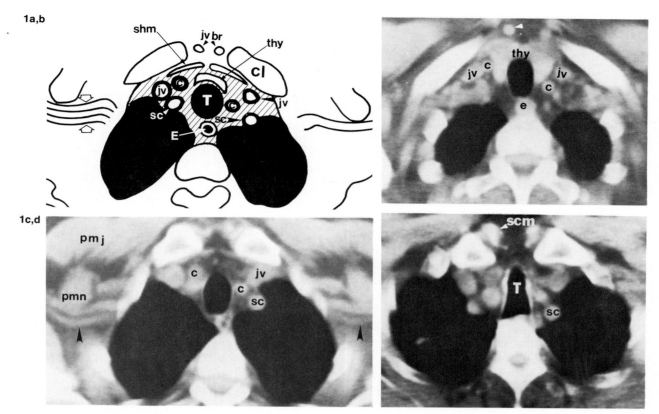

FIG. 1. Normal anatomy—sternal notch. **a:** At this level through the lung apices six major mediastinal vessels usually can be defined: the paired carotid arteries, jugular veins, and subclavian arteries. The carotid arteries (c) are round discrete structures adjacent to the trachea (T); frequently the right carotid artery is anterior to that on the left, although they may be in the same coronal plane. The internal jugular veins (jv) usually are anterior to the subclavian arteries (sc) and may be quite large. Depending on the exact scan level the subclavian arteries may be seen in cross section or in a somewhat longitudinal orientation proceeding along the anteromedial surface of the lung apex toward the axilla. The axillary vessels can be seen in longitudinal orientation lateral to the rib cage (open arrows). The thyroid (thy), which is intimately applied to the anterolateral aspect of the trachea, may have an attenuation value substantially higher than muscle. Within the sternal notch, medial to the heads of the clavicle (cl), the anterior branch of the jugular vein (jv br) may be seen. Other structures are the esophagus (E), and sternohyoid/sternothyroid muscle (shm). **b:** The thyroid (thy) is seen anterolateral to the trachea, just posterior to the anterior branch of the jugular vein (arrowhead). **c:** In another patient at the same level the left subclavian artery (sc) is quite prominent and projects into the anteromedial lung apex. This vessel normally is approximately twice the diameter of the left carotid artery. The axillary vessels (black arrowheads) are seen posterior to the pectoralis major (pmj) and the pectoralis minor (pmn) muscles. **d:** A sabre-sheath configuration of the trachea (T), an anatomic variation characterized by an enlarged anteroposterior dimension and a narrow width, may be seen in individuals with chronic obstructive lung disease. Note the head of the sternocleidomastoid muscle (scm) in the sternal notch and the posterolateral position of a tortuous left subclavian artery (sc).

The superior vena cava, which has an ovoid shape or elliptical configuration oriented in the anteroposterior direction, produces a slight convexity to the right superior mediastinum. The azygous vein intimately contacts the trachea as it arches anteriorly to enter the dorsal aspect of the superior vena cava. The presence of an azygous lobe, found in approximately 1% of the population, may cause some alteration to the contour of the right mediastinum (40). In such instances the azygous arch is laterally displaced and usually more cephalad than normal, and enters the posterolateral aspect of the superior vena cava. Lung inserts medially to the azygous vein and may contact and outline the posterolateral tracheal wall as well as the posterior aspect of the superior vena cava (Fig. 3e).

The mediastinal lymph nodes are reliably imaged by CT. Normal lymph nodes, usually oval or round in shape, can be seen in up to 90% of patients, especially in the middle mediastinum (Fig. 12) (37). Lymph nodes less than 1 cm in cross-sectional diameter are considered normal by CT criteria, although such a normal size node may be involved with microscopic disease. The mediastinal lymph nodes cannot be evaluated by conventional radiography until they become so grossly enlarged that they contact and displace the pleuropulmonary interface with the mediastinum. Of particular importance are those lymph nodes in the pre- and paratracheal area accessible to biopsy through the transcervically inserted mediastinoscope. Additionally, nodes in the anterior mediastinum, in the aor-

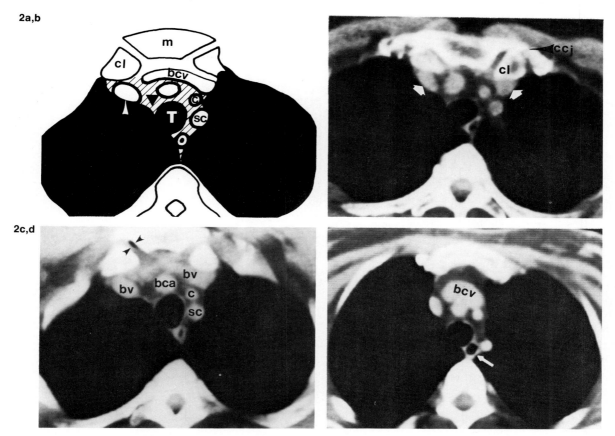

FIG. 2. Normal anatomy—sternoclavicular junction. **a:** Through the manubrium (m) and its articulation with the head of the clavicle (cl), five vessels are usually noted anterior and lateral to the trachea (T): the right brachiocephalic vein (white arrowhead), brachiocephalic artery (bca) (black arrowhead), left carotid artery (c), and left subclavian artery (sc) are virtually always seen in cross section; the left brachiocephalic vein (bcv or bv) may be seen in longitudinal orientation as it crosses the midline to join the right brachiocephalic vein before it forms the superior vena cava at a slightly lower level. The brachiocephalic artery is normally the largest of the three vessels off the aortic arch and the left carotid the smallest. **b:** All five major mediastinal vessels are seen in cross section; the brachiocephalic veins (white arrows) appear as symmetrical structures, posteromedial to the clavicular heads (cl) and the costochrondral junction (ccj). **c:** Air within the sternoclavicular joint (black arrowheads) is a normal finding with the arms positioned above the head. **d:** At a slightly lower level, the left brachiocephalic vein (bcv) is seen oriented longitudinally. Air within the esophagus (arrow), even the considerable amount shown here, is normal.

topulmonary window, in the subcarinal area, and in the hilum are well depicted (Fig. 13). Surgical sampling of the anterior mediastinal, aortopulmonary window, or hilar lymph nodes requires a limited anterior parasternal approach.

The pulmonary hilar anatomy is relatively constant, and five consecutive sections usually provide the required information (Figs. 4–8). The major pulmonary arteries and veins and the trachea and major bronchi, including most of the segmental orifices, can be clearly depicted on contiguous CT scans (29,32,42). Understanding the basic anatomic relationships facilitates CT diagnosis of hilar lymph node enlargement, and can permit the CT localization of bronchial obstructing lesions (31).

In the thorax an extremely wide range of attenuation values must be imaged. In order to assess the lungs, a substantially lower window level and wider window width than used to evaluate the mediastinum are optimal. At the appropriate setting, it is possible to demonstrate the normal moderate size bronchi, the intrapulmonary vessels, the pulmonary parenchyma, and the major interlobar septa (Figs. 14–16). When 5-mm collimation is used, the major fissures can be identified as discrete thin curvilinear white lines surrounded by relatively avascular lung; on the usual 10-mm collimated scans the fissures are less well defined and appear as a thicker hazy band within the pulmonary parenchyma. The region of the minor fissure, usually at the level of the bronchus intermedius, lies within an area of relative paucity of vessels in the right midlung field. Analogous to the standard chest radiograph, preferential blood flow to the dependent portion of the lung is recognizable with CT. On scans performed in the usual supine position, the dorsal portion of the lung receives the most blood flow (Fig. 17).

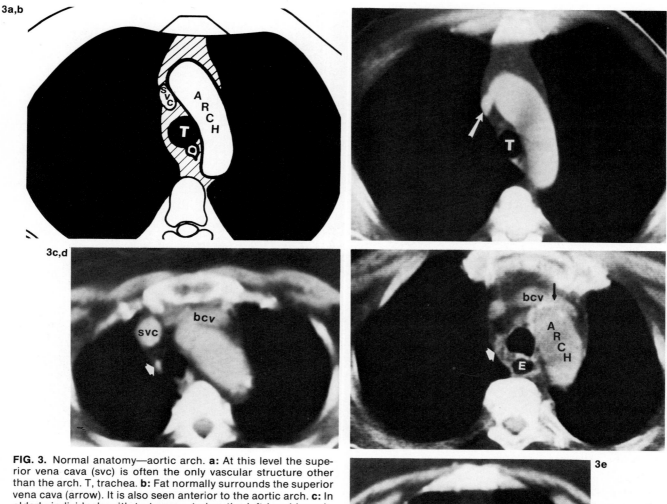

FIG. 3. Normal anatomy—aortic arch. **a:** At this level the superior vena cava (svc) is often the only vascular structure other than the arch. T, trachea. **b:** Fat normally surrounds the superior vena cava (arrow). It is also seen anterior to the aortic arch. **c:** In elderly individuals with tortuous arteries, the left brachiocephalic vein (bcv) may lie just anterior to the aortic arch. Portions of the azygous arch (arrow) may be visualized at this level. **d:** If there is calcification within the aortic arch adjacent to a tortuous left brachiocephalic vein, an aortic dissection with inwardly displaced intimal calcification (black arrow) may be simulated. Serial scanning after bolus injection of intravenous contrast medium into a left medial antecubital vein could clarify the situation if confusion persists. A portion of the azygous arch (white arrow) is seen lateral to the trachea and esophagus (E). **e:** The azygous arch is seen most commonly just caudad at the level of the aortopulmonary window (Fig. 4). However, when an azygous fissure and lobe (al) are present, the azygous vein (arrow) arches further cephalad.

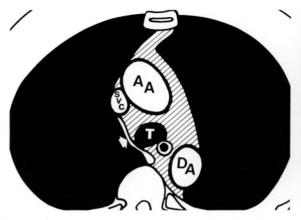

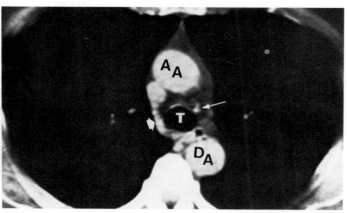

FIG. 4. Normal anatomy—aortopulmonary window. **Left:** Just cephalad to the carina and immediately caudad to the aortic arch, the oval distal trachea (T) is frequently flanked by the azygous arch (arrow) on the right and fat in the aortopulmonary window on the left. The azygous vein arches anteriorly from its prevertebral location and courses intimately around the trachea to enter the superior vena cava (svc) posteriorly. AA, ascending aorta; DA, descending aorta. **Right:** A few small lymph nodes (thin arrow) are seen within fat in the aortopulmonary window.

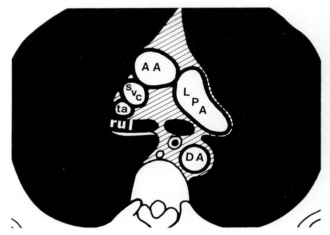

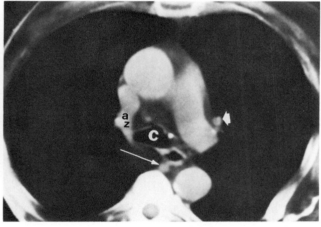

FIG. 5. Normal anatomy—left pulmonary artery. **Left:** The left pulmonary artery (LPA), proceeding posteriorly just cephalad to the left main stem bronchus, forms the left lateral margin of the mediastinum at this cross-sectional level. The right upper lobe bronchus (rul) is usually clearly seen at this level. The following vascular structures may be appreciated: ascending aorta (AA), descending aorta (DA), superior vena cava (svc), and the right upper lobe pulmonary artery or truncus anterior (ta). **Right:** The left pulmonary artery may be at the level of the carina (c). The azygous vein arch (az) is partially imaged as it enters into the superior vena cava. The prevertebral portion of the azygous vein (thin arrow) can also be seen. The thick arrow defines the left superior pulmonary vein.

Because it sometimes blends in with other mediastinal structures, especially in the asthenic individual, the esophagus may be difficult to evaluate. A small amount of air may be seen within the esophageal lumen in approximately 80% of normal patients (Figs. 2, 3d, and 5b). The esophagus usually is posterior and slightly to the left of the trachea, but occasionally the esophagus may lie totally to the left of the trachea. This variation could simulate mediastinal emphysema or tracheomegaly on conventional radiography, or mimic displacement by a mediastinal mass on a barium esophagogram (10).

Recognition of the variations in size, shape, and density of the normal thymus on CT is of paramount

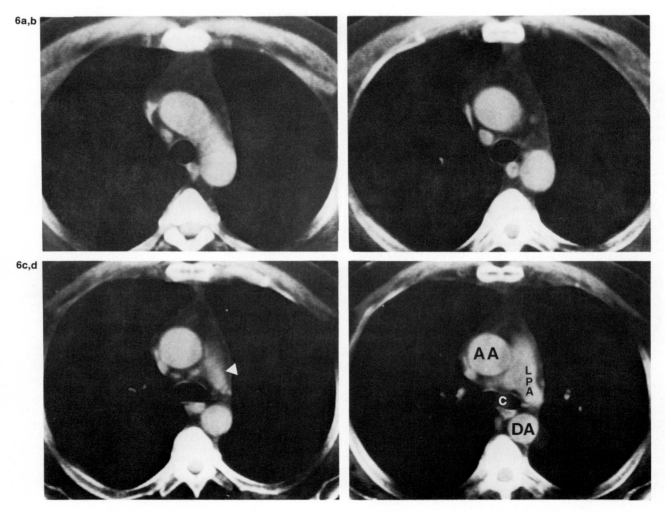

FIG. 6. Normal anatomy. Contiguous scans in a single patient from the aortic arch to the left pulmonary artery at 1-cm intervals demonstrate the changing anatomical relationships of the major mediastinal vessels. **a:** Aortic arch level. **b:** Aortopulmonary window level. **c:** The top of the left pulmonary artery is partly visible (arrowhead) as it is partially averaged with fat in the aor-topulmonary window. **d:** The main pulmonary artery and the left pulmonary artery (LPA) are well defined at the level of the carina (C), although the most proximal portion of the right pulmonary artery is barely visible. AA, ascending aorta; DA, descending aorta.

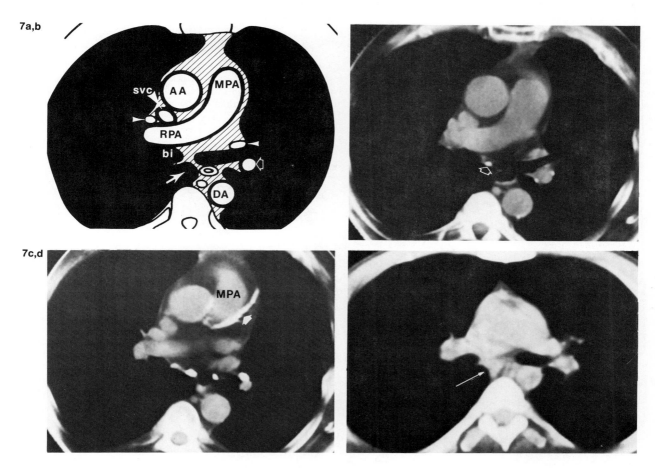

FIG. 7. Normal anatomy—right pulmonary artery. **a:** At this level, the right pulmonary artery (RPA) is seen extending posteriorly and to the right from the main pulmonary artery (MPA) to course just posterior to the superior vena cava (svc) and anterior to the bronchus intermedius (bi). The left lower lobe pulmonary artery (open arrow) is posterior to the left main stem bronchus. Lung inserts into the azygoesophageal recess (arrow) immediately behind the bronchus intermedius. Also, lung frequently inserts into a notch between the left lower lobe pulmonary artery (open arrow) and the descending aorta (DA). Arrowheads, superior pulmonary veins; AA, ascending aorta. **b:** A small calcified lymph node (arrow) is present in the subcarinal region just behind the right pulmonary artery. **c:** The course of a calcified left coronary artery can be visualized (arrow) just lateral to the main pulmonary artery (MPA). Calcified lymph nodes are seen in the subcarinal area and the inferior left hilum. **d:** In children the deep lung concavity in the azygoesophageal recess (arrow) behind the right main pulmonary artery is not found, and the area may rarely display a convexity medially.

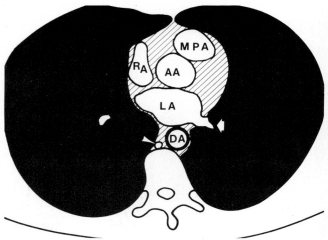

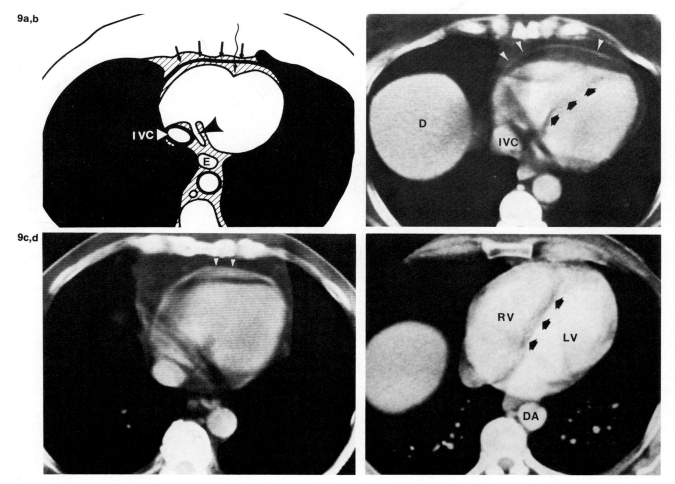

FIG. 8. Normal anatomy—left atrium. **Left:** The right atrium (RA) as well as the root of the aorta (AA) and the main pulmonary artery (MPA) are seen at this level. The inferior pulmonary veins (arrow) may be seen coursing into the left atrium (LA). The azygous vein (arrowhead) and descending aorta (DA) are visible. **Right:** The main pulmonary artery (MPA) is usually somewhat anterior to the ascending aorta (AA) as shown here, but the two structures may be seen in the same coronal plane. Intimal calcification is noted in the anterior wall of the descending aorta (DA). The esophagus (arrowhead) is seen just behind the left atrium (LA).

FIG. 9. Normal anatomy—cardiac ventricles. **a:** At the ventricular level the anterior pericardium (arrows) is virtually always identified as a thin line of soft tissue density between the pericardial (mediastinal) fat anteriorly and the epicardial fat posteriorly. The septal groove (thin arrow) is often visible and identifies the region of the interventricular septum. The coronary sinus (arrowhead), the main venous drainage of the cardiac muscle, may be seen as a tongue-like structure posterior to the right ventricle and adjacent to the inferior vena cava (IVC). The distal esophagus (E) is anterior and sometimes medial to the descending aorta. **b:** The thin line of the anterior pericardium (arrowheads) flanked by fat is easily identified. The ventricular septum (arrows) is visualized due to sufficient surrounding fat. D, right hemidiaphragm; IVC, inferior vena cava. **c:** Just before its insertion into the central tendon of the diaphragm, there may be apparent thickening anteriorly of the pericardium (arrowheads) as it continues around the heart. **d:** Scan during the levophase after bolus administration of intravenous contrast media has opacified both the left (LV) and right (RV) ventricles and the descending aorta (DA). The interventricular septum (arrows) is well demarcated between the opacified ventricles.

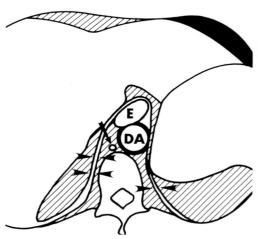
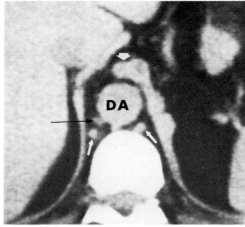
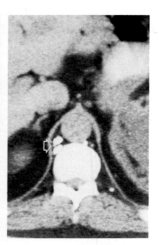

FIG. 10. Normal anatomy—retrocrural space. **Left:** The diaphragmatic crura (arrowheads) demarcate the inferior extent of the posterior mediastinum. In the retrocrural space lie the distal esophagus (E), the descending aorta (DA), azygous (arrow) and hemiazygous veins, and surrounding fat. **Center:** The azygous vein (white arrow) on the right, the hemiazygous vein (white arrow) on the left, and the thoracic duct (thin black arrow) are seen posterior to the descending aorta (DA). The lobulations in the medial portion of the left diaphragmatic crus are normal variations. The esophagus (thick white arrow) is anterior to the aorta and blends in with the left crus. **Right:** In a scan obtained after a previous lymphangiogram, opacified lymph nodes (open arrow) are seen in the retrocrural space.

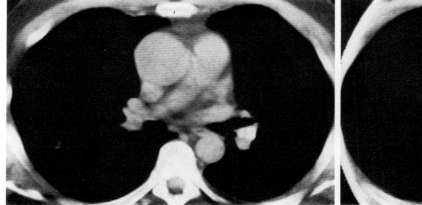
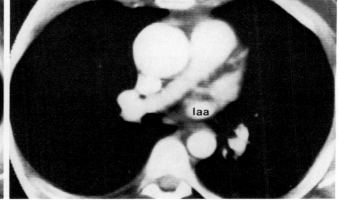

FIG. 11. Normal anatomy—value of intravenous contrast. **Left:** In this individual whose chest roentgenogram showed a prominent right hilum, the precontrast scan was thought to be normal. **Right:** A scan after the intravenous administration of contrast medium confirms that only normal vascular structures are present in the right hilum. The top of the left atrial appendage (laa) is noted at this level.

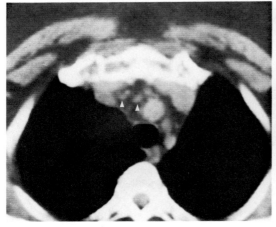
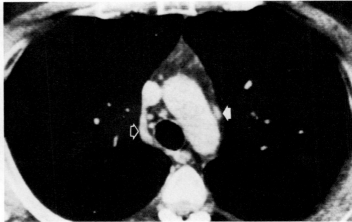

FIG. 12. Normal lymph nodes. **Left:** Multiple small lymph nodes (arrowheads), all less than 5 mm in diameter, are seen within the mediastinal fat adjacent to the five mediastinal vessels at the level of the manubrium. **Right:** At the level of the aortic arch, three small lymph nodes are seen in the pretracheal space just medial to the arch of the azygous vein (open arrow). The so-called azygous node(s) may range from 1 to 3 in number. A lateral aortic node (closed arrow) is also visible.

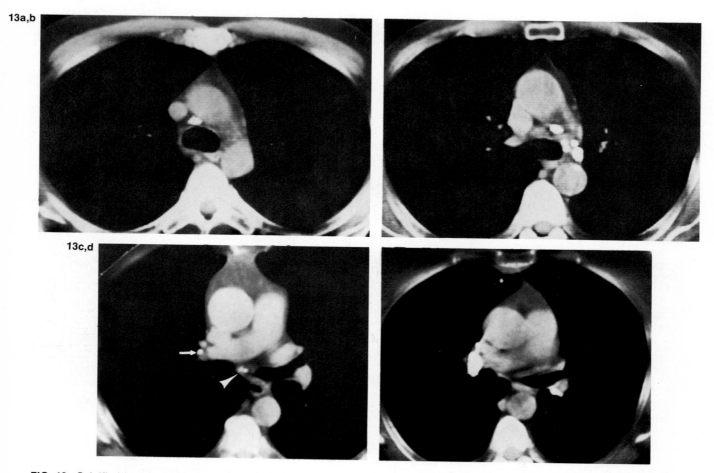

FIG. 13. Calcified lymph nodes demonstrating sites of normally occurring lymph nodes. **a:** A calcified lymph node is present in the pretracheal region just below the level of the aortic and azygous arches. **b:** Calcified lymph nodes in the aortopulmonary window. **c:** Small calcified lymph nodes are present in the right hilum (arrow) and the subcarinal (arrowhead) regions. **d:** A large clump of calcified lymph nodes in the right hilum and a smaller calcified node in the left hilum medial to the left lower lobe pulmonary artery are seen.

14a,b

14c,d

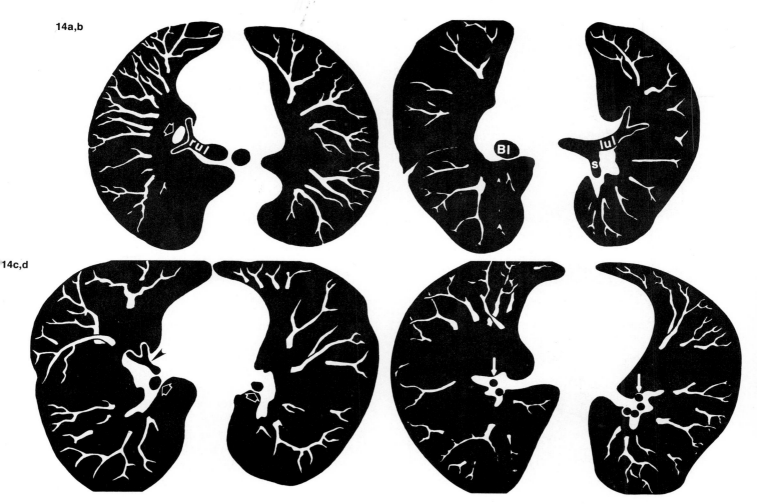

FIG. 14. Normal anatomy—diagrammatic lung images of the hilar regions. Viewed at window settings optimized for the lung, bronchial anatomy of the pulmonary hila can be defined and related to vascular structures. **a:** Corresponding to the left pulmonary artery level the main stem bronchi and the right upper lobe bronchus (rul) can be demonstrated. The anteroposterior dimensions of the main stem bronchi should be equal. The vessel (open arrow) seen in cross section between the anterior and posterior divisions of the right upper lobe bronchus is the right superior pulmonary vein. The apical segmental bronchi and accompanying vessels (not shown here) can almost always be seen in cross section on a more cephalad section at the level of the aortic arch. **b:** One centimeter inferiorly, the bronchus intermedius (BI), left upper lobe bronchus (lul), and superior segment bronchus to the left lower lobe (s) can all be visualized. Note the relative paucity of vessels in the right midlung field in the region of the minor fissure. **c:** At the atrial level, the right middle lobe bronchus (arrowhead) with its medial and lateral segments and the lower lobe bronchi (open arrows) are seen. Frequently the middle lobe artery (not shown) is seen between the segmental bronchi of the right middle lobe. The inferior pulmonary veins are located posterior and medial to the lower lobe bronchi, whereas the lower lobe arteries are just lateral to the bronchi. **d:** At the ventricular level the basilar segment bronchi (arrows) are visible. The basilar segmental bronchi are not consistently seen due to the oblique course they frequently take. Pulmonary arteries and veins account for the soft tissue structures seen adjacent to the segmental bronchi.

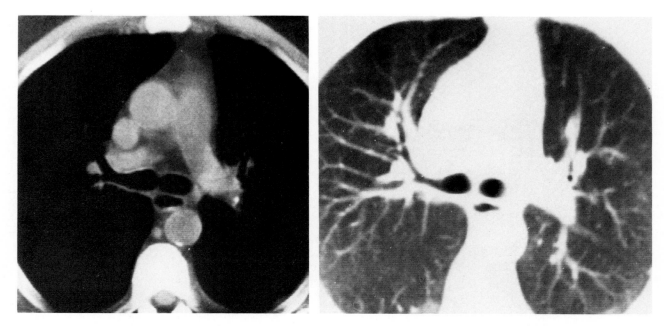

FIG. 15. Normal anatomy—image manipulation. **Left:** Window width and level optimized for demonstration of the mediastinal structures at the level of the left pulmonary artery and right upper lobe bronchus. **Right:** The same scan at a window setting optimal for visualizing lung structure.

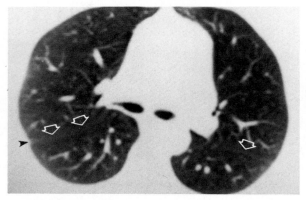

FIG. 16. Normal anatomy—interlobar fissures. The oblique or major fissures (open arrows) are seen as a thin white line. On the right a pleural notch (black arrowhead) also marks the location of the fissure.

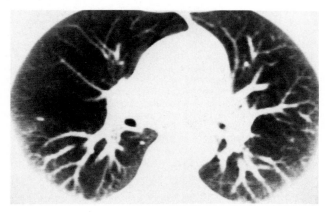

FIG. 17. Normal anatomy—gravity dependent blood flow. The dorsal dominance of pulmonary blood flow commonly seen on CT scans performed in the usual supine position is demonstrated. Note also the sparse vascularity in the right midlung field in the region of the minor fissure.

importance lest it be misinterpreted as an abnormal mediastinal mass. Using contemporary CT scanners, the normal thymus can be recognized in a large percentage of patients, especially those younger than 40 years of age (Fig. 18) (3). Prior to puberty, this bilobed structure fills most of the anterosuperior mediastinum in front of the great vessels. The thymus may extend inferiorly from the lower end of the thyroid gland to the upper portion of the pericardial sac. The two lobes usually make contact superiorly near the midline, and then diverge inferiorly. The left lobe is usually slightly larger and situated slightly higher than the right lobe. Up to 30% of individuals have a fat cleft distinctly dividing the thymus into two lobes on CT. In most of the remainder the lobes are confluent and the thymus assumes an arrowhead (or triangular) configuration. The width and thickness of each lobe can be easily measured on CT (Fig. 19). Although the width of the thymus is quite variable among different age groups, the thickness of the thymus shows a definite decrease in size with advancing age. The maximum thickness of either lobe is 1.8 cm prior to age 20; thereafter, 1.3 cm is a maximal thickness although most normal lobes are less than 0.8 cm in thickness. In the pediatric and adolescent age group the density of the thymus is similar to that of the chest wall muscles (3,12). After puberty a gradual progressive infiltration of fat into the thymic parenchyma occurs. Usually after the age of 40 the organ approaches pure fat in attenuation value; only sparse small nodular densities of thymic parenchyma may remain as subtle reminders of the involuted atrophic thymus still present. In thin patients no recognizable thymic remnant may be visible.

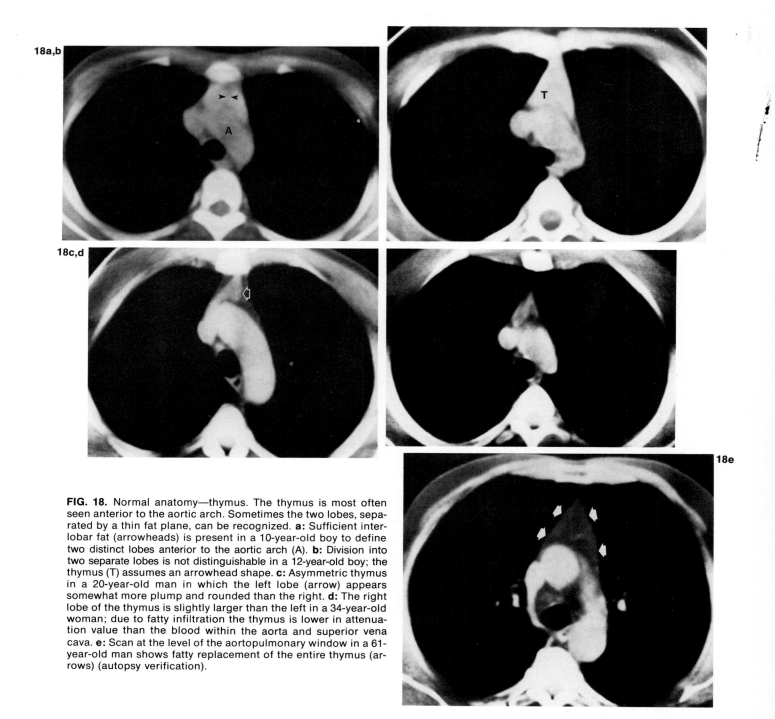

18a,b

18c,d

18e

FIG. 18. Normal anatomy—thymus. The thymus is most often seen anterior to the aortic arch. Sometimes the two lobes, separated by a thin fat plane, can be recognized. a: Sufficient interlobar fat (arrowheads) is present in a 10-year-old boy to define two distinct lobes anterior to the aortic arch (A). b: Division into two separate lobes is not distinguishable in a 12-year-old boy; the thymus (T) assumes an arrowhead shape. c: Asymmetric thymus in a 20-year-old man in which the left lobe (arrow) appears somewhat more plump and rounded than the right. d: The right lobe of the thymus is slightly larger than the left in a 34-year-old woman; due to fatty infiltration the thymus is lower in attenuation value than the blood within the aorta and superior vena cava. e: Scan at the level of the aortopulmonary window in a 61-year-old man shows fatty replacement of the entire thymus (arrows) (autopsy verification).

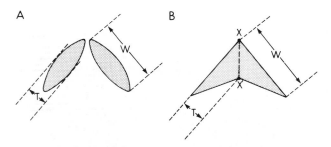

FIG. 19. Determining thymic size. **a:** In a bilobed organ the short axis or thickness (T) is measured perpendicular to the long axis or width (W). **b:** When the two lobes are confluent, creating an arrowhead shape, the thymus is divided in half by a line (X—X¹) through the apex of the organ. The width (W) and thickness (T) are then measured as above. (From ref. 3, with permission from the publisher.)

At least a portion of the normal pericardium, a double-layered fibroserous sac enveloping the heart and origin of the great vessels, is visible on CT in almost all patients. Identification of the normal pericardium as a separate structure is possible only in areas where subepicardial fat is present; young children or emaciated adults may lack such fat. The caudal half is most commonly imaged, and appears as a thin curvilinear density 1 to 2 mm in thickness overlying the anterolateral cardiac surface where the pericardium is surrounded by fat in the mediastinum and in the epicardial layer of the heart (Fig. 9). The most distal portion of the pericardium in front of the right ventricle, just before its insertion into the central tendon of the diaphragm, may measure up to 3 to 4 mm in thickness. The dorsal aspect and the cephalad portion of the pericardium are seen in only a very few patients because of the lack of sufficient surrounding fat in these areas.

The diaphragmatic crura, rarely seen on conventional chest radiographs, can be clearly distinguished on almost all CT studies (Fig. 10) (8). The enclosed retrocrural space, the most inferior extension of the posterior mediastinum, is the major connecting route between the thorax and abdomen. The retrocrural space at the level of the aponeurotic hiatus in the diaphragm for the esophagus and aorta is demarcated by the diaphragmatic crura anteriorly and laterally and the vertebral column posteriorly. Normally seen constituents of this space include fat, the aorta, the azygous and hemiazygous veins, the thoracic duct, and associated lymph nodes. Normal lymph nodes in this area probably do not exceed 6 mm in cross-sectional diameter (9). Rarely, gas may appear to be within the retrocrural space on CT (39). This is due to aerated normal lung extending especially deep into the posterior costophrenic sulci and insinuating medial to the decussating diaphragmatic crura. This lung tissue should

not be confused with retroperitoneal or mediastinal air caused by an abscess.

TECHNIQUE

Computed tomography of the thorax is performed in suspended inspiration at total lung capacity. Short scanning times (5 sec or less) are particularly important in the thorax, and in conjunction with breath holding, markedly reduce artifacts due to respiratory and cardiac motion.

A mediastinal CT examination need not be performed in a stereotyped fashion; each study is best tailored to the clinical problem being evaluated. Patients are usually examined in the supine position; decubitus or prone views may be readily obtained when indicated. Most scans are performed at 1-cm serial intervals with a slice thickness of 10 mm; narrower collimation is reserved for questionable small lesions (e.g., query thymoma or parathyroid adenoma). The entire thorax is not surveyed in every patient. Focal abnormalities detected on a plain chest radiograph may be completely evaluated in less than 10 min; scanning the entire thorax takes approximately 30 min to accomplish.

Intravenous iodinated contrast medium is administered at the discretion of the radiologist when deemed potentially valuable to differentiate a vascular from a nonvascular mass or to depict the relationship of a mass lesion to the mediastinal vessels or the heart. When a large area of the mediastinum is being evaluated, sustained enhancement of the major vessels can be achieved by the rapid intravenous infusion of 150 ml of 60% iodinated contrast medium immediately following a priming bolus of 50 ml of 60% iodinated contrast medium (Fig. 20). For study of focal regions in detail, serial scanning following a 25- to 50-cc bolus of 60% iodinated contrast medium is optimal (Figs. 21–23). A medially directed antecubital vein should always be chosen as the site for injection since drainage is directly to the basilic system and the superior vena cava. If a laterally directed vein is used, since this system drains to the cephalic vein, valves often impede immediate flow to the cava when the arms are placed over the head in the usual position for scanning. If possible, obtaining multiple repetitive scans ("dynamic scanning") at the same level after a bolus injection is advantageous. This ensures that the arrival of the bolus in the desired vessels will be coincident with one or more scan exposures. Guesswork that otherwise might be necessary because of individual variations in circulation time is reduced and consequently the volume of contrast medium necessary for a study is diminished. Three scans—at approximately 8, 15, and 22 sec after initiation of the bolus

20a,b

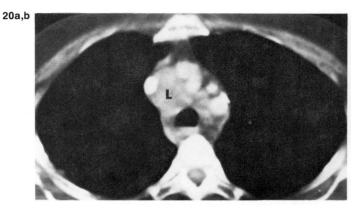

20c

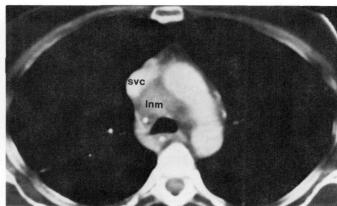

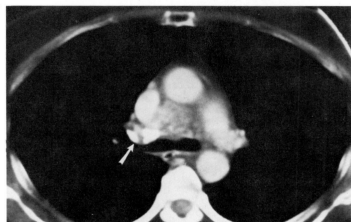

FIG. 20. Intravenous contrast medium administration—infusion technique. Mediastinal widening was noted on a plain chest radiograph in a 48-year-old woman. Scanning during a rapid infusion of iodinated contrast medium permitted excellent vascular opacification throughout the mediastinum. **a:** Lymphoma (L) involving lymph nodes in the superior mediastinum is clearly distinguished from opacified vessels. **b:** The lymph node mass (lnm) displaces and compresses the superior vena cava (svc). **c:** Neoplasm extends to the precarinal level. Calcified lymph nodes (arrow) anterior to the right upper lobe bronchus are incidentally noted.

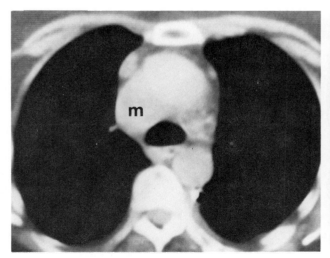

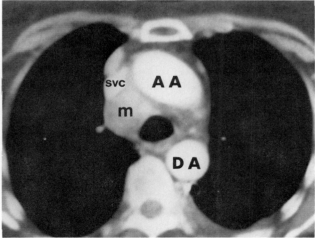

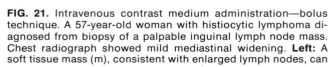

FIG. 21. Intravenous contrast medium administration—bolus technique. A 57-year-old woman with histiocytic lymphoma diagnosed from biopsy of a palpable inguinal lymph node mass. Chest radiograph showed mild mediastinal widening. **Left:** A soft tissue mass (m), consistent with enlarged lymph nodes, can be recognized in the right paratracheal area. **Right:** Repeat scan at same level following bolus injection of intravenous contrast medium more clearly defines the lymph node mass (m) from the superior vena cava (svc) and the ascending aorta (AA). DA, descending aorta.

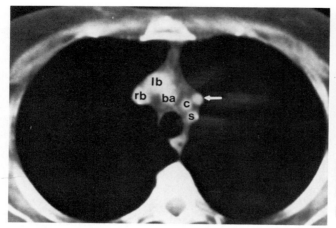
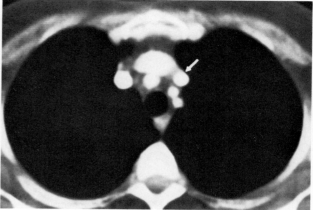

FIG. 22. Intravenous contrast medium administration—bolus technique. A 68-year-old woman with a carcinoma of the left upper lobe. CT examination was requested to assess the mediastinum before contemplated resection. **Left:** An extra round density (arrow) is seen lateral to the major arterial branches of the aorta. rb, right brachiocephalic vein; lb, left brachiocephalic vein; ba, brachiocephalic artery; c, carotid artery; s, left sub-clavian artery. **Right:** After an intravenous bolus injection of iodinated contrast medium, the lesion in question (arrow) enhances to a density similar to that of the nearby vascular structures. Sequential scans showed that this anatomic vascular variation represents a prominent left superior intercostal vein that drained into the left brachiocephalic vein at a more cephalad level ("a persistent left superior vena cava").

injection—usually suffice to see the peripherally injected contrast agent passing progressively through the various mediastinal venous and arterial structures. Late in the serial scan sequence a low-density intraluminal region in the superior vena cava should not be mistaken for a thrombus (Fig. 24); this phenomenon of laminar flow is due to residual opacified blood moving slowly near the periphery while more rapidly moving unopacified blood occupies the center of the vessel. Filling defects in the superior vena cava, especially anteriorly, may also result from incomplete mixing of opacified and unopacified blood from the two brachiocephalic veins, with the high-density contrast medium layering posteriorly. These flow-related filling defects usually disappear on scans obtained during the maximal concentration of the bolus in the superior vena cava. Differentiation of flow phenomena from a true filling defect, however, could be difficult or impossible if only a single image were obtained after injection.

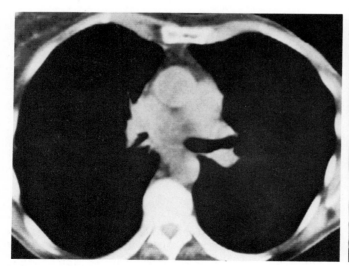
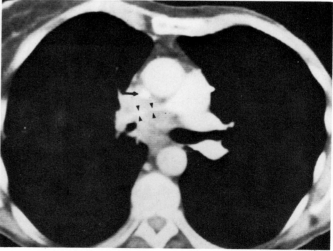

FIG. 23. Intravenous contrast medium administration—bolus technique. A 58-year-old woman with facial swelling. A carcinoma involving the bronchus intermedius was documented bronchoscopically. **Left:** Scan at the level of the right pulmonary artery shows narrowing of the bronchus intermedius and a probable soft tissue mass in the precarinal region. **Right:** Repeat scan at the same level following a bolus injection of contrast medium demonstrates neoplasm extending deep into the mediastinum, surrounding and narrowing the superior vena cava (arrow) and the right pulmonary artery (arrowheads).

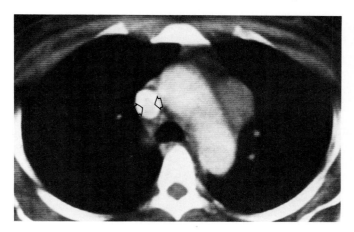

FIG. 24. Flow artifact in superior vena cava. A 67-year-old man with a large mass noted lateral to the aortic arch on a plain chest radiograph. CT performed to exclude the possibility of an aneurysm. Following a bolus injection of intravenous contrast medium, there is inhomogeneous opacification of the superior vena cava simulating a central thrombus. This artifactual filling defect (open arrows), due to laminar flow, is typically seen on the last serial scans following a bolus injection.

Reconstructed sagittal, coronal, or oblique images are only rarely of clinical value; sufficient information for correct interpretation usually is available from the standard cross-sectional images. Reformatted images may be useful in very selected cases to facilitate definitive diagnosis when the routine transverse sections are ambiguous and sometimes as an adjunct to radiation therapy planning. Reconstructions sometimes are helpful in conceptualizing pathologic lesions in a three-dimensional fashion and to demonstrate interrelationships that may be difficult to comprehend from the standard format.

Unlike conventional X-ray equipment, the CT beam is narrowly collimated and results in a skin dose of approximately 0.3 to 2 rems per examination. Although this dose greatly exceeds that of a plain chest radiograph, it is less than the overall dose from conventional chest tomography or angiography (25).

INDICATIONS

The relatively inexpensive and universally available standard chest roentgenogram continues to serve well as the initial radiologic examination in patients with suspected chest disease. But a wide range of applications for CT has emerged in the evaluation of chest problems. Computed tomography of the mediastinum is used most often as a supplementary or "problem-solving" technique when the etiology of a definite or questionable abnormality demonstrated on the plain chest radiograph cannot be determined by conventional noninvasive radiologic methods (e.g., fluoroscopy, decubitus views) or clinical correlation. The question of whether a mediastinal abnormality detected on a plain chest radiograph represents a pathological finding is a commonplace occurrence. Sometimes a mediastinal lesion is suspected on a frontal or lateral radiograph, but not on both, so that accurate localization of a potential pathologic process within the mediastinum is difficult. Computed tomography is a superb noninvasive modality for clarifying such problems, and has replaced conventional tomography in the evaluation of most mediastinal problems.

Lesion Seen or Questioned on Plain Chest Radiograph

Attenuation Value of a Mediastinal Mass

Determination of the relative attenuation value [now predominantly expressed in Hounsfield units (HU)] of a mediastinal mass by CT may permit a definite diagnosis noninvasively. This measurement of the capacity of the tissue in question to absorb X-rays bears a close linear relationship to the physical density (attenuation coefficient) of the lesion (Fig. 25). Computed tomography usually permits rapid and confident identification of air, fat, serous fluid, iodinated contrast material, and calcium within suspicious tissues. Minute calcifications, fatty deposits, or necrotic areas within a mass may not be identifiable on standard chest radiographs or conventional tomography.

Local or diffuse benign mediastinal fat collections can be diagnosed with almost absolute certainty (5,19,26,35). Homogeneous lesions that present with attenuation values characteristic of benign fatty tissue (approximately −80 HU) include a pericardial fat pad, omental herniations through the foramens of Morgagni or Bochdalek, or focal mediastinal fat deposition (Fig. 26). In such cases the CT diagnosis is usually conclusive and no further diagnostic work-up is indicated. A teratoma should be suspected when fat, and perhaps calcification, is seen intermixed within an anterior mediastinal mass (Fig. 27). Malignant fatty tumors tend to be inhomogeneous, and even the well-differentiated liposarcomas contain some soft tissue density elements in addition to the areas of fat density. In fact, most liposarcomas have a near soft tissue attenuation value.

Most benign cystic lesions of the mediastinum have a homogeneous near-water equivalent density (Fig. 28); they do not enhance after intravenous contrast administration (21,34). Pericardial cysts are most commonly located in the right cardiophrenic angle, whereas the foregut cysts (bronchogenic or enterogenous) usually are near the main bronchi or in a subcarinal location. Generally, the appearance and attenuation values are so characteristic that surgery may be

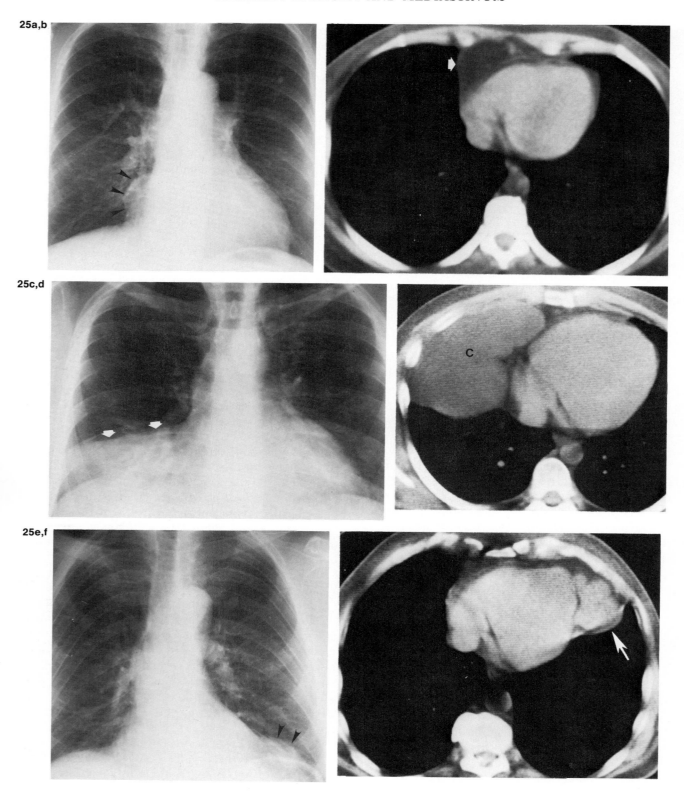

FIG. 25. Cardiophrenic angle masses of different etiologies. **a:** Chest radiograph demonstrates a right cardiophrenic angle mass (arrowheads) in a 49-year-old woman with melanoma of the left shoulder. **b:** A CT scan shows that the mass (arrow) is simply a benign pericardial fat pad of no clinical significance. **c:** Chest radiograph in a 19-year-old man, initially evaluated 2 weeks earlier for possible pneumonia, shows a large poorly defined density (arrows) in the region of the right middle lobe. **d:** CT shows a large homogeneous near-water density mass (C) in the right cardiophrenic angle consistent with a pericardial (duplication) cyst. **e:** Chest radiograph demonstrates a new left cardiophrenic angle mass (arrowheads) in a 66-year-old man previously treated for histiocytic lymphoma. Recurrence of lymphoma and the development of a pericardial fat pad due to steroid treatment were the primary considerations. **f:** CT shows that the mass is of soft tissue density (arrow), consistent with enlarged pericardial lymph nodes due to recurrent malignancy.

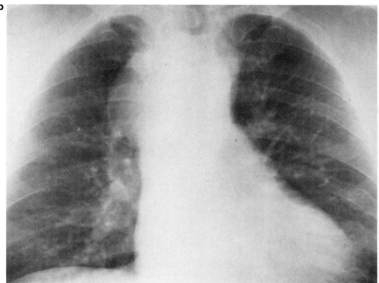
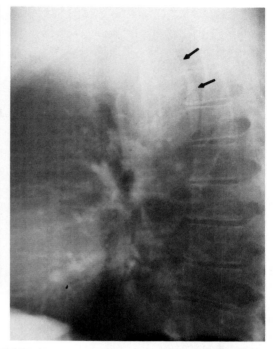

26a,b

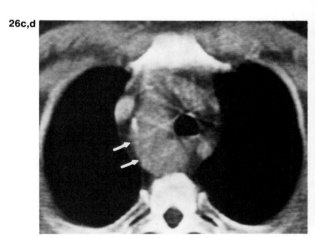
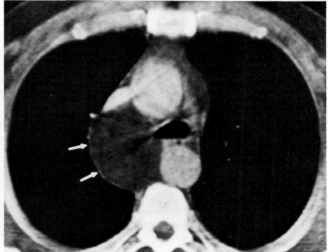

26c,d

FIG. 26. Mediastinal mass—right aortic arch and lipoma. **a,b:** Posteroanterior and lateral chest radiographs of a 63-year-old man admitted for facial burns show superior mediastinal widening and a retrotracheal density (arrows). **c:** CT scan demonstrates a right aortic arch (arrows) accounting for a portion of the mediastinal mass. **d:** A scan 2 cm inferiorly demonstrates a focal mediastinal mass with an attenuation value characteristic of benign fat (arrows) accounting for much of the widening. The descending portion of the right aortic arch is responsible for the retrotracheal density. This case illustrates the value of CT, not only in obviating an aortogram, but probably in preventing a thoracotomy. Had an aortogram been done, an unexplained mediastinal mass still would have been present.

avoided, and only roentgenographic follow-up is necessary in asymptomatic patients. Operation may be reserved for patients with symptoms or those unusually large cysts potentially capable of compressing a major mediastinal structure. On occasion, bronchogenic cysts may be filled with thick viscid secretions, resulting in a higher attenuation value, thus simulating a solid neoplasm (Fig. 29) (24). In such circumstances surgery is usually required for definitive evaluation. In mediastinal abscess, CT may demonstrate

the fluid content of the mass, and, not infrequently, air within it that cannot be seen on plain radiographs.

When a mediastinal mass has an attenuation density of approximately 30 to 80 HU and enhances only minimally in comparison to surrounding vessels after intravenous contrast medium administration, neoplasm is the most likely cause. Such soft tissue density tumors may contain areas of necrosis that superficially resemble cysts on CT. However, these neoplastic lesions always have a thick wall, an irregular margin, or

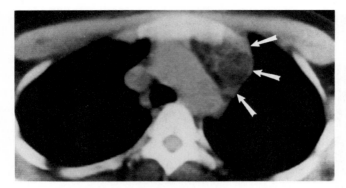

FIG. 27. Mediastinal mass—teratoma. An inhomogeneous mass (arrows) lateral to the aortic arch—containing fat, near water, and some tissue densities—represents a benign teratoma arising from the left lobe of the thymus in a 25-year-old woman.

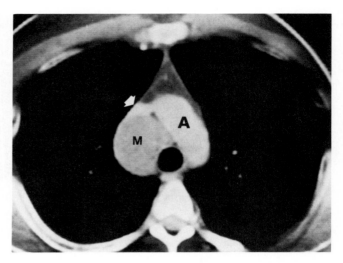

FIG. 28. Mediastinal mass—duplication cyst. CT defines a well-circumscribed, homogeneous paratracheal mass (M) with an attenuation value slightly above water, consistent with a benign duplication cyst in a 48-year-old man. The mass has not changed in size during a 3-year follow-up period on subsequent chest radiographs. Arrow, superior vena cava; A, aorta.

a soft tissue density component that allows their distinction from a benign cyst. Although CT may be valuable in determining the extent or origin of a soft tissue density mass and its relationship to other mediastinal structures, histologic diagnosis is not possible. If the interface between the mass and the surrounding mediastinal structures and fat is sharply preserved, the tumor is probably benign, although malignant lymphadenopathy may display such characteristics. Demonstration of invasion of the mediastinal fat or extension to involve the pleura, pericardium, or adjacent lung, however, strongly suggests malignant neoplasm. But mediastinitis secondary to granulomatous infection may produce identical changes.

Computed tomography is capable of specifically diagnosing a mediastinal thyroid as the cause of a mediastinal mass (6,14). Thoracic goiters almost al-

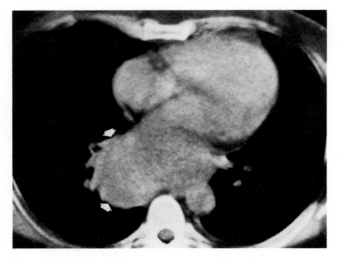

FIG. 29. Mediastinal mass—duplication cyst. CT scan in a 35-year-old man demonstrates a large posterior mediastinal mass (arrows) of soft tissue density; at surgery this proved to be an esophageal duplication cyst filled with thick viscid fluid.

ways arise from one or both lower poles of the thyroid or from the isthmus and are contiguous with the cervical portion of the gland on serial scans (Fig. 30), rather than separate ectopic lesions. Due to an increased iodine content, retrosternal thyroid tissue typically appears denser (sometimes above 100 HU) than surrounding mediastinal structures or the thoracic wall muscles (Fig. 31). After the intravenous administration of urographic contrast material, a prolonged (often greater than several minutes) rise in CT numbers characteristically occurs; this enhancement may be uniform or inhomogeneous throughout the gland. Since retrosternal thyroid frequently represents a form of multinodular goiter pathologically, focal calcifications or low-density cystic portions or areas of necrosis may be detected on CT. Intrathoracic goiters may extend caudally as low as the carina. The relationship of the thyroid mass to the subclavian arteries and innominate veins, as well as the trachea and esophagus, can be established much more precisely with CT than with conventional radiography or radionuclide imaging (Fig. 32). Although most of these goiters are located in the anterior mediastinum and deviate the brachiocephalic vessels posteriorly or laterally, those lesions posterior to the great vessels usually require a combined neck and thoracic surgical approach for resection. The area of the thoracic inlet near the thyroid should be scrutinized closely as incidental masses may be discovered (Fig. 33).

The use of CT can greatly expedite the diagnostic process by supplanting multiple, previously used imaging studies (conventional tomography, barium

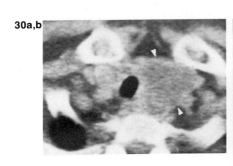
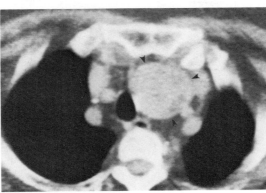

FIG. 30. Intrathoracic multinodular goiter. Plain radiographs in a 54-year-old man showed a superior mediastinal mass associated with deviation of the trachea thought to represent an enlarged retrosternal thyroid. **a,b:** CT scans at the sternal notch and sternoclavicular junction levels show that the mass (arrowheads), which contains several areas of low attenuation, arises from the left lobe of the thyroid and extends inferiorly and posteromedially to the mediastinal vessels.

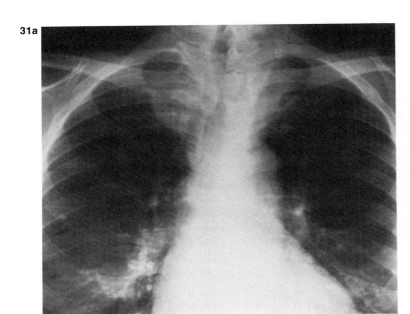

FIG. 31. Intrathoracic goiter. **a:** Chest radiograph demonstrates marked tracheal narrowing, probably in association with a superior mediastinal mass, in a 67-year-old man with stridor. **b:** CT scan at a level just above the sternal notch shows an enlarged thyroid (arrows). The gland can be confidently identified not only by its shape and location, but also because the majority of it is of relatively high density due to its iodine content. **c:** One centimeter inferiorly, the enlarged gland extends around and markedly compresses the trachea. The goiter contains some areas of low attenuation and calcification.

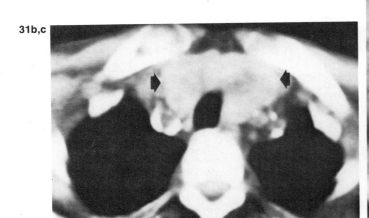
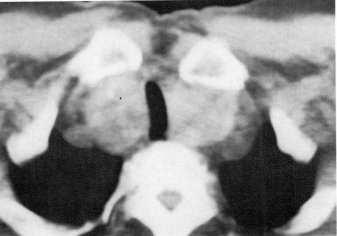

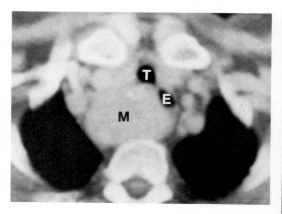

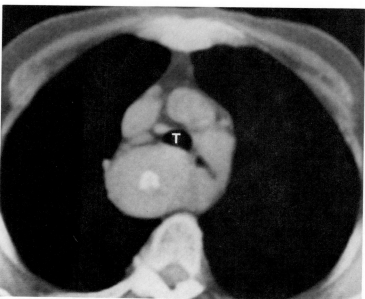

FIG. 32. Intrathoracic goiter. Scans at the level of the sternal notch and aortic arch demonstrate a large soft tissue mass (M) containing foci of calcification, extending behind and impinging on both the trachea (T) and the esophagus (E). A combined neck and thoracic surgical approach was required to remove the mass.

esophagography, radionuclide scintigraphy, and angiographic procedures such as cavography, pulmonary arteriography, and aortography), which in many cases even together accomplished only localization of the mass.

Mediastinal Widening

When mediastinal widening is detected on the plain chest radiograph, the cause may be a normal variant (such as abundant fat deposition or tortuous vessels) or a pathologic lesion. The latter may be vascular in etiology (such as an aneurysm) or be caused by a primary neoplasm or enlarged lymph nodes. Fluoroscopy, conventional laminography, or a barium esophagogram may confirm the presence of a pathologically widened mediastinum, but rarely aid in defining the etiology. Computed tomography is ideally

suited for analysis of the widened mediastinum (4,27,36). It can differentiate vascular from nonvascular causes, and often provides a specific and conclusive diagnosis. Invasive diagnostic procedures such as mediastinoscopy or aortography may be reserved for those situations in which additional clinical information is required or rarely when the CT findings are equivocal.

The mediastinum is frequently widened by innocuous abundant fat deposition and, in older patients, by tortuous or dilated great vessels. These changes may be difficult to distinguish from other disease entities on conventional radiography. Computed tomography can easily separate such an innocently widened mediastinum from truly pathologic conditions in a simple and unequivocal fashion, eliminating the need for any further investigation. Mediastinal lipomatosis can be confidently diagnosed with CT. Smoothly marginated homogeneous low-density areas surround the great ves-

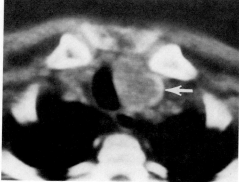

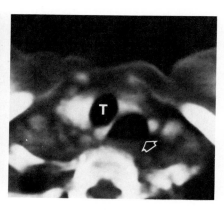

FIG. 33. Thoracic inlet masses. **a:** In a 33-year-old woman with a pulmonary nodule, a mass was discovered in the left lobe of the thyroid. Normal thyroid tissue of higher attenuation value (arrow) is seen peripheral to the mass, which deviates and compresses the trachea. Surgical resection disclosed histiocytic lymphoma. **b:** An incidental Zenker's diverticulum (open arrow), containing an air-fluid level, is demonstrated at the level of the thoracic inlet in a 77-year-old woman. T, trachea.

34a

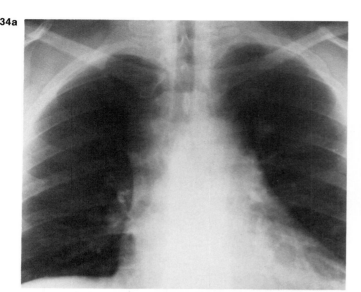

FIG. 34. Mediastinal widening—mediastinal lipomatosis. **a:** Routine chest radiograph in a 30-year-old man with an inguinal hernia shows widening of the mediastinum. **b,c:** Scans at levels of the manubrium and aortic arch respectively demonstrate abundant fat throughout the mediastinum accounting for the widening. A mildly enlarged paratracheal lymph node is seen, presumably secondary to old granulomatous disease (no change on repeat scans 4 months later).

34b,c

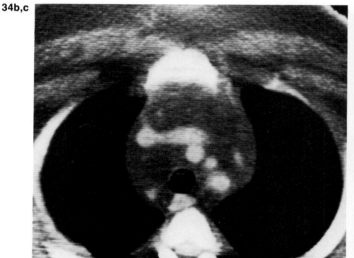

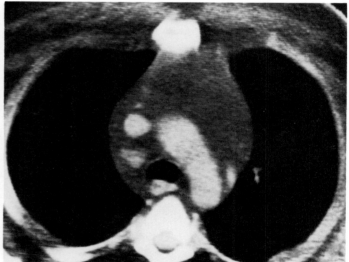

sels in the superior mediastinum, sometimes causing them to be situated more laterally than normal (Fig. 34). Displacement of the trachea or esophagus does not occur. Whereas mediastinal lipomatosis may be associated with obesity, corticosteroid ingestion, or Cushing's syndrome, these factors often are not present. In the elderly, a tortuous innominate artery frequently displaces the superior vena cava or right innominate vein laterally to cause mediastinal widening on the plain chest roentgenogram (Fig. 35).

The transverse plane CT images usually have proven more valuable in assessing the questionably pathologic mediastinum than oblique or lateral radiographs or conventional tomography, because these latter techniques often fail to project the abnormality away from superimposed normal mediastinal contents (Fig. 36). Computed tomography has emerged as the most valuable radiologic technique for evaluating the mediastinal

lymph nodes. When a lymph node exceeds 1.5 cm in diameter, it is considered pathologic; such enlargement may be caused by either a neoplastic or inflammatory process. It cannot be overemphasized that lymph node enlargement detected on CT is not specific for neoplastic involvement, although expansion above 2 cm in diameter most frequently is caused by neoplastic disease. Also, neoplasm that replaces the normal nodal architecture but does not cause enlargement will not be discerned on CT scanning. Despite this limitation, CT allows detection of lymph node enlargement at an earlier stage than is possible with any other radiologic method. By precisely depicting which group of lymph nodes are involved, CT is valuable in assessing whether patients are likely to benefit from tissue sampling via a transcervical mediastinoscopy or a parasternal mediastinotomy (Fig. 37).

Vascular anomalies or dilatation, including aneu-

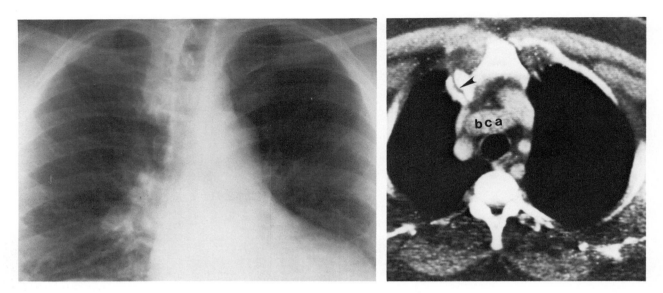

FIG. 35. Mediastinal widening—tortuous innominate artery. **Left:** Chest radiograph in a 73-year-old man demonstrates widening of the superior mediastinum. **Right:** The brachiocephalic artery (bca) on this and adjacent scans is quite tortuous and deviates the brachiocephalic veins laterally. Additionally, hypertrophic spurring about the sternoclavicular joint (arrowhead) creates a further increase in density along the right superior mediastinum.

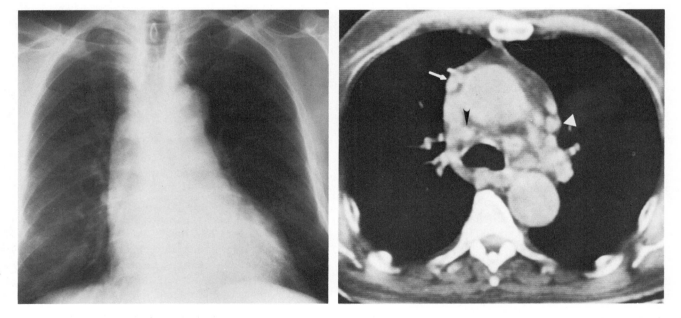

FIG. 36. Mediastinal widening—lymphoma. **Left:** Chest radiograph of a 78-year-old man with fatigue and weight loss shows widening of the mediastinum, thought most likely to represent only tortuous vessels. **Right:** CT scan demonstrates enlarged lymph nodes in the anterior mediastinum (white arrow), in the pretracheal region in the plane of mediastinoscopy (black arrowhead), and in the aortopulmonary window (white arrowhead). Mediastinoscopy disclosed histiocytic lymphoma.

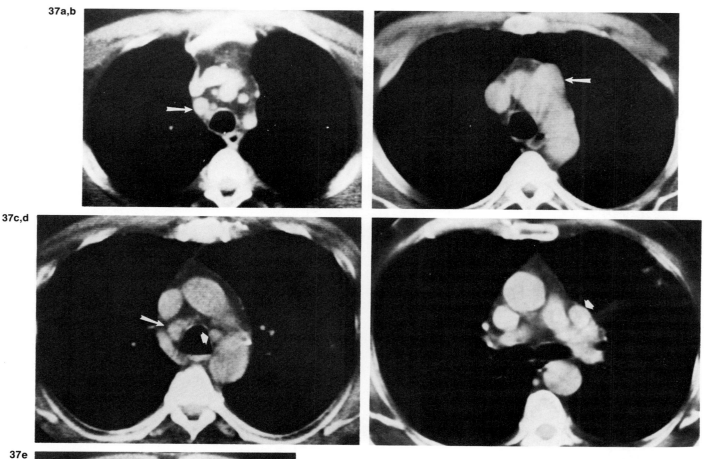

37a,b

37c,d

37e

FIG. 37. Lymph node enlargement in various regions. **a:** Right paratracheal lymphadenopathy (arrow) in the plane of mediastinoscopy. **b:** Lymphadenopathy anterolateral to the aortic arch (arrow); these nodes cannot be sampled by transcervical mediastinoscopy but may be reached by an anterior parasternal mediastinotomy. **c:** Lymphadenopathy in the aortopulmonary window (thick short arrow) as well as pretracheal adenopathy (thin arrow) medial to the azygous vein. **d:** Left hilar adenopathy (arrow) anterior to the left pulmonary artery. **e:** Nodes in the subcarinal region (arrow) produce a convex mediastinal margin between the bronchus intermedius (black arrowheads) and the azygous vein (arrowhead). *Continued on following page.*

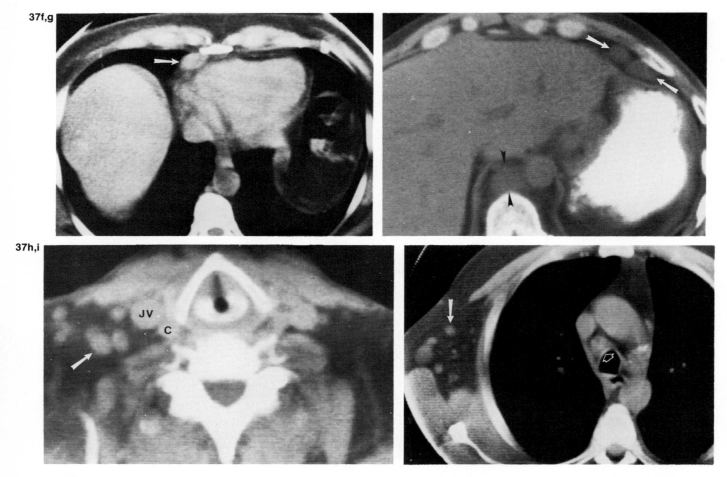

FIG. 37 *(cont.)* Lymph node enlargement in various regions. **f:** Pericardial lymphadenopathy (arrow) in the right cardiophrenic angle. **g:** Juxtadiaphragmatic lymphadenopathy (white arrows) as well as retrocrural adenopathy (black arrowheads). **h:** Lymphadenopathy in the right supraclavicular region (arrow) lateral to the carotid artery (c) and jugular vein (jv). **i:** Normal and enlarged lymph nodes (arrow) in the right axilla plus paratracheal adenopathy (open arrow).

rysm formation, responsible for mediastinal widening should be diagnosable by CT in almost all cases (1,4). Generally, the distinction between a mass lesion and a vascular structure—including normal vessels, aneurysms, and ectatic or aberrant arteries—can be made by following the anatomy of the great vessels on serial scans. Curvilinear areas of calcification can be seen peripherally surrounding most atherosclerotic aneurysms. Intravenous contrast enhancement is frequently employed to more confidently delineate a vascular structure (Fig. 38). Following a bolus injection of intravenous contrast medium, the attenuation value of the shadow in question should enhance to the same extent as adjacent normal vessels if it is vascular in etiology. Solid mediastinal lesions never enhance to such a degree. Aneurysms can be confidently diagnosed, their size determined, and intramural thrombi identified with precision by CT (Figs. 39 and 40). Some caution is advised in evaluating a tortuous aorta. The cross-sectional scan analyzed may incorporate both

portions of a kink in the aorta, imaging them as a single structure and appearing much larger than the actual diameter of either limb of the tortuous aorta. Also, it should be emphasized that an aneurysm entirely filled with thrombus will not enhance on CT and a solid soft tissue neoplasm would be simulated; a similiar pitfall could occur with angiography. Usually, ancillary findings are present on CT, such as changing caliber of the aortic lumen or surrounding calcification, to strongly suggest the correct diagnosis. An additional caveat is that some highly vascular lesions (e.g., leiomyosarcoma, angiofollicular lymph node hyperplasia, or an intrathoracic goiter) may show striking enhancement (Fig. 41). Especially with the infusion technique, the degree of opacification may simulate an aneurysm. Rapid serial scanning after bolus injection usually can clarify the problem. If surgical resection of an aneurysm is contemplated, the information provided by CT alone may not suffice for proper preoperative planning; angiography also may be re-

38a,b

38c,d

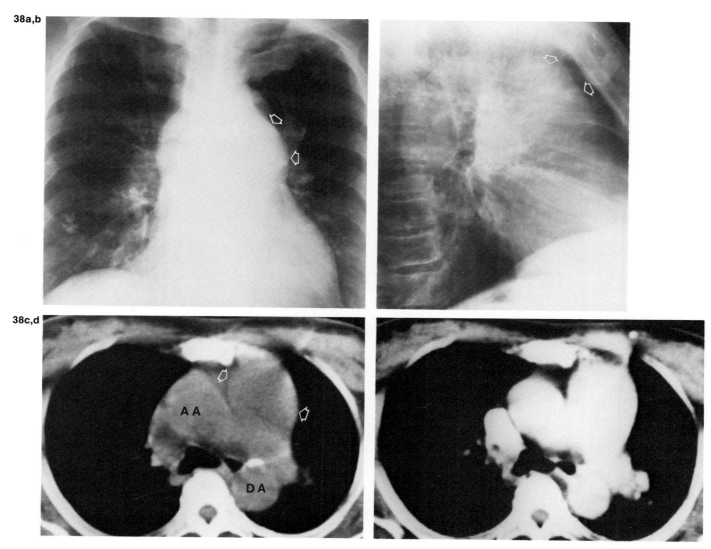

FIG. 38. Idiopathic dilatation of the pulmonary outflow tract. **a,b:** Posteroanterior and lateral chest radiographs in a 62-year-old woman demonstrate an apparent mass (arrows) in the region of the pulmonary artery. There was no clinical evidence of pulmonary hypertension nor was a murmur audible. Definite distinction between a vascular structure and a mass could not be made. **c:** On a noncontrast enhanced scan the suspected mass (open arrows) appears to represent a dilated pulmonary artery. Ascending aorta, AA; descending aorta, DA. **d:** CT scan during a rapid infusion of contrast medium confirms that the "mass" is due to dilatation of the pulmonary artery and outflow tract.

quired in the infrequent case when CT is unable to clearly differentiate a vascular from nonvascular lesion.

Computed tomography is a valuable screening test in the patient with suspected aortic dissection (16,23). Dissection of the aorta, which may have a catastrophic or insidious clinical presentation, usually begins as an intimal tear near the aortic root. The anatomic site of the tear influences both treatment and prognosis. Hence, it is necessary to diagnose the condition rapidly and to classify it into one of two types. Type A affects the ascending aorta or the arch or both and is usually treated by surgery. Type B involves only regions of the aorta distal to the left subclavian artery; medical manage-

ment usually suffices with elective surgery occasionally performed at a later time. Computed tomography is a reliable, noninvasive technique that generally can diagnose (Figs. 42 and 43) or reasonably exclude aortic dissection, obviating aortography in most cases. An increase in aortic caliber may be present on scans at the site of the dissection; usually the involved length is longer than with an atherosclerotic aneurysm. Internal displacement of intimal calcification may be seen on precontrast scans. A separate false lumen may be recognizable and appear denser than the flowing blood in the true lumen if the dissecting hematoma is acute. The false lumen may have a lower attenuation value if the dissection is chronic. Distinct separation

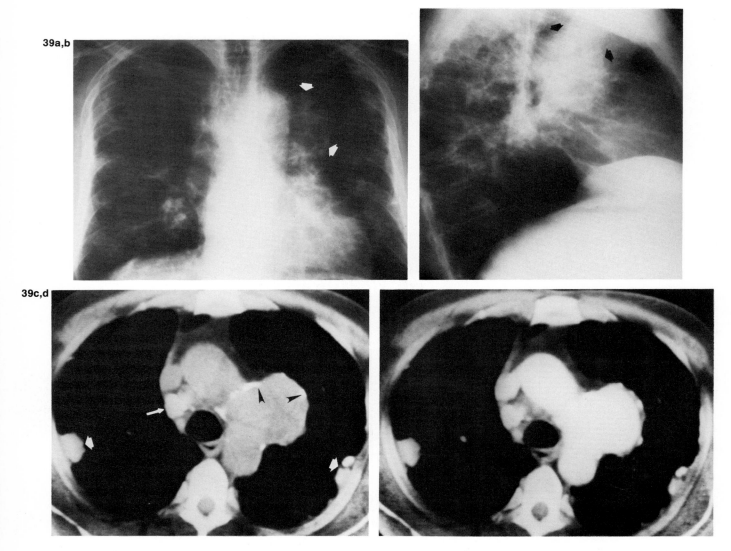

FIG. 39. Atherosclerotic aortic aneurysm. **a,b:** Posteroanterior and lateral chest radiographs in a 63-year-old man with extensive exposure to asbestos demonstrate a left thoracic mass (arrows) adjacent to the aortic arch. Bronchogenic carcinoma and possibly an aortic aneurysm were considered the likely diagnostic possibilities. **c:** On a noncontrast CT, atherosclerotic calcification (black arrowheads) extends from the aortic arch around the mass, compatible with a diagnosis of an aneurysm. Calcified paratracheal lymph nodes (thin white arrow) and calcified pleural plaques (thick white arrows) also are noted. **d:** CT scan following a bolus injection of contrast medium confirms a localized saccular aortic aneurysm as the cause of the mass.

of the false from the true lumen may require scanning after the administration of iodinated intravenous contrast material, at which time the separating intimal flap usually is optimally demonstrated. If only the true lumen enhances, it may be deformed and narrowed, and the aortic wall may appear eccentrically thickened. Delayed opacification and washout of the false lumen may sometimes occur. Enhancement of granulation tissue around a subacute or chronic dissection may occur. Angiography usually is still required for a patient being considered for surgery in order to assess involvement of the branch vessels and to determine exactly the sites of intimal tear and reentry. Easily

repeatable CT also has proven valuable in the follow-up of patients with aortic dissection (17). Persistent patency of the false lumen occurs in a high percentage of patients after medical or surgical therapy; the success of surgery relates to prevention of proximal extension and removal of a weakened portion of the wall. The presence of a persistent false lumen predisposes to further complications; CT can demonstrate redissection, extension of the dissection, or aneurysm formation with the danger of future rupture.

Computed tomography can play an important diagnostic role in an array of congenital vascular anomalies of the aortic arch and major mediastinal vessels (1).

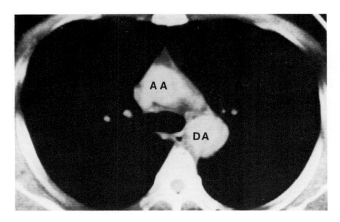

FIG. 40. Traumatic aortic aneurysm. The proximal descending aorta (DA) is pathologically enlarged in diameter compared to the ascending aorta (AA) in a 28-year-old who had been in an automobile accident 3 months previously.

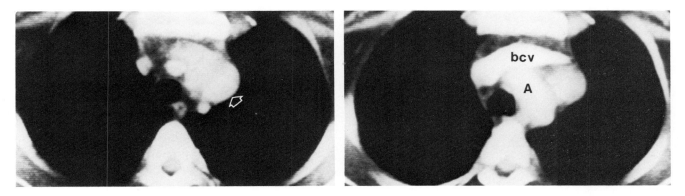

FIG. 41. Contrast enhancement of a highly vascular neoplasm (leiomyosarcoma). **Left:** CT scan during an infusion of contrast medium demonstrates enhancement of a soft tissue mass (arrow) to nearly the same degree as the adjacent normal vessels, simulating an aneurysm. **Right:** Repeat CT scan at a slightly lower level after a bolus injection of contrast medium into a left medial antecubital vein again demonstrates enhancement of the mass, but it is not as marked as in the adjacent left brachiocephalic vein (bcv) or the aortic arch (A).

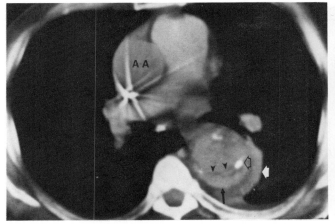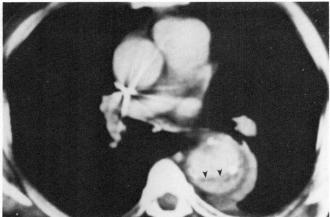

FIG. 42. Aortic dissection—type B. A 69-year-old man with chronic cardiac problems and an indwelling transvenous pacemaker presented with acute chest pain. **Left:** Following a bolus injection of contrast medium, an early sequential scan demonstrates some opacification of the main and right pulmonary arteries and some artifactual streaking from the pacemaker in the superior vena cava. The unenhanced ascending aorta (AA) appears normal. The descending aorta is enlarged, and there is internal displacement of intimal calcification (open arrow) with a faintly visible curvilinear intimal flap (arrowheads) separating the true lumen from the false lumen posteriorly, consistent with a type B dissection. Note that the density of the blood in the false lumen (black arrow) is higher than the blood in the true lumen. The cresentic density (white arrow) external to the aorta most likely represents some hemorrhage into the mediastinum or the pleural space. **Right:** Later in the scan sequence when opacified blood has reached the aorta, the intimal flap (arrowheads) in the descending aorta is more convincingly demonstrated. Note that the blood in the true lumen is now denser than that in the false lumen. The ascending aorta remains normal.

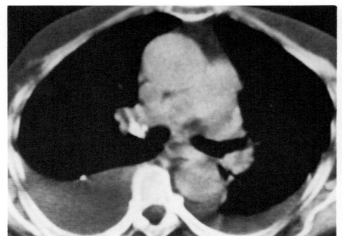 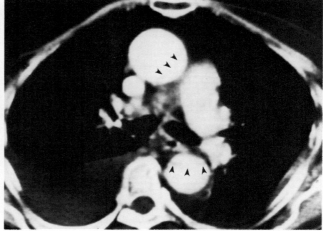

FIG. 43. Aortic dissection—type A. **Left:** No definite aortic abnormality can be seen on a precontrast scan in a 48-year-old woman with chest pain. Bilateral pleural effusions are present. **Right:** Following a bolus injection of contrast medium, intimal flaps (arrowheads) can be seen in both the ascending and descending aorta. Slightly greater enhancement of the true lumen is noted.

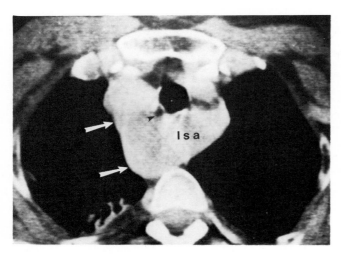

FIG. 44. Right aortic arch. A right aortic arch (arrows) accounted for mediastinal widening seen on a plain chest radiograph in a 53-year-old man. Dilatation of the origin of the aberrant left subclavian artery (lsa) displaces the trachea forward and the esophagus (arrowhead) forward and to the right.

Such mediastinal vascular anomalies may be mistaken for a mass lesion on plain chest radiographs and CT; alternatively an anomaly may be detected incidentally on scans performed for another reason. With a right aortic arch, the ascending and arch portions of the aorta lie in the right anterior mediastinum with the proximal descending aorta positioned to the right of the spine. Most frequently, an aberrant left subclavian artery with its dilated origin (diverticulum of Kommerell) is seen extending posterior to the esophagus (Fig. 44). Some vascular anomalies may be encountered while studying the mediastinum for other reasons, such as the staging of bronchogenic carcinoma or lymphoma. These include an aberrant right subclavian artery (Fig. 45), the most common anomalous arrangement of the aortic arch vessels, or a persistent left superior vena cava (20) (Fig. 22), the most common variant of systemic venous return to the heart. In selected clinical instances, CT may serve as an efficient screening ex-

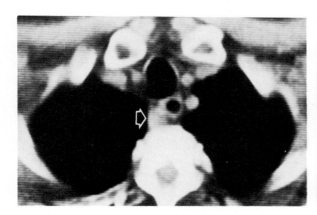 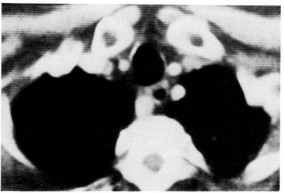

FIG. 45. Aberrant right subclavian artery. **Left:** A round prevertebral soft tissue structure (arrow) is seen adjacent to the esophagus at the level of the sternal notch. This "mass" could be traced caudally on sequential scans to merge with the top of the aortic arch posteriorly. **Right:** Following bolus administration of contrast medium, the "mass" enhances to the same degree as the other major superior mediastinal vessels.

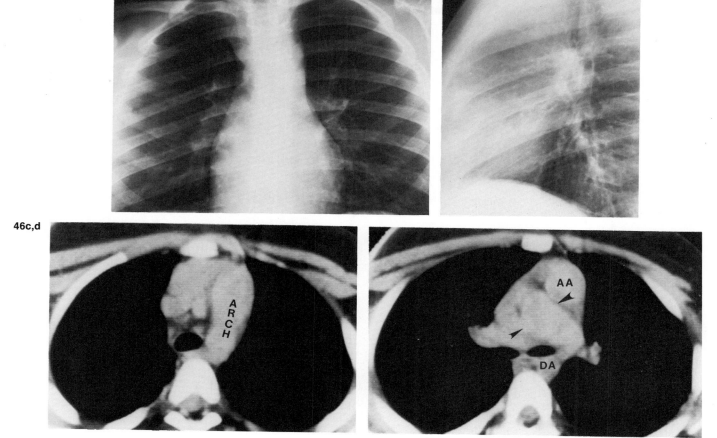

FIG. 46. Transposition of the great vessels. An 11-year-old boy with a systolic heart murmur. **a,b:** Posteroanterior and lateral chest radiographs demonstrate widening of the superior mediastinum and an increase in density in the retrosternal clear space. **c:** The arch of the aorta (ARCH) has an anteroposterior orientation rather than the usual curved right-to-left configura-tion. **d:** At the level of the carina, the ascending aorta (AA) is positioned in front of and to the left of the pulmonary artery trunk (arrowheads). Note that the main and left pulmonary arteries are larger in diameter than the ascending aorta; this is caused by poststenotic dilatation from associated pulmonic valvular stenosis. DA, descending aorta.

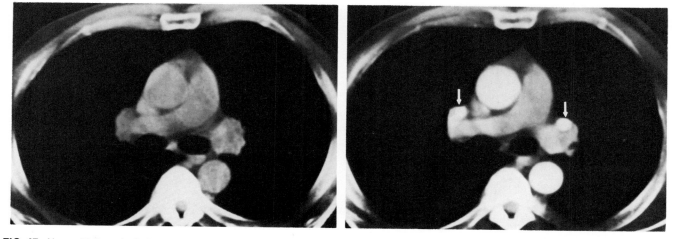

FIG. 47. Normal hilum. **Left:** In a 48-year-old man, both hilar regions appear prominent on conventional chest radiographs and on this noncontrast scan at the level of the right pulmonary artery. **Right:** Following bolus injection of contrast medium, the hilar structures completely opacify. Arrows indicate the superior pulmonary veins.

amination or as a complement to angiography, such as in transposition of the great vessels (Fig. 46) or co-arctation of the aorta (1,15). Computed tomography can be beneficial in the assessment of surgically treated patients with coarctation of the aorta to detect residual or recurrent narrowing, complicating dissection, or aneurysm formation. With a pseudocoarctation, which usually presents as a mediastinal mass on a plain chest radiograph in a hypertensive middle-aged man, CT shows that the mass is clearly part of the aorta. The aortic arch rises quite high in the mediastinum, and the proximal descending aorta is located ventral to the spine producing a kinked appearance (13).

Further assessment of an enlarged or questionably prominent hilum noted on a plain chest radiograph is a common radiologic problem. Usually, the major decision to be made is whether the prominence is due to a normal variation (Fig. 47), enlargement of the pulmonary artery (Fig. 48), enlarged lymph nodes, or to a tumor (Fig. 49). Although CT certainly is capable of resolving this dilemma, generally, we believe the more readily available and less expensive conventional tomography (often in the 55° posteror oblique projection) suffices for this differentiation. However, when such techniques fail, CT usually can determine the etiology of the hilar prominence (30,41). Evaluation of the

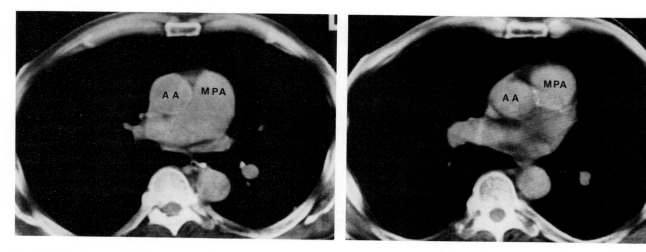

FIG. 48. Pulmonary arterial hypertension. **Left:** The main pulmonary artery (MPA) and the proximal horizontal, intrapericardial portion of the right pulmonary artery are markedly dilated in comparison to the ascending aorta (AA). **Right:** One centimeter inferiorly, the hilar portion of the right pulmonary artery is seen to be dilated. Note that the pulmonary artery (MPA) is equivalent in size to the ascending aorta (AA) and thus abnormally large.

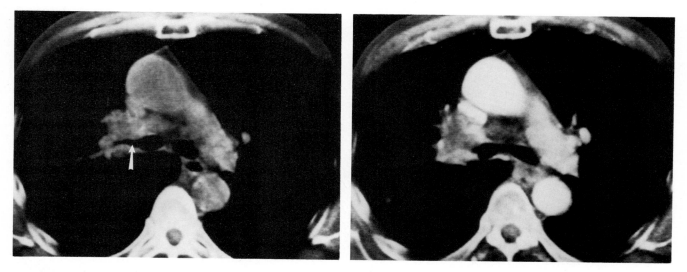

FIG. 49. Bronchogenic carcinoma of the right hilum. Plain chest radiographs in a 62-year-old man showed a prominent right hilum. **Left:** A soft tissue mass is present surrounding and narrowing the right upper lobe bronchus (arrows). **Right:** Following a bolus injection of intravenous contrast medium, the nonenhancing neoplasm is better defined. Posterior compression of the superior vena cava indicates extension of the neoplasm into the mediastinum.

50a,b

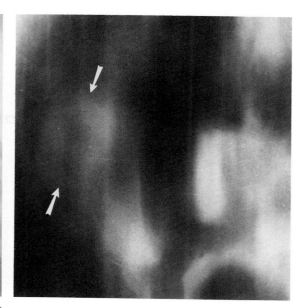

50c

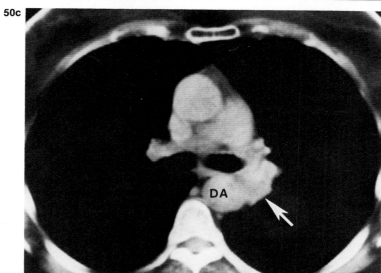

FIG. 50. Bronchogenic carcinoma of left hilum. **a:** A routine chest radiograph in a 52-year-old woman suggested an enlarged left hilum. **b:** Tomogram of the left hilum in the 55° posterior oblique projection demonstrates a mass (arrows) posterior to the trachea. **c:** CT scan shows a mass (arrow) in the superior segment of the left lower lobe infiltrating into the space between the descending aorta (DA) and the left pulmonary artery.

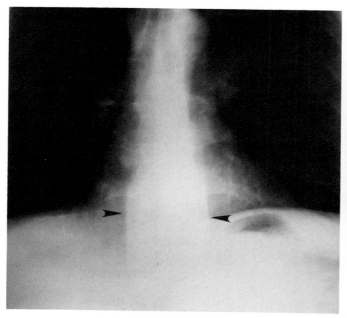

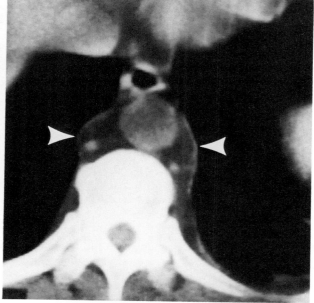

FIG. 51. Abundant retrocrural fat. **Left:** Chest radiograph shows widening of the paraspinal lines (arrowheads). **Right:** CT scan shows abundant fat in the paraspinal region laterally (arrowheads).

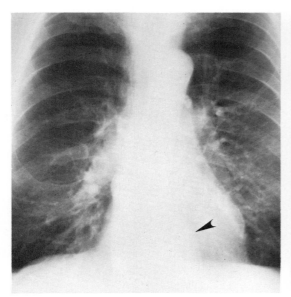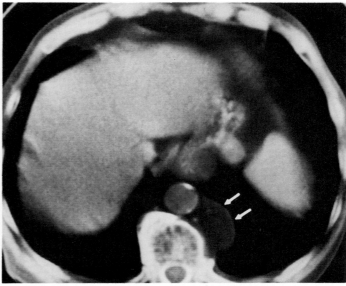

FIG. 52. Unilateral paraspinal fat. **Left:** A left paraspinal mass (arrowhead) is noted on a routine chest radiograph in a 79-year-old man. **Right:** CT demonstrates a localized benign fat collection (arrows), which may represent herniation of retroperitoneal fat or a lipoma.

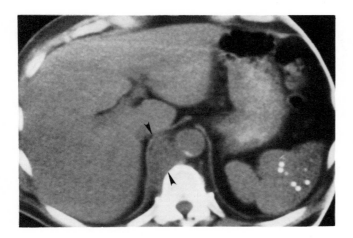

FIG. 53. Retrocrural lymphadenopathy. Enlarged lymph nodes (arrowheads) due to histiocytic lymphoma have replaced the fat in the right retrocrural space and have pushed the right diaphragmatic crus laterally, accounting for right paraspinal line widening noted on a plain chest radiograph.

hilum can be accomplished more quickly with CT than conventional tomography, and CT may provide additional valuable information about the lung and remaining mediastinum (Fig. 50). When the entire mediastinum needs to be assessed (e.g., staging of bronchogenic carcinoma), CT is the preferred initial technique. Even without contrast medium injection, if the intrapericardial portion of the main pulmonary artery or its two major branches are enlarged, it is reasonable

to assume that the extrapericardial portion of the vessel likewise is increased in size. The diameter of the intrapericardial segment of the right pulmonary artery can be easily measured on CT; values above 16 mm suggest the presence of pulmonary arterial hypertension (33). In problem cases marked increase in the attenuation value of the hilar mass density following intravenous contrast enhancement indicates that the mass is the pulmonary artery.

Paraspinal Line Widening

When the etiology of paraspinal line widening seen on a plain chest radiograph cannot be resolved by conventional radiologic techniques (e.g., barium esophagogram, detailed spine views), CT is an excellent tool to clarify the cause (8,11,18). It can readily distinguish enlarged lymph nodes from abnormal vessels as well as a wide range of anatomic variants that may simulate disease.

Normal processes of aging can result in displacement of the paraspinal lines, the most common being lateral osteophyte formation. Only slightly less frequent is a tortuous descending aorta. Extensive fat deposition, sometimes associated with obesity or glucocortocoid excess, in the retrocrural space can result in lateral displacement of the diaphragmatic crura and subsequent widening of the paraspinal lines (Figs. 51 and 52). Pathological processes that can cause displacement of these lines can originate in any of the

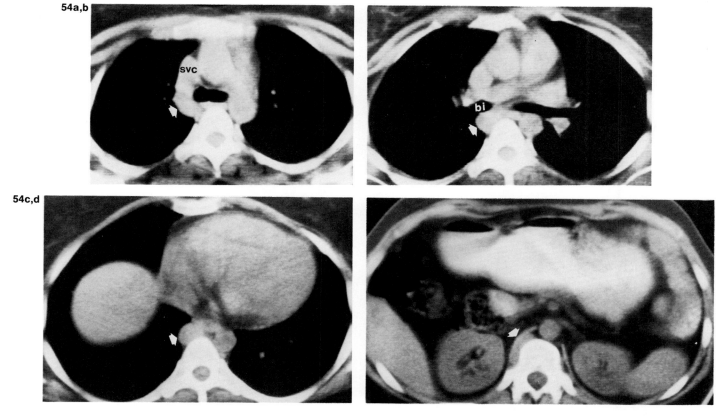

FIG. 54. Azygous continuation of the inferior vena cava. **a:** An enlarged azygous arch (arrow) is seen coursing lateral to the right main stem bronchus. svc, superior vena cava. **b:** At the level of the bronchus intermedius (bi), the dilated azygous vein (arrow) fills in the azygoesophageal recess. **c:** At the ventricular level, the enlarged azygous vein (arrow) is seen, accounting for bulging of the right paraspinal line noted on a chest radiograph. **d:** At the level of the L-2 vertebral body, an enlarged ascending lumbar vein (arrow) is seen in the right paravertebral space. No inferior vena cava is identified.

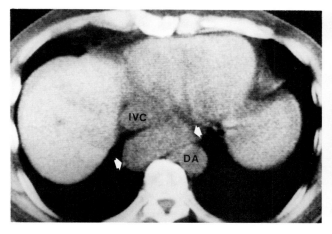

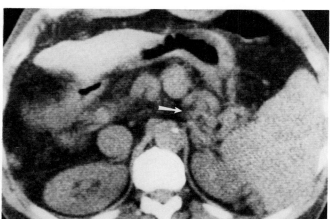

FIG. 55. Esophageal varices. A 57-year-old man with clinical findings attributed to hypersplenism. A chest radiograph demonstrated right paraspinal line widening. **Left:** A large paraesophageal mass (arrows) adjacent to the inferior vena cava (IVC) and the descending thoracic aorta (DA). **Right:** A scan through the abdomen demonstrates myriad enlarged vessels (arrow) medial to an enlarged spleen consistent with portal hypertension. A lobulated contour of the liver, consistent with cirrhosis, was seen on intermediate level scans. The paraesophageal mass showed enhancement on scans after the administration of intravenous contrast medium, and a barium swallow confirmed esophageal varices to be the cause of the paraspinal mass.

56a,b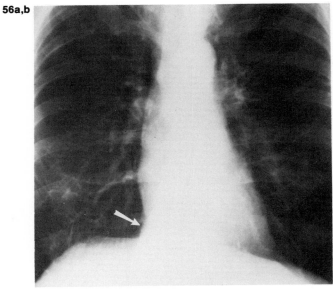

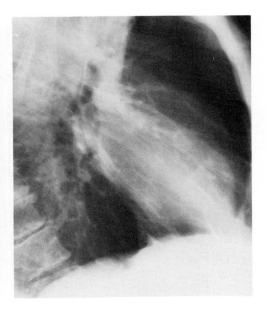

56c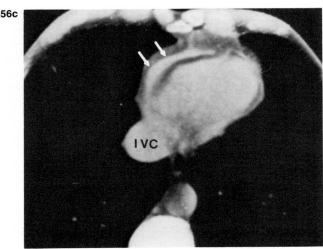

FIG. 56. Constrictive pericarditis. A 70-year-old man with dyspnea and fatigue. **a,b:** Posteroanterior and lateral chest radiograph were interpreted as showing changes consistent with chronic obstructive pulmonary disease. A paraspinal mass (arrow) was noted on the frontal projection. **c:** CT scan at the ventricular level shows a markedly enlarged inferior vena cava (IVC) accounting for the paraspinal mass, associated with substantial pericardial thickening (arrows).

retrocrural structures or extend from disease of the spine. Lymph node enlargement due to lymphoma (Fig. 53) or metastatic neoplasm, or rarely to inflammatory disease, is most frequent. Descending thoracic aortic aneurysms, dilatation of the azygous-hemiazygous venous system (Fig. 54), periesophageal varices (Fig. 55), or other venous abnormalities (Fig. 56) are less common. Diseases of the spine—such as a pyogenic or tuberculous abscess (Fig. 57), metastatic carcinoma, and compression fractures, with extension of the process or a concomitant hematoma into the paraspinal soft tissues—also may cause bulging of the paraspinal lines. These entities can be recognized by changes in the vertebral bodies themselves as well as the adjacent soft tissues. Certainly a simple esophageal hiatal hernia may frequently cause paraspinal line widening (Fig. 58), but CT should not be required for its diagnosis.

Detection of Occult Disease

Because of the remarkable ability of CT to display discrete structures within the mediastinum, on occasion CT may be useful in evaluating patients in whom this area appears normal on a plain chest radiograph when there is strong clinical suspicion of disease in this location (Fig. 59). Nodal enlargement, especially in pretracheal and innominate vein areas, may be detected before such nodes increase sufficiently in size to contact the lung and produce conventional radiographic abnormalities.

Thymus

Computed tomography of the mediastinum should be the imaging procedure of choice following standard

57a,b

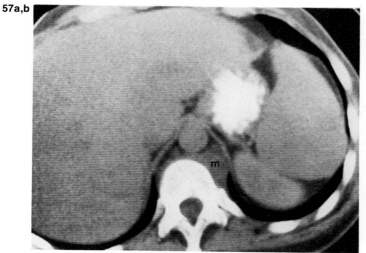

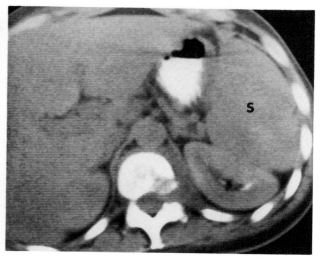

57c

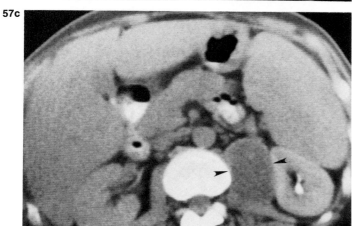

FIG. 57. Tuberculous paraspinal abscess. A 47-year-old man with lower thoracic back pain. Chest and thoracolumbar spine radiographs showed widening of the left paraspinal line without any osseous abnormality. **a:** A retrocrural soft tissue mass (m) is seen deviating the left diaphragmatic crus laterally. **b:** One centimeter inferiorly destruction of a portion of the L-1 vertebral body is noted in addition to the paravertebral soft tissue density. Splenomegaly (S) also is present. **c:** Two centimeters more inferiorly, the abscess extends into the psoas muscle (arrowheads) and deviates the left kidney laterally.

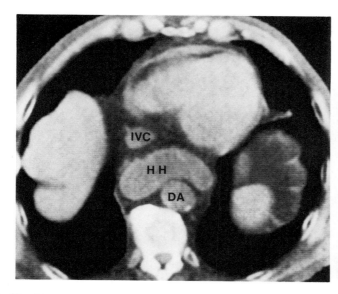

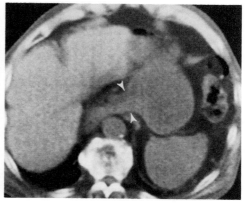

FIG. 58. Hiatal hernia. **Left:** Paraspinal widening caused by a hiatal hernia (HH) between the descending aorta (DA) and inferior vena cava (IVC). **Right:** Farther caudad, contiguity with the gastric fundus (arrowheads) confirms that the near-water density retrocrural mass represents a hiatal hernia.

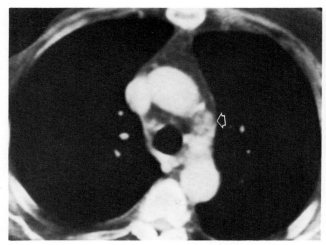

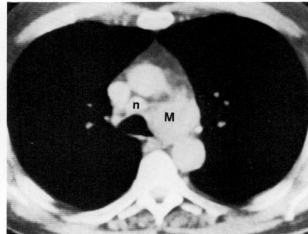

FIG. 59. Lymphadenopathy in the aortopulmonary window. **Left:** A 56-year-old woman presented with hoarseness 6 years following a right radical mastectomy. Laryngoscopy disclosed left vocal cord paralysis without an intrinsic laryngeal lesion. No mediastinal abnormality was detectable prospectively or retrospectively on the plain chest radiographs. CT defines lymph nodes (open arrow) in the aortopulmonary window. Biopsy at thoracotomy revealed metastatic breast carcinoma. **Right:** A 51-year-old man with a paralyzed left true vocal cord. A large lymph node mass (M) in the aortopulmonary window is seen, in addition to pretracheal adenopathy (n). Mediastinoscopy disclosed oat cell carcinoma.

60a,b

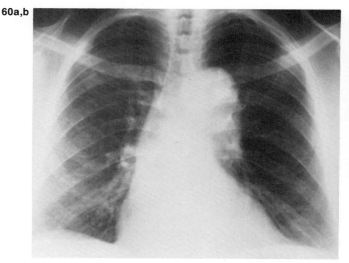

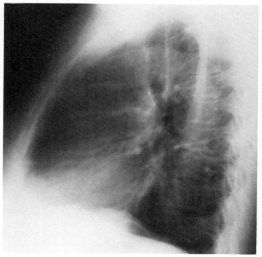

60c

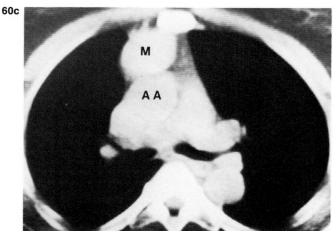

FIG. 60. Thymoma. A 75-year-old woman with recent onset of myasthenia gravis. **a,b:** Posterior and lateral chest radiographs are negative except for a tortuous aorta. No mediastinal mass is seen. **c:** CT demonstrates a 4-cm mass (M) in the vicinity of the inferior right lobe of the thymus, anterior to the ascending aorta (AA). Clinical symptoms abated after surgical removal of the thymoma.

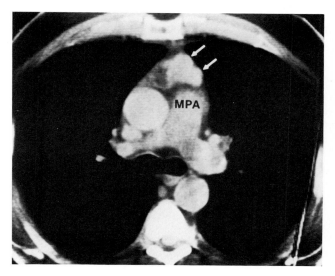

FIG. 61. Thymoma. A slightly lobulated mass (arrows) anterior to the main pulmonary artery (MPA) proved to be a thymoma in a 47-year-old man with myasthenia gravis and a questionable density in the anterior mediastinum on a lateral chest radiograph.

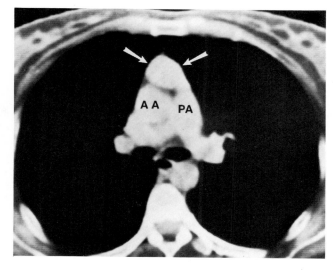

FIG. 63. Thymic hyperplasia, dominant nodule. A 2.5-cm mass (arrows) is seen in the inferior portion of the right lobe of the thymus in a 45-year-old woman with myasthenia gravis. AA, ascending aorta; PA, pulmonary artery. Histologically the mass was interpreted as thymic hyperplasia rather than a thymoma.

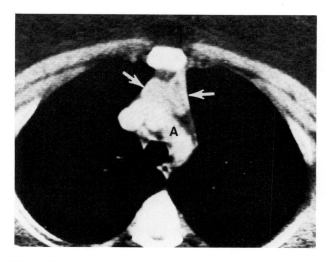

FIG. 62. Thymic hyperplasia. Anterior to the aortic arch (A) there is an increase in size of both lobes (arrows) of the thymus in a 40-year-old woman with myasthenia gravis.

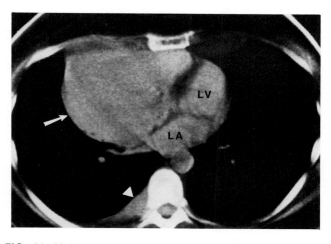

FIG. 64. Malignant ("invasive") thymoma. A large anterior mediastinal mass (arrow) merges with the right cardiac border. A metastatic deposit (arrowhead) is seen along the paraspinal pleura. LA, left atrium; LV, left ventricle.

chest radiography when thymic pathology is suspected (2).

Thymomas are solid neoplasms that occur in association with myasthenia gravis or other less common conditions (red cell aplasia, hypogammoglobulinemia), or sporadically. Because of the proximity of the thymus to the major mediastinal vascular structures, small thymic lesions often are not detectable on plain chest radiography or conventional tomography (Fig. 60). The 10 to 15% incidence of thymomas in patients with myasthenia gravis has led to routine CT screening of the anterosuperior mediastinum in many of these patients, especially if they are young or with recently

exacerbated symptoms. Computed tomography also is recommended to search for a thymic carcinoid whenever there is clinical suspicion of ectopic adrenocorticotropic hormone (ACTH) production causing Cushing's syndrome (7).

Computed tomography evaluation of the thymus is optimally performed using contiguous 10-mm thick sections from the level of the brachiocephalic veins inferiorly to the root of the ascending aorta. Scanning at 5-mm intervals using 5-mm collimation, sometimes after intravenous contrast medium administration, may be valuable in selected problem cases.

Computed tomography is a sensitive and specific

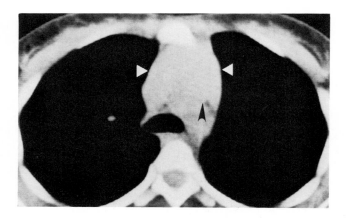

FIG. 65. Thymic hyperplasia associated with Graves' disease. Chest radiographs in a 23-year-old woman suggested a mass in the anterior mediastinum. Diffuse enlargement of the thymus (arrowheads) fills the anterior mediastinum. A follow-up chest radiograph 1 year later has shown no change in this anterior mediastinal mass attributable to thymic hyperplasia.

diagnostic procedure for the detection of thymoma in patients with myasthenia gravis; lesions as small as 1 cm in diameter can be depicted (2,28). Thymomas produce a distinct focal soft tissue density bulge along the normally smooth outer margin of the thymus, or, when large, totally replace the organ with a round or ovoid mass (Fig. 61). Thymic lymphoid hyperplasia may sometimes be recognizable on CT as diffuse enlargement, especially in thickness (Fig. 19), of the organ with maintenance of its normal shape (Fig. 62). This condition is present in many patients with myasthenia gravis. Whereas the histology is not distinctive, it is

characterized by numerous lymphoid follicles with active germinal centers in the medulla surrounded by a plasma cell and lymphocytic infiltration. The thymus may or may not be diffusely expanded. On rare occasion thymic lymphoid hyperplasia may present as a dominant nodule, simulating a thymoma (Fig. 63). Although CT generally can confidently diagnose or exclude a thymoma, it can only diagnose but never exclude lymphoid hyperplasia. A false negative diagnosis of thymic hyperplasia is of doubtful clinical significance since no convincing data exist that removing a hyperplastic thymus will improve the symptoms of myasthenia gravis. In the absence of a thymoma, surgery generally is reserved for medical treatment failures.

Approximately 15% of thymomas are classified as malignant. Since the histological appearance of a thymoma does not permit reliable differentiation between the benign and malignant forms, the term "invasive" thymoma generally is preferred to "malignant" thymoma. Such an invasive thymoma may extend locally into adjacent mediastinal structures or implant along the pleural or pericardial surfaces. Rarely this neoplasm may grow directly through the chest wall or the visceral pleura into the lung. These patterns of spread may be detected by CT (43). An invasive thymoma should be suspected when, in addition to an anterior mediastinal mass in the vicinity of the thymus, widespread infiltration into the surrounding mediastinal fat and fascia or soft tissue masses along the pleural or pericardial surface are seen (Fig 64). Computed tomography is far more valuable than conventional

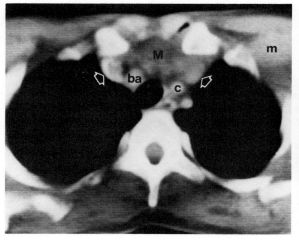

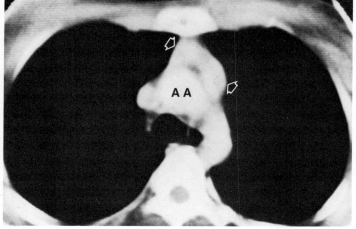

FIG. 66. Hodgkin's disease involving the thymus. A 30-year-old woman with malaise, low grade fever, and a left supraclavicular mass. Biopsy of the mass disclosed only a necrotic lymph node. Standard chest radiographs were normal. CT was obtained to determine if any occult enlarged mediastinal lymph node accessible to mediastinoscopy was present. **Left:** Postcontrast scan shows an anterior mediastinal mass (M) medial to the opacified brachiocephalic veins (open arrows) and in front of the brachiocephalic artery (ba) and the left carotid artery (c).

Incidental air in the left sternoclavicular joint is present. The supraclavicular mass (m) is seen laterally. **Right:** Caudally at the level of the distal trachea, there is a bilobed soft tissue mass (arrows) anterior to the ascending aorta (AA), compatible with an enlarged thymus (the thickness of the left lobe measures 1.8 cm). Histologic examination of specimens obtained at thoracotomy disclosed nodular sclerosing Hodgkin's disease infiltrating the thymus and some anterior mediastinal lymph nodes.

67a,b

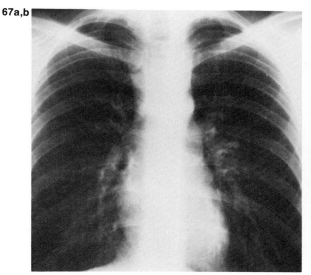
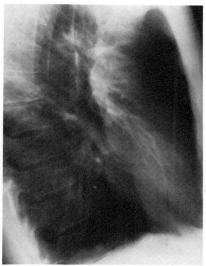

67c,d

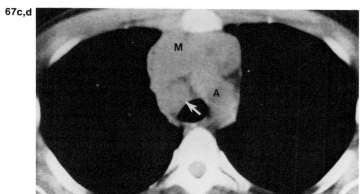
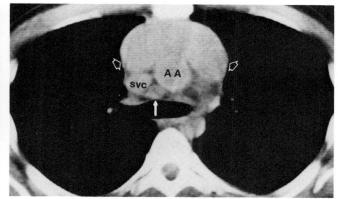

FIG. 67. Hodgkin's disease involving the thymus. **a.** Posteroanterior chest radiograph demonstrates superior mediastinal widening in a 47-year-old man with fever, weight loss, and pruritus. **b.** Lateral radiograph shows increased soft tissue density anterior to the trachea. **c.** CT shows a large soft tissue mass (M) filling the anterior mediastinum anterior to the aortic arch (A). Pretracheal adenopathy (arrow) is also present. **d.** Two centimeters inferiorly, the mass (open arrows) drapes around the ascending aorta (AA) and superior vena cava (svc). A precarinal lymph node (arrow) is also noted. Autopsy disclosed mixed cellularity Hodgkin's disease markedly enlarging the thymus, as well as involving pretracheal lymph nodes. Based on plain chest radiographic findings above, such involvement of the thymus has frequently been interpreted as anterior mediastinal lymphadenopathy.

radiography in defining the precise extent of disease, directing operative intervention or radiotherapy planning, evaluating treatment response, and monitoring for disease recurrence. Invasive thymomas are radiosensitive neoplasms with good prospects for long-term control.

In Graves' disease a true thymic hyperplasia involving the cortex and medulla may occur; the weight and size of the organ are increased and the changes are recognizable by CT (Fig. 65). Some lymphoreticular neoplams may infiltrate the thymus and produce relatively symmetric enlargement on CT (Fig. 66). Associated mediastinal lymph node enlargement is frequent (Fig. 67).

Thymic cysts, although not common, occasionally could simulate a lymphoma or thymoma on conventional radiographs. On CT, a conclusive diagnosis of benign thymic cyst should be possible based on finding a homogeneous near-water density mass with an imperceptible wall. Rarely, such cysts can result from prior radiation treatment for mediastinal Hodgkin's disease (2). Although some lymphomas or thymomas may be predominantly cystic, they always have a soft tissue component or a thick wall.

Parathyroid

An aberrantly located superior mediastinal parathyroid adenoma or hyperplastic gland may be the cause of hyperparathyroidism. The use of CT for such assessment is particularly valuable in patients in whom neck exploration failed to demonstrate an adenoma (22). The use of contiguous 5-mm collimated sections is often advantageous for demonstrating these generally small (6–15 mm) lesions. Concomitant infusion of urographic contrast medium also may be helpful to opacify the lower neck and mediastinal vessels and the thyroid gland and avoid confusing these structures with an adenoma.

CONCLUSION

When a further radiologic study is clinically indicated to evaluate a definite or suspected mediastinal abnormality discovered on a plain chest radiograph, CT generally is the preferred initial method. Mediastinal CT frequently provides diagnostic information unavailable from alternative noninvasive radiologic or clinical techniques. Computed tomography can determine whether the etiology is a benign anatomic variation or pathologic alteration of a mediastinal vascular structure, ascertain the attenuation value of a detected lesion, depict the presence and extent of a mass and its anatomic relationship to normal structures, and sometimes direct biopsy procedures. Not infrequently, further diagnostic evaluation—including such invasive procedures as angiography, mediastinoscopy, or thoractomy—may be averted. When CT indicates a benign process and the patient has no intrathoracic symptoms, the maximal requirement may be only follow-up chest roentgenograms.

REFERENCES

1. Baron RL, Gutierrez FR, Sagel SS, Levitt RG, McKnight RC: CT of anomalies of mediastinal vessels. AJR 137:571–576, 1981
2. Baron RL, Lee JKT, Sagel SS, Levitt RG: Computed tomography of the abnormal thymus. *Radiology* 142:127–134, 1982
3. Baron RL, Lee JKT, Sagel SS, Peterson RR: Computed tomography of the normal thymus. *Radiology* 142:121–125, 1982
4. Baron RL, Levitt RG, Sagel SS, Stanley RJ: Computed tomography in the evaluation of mediastinal widening. *Radiology* 138:107–113, 1981
5. Bein ME, Mancuso AA, Mink JR, Hansen GC: Computed tomography in the evaluation of mediastinal lipomatosis. *J Comput Asst Tomogr* 2:379–383, 1978
6. Binder RE, Pugatch RD, Faling LJ, Kanter RA, Sawin CT: Diagnosis of posterior mediastinal goiter by computed tomography. *J Comput Assist Tomogr* 4:550–552, 1980
7. Brown LR, Augenbaugh GL, Wick MR, Baker BA, Salassa RM: Roentgenologic diagnosis of primary corticotropin-producing carcinoid tumors of the mediastinum. *Radiology* 142:143–148, 1982
8. Callen PW, Filly RA, Korobkin M: Computed tomographic evaluation of the diaphragmatic crura. *Radiology* 126:413–416, 1978
9. Callen PW, Korobkin M, Isherwood I: Computed tomographic evaluation of the retrocrural prevertebral space. AJR 129:907–910, 1977
10. Cimmino CV: The esophageal-pleural stripe: An update. *Radiology* 140:607–613, 1981
11. Crowe JR, Brown LR, Muhm JR: Computed tomography of the mediastinum. *Radiology* 128:75–87, 1978
12. Dixon AK, Hilton CJ, Williams GT: Computed tomography and histological correlation of the thymic remnant. *Clin Radiol* 32:255–257, 1981
13. Gaupp RJ, Fagan CJ, Davis M, Epstein ME: Pseudocoarctation of the aorta. *J Comput Asst Tomogr* 5:571–573, 1981
14. Glazer GM, Axel L, Moss AA: CT diagnosis of mediastinal thyroid. AJR 138:495–498, 1982
15. Godwin JD, Herfkens RJ, Brundage BH, Lipton MJ: Evaluation of coarctation of the aorta by computed tomography. *J Comput Asst Tomogr* 5:153–156, 1981
16. Godwin JD, Herfkens RJ, Skiolderbrand CG, Federle MP, Lipton MJ: Evaluation of dissections and aneurysms of the thoracic aorta by conventional and dynamic CT scanning. *Radiology* 136:125–133, 1980
17. Godwin JD, Turley K, Herfkens RJ, Lipton MJ: Computed tomography for follow-up of chronic aortic dissections. *Radiology* 139:655–660, 1981
18. Heitzman ER: Computed tomography of the thorax: Current perspectives. AJR 136:2–12, 1981
19. Homer MJ, Wechsler RJ, Carter BL: Mediastinal lipomatosis: CT confirmation of a normal variant. *Radiology* 128:657–661, 1978
20. Huggins TJ, Lesar ML, Friedman AC, Pyatt RC, Thane TT: CT appearance of persistent left superior vena cava. *J Comput Asst Tomogr* 6:294–297, 1982
21. Jost RG, Sagel SS, Stanley RJ, Levitt RG: Computed tomography of the thorax. *Radiology* 126:125–136, 1978
22. Krudy AG, Doppman JL, Brennan MF, Marx SJ, Speigel AM, Stock JL, Aurbach GD: The detection of mediastinal parathyroid glands by computed tomography, selective arteriography, and venous sampling. *Radiology* 140:739–744, 1981
23. Larde D, Belloir C, Vasile N, Frija J, Ferrane J: Computed tomography of aortic dissection. *Radiology* 136:147–151, 1980
24. Marvasti MA, Mitchell GE, Burke WA, Meyer JA: Misleading density of mediastinal cysts on computerized tomography. *Ann Thorac Surg* 31:167–170, 1981
25. Maue-Dickinson M, Trefler M, Dickson DR: Comparison of dosimetry and image quality in computed and conventional tomography. *Radiology* 131:509–514, 1979
26. Mendez G, Isikoff MB, Isikoff SK, Sinner WN: Fatty tumors of the thorax demonstrated by CT. AJR 133:207–212, 1979
27. McCloud TC, Wittenberg J, Ferrucci JT, Jr: Computed tomography of the thorax and standard radiographic evaluation of the chest: A comparative study. *J Comput Asst Tomogr* 3:170–180, 1979
28. Moore AV, Korobkin M, Powers B, Olanow W, Ravin CE, Putman CE, Breiman RS, Ram PC: Thymoma detection by mediastinal CT: Patients with myasthenia gravis. AJR 138:217–222, 1982
29. Naidich DP, Khouri NF, Scott WW, Wang K, Siegelman SS: Computed tomography of the pulmonary hila: 1. Normal anatomy. *J Comput Assist Tomogr* 5:459–467, 1981
30. Naidich DP, Khouri NF, Stitik FP, McCauley DI, Siegelman SS: Computed tomography of the pulmonary hila: 2. Abnormal anatomy. *J Comput Assist Tomogr* 5:468–475, 1981
31. Naidich DP, Stitik FP, Khouri NF, Terry PB, Siegelman SS: Computed tomography of the bronchi: 2. Pathology. *J Comput Assist Tomogr* 4:754–762, 1980
32. Naidich DP, Terry PB, Stitik FP, Siegelman SS: Computed tomography of the bronchi: 1. Normal anatomy. *J Computed Assist Tomogr* 4:746–753, 1980
33. O'Callaghan JP, Heitzman ER, Somogyi JW, Spirt BA: CT evaluation of pulmonary artery size. *J Comput Asst Tomogr* 6:101–104, 1982
34. Pugatch RD, Braver JH, Robbins AH, Faling LJ: CT diagnosis of pericardial cysts. AJR 131:515–516, 1978

35. Pugatch RD, Faling LJ, Robbins AH, Spira R: CT diagnosis of benign mediastinal abnormalities. *AJR* 134:685–694, 1980
36. Robbins AH, Pugatch RD, Gerzof SG, Faling LJ, Johnson WC, Spira R, Gale WR: Further observations on the medical efficacy of computed tomography of the chest and abdomen. *Radiology* 137:719–725, 1980
37. Schnyder PA, Gamsu G: CT of the pretracheal retrocaval space. *AJR* 136:303–308, 1981
38. Siegel MJ, Sagel SS, Reed K: The value of computed tomography in the diagnosis and management of pediatric mediastinal abnormalities. *Radiology* 142:149–155, 1982
39. Silverman PM, Godwin JD, Korobkin M: Computed tomographic detection of retrocrural air. *AJR* 138:825–827, 1982
40. Speckman JM, Gamsu G, Webb WR: Alterations in CT mediastinal anatomy produced by an azygous lobe. *AJR* 137:47–50, 1981
41. Webb WR, Gamsu G, Glazer G: Computed tomography of the abnormal pulmonary hilum. *J Comput Assist Tomogr* 5:485–490, 1981
42. Webb WR, Glazer G, Gamsu G: Computed tomography of the normal pulmonary hilum. *J Comput Assist Tomogr* 5:476–484, 1981
43. Zerhouni EA, Scott WW, Baker RR, Wharam MD, Siegelman SS: Invasive thymomas: Diagnosis and evaluation by computed tomography. *J Comput Assist Tomogr* 6:92–100, 1982

Chapter 5

Lung, Pleura, Pericardium, and Chest Wall

Stuart S. Sagel

LUNG

Solitary Pulmonary Nodule

The definite evaluation of a solitary pulmonary nodule newly detected on a plain chest radiograph is a common clinical problem. The presence of calcification within such a pulmonary lesion generally is a reliable sign that the nodule is benign. Low kilovoltage spot roentgenograms and/or conventional tomograms should be employed first to discover any calcification and determine its pattern within the nodule. The detection of a significant calcium content by these standard radiologic techniques, however, is not always a simple matter. Calcium is easy to recognize when it is deposited in a distinctive pattern—such as a central nidus, in concentric rings, or in a popcorn-like configuration—because of the contrast difference with noncalcified areas of the nodule. But it is much more difficult to ascertain when the calcium is distributed diffusely throughout the lesion in a homogeneous fashion. Since density on a radiographic film is an imprecise parameter, the determination of the calcium content of a nodule that appears homogeneous on standard radiography is often quite subjective. In such cases in which the conventional studies are inconclusive—a well-circumscribed nodule with equivocal or no definite calcification—CT can serve as a more objective and sensitive ancillary method to assess its nature (16,35). Without CT, because sputum cytology usually is negative and bronchoscopy unrewarding with small pulmonary nodules, the only alternatives are thoracotomy, needle biopsy, or frequent serial radiographs to determine possible growth of the lesion. Computed tomography may provide conclusive evidence of diffuse calcification within the nodule and justify conservative clinical management. Calcium with its higher atomic number relative to other body tissues attenuates X-rays to a greater extent and produces a higher CT number within any tissue containing an appreciable amount.

The major technical problem inhibiting easy application of CT to measure the attenuation value of a solitary pulmonary nodule is the partial volume effect (Fig. 1). Although the pictorial representation of the CT scan slice is two dimensional, the data summarized in the image are derived from a three-dimensional slice of tissue. Thus, if a nodule 8 mm in diameter is imaged on a CT scan with a collimated thickness of 10 mm, the CT number readings from the area of interest will receive an important contribution from the air in the lung cephalad and caudad to the lesion. Consequently, a small amount of air-filled lung within the depicted volume will markedly lower the calculated attenuation value. With the newer scanners, this partial volume effect may be minimized or eliminated by obtaining thinly collimated (2–5 mm) slices to provide more precise data about smaller lesions (Fig. 2). However, such thin sections introduce another technical problem—that of registration. Because considerable variation in diaphragmatic position (sometimes greater than 1 cm) can occur during successive breath-holding in either inspiration or expiration even in very cooperative patients, it may be exceedingly difficult to suspend respiration at the exact same degree. Thus getting small pulmonary nodules, especially those near the diaphragm, to fall exactly within a thinly collimated slice without incorporating surrounding lung can be a very time consuming process requiring many repetitive scans.

The preferred technique in the CT evaluation of the "density" of a solitary pulmonary nodule is to first localize the lesion on a preliminary scannogram. Then 1-cm collimated scans in the appropriate location are obtained at resting lung (end tidal) volume (instructions to the patient are breathe in, breathe out, relax, and hold your breath) until the nodule is identified. After locating the nodule, additional more thinly collimated scans are obtained. The slice thickness of such scans should be less than one-half the diameter of the nodule under evaluation. For practical purposes,

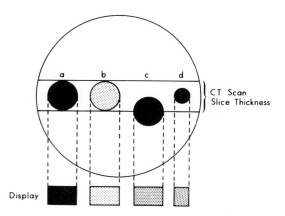

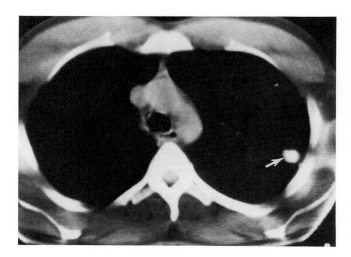

FIG. 1. Schematic representation of the partial volume effect. If a 1 cm in diameter calcified pulmonary nodule (a) entirely occupies a 1-cm collimated slice, its central displayed attenuation values will reflect its high calcium content. Likewise, if a 1-cm noncalcified nodule (b) is encompassed within the 1-cm slice thickness, its displayed value will be that of soft tissue. However, if a 1-cm calcified nodule (c) only partially occupies the collimated slice or if the nodule (d) is notably smaller than 1 cm, its displayed density will be substantially lowered because its contents will be calculated together (partially averaged) with the very low density surrounding lung tissue.

FIG. 3. Calcified pulmonary nodule. Calcification could not be confidently identified within this left lung nodule on low kilovoltage spot radiographs or conventional tomograms. Diffuse calcification throughout the 1.2-cm nodule (arrow) is clearly depicted on a 5-mm collimated scan.

5-mm collimation generally is used for nodules greater than 1 cm in diameter, and 2-mm collimation with nodules 1 cm or less in size. The patient is moved cephalad and caudad to obtain sequential sections through the lesion; in cooperative patients several scans are often performed during a single breath-holding maneuver. The section in which the nodule appears largest is chosen for analysis. If the nodule contains visible diffuse calcifications, no further evaluation is necessary (Fig. 3). Similarly, on occa-

sion, an apparent solitary pulmonary nodule on conventional radiography may be shown on CT to represent a linear scar or benign rib lesion on CT rather than a true lung nodule. Otherwise, the attenuation values within the nodule are determined (Fig. 4). All solid pulmonary nodules should show a mean attenuation value of at least 60 Hounsfield units (HU). If the number is less, then the slice thickness used was too large or the thin section analyzed was not taken sufficiently close to the center of the nodule.

Using our scanner at the 120 kVp setting, we have found that a mean CT number, or 5 central voxels,

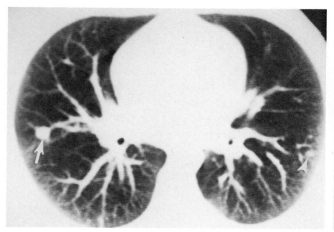

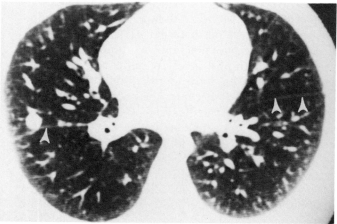

FIG. 2. Advantages and disadvantages of thin collimation. **Left:** A 1-cm collimated section demonstrates an 11 mm in diameter right lung nodule (arrow) and a 4 mm in diameter left lung nodule (arrowhead). **Right:** A 2-mm collimated scan at a similar level shows the right lung nodule; determined attenuation values were free of partial volume averaging with the surrounding lung. The left lung nodule, however, is not seen on this slice,

emphasizing the difficulty frequently encountered of trying to get small lung nodules to fall within a very narrow collimated scan. Note that on this thin slice the oblique interlobar fissures (arrowheads) are clearly depicted. However, it is much more difficult to trace the pulmonary vessels in their entirety and many resemble small nodules at the lung periphery.

4a,b

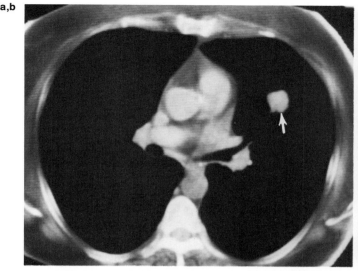

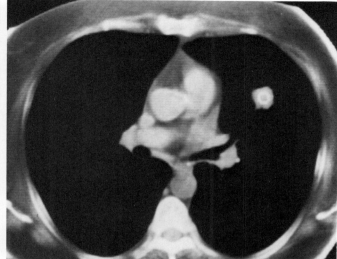

4c

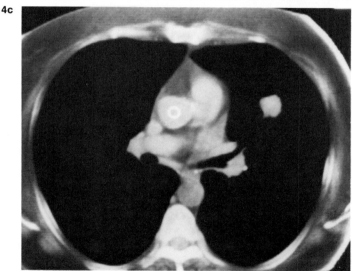

FIG. 4. Attenuation value measurements. **a:** A left lung nodule (arrow) 2.5 cm in diameter. **b:** Cursor circle placed within the nodule to determine the contained attenuation values. **c:** Same size cursor circle placed on the ascending aorta to determine a comparative reference standard for soft tissue density within the slice in a nonanemic patient.

greater than 140 HU, or double that expected from a solid noncalcified soft tissue lesion (60–80 HU), is a reliable predictor of the benignancy of a lesion. Since thinly collimated scans are noisier and subject to greater statistical variation, follow-up chest radiographs in 6 to 12 months are recommended to corroborate that the nodule is stable.

A point that cannot be overemphasized is that the attenuation values obtained from the same lesion may vary considerably when the images are generated by machines from different manufacturers with discordant software and hardware. Also, variations of as much as ±15 HU can occur on exactly the same scanner from day to day because of kilovoltage or detector drift. Because of these technological problems, in addition to inherent limitations in determining CT numbers (which quantiatively are relative and not absolute values largely related to artifacts created by beam hardening), it is difficult to establish universal values for

detection of calcification within a pulmonary nodule. It is advisable for each radiology department to determine its own values for confidently separating a benign from an indeterminate lesion. Using our technique and diagnostic criteria, approximately 15% of solitary pulmonary nodules not definitely calcified on conventional radiography have been diagnosed as benign. The remaining 85%, subsequently determined to be almost evenly divided between benign lesions and malignant neoplasms, fell into the indeterminate category; such indeterminate results are higher than previously reported (35). Perhaps the use of dual energy scanning, to more precisely determine the amount of a high atomic number material present in small quantities, will overcome the problems described in CT scanning at a single kilovoltage level.

Computed tomography following the bolus administration of iodinated intravenous contrast media may on rare occasion be helpful in differentiating a vascular

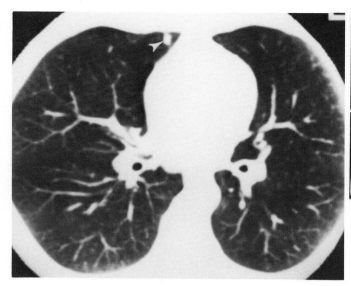

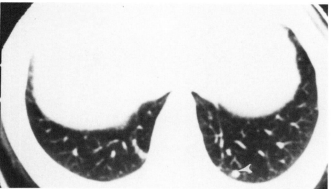

FIG. 5. Occult pulmonary metastasis. **Left:** A lung metastasis (arrowhead), 8 mm in diameter, is seen anterior to the right atrium in a 30-year-old man with melanoma and no pulmonary lesion recognizable on conventional tomography. **Right:** A solitary pulmonary metastasis (arrowhead) is demonstrated in a subpleural location caudad to the dome of the left hemidiaphragm in a 9-year-old boy with osteosarcoma.

(e.g., arteriovenous malformation or sequestration) from a nonvascular lung lesion (12).

Occult Pulmonary Metastases

In patients with primary extrapulmonary malignancy, CT provides a sensitive method for identifying small lung metastases, which are undetectable or poorly seen by standard chest radiography or tomography (20,23,25,33). Pulmonary parenchymal lesions smaller than 6 mm generally will not be seen with conventional radiologic techniques, and the visibility of nodules 6 to 15 mm in diameter is influenced by several factors. Not only are the size and density of the lesion important, but also the nature of surrounding structures greatly affects detection. When bones, blood vessels, or the heart is adjacent, it often obscures the details of the outline of a nodule. The vast majority of

pulmonary metastases occur in the outer one-third of the lung parenchyma, frequently in a subpleural location (34). These subpleural nodules often are difficult to detect on conventional tomography, as the blurring produced by this technique frequently is insufficient to erase the obscuring densities of the overlying chest wall. The transverse cross-sectional display of CT affords an ideal demonstration of these peripherally situated lung lesions unobscured by the overlying and confusing shadows of the chest wall (Fig. 5). In addition, CT improves visualization of lesions in the lung apex, in the retrocardiac and retrosternal regions, and in the posteroinferior lung recesses near the diaphragm (Fig. 6). The better photographic contrast of CT also decreases the observer error in which pulmonary nodules are frequently overlooked on conventional

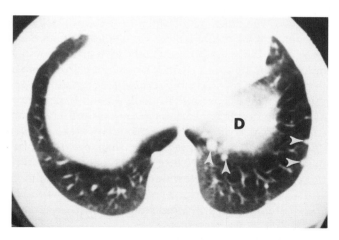

FIG. 6. Multiple small pulmonary metastases (arrowheads) are demonstrated in the lung periphery and adjacent to the left hemidiaphragm (D).

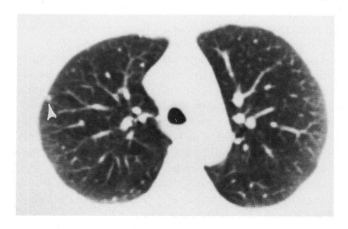

FIG. 7. A pulmonary nodule (arrowhead), 3 mm in diameter, identified on CT was the only manifestation suggestive of metastatic disease in this 53-year-old woman with a groin melanoma being considered for a radical retroperitoneal lymph node dissection. Intraabdominal surgery was deferred; a follow-up plain chest radiograph 6 weeks later demonstrated numerous new small lung nodules.

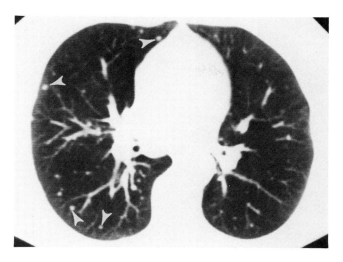

FIG. 8. Multiple peripheral lung metastases (arrowheads) can be confidently identified because they are larger than the corresponding pulmonary vessels in the same region.

tomography because they lack a marked contrast difference from the surrounding lung. The ability to display pulmonary nodules on the CT console as a white structure against the black background of the lung, rather than as a light gray nodule against a darker gray background of the pulmonary parenchyma on conventional tomography, enhances their density difference and consequently their detectability. Particularly with lesions 3 to 6 mm in size, CT frequently identifies one or more lung nodules when conventional tomography shows none (Fig. 7), two or more nodules when tomography reveals only one, or bilateral nodules when tomography shows only unilateral disease.

Identifying pulmonary nodules on CT generally is quite straightforward. If the nodular density is in the periphery of the lung and is separate from, and larger than, adjacent vascular structures located a similar distance from the chest wall, then the density represents a nodule (Fig. 8). When pulmonary nodules are similar in size or smaller than vessels in the same area, interpretation is more difficult. Viewing sequential scans is imperative; if the suspected lesion is continuous with a vascular structure on adjacent scans, the density is probably a vessel rather than a nodule. Repeating scans of the area with the patient in an alternative position (prone, decubitus) sometimes is valuable in clarifying a suspicious nodular density; a vessel often changes its size and shape whereas a true nodule is unaltered.

Occasionally, the CT examination will detect a small irregular linear density in the periphery of the lung. Such a shape is not characteristic of a metastasis, which is invariably round, but rather is more consistent with a scar or focal atelectasis. A repeat scan in approximately 2 months may be helpful if further clarification is required.

Although CT is more sensitive than conventional radiological studies in detecting small pulmonary nodules, a major limitation of CT is that it lacks specificity in distinguishing benign from malignant lesions, unless the nodule is diffusely calcified. Many of the nodules identified by CT prove to be benign granulomas or pleural-based lymph nodes; granulomas may constitute approximately 25% of the occult nodules in endemic areas. Thus, the demonstration of single or multiple nodules, even in the patient with a known primary malignancy, is by no means diagnostic of metastasis (33). Nevertheless, most pulmonary nodules detected on CT, particularly in the pediatric age group or the older patient with an entirely normal plain chest radiograph, do represent metastases. Short of performing a CT-guided limited thoracotomy for definitive histologic diagnosis, a repeat CT examination after waiting a period of approximately 6 weeks may be required before a definitive distinction between metastasis or granuloma is attempted. An increase in size or number of the nodule(s) on a follow-up CT study may be assumed to represent *de facto* evidence of metastatic disease.

Because of the problem with tissue specificity, plus additional constraints related to the availability and expense of CT machine time, if the overall incidence of lung metastases in the disease being evaluated is very low (e.g., stage 1 carcinoma of the cervix), then the extra effort and cost to detect occult metastases by CT are not justified. But there are patients with primary neoplasms that have a high propensity for lung metastases (osteosarcoma, malignant melanoma, testicular carcinoma) or in whom the likelihood of discerning additional lesions is great (presumed solitary or closely grouped pulmonary metastases). Whole lung CT can have a major clinical impact and is warranted in such patients when detection of an otherwise occult pulmonary nodule(s) would alter the course of treatment, particularly cancellation of planned extensive surgery (e.g., radical amputation, retroperitoneal lymph node dissection, or resection of lung metastases) or justify institution of chemotherapy. In addition, CT of the lung may be valuable in a patient with malignant cells detected on sputum cytology or with a paraneoplastic syndrome, and no lesion demonstrable on plain chest radiographs or fiberoptic bronchoscopy. In this small group of patients, CT can be useful in localizing a primary pulmonary neoplasm. These carcinomas are frequently situated in areas poorly visualized by standard techniques, such as the lung apices, the paramediastinal areas, or the juxtadiaphragmatic regions.

Other Occult Pulmonary Processes

Some lung lesions may be difficult to see or characterize on conventional radiographs because they are partially obscured or hidden by superimposed struc-

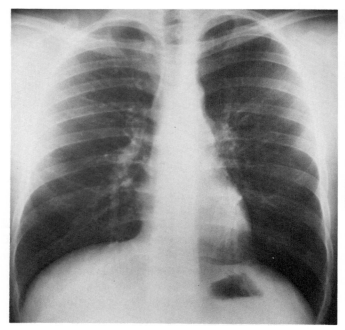

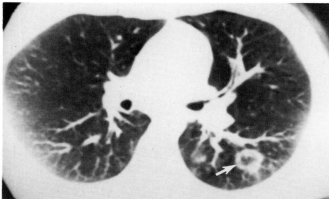

FIG. 9. Occult lung cavity. An 18-year-old man with several episodes of unexplained hemoptysis during a 1-week period. Fiberoptic bronchoscopy was normal. **Left:** Posteroanterior and lateral (not shown) chest radiographs disclosed no lung abnormality. **Right:** A small cavitary lesion (arrow) is demonstrated on CT in the superior segment of the left lower lobe. Subsequent serological tests revealed a rising histoplasmin titer; the patient made an uneventful recovery without therapy. A follow-up CT examination 4 weeks later was normal.

tures—such as tortuous mediastinal vessels, the heart, or the musculoskeletal chest wall. Sometimes technical factors, such as marked obesity or the inability of the patient to sit or stand, preclude optimal radiological evaluation of a pulmonary process.

Pathological processes involving the lung parenchyma may be detectable on CT despite a normal chest roentgenogram. These include small pulmonary cavities (18) (Fig. 9), subsegmental atelectasis (36), emphysematous changes, and interstitial lung disease due to a variety of causes.

Since the CT or Hounsfield number is linearly proportional to physical and electron density, it has been postulated that CT might have a potential role in the detection of diffuse pulmonary diseases that affect lung density (32,39). Theoretically, such pathological processes might be diagnosed before they produce changes that are visible on conventional chest radiographs and possibly before they are evident by sophisticated pulmonary function testing. The diffuse intersti-

tial lung diseases caused by inorganic dust, drugs, or opportunistic infection increase lung density whereas emphysema and possibly pulmonary thromboembolism, decrease it.

In normal adults, the attenuation value of the lung varies from approximately −700 to −860 HU; lung densities are somewhat higher in children below the age of 10. The attenuation values may be up to 200 HU higher in the posterior dependent portions of the lung because of the preferential blood flow received in the supine position. This gradient is reduced at full inspiration, which also causes all values to become more negative.

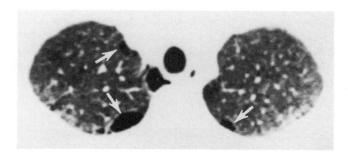

FIG. 10. Bullous areas (arrows) devoid of pulmonary vessels are seen in the lung apices of a 63-year-old man with a normal plain chest roentgenogram.

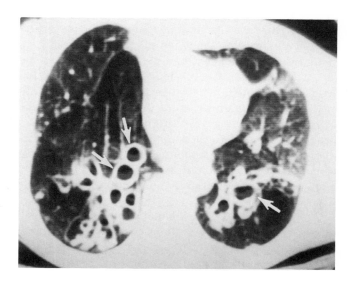

FIG. 11. Cystic bronchiectasis. Dilated thick-walled bronchi (arrows), many containing air-fluid levels, are clustered together in both lower lobes.

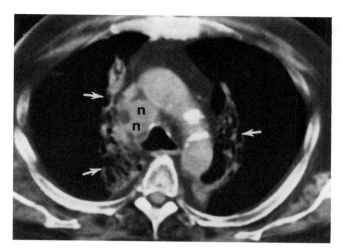

FIG. 12. A 63-year-old man, treated with irradiation 1 year previously for an oat cell carcinoma of the right upper lobe; returned with malaise and weight loss. Plain chest radiographs showed only changes due to radiation fibrosis. A CT scan demonstrates new enlarged lymph nodes (n) in the pretracheal area, in addition to the paramediastinal fibrosis (arrows) resulting from radiation therapy. Recurrent carcinoma was diagnosed from mediastinoscopic biopsy.

Currently, major limitations exist in determining lung density for comparison between patients. It is impossible to obtain absolute attenuation values for each individual. Determination of the CT numbers is affected by beam hardening artifacts caused by differences in patient size, habitus, shape, and position in the scan field. Additional problems in obtaining true densitometric values are created by the partial volume effect and technical machine variables such as kilo-

voltage drift and photomultiplier gain. Some useful information may be provided by assessing the patient's anteroposterior gradient or by comparing the two lungs or the values obtained with a previous study. Consequently, at present the use of CT to determine lung density is limited to physiological investigations of derangements involving pulmonary perfusion or ventilation; further studies are required to determine if CT will ever have an established clinical role.

Bullous areas in the lung are commonly detected on CT examinations in patients with or without known chronic obstructive pulmonary disease. Such lesions, especially when small, frequently cannot be recognized on the plain chest radiograph (Fig. 10). On rare occasion, CT can provide information about the extent of bullous disease that may be helpful if resection of apparently localized bullae is being contemplated in an attempt to improve pulmonary function (10). Also, CT may be useful in distinguishing large peripheral lung bullae from a loculated pneumothorax.

Computed tomography may be used to confirm a diagnosis of bronchiectasis suspected on the basis of plain radiographic or clinical findings (27). Dilated thick-walled bronchi extending toward the periphery of the lung, sometimes containing air-fluid levels, may be seen (Fig. 11). Such distended bronchi usually can be distinguished from emphysematous blebs because the latter typically have no definable wall thickness, are not dispersed linearly, and do not have recognizable accompanying vessels. By establishing the presence and anatomic extent of bronchiectasis, CT may eliminate the need for bronchography in selected cases.

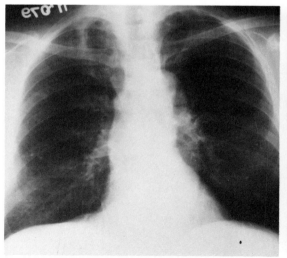

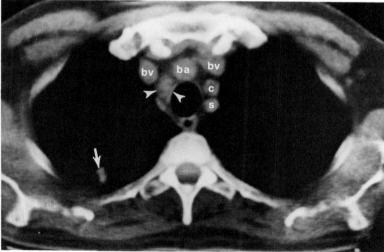

FIG. 13. Left: Routine chest radiograph in a 57-year-old man demonstrates a nodular infiltrate in the right lung apex. A prominent soft tissue density is also seen in the azygous vein area. Sputum analysis and fiberoptic bronchoscopy including washings were negative. A needle aspiration biopsy of the pulmonary lesion was requested for further evaluation. **Right:** A CT examination was performed to help decide the next appropriate tissue sampling technique. In addition to the apical nodular infiltrate (arrow), an enlarged lymph node (arrowheads) in the pretracheal plane is seen. Mediastinoscopy rather than needle biopsy was recommended; biopsy via the former technique disclosed metastatic poorly differentiated squamous cell carcinoma. bv, brachiocephalic veins; ba, brachiocephalic artery; c, carotid artery; s, subclavian artery.

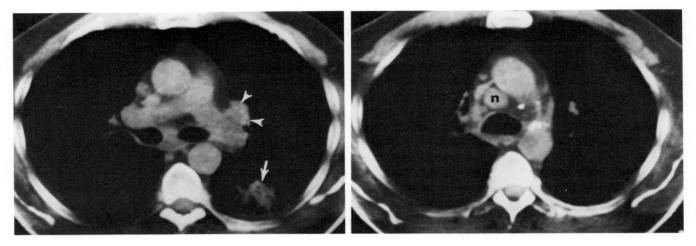

FIG. 14. Chest radiographs in a 58-year-old man showed a mass in the superior segment of the left lower lobe and an enlarged left hilum. Slight widening of the mediastinum was apparent. **Left:** Scan just below the carina demonstrates the primary bronchogenic carcinoma (arrow) in the left lower lobe and left hilar lymph node enlargement (arrowheads). **Right:** Scan 2 cm cephalad demonstrates an enlarged lymph node (n) in the pretracheal plane, consistent with unresectable mediastinal spread. Mediastinoscopy confirmed nodal metastasis.

Patchy, confluent areas of increased pulmonary attenuation due to acute radiation pneumonitis may be recognizable when conventional radiographs are normal (26,28). Chronic radiation changes may produce paramediastinal fibrosis, often resulting in a straight lateral margin with the adjacent aerated lung. Volume loss and distortion of the tracheobronchial tree, mediastinal vessels, and the esophagus may occur. Development of a discrete mass in the lung or mediastinum (Fig. 12) or focal pulmonary cavitation after stabilization of the radiation changes suggests recurrent neoplasm or infection.

Computed tomography on occasion may be valuable in diagnosing atelectasis of a lobe when the plain chest radiographic findings are not definitive. The cross-sectional CT images can demonstrate strikingly the volume loss within a hemithorax as well as the collapsed lobe.

Bronchogenic Carcinoma

Computed tomography can substantially influence the diagnostic evaluation and therapeutic plan in many patients with known or suspected bronchogenic carcinoma (4,20,21,31). Because CT provides a detailed view of the segmental and subsegmental bronchi in

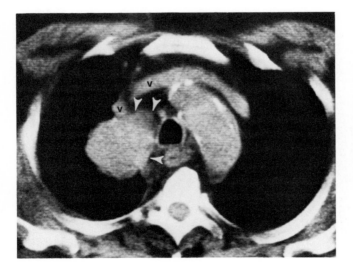

FIG. 15. A 63-year-old man with large cell undifferentiated carcinoma of the right upper lobe. The carcinoma extends into the mediastinal fat (arrowheads) posteromedial to the junction of the two brachiocephalic veins (v).

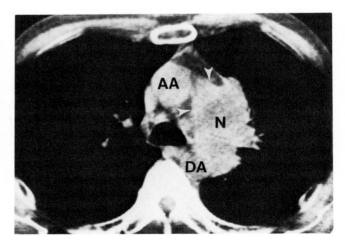

FIG. 16. A 71-year-old man with squamous cell carcinoma of the left upper lobe. Invasion of the mediastinal fat (arrowheads) in the area of the aortopulmonary window by the primary neoplasm (N) is demonstrated. AA, ascending aorta; DA, descending aorta.

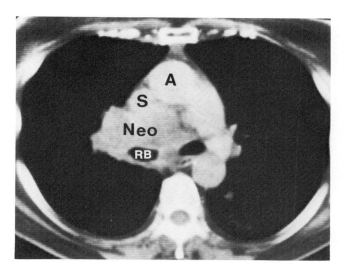

FIG. 17. A 54-year-old woman with squamous cell carcinoma of the right upper lobe. Neoplasm (Neo) extends deep into the mediastinum behind the superior vena cava (S) and the ascending aorta (A), and around the right main stem bronchus (RB).

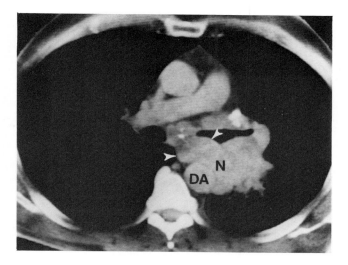

FIG. 18. A 67-year-old man with squamous cell carcinoma of the left lower lobe. Not only is the fat plane around the descending aorta (DA) obliterated by the adjacent neoplasm (N), but tumor is seen extending deep into the mediastinum (arrowheads) behind the left main stem bronchus and in front of the descending aorta.

cases where the suspected neoplasm is relatively small, precise depiction of the location of an endobronchial mass may be a helpful adjunct in directing the bronchoscopist to the appropriate biopsy site. When sputum analysis and fiberoptic bronchoscopy both yield negative results in a patient with a pulmonary mass, the findings on the CT examination can be valuable in directing further diagnostic evaluation. The next appro-

priate test may be suggested (Figs. 13 and 14), be it a transcervical mediastinoscopy, anterior parasternal mediastinotomy, percutaneous needle biopsy, or conventional thoracotomy.

Computed tomography has a very high accuracy in predicting the likelihood of curative surgical resection in the majority of patients with bronchogenic carcinoma (4,31). Staging by CT is clearly superior to conventional radiologic techniques for the demonstration of direct extension of the primary neoplasm into the mediastinum or chest wall and the detection of en-

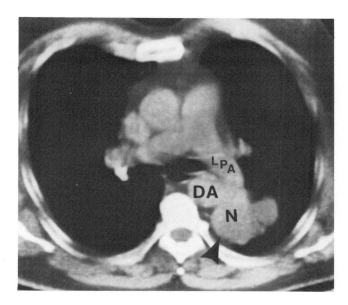

FIG. 19. A 67-year-old woman with squamous cell carcinoma of the superior segment of the left lower lobe. Neoplasm (N) is seen abutting the descending aorta (DA), the left pulmonary artery (LPA), and the pleura (arrowhead) but no definite invasion of the mediastinum (compare to Fig. 18) or chest wall is present. At surgery, the neoplasm was confined to the left lower lobe and easily resected.

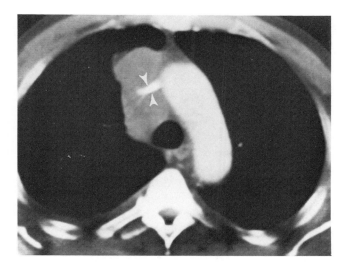

FIG. 20. Scan following a bolus injection of iodinated contrast material demonstrates a right upper lobe undifferentiated carcinoma invading the mediastinum and compressing the superior vena cava (arrowheads).

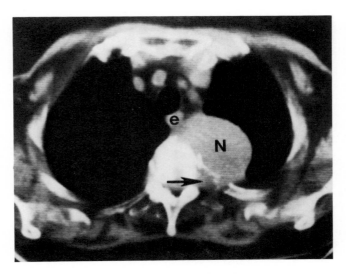

FIG. 21. A 57-year-old woman with squamous cell carcinoma of the left upper lobe diagnosed by needle aspiration biopsy. A CT scan demonstrates invasion of the chest wall with rib destruction (arrow) by the primary neoplasm (N), which also extends into the mediastinal fat adjacent to the esophagus (e). The patient was considered unresectable for cure and treated with radiation therapy.

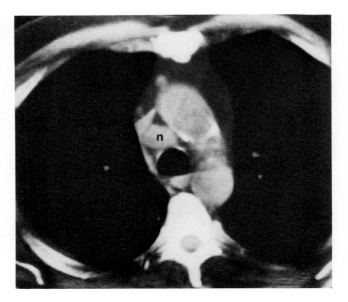

FIG. 22. Enlarged (2.8 cm in diameter) pretracheal lymph node (n) shown by mediastinoscopy to be involved with metastatic poorly differentiated squamous cell carcinoma.

larged mediastinal lymph nodes (20,23,38). However, a staging CT examination need not be performed in all patients with bronchogenic carcinoma. Those with clinically evident metastatic disease or such marked abnormalities on the plain chest radiograph precluding resection usually do not require a study. Also, the patient with a newly discovered small, irregular, peripheral pulmonary nodule and a normal appearing mediastinum on plain chest radiographs is unlikely to benefit from a CT examination. In this circumstance, mediastinal metastases are very uncommon, and proceeding directly to thoracotomy or needle biopsy generally is justified providing there are no clinical contraindications.

Contiguous extension of a primary bronchogenic carcinoma into the mediastinum, particularly when mediastinal vascular invasion has occurred, precludes successful surgical resection for cure. With conventional tomography, it is frequently difficult to determine whether a centrally situated pulmonary mass invades the mediastinum or merely lies in close proximity to it. Computed tomography can establish that the mediastinum is involved by direct extension when invasion of the mediastinal fat (Figs. 15 and 16) or around the mediastinal vessels (Figs. 17 and 18) is demonstrated. Computed tomographic demonstration of such involvement predicting incurable disease can influence the decision against thoracotomy. It should be emphasized that a neoplastic mass simply contacting the mediastinal pleura, with the lack of a well-defined fat plane between the lesion and the mediastinum, does not necessarily indicate mediastinal invasion (Fig. 19). The

tumor mass must infiltrate into (interdigitate with) the mediastinal fat or extend around the great vessels or major bronchi before extension can be confidently diagnosed. Scanning after a bolus injection of contrast media is often beneficial in confirming mediastinal vascular involvement (Fig. 20).

Similar to the mediastinum, care must be taken in not overdiagnosing invasion of the chest wall. When neoplasm simply abuts the pleura, even if associated with local pleural thickening or a pleural effusion, real

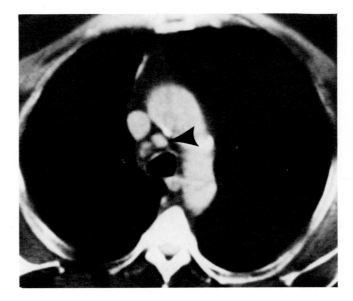

FIG. 23. A 57-year-old man with large cell carcinoma of the right upper lobe. An enlarged (1.7 cm in diameter) pretracheal lymph node (arrowhead) was shown to be due to reactive hyperplasia by mediastinoscopy.

24a,b

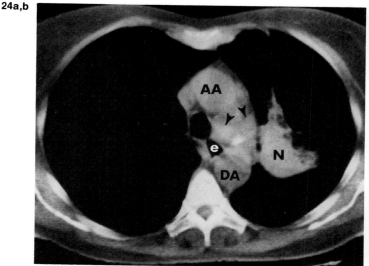
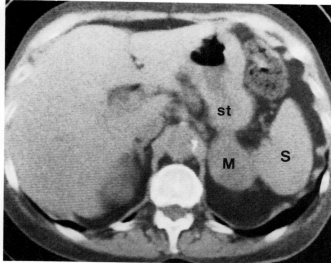

24c

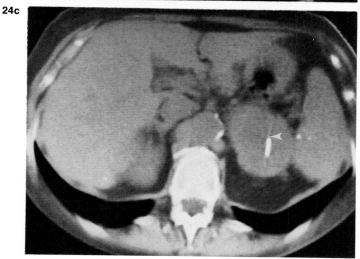

FIG. 24. A 56-year-old woman with bronchoscopically diagnosed squamous cell carcinoma of the left upper lobe. **a:** Scan through the primary neoplasm (N) strongly suggests lymph node metastases (arrowheads) in the aortopulmonary window. AA, ascending aorta; DA, descending aorta; e, esophagus. **b:** Scan through the upper abdomen demonstrates a mass (M) enlarging the left adrenal. S, spleen; st, stomach. **c:** Scan, performed in prone position at the time of percutaneous needle biopsy done to document disseminated disease, confirms that the tip of the biopsy needle (arrowhead) with its associated artifact is properly positioned within the mass. The aspirate yielded metastatic squamous cell carcinoma.

invasion may not be present. Associated inflammatory changes can result in these findings. A definite diagnosis of chest wall invasion requires the demonstration of bony (rib or vertebral body) destruction (Fig. 21) or a discrete extrapleural mass. Even direct invasion of the chest wall by a peripheral bronchogenic carcinoma, although a very poor prognostic sign, may not connote absolutely that the lesion is unresectable.

The presence of mediastinal lymph node metastases secondary to bronchogenic carcinoma presages a very poor prognosis and usually indicates incurable disease. Patients with low ipsilateral mediastinal lymph node metastases without capsular invasion from a well-differentiated squamous cell carcinoma have some chance of surgical salvage. Computed tomography can be very valuable in detecting mediastinal lymph node enlargement (Fig. 22) and can serve as a useful guide for selection of an invasive staging procedure before attempting curative resection of a bronchogenic carcinoma. Enlarged lymph nodes around the innominate

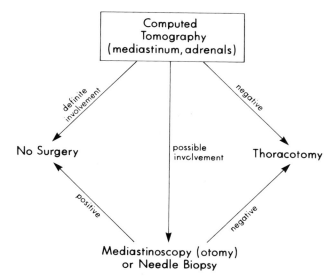

FIG. 25. Schematic diagram demonstrating the effect of the CT findings on the management of patients with bronchogenic carcinoma.

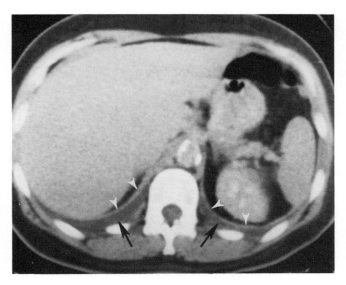

FIG. 26. Bilateral pleural effusions (arrows) are noted on a scan through the upper abdomen. Their intrathoracic location is certain because these near-water density collections are posterior to the diaphragmatic crura (arrowheads).

vessels, in the pretracheal and aortopulmonary region, in the internal mammary chain, and in the subcarinal area around the azygoesophageal recess can be more easily seen than with the standard roentgenographic techniques. But CT, like all radiologic methods, does not provide a histologic diagnosis. The demonstration of enlarged mediastinal lymph nodes in the patient with bronchogenic carcinoma does not automatically imply metastatic disease. Computed tomography cannot distinguish lymph node enlargement due to inflammatory disease from that due to neoplasm (Fig. 23). Also, CT will fail to detect microscopic metastatic disease in normal size lymph nodes. Recognizing these limitations, our diagnostic criteria on CT scans are that

mediastinal lymph nodes less than a centimeter in diameter are considered unlikely to harbor metastatic disease. Those nodes 1 to 2 cm in diameter are considered indeterminate; such mild enlargement can be caused by either neoplasm or granulomatous disease. Mediastinal lymph nodes more than 2 cm in diameter in a patient with a known primary bronchogenic carcinoma almost certainly are due to neoplastic involvement. In general, histologic confirmation of neoplasm within the mediastinal lymph nodes shown to be enlarged on CT is recommended in patients otherwise considered operative candidates. In many cases, this determination can be made by mediastinoscopy or anterior parasternal mediastinotomy. These staging techniques usually can be avoided prior to thoracotomy when the mediastinum appears normal on CT.

Although mediastinoscopy generally is regarded as the gold standard for preoperative mediastinal evaluation, and has greatly decreased the incidence of thoracotomies done for surgically noncurable neoplasms, definite limitations to the technique exist. The mediastinoscope does not evaluate all of the mediastinal compartments and a notable percentage of patients with bronchogenic carcinoma and a negative mediastinoscopy have mediastinal lymph node metastases at surgery. Only the middle mediastinum, anterior and lateral to the trachea and posterior to the major vessels (innominate artery and veins, superior vena cava, and ascending aorta), is accessible for biopsy. The pretracheal lymph nodes, nodes in the anterior subcarinal space, and nodes extending down the right main stem bronchus can be sampled with this technique. However, lymph nodes in the anterior mediastinum (prevascular space), aortopulmonary window, left tracheobronchial angle, and posterior portion of the mediastinum are inaccessible. Computed tomography allows

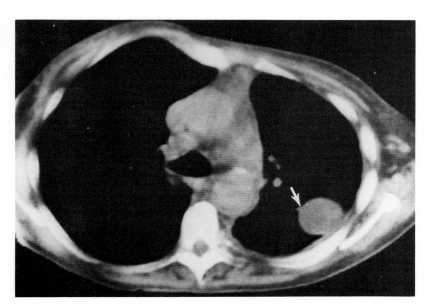

FIG. 27. Small left exudative pleural effusion due to metastatic breast carcinoma, partially accumulating in the oblique interlobar fissure (arrow) in the supine position assumed for the scan. Such a collection should not be confused with a solid lung or pleural mass. Note an enlarged pretracheal lymph node and the reduced volume of the left hemithorax resulting from prior radiation therapy.

28a,b

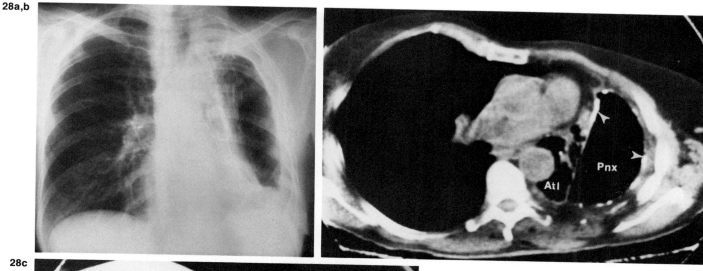

28c

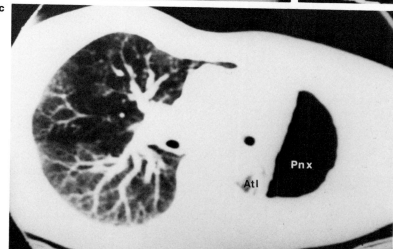

FIG. 28. A 66-year-old woman with fever who was treated many years previously with repetitive pneumothoraces for tuberculosis. **a:** Chest radiograph was interpreted as showing marked pleural thickening and calcification and volume loss in the left lung. **b,c:** CT scans, at soft tissue and lung window settings, respectively, demonstrate that there is atelectasis of the left lung (Atl) as well as pleural thickening and calcification (arrowheads). In addition, an unsuspected chronic pneumothorax space (Pnx) persists.

assessment of all of these areas and can serve as a guide as to whether parasternal mediastinotomy or needle aspiration biopsy would be useful to assess enlarged lymph nodes in the anterior mediastinum or the ipsilateral hilar area.

Controversy exists regarding the best radiologic technique for detecting hilar lymph node enlargement. Although some previous reports maintain that conventional tomography, especially in the 55° posterior oblique projection, is superior to CT (20,23), these studies all were conducted with older CT equipment, more limited knowledge of CT anatomy, and often less than optimal technique (intravenous contrast media were not used in problem cases). The argument is probably moot in patients with bronchogenic carcinoma at most medical centers. Ipsilateral hilar lymph node involvement alone does not mean that the patient is unresectable for cure; it merely indicates that a pneumonectomy will be required if surgical resection is attempted. It is the presence of mediastinal metastat-

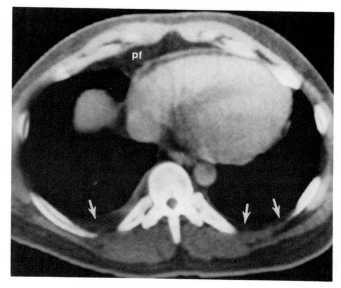

FIG. 29. Extrapleural fat (arrows). Note that the density of this collection is similar to that of the pericardial fat (pf).

30a,b

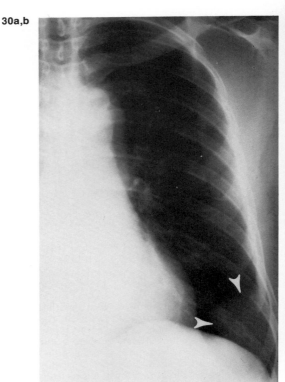

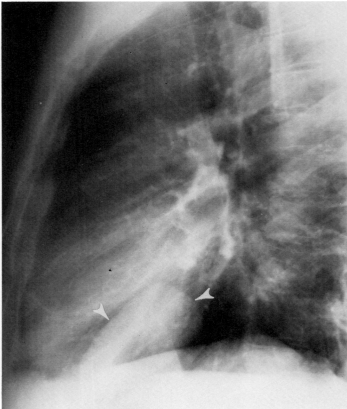

30c

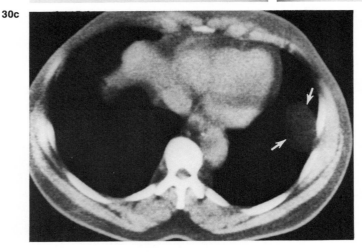

FIG. 30. Interfissural lipoma. **a,b:** Mass (arrowheads) in left lower hemithorax discovered on routine chest radiographs in a 71-year-old man. **c:** CT demonstrates a homogeneous, well-circumscribed, fat-density mass (arrows) in the location of the inferior portion of the left major fissure.

ic disease (in the form of direct extension of the primary neoplasm or lymph node metastases) that contraindicates surgery. The ability to more precisely evaluate the mediastinum and determine the relationship between tumor and various mediastinal structures makes CT far more valuable than conventional tomography in staging bronchogenic carcinoma.

The staging CT examination for bronchogenic carcinoma should be extended into the upper abdomen to include scans for assessment of the adrenals. Bronchogenic carcinoma has a propensity to metastasize to

these glands, and CT is quite sensitive in detecting small adrenal masses. The majority of patients with demonstrable adrenal metastases do not have clinical signs of adrenal insufficiency. Only rarely is the adrenal the only site of metastatic disease from bronchogenic carcinoma to contraindicate surgery. Even though almost all patients with metastatic enlargement of the adrenals have CT evidence of mediastinal involvement, in a few cases the depiction of an adrenal mass does increase the confidence of the interpreter in diagnosing widespread disease. A small adrenal mass in a patient with

31a,b

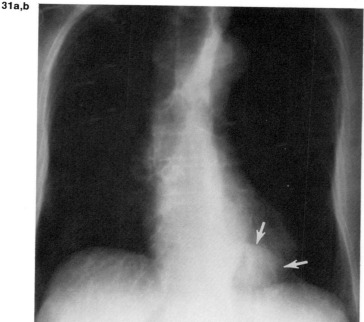

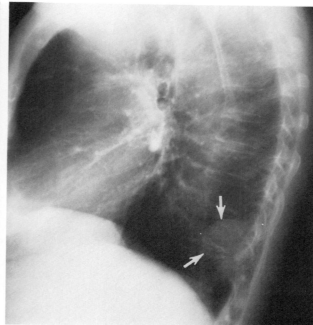

31c

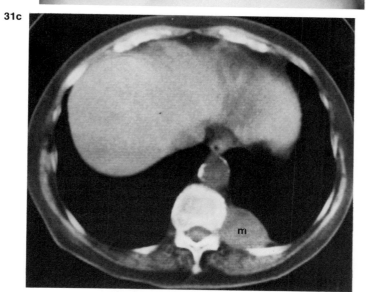

FIG. 31. a,b: Routine chest radiographs in a 67-year-old woman demonstrate a pleural based mass (arrows). **c:** CT shows that the mass (m) is of soft tissue density. Surgical resection disclosed a neurofibrosarcoma.

bronchogenic carcinoma and a normal mediastinum likely represents an incidental adenoma rather than metastasis. Percutaneous needle biopsy of an adrenal mass under CT-directed guidance may be useful in selected instances to confirm dissemination (Fig. 24).

The absence of lymph nodes in the mediastinum greater than 1 cm in diameter and clear separation of the primary neoplasm from the mediastinum have an exceedingly high predictive value that surgical resection for cure could be successfully attempted (Fig. 25). The presence of mediastinal lymph nodes greater than 2 cm in diameter or invasion of tumor into the mediastinal fat or encasing the mediastinal vessels is an al-

most absolute predictor of the nonresectability for cure of bronchogenic carcinoma (4). Since nonneoplastic enlargement of mediastinal lymph nodes greater than 2 cm in diameter certainly can occur, and might coexist incidently in a patient with bronchogenic carcinoma, the former criterion is not likely to prove infallible. The findings of a mediastinal lymph node(s) between 1 and 2 cm in diameter, neoplasm abutting but not definitely invading the mediastinum, pleural or pericardial thickening, or unsuspected noncalcified lung nodules place approximately one-third of patients with bronchogenic carcinoma into an indeterminate category regarding resectability for cure. But even

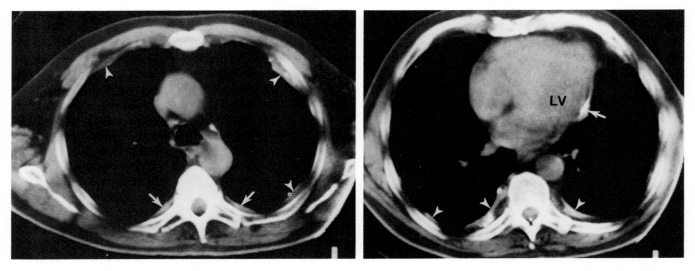

FIG. 32. A 42-year-old man with sustained exposure to asbestos. **Left:** Soft tissue density pleural plaques, some containing foci of calcification (arrowheads), are seen beneath the chest wall. Location of such plaques in the paravertebral area (arrows) is frequent. **Right:** Focally thickened and calcified pleura (arrow) is seen adjacent to the left ventricle (LV), in addition to the plaques posteriorly (arrowheads).

in this circumstance, the CT findings can alert the surgeon to the need for histologic assessment of the mediastinum prior to thoracotomy and often provide information as to whether this would be best accomplished by transcervical mediastinoscopy, anterior parasternal mediastinotomy, or guiding a percutaneous needle to sample suspected metastatic disease.

Computed tomography also has proven extremely useful in radiotherapy treatment planning for bronchogenic carcinoma (9,29). Computed tomography is often essential for clear delineation of the extent of the neoplastic disease and its relationship to surrounding structures. The information derived from the scans has often resulted in altering the design of the planned dose distribution, to either a greater or lesser volume, in order to improve tumor coverage and spare uninvolved areas. Care must be taken not to confuse consolidation or atelectasis distal to an endobronchial lesion with an extensive neoplastic mass.

PLEURA

Pleural abnormalities are frequently detected on CT examinations of the thorax and upper abdomen performed for other indications (Figs. 26–28). In the obese patient, abundant extrapleural fat (Fig. 29) should not be mistaken for pleural disease.

Conventional reoentgenographic techniques, in-

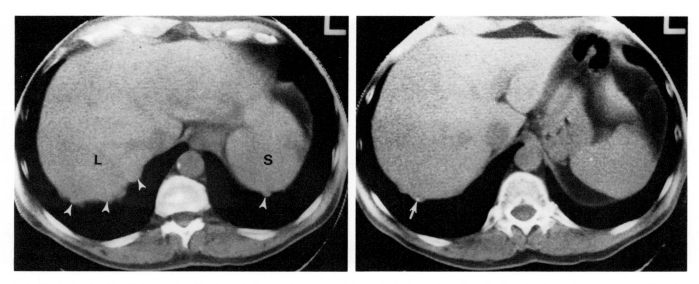

FIG. 33. Left: Small soft tissue density pleural plaques (arrowheads) create bulges along the diaphragmatic surface above the liver (L) and spleen (S) in a 54-year-old man exposed to asbestos many years before. **Right:** One pleural plaque (arrow) contains calcification.

34a,b

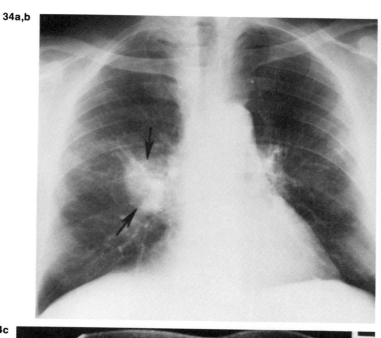

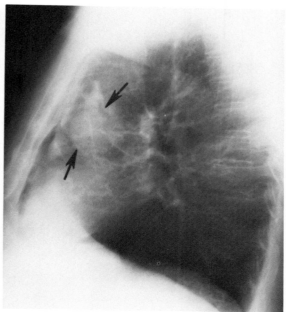

34c

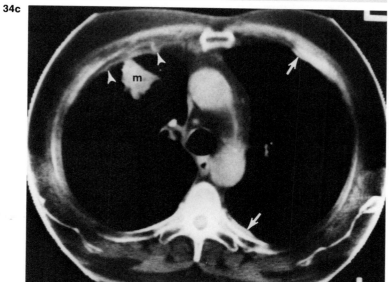

FIG. 34. "Round" atelectasis. **a,b:** Chest radiographs in a 57-year-old man with laryngeal carcinoma show an irregular mass (arrows) in the right lung anteriorly. **c:** CT shows that the lung mass (m) is adjacent to an area of focal pleural thickening (arrowheads). The volume of the right hemithorax is slightly smaller than the contralateral side. Pleural plaques (arrows) are seen in the left hemithorax. **d,e:** Scans at lung window settings demonstrate the surrounding pulmonary vessels (arrowheads) converging around the atelectatic lung. A history of exposure to asbestos was subsequently obtained.

34d,e

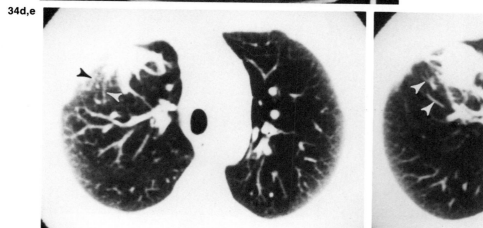
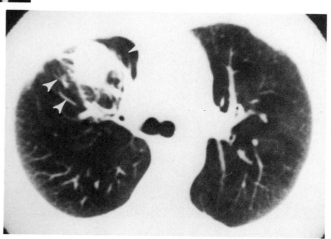

35a

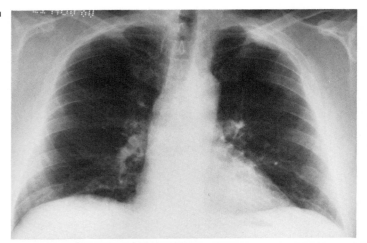

FIG. 35. Malignant mesothelioma. **a:** Chest radiograph in a 61-year-old man with weight loss demonstrates thickening along the left superolateral pleural surface. **b,c:** CT shows lobulated pleural thickening of soft tissue density (arrowheads) without any areas of calcification. Surgery disclosed a malignant mesothelioma and decortication was attempted.

35b,c

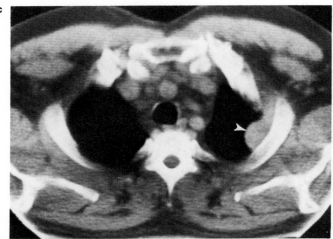

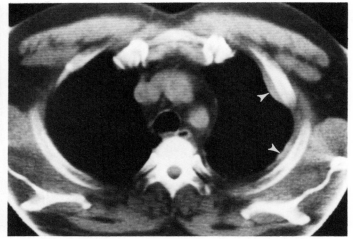

cluding lateral decubitus and oblique views, remain the primary procedures for detection of pleural effusion and pneumothorax. At times, pleural lesions can be difficult to evaluate on posteroanterior and lateral chest radiographs because they do not present in pro-file to the X-ray beam. When the standard techniques, including fluoroscopy with spot filming in oblique projections, fail to provide conclusive information, CT is an ideal method for the assessment of pleural lesions. On the transverse CT images, no overlying

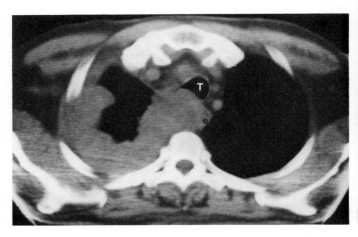

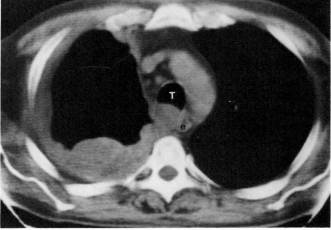

FIG. 36. Malignant mesothelioma. Extensive, lobulated neoplasm encompassing the right lung is seen extending into the mediastinum and compressing the trachea (T) and esophagus (e) in a 43-year-old man.

37a,b

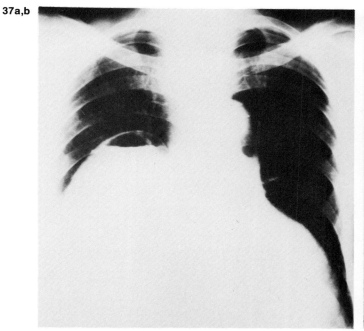

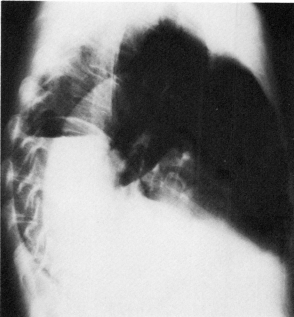

37c

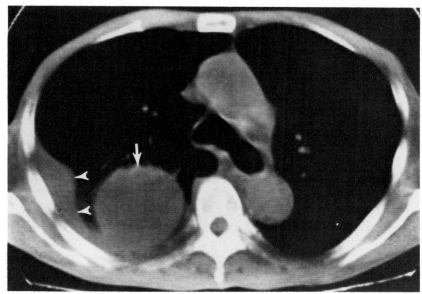

FIG. 37. Empyema with bronchopleural fistula. **a,b:** Chest radiographs in a febrile 79-year-old man obtained at the referring hospital demonstrate a large air-fluid collection posteriorly in the right hemithorax. **c:** CT shows a smooth mass (arrow) in the posterior portion of the major fissure, which is sharply demarcated from the adjacent lung. Additional contiguous pleural disease (arrowheads) of similar density is present.

structures obscure visualization of the pleural-parenchymal interface and there is inherent sharp contrast between the underlying low-density lung parenchyma and the adjacent much denser chest wall and mediastinum.

Computed tomography may show abnormalities of the pleura at an earlier stage than conventional radiological techniques. Small pleural effusions and pleural-based tumor nodules are readily seen. Based on differences in density, loculated pleural fluid usually can be distinguished from a neoplasm involving the pleura or chest wall (Figs. 30 and 31). Attenuation value determinations generally are not specific enough to distinguish the composition of the various pleural

fluid collections, and sometimes a homogeneous pleural mass cannot be distinguished from loculated pleural fluid. Ultrasonography may be valuable for this latter distinction.

Confirmation of Pleural Disease

Pleural plaques associated with asbestos exposure must attain a diameter close to 5 mm before they are visible on conventional roentgenograms. Computed tomography is more sensitive than plain chest radiography in the detection of both calcified and noncalcified pleural plaques, and can be helpful in distinguishing plaques from confusing normal soft tissue

38a,b

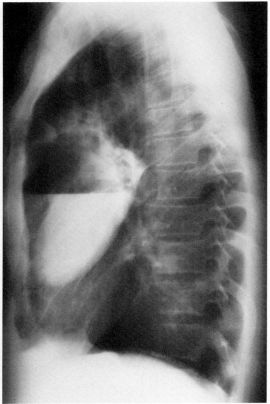

38c

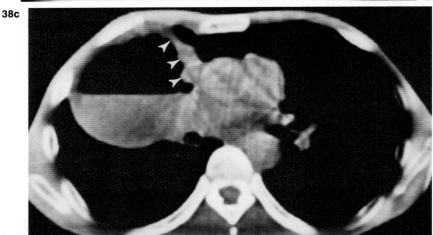

FIG. 38. Lung abscess. **a,b:** Chest radiographs in a febrile 64-year-old man demonstrate a large air-fluid collection anteriorly in the right hemithorax. **c:** CT shows an irregular, thick-walled (arrowheads) cavity in the right middle lobe.

companion shadows (17). Plaques appear on CT as areas of soft tissue thickenings, sometimes with linear or focal internal or peripheral calcification, immediately beneath the ribs and chest wall (Figs. 32 and 33).

In addition, CT can be valuable in confirming a diagnosis of ''round atelectasis'' when conventional roentgenographic studies are equivocal (22,37). The third dimension provided by CT makes it excellent for evaluating simultaneously the pleural and parenchymal components of this intrathoracic mass, and can help in more confidently excluding a malignant neo-

plasm. The lesion consists of condensed atelectatic lung parenchyma with marked thickening of the adjacent pleura (Fig. 34). Pulmonary vessels converge around the mass, and the surrounding lung parenchyma usually is hyperinflated. The excellent evaluation of the entire thorax provided by CT can be important because this condition, which is commonly associated with asbestos exposure, frequently is but one manifestation of extensive intrathoracic disease with pleural plaques and pulmonary fibrosis. On occasion, these lesions can grow very slowly, probably second-

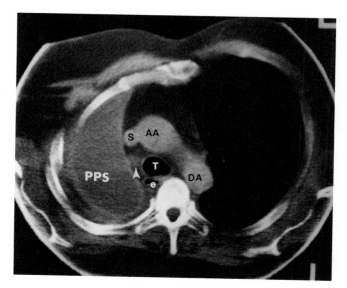

FIG. 39. Normal postpneumonectomy space. In a 58-year-old woman 18 months after a right pneumonectomy, the moderate size residual postpneumonectomy space (PPS) is substantially lower in density than the blood in the superior vena cava (S) and in the ascending (AA) and descending (DA) aorta. The right hemithorax is reduced in size, and the mediastinum is shifted toward that side. A normal size pretracheal lymph node (arrowhead) is noted. T, trachea; e, esophagus.

ary to increasing fibrosis in the surrounding pleura and parenchyma.

Computed tomography also can provide useful information about the extent of a malignant mesothelioma, which is frequently underestimated based

on plain chest radiographs alone (1). This neoplasm can appear on CT as an irregular, pleural-based mass(es) or soft tissue thickening surrounding the lung (Fig. 35); spread into the fissures and mediastinum (Fig. 36) is common. Extension into the chest wall, the contralateral hemithorax, or the upper abdomen may be present.

Pleural Versus Parenchymal Disease

Generally, fluoroscopy, in conjunction with decubitus and oblique radiographs, suffices to distinguish a parenchymal process from a pleural or extrapleural lesion. Ultrasound, although helpful in assessing pleural collections, is of little value in diagnosing parenchymal lung disease. Conventional tomography only rarely provides useful information to distinguish a peripheral parenchymal lesion from a pleural process or to determine if a peripheral lung lesion has involved the pleura or chest wall. On occasion, CT may be valuable in the distinction of a peripheral pulmonary nodule from localized pleural thickening, or a pleural process (empyema or hydropneumothorax) from a parenchymal lesion (lung abscess or cavitating carcinoma).

Differentiation of a pyopneumothorax from a lung abscess, both of which may appear on roentgenograms as a "cavitary" lesion with an air-fluid lesion adjacent to the chest wall, may be a difficult diagnostic problem. An accurate diagnosis is critical because of the seriousness of the lesions and their disparate treatments. Em-

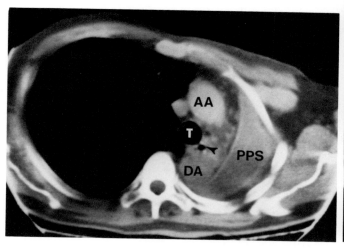

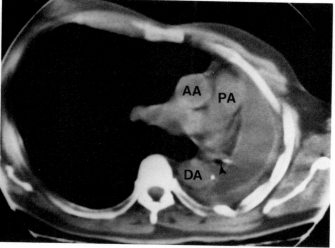

FIG. 40. Normal postpneumonectomy changes. **Left:** In a 53-year-old man 1 year after a left pneumonectomy, the mediastinum has shifted toward the contracted left hemithorax. The postpneumonectomy space (PPS) is lower in density at comparable anteroposterior levels than the blood in the ascending (AA) and descending (DA) aorta. The lower density apparent in the posterior half of this space is artifactually related to beam hard-

ening caused by greater attenuation of the X-rays as they pass through the shoulder girdle and scapula. Normal size lymph nodes are probably present in the mediastinal fat lateral to the aorta. T, trachea; arrowhead, esophagus. **Right:** Lung from the contralateral side has herniated anteriorly in front of the ascending aorta (AA) and posteriorly in front of the descending aorta (DA). PA, pulmonary artery; arrowhead, esophagus.

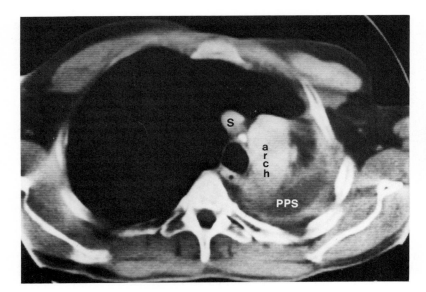

FIG. 41. Very small residual left postpneumonectomy space (PPS). Lung from the contralateral side has herniated only anteriorly in front of the superior vena cava (S) and aortic arch (arch).

pyemas are managed by drainage through a thoracostomy tube; lung abscesses are appropriately treated with antibiotic therapy and postural drainage. When conventional radiographic methods fail to differentiate a loculated pyopneumothorax with a bronchopleural fistula from a peripheral lung abscess, CT can be effective in distinguishing between them (2,30). The cross-sectional CT image demonstrates the three-dimensional shape of the lesion as well as the pleural-parenchymal interface, permitting more accurate localization. A pyopneumothorax characteristically has a regular smooth shape with a sharply defined border between the lesion and the lung (Fig. 37). Scanning the patient in different positions (prone, decubitus) usually demonstrates a change in the configuration of the cav-

ity and unequal fluid levels which closely approximate the chest wall. In contradistinction, a lung abscess typically is round with an irregular thick wall, and lacks a discrete boundary between the lesion and the lung parenchyma (Fig. 38). It may be separated from the pleura by a thin rim of diminished attenuation. When the patient is scanned in different positions, the air-fluid level remains of equal length in all dimensions.

It is often difficult to evaluate parenchymal lung disease with plain radiographs when there is extensive pleural disease. The pleural, chest wall, or parenchymal contributions to a plain chest radiographic abnormality can be assessed with CT (30). Important information can be provided regarding the presence, lo-

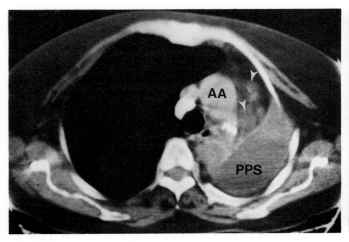
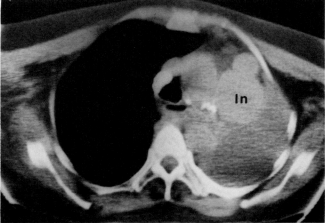

FIG. 42. A 56-year-old woman with weight loss and malaise 9 months following a left pneumonectomy for bronchogenic carcinoma. Chest radiographs showed only an opaque left hemithorax. **Left:** This scan was initially interpreted as unremarkable. In retrospect, enlarged lymph nodes (arrowheads) are identifiable in the mediastinal fat lateral to the ascending aorta (AA) and anteromedial to the postpneumonectomy space (PPS). **Right:** Follow-up scan 3 months later when symptoms persisted shows marked interval enlargement of the paraaortic lymph nodes (In). Metastatic recurrence was confirmed by percutaneous needle biopsy.

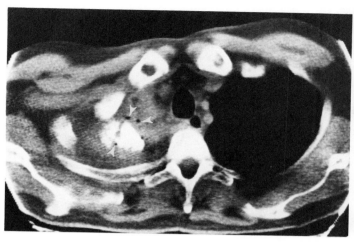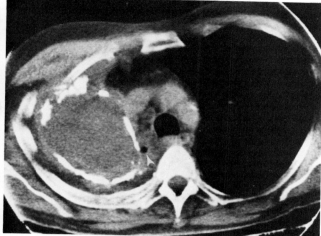

FIG. 43. A 67-year-old man with an unexplained fever 18 years after a previous right pneumonectomy. Chest radiographs were unchanged and noncontributory. CT scans show several small air bubbles (arrowheads) clustered about the peripherally calcified postpneumonectomy space. Subsequently 500 cc of purulent material were drained from the right hemithorax.

calization, and extent of any concomitant lung or mediastinal abnormality obscured by substantial pleural disease, be it thickening or a free or loculated pleural effusion, especially when the fluid cannot be removed by thoracentesis. With free pleural fluid, scans taken in the decubitus or prone position may facilitate evaluation of the parenchymal disease component.

Postpneumonectomy Space

When a hemithorax is opaque on conventional radiography as a result of a previous pneumonectomy,

ipsilateral recurrence of disease cannot be detected by chest roentgenograms unless it is so gross that mediastinal shift occurs. Computed tomography can be helpful in detecting recurrent neoplasm in the postpneumonectomy space at an earlier stage. Knowledge of the alterations in normal anatomy following a pneumonectomy is essential so as to not confuse the distorted and displaced great vessels or heart for an abnormal soft tissue mass. In only approximately 40% of patients does the postpneumonectomy space become completely obliterated and occupied by the relocated mediastinal structures. In the remainder, a postpneumonectomy space persists that is relatively ho-

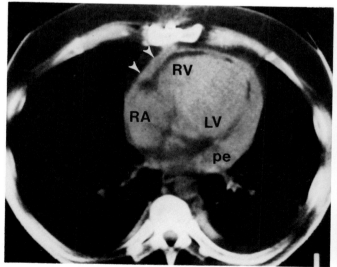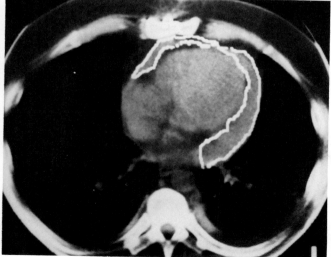

FIG. 44. Pericardial effusion in a 42-year-old woman 2 weeks following a sternotomy. **Left:** In the supine position, a moderate size serosanguinous pericardial effusion (pe) collects predominantly dorsolateral to the left ventricle (LV), while a smaller amount (arrowheads) extends anterior to the right atrium (RA) and right ventricle (RV). **Right:** Quantitative approximation of the amount of pericardial fluid can be accomplished by summing the volumes of fluid traced out (white highlights) on the serial scans.

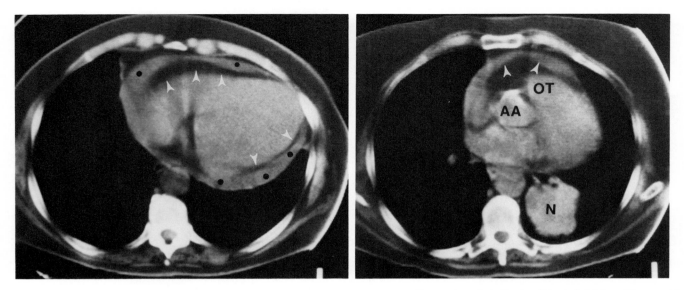

FIG. 45. Left: The epicardial fat (arrowheads) separates the heart from a surrounding pericardial effusion (black dots) in a 47-year-old woman with a bronchogenic carcinoma. **Right:** Fluid in the pericardial sac (arrowheads) extends cephalad in front of the ascending aorta (AA) and the outflow tract of the right ventricle (OT). The primary neoplasm (N) is seen in the left lower lobe.

mogeneous and of lower density than soft tissue (Fig. 39), presumably because it contains residual fluid, even many years following surgery (5). The space can vary from 1 to 5 cm in transverse diameter. The mediastinum tends to rotate following a right pneumonectomy, with a resultant transverse orientation of the aortic arch, and usually shifts following a left pneumonectomy with an anteroposterior orientation of the aortic arch. The contralateral lung herniates anteriorly following a right pneumonectomy; after a left pneumonectomy it may herniate posteriorly as well as anteriorly (Fig. 40). In general, the greater the lung herniation, the smaller is the postpneumonectomy space

(Fig. 41). Recurrence of neoplasm can be identified as a soft tissue mass projecting into this lower density space or as enlarged lymph nodes in the mediastinum (Fig. 42). Computed tomography may also be of value in confirming infection in the postpneumonectomy space (Fig. 43).

PERICARDIUM

Congenital Absence of the Left Pericardium

Most patients with this anomaly who do not have associated cardiac defects are asymptomatic. Com-

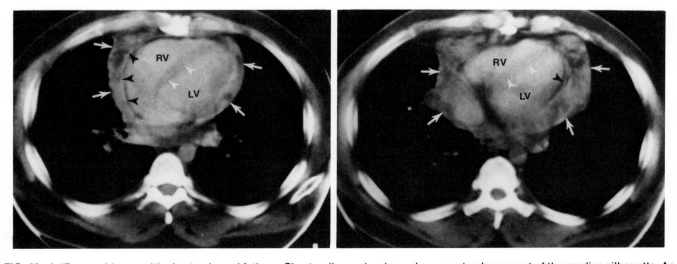

FIG. 46. A 47-year-old man with chest pain and fatigue. Chest radiographs showed apparent enlargement of the cardiac silhouette. An echocardiogram was interpreted as showing a pericardial effusion, but no fluid was obtained by pericardiocentesis. The postcontrast CT scans above demonstrate a normal pericardium (black arrowheads) just external to the epicardial fat, without any evidence of a pericardial effusion. However, an irregular inhomogeneous soft tissue mass (arrows) totally surrounds the heart and pericardium. Biopsy at thoracotomy disclosed Kaposi's sarcoma. RV, right ventricle; LV, left ventricle; white arrowheads, interventricular septum.

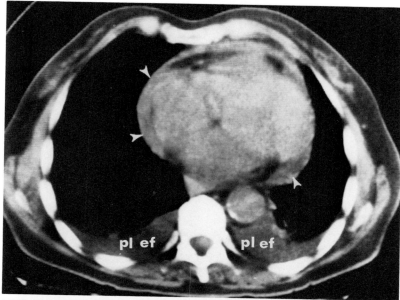

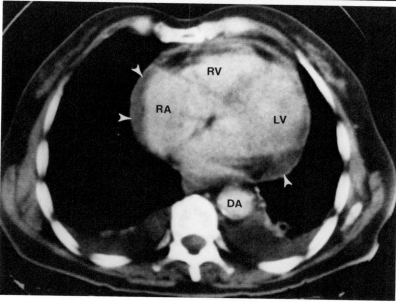

FIG. 47. Pericardial effusion. **Above:** Surrounding the heart is a slightly lower density pericardial effusion (arrowheads) in a 53-year-old woman in whom the echocardiogram was equivocal. Bilateral pleural effusions (pl ef) are present. **Below:** Scan at the same level following an infusion of iodinated contrast material demonstrates enhancement of the blood in the intracardiac chambers and in the descending aorta (DA). There is no enhancement of the pericardial effusion (arrowheads), which is now more clearly demarcated from the heart. RA, right atrium; RV, right ventricle; LV, left ventricle.

puted tomography may be of some value in confirming a diagnosis of complete absence of the left pericardium when a hilar or mediastinal lesion is suggested on plain chest radiography (3). The diagnostic findings on CT include nonvizualization of the pericardium around the left anterolateral aspect of the heart, with lung directly contacting the myocardium, and a change in the axis of pulmonary artery with lateral protrusion of the main pulmonary artery.

Pericardial Effusion

A pericardial effusion generally is recognizable on CT as an increase in thickness of the normal band-like pericardium; the underlying epicardial fat may be compressed (14,15,19,24). Most commonly, the fluid has a near-water density value and represents a transudate, or rarely a chylous effusion. Near soft tissue density collections may occur with an exudative effusion or a hemopericardium. Pericardial fluid initially tends to accumulate in the most caudal portions of the pericardial sac. In the supine position, a small effusion usually collects dorsal to the left ventricle and behind the left lateral aspect of the left atrium. When the volume is larger, the fluid extends ventrally in front of the right ventricle and atrium (Fig. 44). In massive pericardial effusions, the heart appears to float within the distended sac, and fluid extends cephalad to surround the origin of the great vessels (Fig. 45). The overdistended pericardium may project caudally and compress the diaphragm and upper abdominal organs. Encapsulated pericardial effusions can occur when fi-

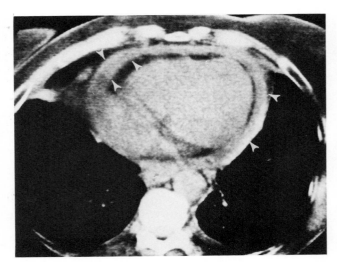

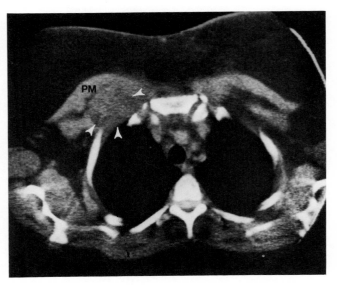

FIG. 48. Pericardial thickening. On a scan performed during an infusion of contrast media, there is enhancement of the soft tissue density pericardium (arrowheads), which measures up to 6 mm in thickness.

brous adhesions seal off portions of the pericardial space; dorsal and right anterolateral loculations are most common. Occasionally, the encapsulated fluid will bulge toward the heart, and can result in the hemodynamics of cardiac tamponade or constrictive pericarditis.

Echocardiography currently remains the method of choice for depicting pericardial effusions. Its major advantages include the ease of the examination and the portability of the equipment, along with the absence of exposure to ionizing radiation. Nevertheless, technical limitations and interpretative pitfalls exist, and CT can be used to supplement or complement ultrasound when diagnostic problems arise (Fig. 46). Computed

FIG. 50. A 27-year-old obese woman previously treated for Hodgkin's disease. A routine chest radiograph was suspicious for new mediastinal widening. CT showed no mediastinal abnormality, but disclosed a chest wall mass (arrowheads) posterior to the pectoralis major muscle (PM). Repeat physical examination confirmed a mass in this area, and a percutaneous needle biopsy demonstrated recurrent Hodgkin's disease.

tomography is especially beneficial in patients requiring evaluation following a thoracic surgical procedure, when pleural effusions are present (Fig. 47), and in the diagnosis of a loculated pericardial effusion (24).

Pericardial Thickening

The pericardium can respond to injury by fibrin production and cellular proliferation in addition to fluid output. All three mechanisms can occur concomitantly

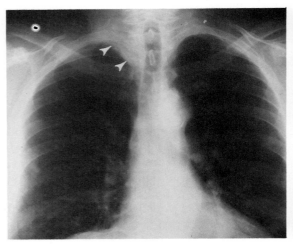

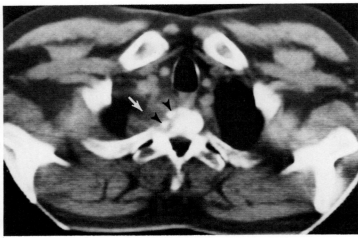

FIG. 49. Left: A routine chest roentgenogram in a 59-year-old man demonstrates some thickening (arrowheads) in the right pulmonary apex. On questioning, the patient admitted to some right shoulder pain, and a superior sulcus bronchogenic carcinoma was considered the likely cause. Cytologic examinations from needle aspiration biopsies of the region were negative. Detailed bone radiographs were normal. **Right:** CT, done to determine if a vessel or fat could account for the roentgenographic apical density, shows a definite soft tissue mass (arrow) surrounding the partially destroyed second thoracic vertebral body, which contains two sequestra (arrowheads). Staphylococcal osteomyelitis was disclosed at thoracotomy.

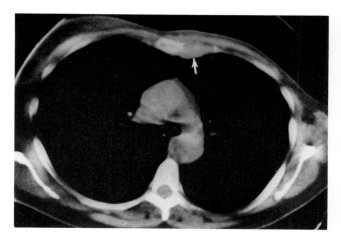

FIG. 51. A lateral chest radiograph demonstrated a suspicious retrosternal soft tissue density in a 48-year-old woman 2 years after a left mastectomy for carcinoma. CT confirmed a definite chest wall mass (arrow); percutaneous needle biopsy disclosed recurrent carcinoma.

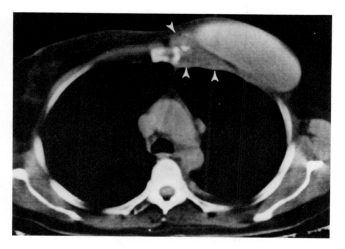

FIG. 52. A 39-year-old woman, 4 years post left mastectomy for carcinoma and 9 months after insertion of a breast prosthesis, developed some anterior chest wall pain. No definite mass was palpable; an infected prosthesis versus recurrent neoplasm was queried. CT demonstrates a soft tissue density chest wall mass (arrowheads) just beneath the prosthesis. Left pleural thickening and a questionably enlarged paraaortic lymph node also are present. Percutaneous needle biopsy under CT guidance of the chest wall mass disclosed recurrent carcinoma.

or independently. Pericardial thickening may result from proliferation of fibrin deposits or organized blood products, or through neoplastic invasion. Detection of pericardial thickening can be accomplished with CT (24). The soft tissue density thickening can range from 0.5 to 2.0 cm, and may be focal or involve the entire pericardium. Generally, the maximal thickening occurs ventrally. The thickened pericardium usually is smooth, but can be nodular in neoplastic disease. Distinction from a small exudative or bloody pericardial effusion may not be possible with CT. A change in its configuration, in the region where pericardial broadening is present, on scans done in a decubitus or prone position would imply fluid accumulation rather than thickening, whereas some enhancement after intravenous contrast medium administration would strongly suggest thickening and not fluid (Fig. 48).

The classical clinical dilemma requires that constrictive pericarditis be distinguished from restrictive or infiltrative cardiomyopathy (e.g., amyloidosis). Both syndromes may have identical clinical manifestations and hemodynamic characteristics. The accurate differentiation of a normal from a thickened pericardium by CT greatly contributes to the solution of this problem. Although echocardiography is an excellent technique for the diagnosis of pericardial effusion, it is less accurate in the recognition or exclusion of pericardial thickening. The finding of a normal pericardium on CT practically excludes the diagnosis of constrictive pericarditis (24). In addition to the pericardial thickening that occurs with constrictive

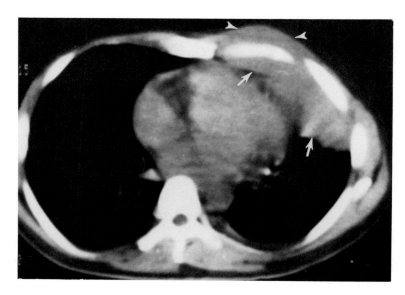

FIG. 53. A 34-year-old man with a persistent lingular pneumonia and left chest pain. CT shows thickening of the chest wall soft tissues (arrowheads) adjacent to the pulmonary consolidation (arrows). A small left pleural effusion also is noted. Needle aspiration biopsy of the lung and chest wall recovered Actinomyces israelii.

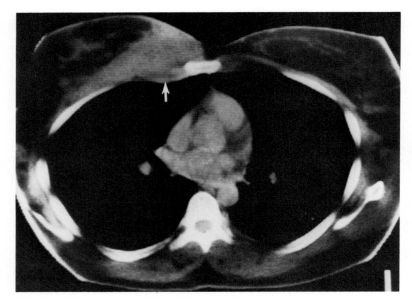

FIG. 54. Right breast carcinoma extending posteriorly into the thoracic wall (arrow).

pericarditis, nonspecific changes indicative of restrictive cardiac filling may be demonstrable on CT (8). Severe systemic venous hypertension can result in dilatation of the inferior vena cava (Fig. 56, Chapter 4), ascites, and pleural effusions. On scans obtained following intravenous contrast medium administration, angulation of the interventricular septum, indicative of abnormal cardiac motion, and external compression and deformity of the right cardiac chambers may be recognizable.

It must be emphasized that focal pericardial thickening or calcifications, sometimes quite large, may be encountered incidently on thoracic CT scans. The former is especially common in patients who have received previous mediastinal irradiation. The mere presence of thickening or calcification may not have any physiological significance. Encasement of large portions of both ventricles is usually necessary to produce hemodynamic consequences.

Neoplastic cells can reach the pericardium by direct invasion from an adjacent organ (carcinomas of the lung and breast are the most frequent neoplasms involving the pericardium), and via hematogenous or lymphatic spread. Accompanying mediastinal lymph node enlargement may be present. Computed tomography is an excellent tool for the diagnosis of neoplastic pericardial disease (24). This most often manifests as an exudative effusion, but plaque-like thickening or nodular masses can occur along the pericardium.

CHEST WALL

Lesions involving the bones and soft tissues of the chest wall sometimes can be difficult to evaluate with the conventional radiographic methods. Again, the ability of CT to distinguish between fat and soft tissue density structures and to display the components of the chest wall in cross section is valuable when assess-

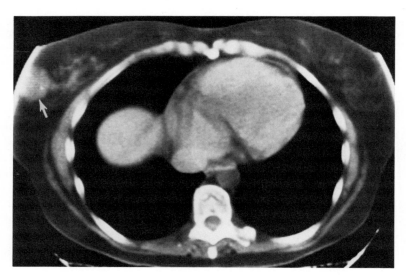

FIG. 55. Breast neoplasm (arrow) initially discovered on CT performed for evaluation of the mediastinum.

56a,b

56c,d

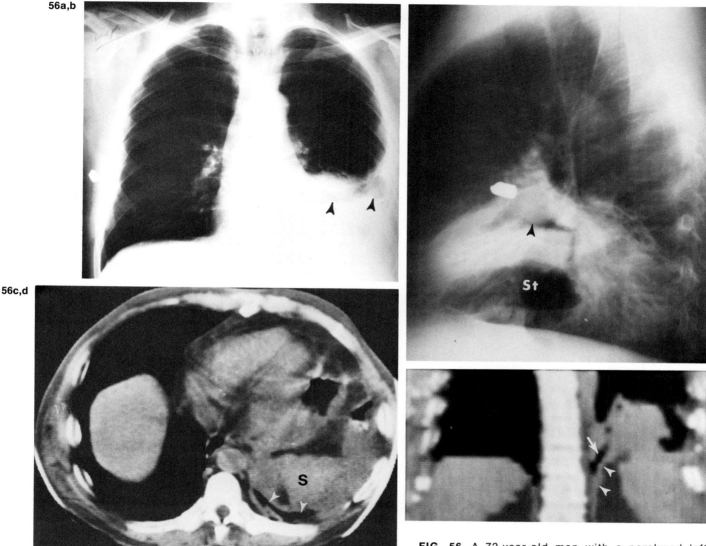

FIG. 56. A 72-year-old man with a paralyzed left hemidiaphragm resulting from a gunshot wound 7 years previously. He developed fever and left upper quadrant abdominal pain 6 months after a colectomy for diverticulitis. A subphrenic abscess was suspected. **a,b:** Chest radiographs demonstrate an air-fluid collection (arrowheads) above the gastric air bubble (St) in the vicinity of the left hemidiaphragm. However, it was uncertain whether this collection was supra- or subdiaphragmatic. Neither decubitus radiographs nor ultrasound was helpful in this distinction. **c:** Transverse CT shows some air (arrowheads) posterior to the spleen (S), but the radiologist was uncertain of its exact location. **d:** Reconstructed coronal scan demonstrates that the air (arrow) is definitely superior to the left crus of the diaphragm (arrowheads) and therefore in the thorax. A 300-cc empyema was subsequently drained at surgery.

ing the location and extent of a disease process involving the bones or soft tissues of the chest wall (11,13) (Figs. 49–52).

Lipomas of the extrapleural space and chest wall can be diagnosed based on their characteristic attenuation values. Osseous, muscular, and subcutaneous tissue invasion can be detected in patients with neoplastic disease or an aggressive infectious process. Extension of a pleural, mediastinal, or pulmonary parenchymal process into the chest wall (Fig. 53) or intrusion of a primary chest wall mass into the thoracic cavity or spinal canal can be visualized. Information

about the extent of such involvement can be crucial when planning surgical resection or radiation therapy of neoplasms of the thorax. Mediastinal lymphoma not infrequently spreads along the pleural and chest wall surface. Documentation of such spread is important in designing proper radiation ports or to support a decision to give adjunctive chemotherapy.

Computed tomography usually is preferable to conventional tomography to further evaluate a known or suspected abnormality of the sternum or sternoclavicular joint seen on standard plain radiographs (7). Assessment of the scapula may be similarly valuable.

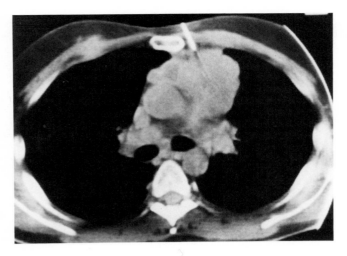

FIG. 57. Chest radiographs in a 26-year-old man previously treated for Hodgkin's disease demonstrated a new anterior mediastinal mass. CT was used to precisely guide a Franseen-type biopsy needle into the mass. The histologic specimen showed recurrent Hodgkin's disease.

Computed tomography may be helpful in selected patients with known or suspected breast carcinoma, especially if the breasts are dense and mammography is equivocal (6). Breast carcinomas usually enhance during a rapid infusion of intravenous contrast media; this characteristic can help distinguish cancer from surrounding fibrocystic tissue. The retromammary space (Fig. 54) and high axilla are well demonstrated on CT, and the findings can be useful if primary radiation therapy is contemplated. On occasion, a breast mass may be discovered incidently on CT (Fig. 55).

Multiplanar reconstruction can be valuable for precise localization of paradiaphragmatic lesions, clearly separating a supra- from a subdiaphragmatic process (Fig. 56).

AID IN PERCUTANEOUS NEEDLE BIOPSY

Computed tomography can be valuable in guiding a needle tip into a chest wall or mediastinal mass (Fig. 57) for tissue sampling. Fluoroscopic guidance, however, is preferred when biopsying most pulmonary lesions because it is quicker, less costly, and usually can be accomplished during a single breath-holding maneuver. In selected cases, when a pulmonary lesion is difficult to see with fluoroscopy (e.g., low in a posterior costophrenic sulcus), or angulation of the needle is required to reach the target tissue (e.g., directly under the scapula or a rib), CT guidance can be very helpful.

REFERENCES

1. Alexander E, Clark RA, Colley DP, Mitchell SE: CT of malignant pleural mesothelioma. *AJR* 137:287–291, 1981
2. Baber CE, Hedlund LW, Oddson TA, Putman CE: Differentiating empyemas and peripheral pulmonary abscesses. *Radiology* 135:755–758, 1980
3. Baim PS, MacDonald IL, Wise DJ, Lankei SC: Computed tomography of absent left pericardium. *Radiology* 135:127–128, 1980
4. Baron RL, Levitt RG, Sagel SS, White MJ, Roper CL, Marbarger, JP: Computed tomography in the preoperative evaluation of bronchogenic carcinoma. *Radiology* (in press)
5. Biondetti PR, Fiore D, Sartori F, Colognato A, Ravasini R, Romani S: Evaluation of the post-pneumonectomy space by computed tomography. *J Comput Assist Tomogr* 6:238–242, 1982
6. Chang, CHJ, Nesbit DE, Fisher DR, Fritz SL, Dwyer SJ, Templeton AW, Lin F, Jewell WR: Computed tomographic mammography using a conventional body scanner. *AJR* 138:553–558, 1982
7. Destouet JM, Gilula LA, Murphy WA, Sagel SS: Computed tomography of the sternoclavicular joint and sternum. *Radiology* 138:123–128, 1981
8. Doppman JL, Rienmuller R, Lissner J, Cyran J, Bolte HD, Strauer BE, Hellwig H: Computed tomography in constrictive pericarditis. *J Comput Assist Tomogr* 5:1–11, 1981
9. Emami B, Melo A, Carter BL, Munzenreider JE, Piro AJ: Value of computed tomography in radiotherapy of lung cancer. *AJR* 131:63–67, 1978
10. Fiore D, Biondetti PR, Sartori F, Calabro F: The role of computed tomography in the evaluation of bullous lung disease. *J Comput Assist Tomogr* 6:105–108, 1982
11. Gautard RD, Dussault RG, Chahlaoui J, Duranceau A, Sylvester J: Contribution of CT in thoracic bony lesions. *J Can Assoc Radiol* 32:29–41, 1981
12. Godwin JD, Webb WR: Dynamic computed tomography in the evaluation of vascular lung lesions. *Radiology* 138:629–635, 1981
13. Gouliamos AD, Carter BL, Emami B: Computed tomography of the chest wall. *Radiology* 134:433–436, 1980
14. Guthaner DF, Wexler L, Harell G: CT demonstration of cardiac structures. *AJR* 133:75–81, 1979
15. Houang MIW, Arozena X, Shaw DG: Demonstration of the pericardium and pericardial effusion by computed tomography. *J Comput Assist Tomogr* 3:601–603, 1979
16. Jost RG, Sagel SS, Stanley RJ, Levitt RG: Computed tomography of the thorax. *Radiology* 126:125–136, 1978
17. Katz D, Kreel L: Computed tomography in pulmonary asbestosis. *Clin Radiol* 30:207–213, 1979
18. Kruglik GD, Wayne KS: Occult lung cavity causing hemoptysis: Recognition by computed tomography. *J Comput Assist Tomogr* 4:407–408, 1980
19. Lackner K, Thurn P: Computed tomography of the heart: ECG-gated and continuous scans. *Radiology* 140:413–420, 1981
20. McCloud TC, Wittenberg J, Ferrucci JT: Computed tomography of the thorax and standard radiographic evaluation of the chest: A comparative study. *J Comput Assist Tomogr* 3:170–180, 1979
21. Metzger RA, Mulhern CB Jr, Arger PH, Coleman BG, Epstein DM, Gefter WB: CT differentiation of solitary from diffuse bronchioalveolar carcinoma. *J Comput Assist Tomogr* 5:830–833, 1981
22. Mintzer RA, Gore, RM, Vogelzang RL, Holz S: Rounded-atelectasis and its association with asbestos-induced pleural disease. *Radiology* 139:567–570, 1981
23. Mintzer RA, Malave SR, Neiman HL, Michaelis LL, Vanecko RM, Sanders JH: Computed vs. conventional tomography in the evaluation of primary and secondary pulmonary neoplasms. *Radiology* 132:653–659, 1979
24. Moncada R, Baker, M, Salinas M, Demos TC, Churchill R, Love L, Reynes C, Hale D, Cardoso M, Pifarre R, Gunnar RM: Diagnostic role of computed tomography in pericardial heart disease. *Am Heart J* 100:263–282, 1982
25. Muhm JR, Brown LR, Crowe JR, Sheedy II PF, Hattery RR, Stephens DH: Comparison of whole lung tomography and computed tomography for detecting pulmonary nodules. *AJR* 131:981–984, 1978

26. Nabawi, P, Mantravadi R, Breyer D, Capek V: Computed tomography of radiation-induced lung injuries. *J Comput Assist Tomogr* 5:568–570, 1980

27. Naidich DP, McCauley DI, Khouri NF, Stitik FP, Siegelman SS: Computed tomography of bronchiectasis. *J Comput Assist Tomogr* 6:437–444, 1982

28. Pagani JJ, Libshitz HI: CT manifestations of radiation-induced change in chest tissue. *J Comput Assist Tomogr* 6:243–248, 1982

29. Prasad S, Pilepich MV, Perez CA: Contribution of CT to quantitative radiation therapy planning. *AJR* 136:123–128, 1981

30. Pugatch RD, Faling LJ, Robbins AH, Snider GL: Differentiation of pleural and pulmonary lesions using computed tomography. *J Comput Assist Tomogr* 2:601–606, 1978

31. Rea HH, Shevland JE, House AJS: Accuracy of computed tomographic scanning in assessment of the mediastinum in bronchial carcinoma. *J Thorac Cardiovasc Surg* 81:825–829, 1981

32. Rosenblum LJ, Mauceri RA, Wellenstein DE: Density patterns in the normal lung as determined by computed tomography. *Radiology* 137:409–416, 1980

33. Schaner EG, Chang AE, Doppman JR, Conkle DM, Flye MW, Rosenberg SA: Comparison of computed and conventional whole lung tomography in detecting pulmonary nodules: A prospective radiologic-pathologic study. *AJR* 131:51–54, 1978

34. Scholten ET, Kreel L: Distribution of lung metastases in the axial plane. A combined radiological-pathological study. *Radiol Clin (Basel)* 46:248–265, 1977

35. Siegelman SS, Zerhouni EA, Leo FP, Khouri NF, Stitik FP: CT of the solitary pulmonary nodule. *AJR* 135:1–13, 1980

36. Toombs BD, Sandler CM, Lester RG: Computed tomography of chest trauma. *Radiology* 140:733–738, 1981

37. Tylen U, Nilsson U: Computed tomography in pulmonary pseudotumors and their relation to asbestos exposure. *J Comput Assist Tomogr* 6:229–237, 1982

38. Webb WR, Jeffrey RB, Godwin JD: Thoracic computed tomography in superior sulcus tumors. *J Comput Assist Tomogr* 5:361–365, 1981

39. Wegener OH, Kaeppe P, Oeser H: Measurement of lung density by computed tomography. *J Comput Assist Tomogr* 2:263–273, 1978

Chapter 6

Normal Abdominal Anatomy

Dennis M. Balfe, Roy R. Peterson, and Joseph K. T. Lee

Since the introduction of ultrasound (US) and CT of the abdomen as clinically applicable techniques, considerable interest in understanding the cross-sectional presentation of normal and pathological anatomy has been aroused (15). Experience from other radiologic studies has made it clear that the full range of normal variation must be completely grasped in order to recognize what is abnormal.

Computed tomographic images display a wealth of information regarding abdominal viscera, fascial planes, muscles, and bony structures in every anatomic section scanned. To digest this information adequately, it is useful to develop an orderly system by which every section can be searched for the presence of a disease process. Accordingly, in the following pages, an effort has been made to present anatomic information stressing key areas, where there are organ-related or musculoskeletal landmarks, and where pathologic processes tend to occur. Thus, the lower abdomen between the hilus of the kidneys and the bifurcation of the aorta will be discussed in one section, whereas upper abdominal sections, particularly in the region of the head of the pancreas, may contain two or more important areas, each of which will be discussed separately.

Additionally, an attempt has been made to include some discussion of anatomy that is not visible on CT images but is nevertheless important to the understanding of pathologic processes. The works of Meyers (12) and Whalen (23) in particular have drawn attention to dynamic features important in interpretation of radiologic studies of the abdomen. Peritoneal effusions, for example, follow well-defined flow patterns because of the influence of gravity, and are restricted by the various peritoneal compartments. Similarly, retroperitoneal effusions are affected by well-defined fascial planes that can, to a limited extent, be delineated by CT. An understanding of these "invisible" anatomic considerations is essential to the understanding of pathologic processes in the abdomen.

AREA I: GASTROESOPHAGEAL JUNCTION

The esophageal hiatus is well imaged on most scans of the upper abdomen (4) (Fig. 1). The distal esophagus can be identified as a round 2- to 3-cm structure of soft tissue attenuation lying immediately anterior to the aorta. Air or orally administered contrast material sometimes may be seen within its lumen. At the level of the esophageal hiatus, there is obvious separation of the diaphragmatic crura; the left crus is shorter and more sagitally oriented, whereas the right crus is longer, thicker, and often coronally oriented. Occasionally, the right crus may extend to the left of the midline (Fig. 2). Not uncommonly, there is a bulbous anterior extension of the right crus that protrudes into the region of gastrohepatic ligament anterior to the esophagus (Fig. 3). This is a reflection of the fact that the esophagus passes anterior to the left crus, which remains in contact with the aorta, but posterior to the medial portion of the right crus, which thus must occupy a more anterior position. The bulbous right crus can be distinguished from a pathologic process, such as lymph node enlargement, by noting its continuity with the remainder of the right crus.

The portion of stomach imaged on this section is the cardia. Several fixed relationships are displayed. A triangular or crescentic space, bounded posteriorly by the esophagus and right crus of the diaphragm, on the right by the left lobe of the liver and on the left by the lesser curvature of the stomach, is occupied by the gastrohepatic ligament, which frequently contains considerable fat (Fig. 4). This ligament extends into the fissure for the ligamentum venosum, commonly seen on the visceral surface of the liver immediately adjacent to the right crus of the diaphragm. Herein are contained the left gastric artery and left gastric (coronary) veins as well as the left gastric group of lymph nodes. These lymph nodes drain the distal esophagus and the lesser curvature of the stomach, and conduct

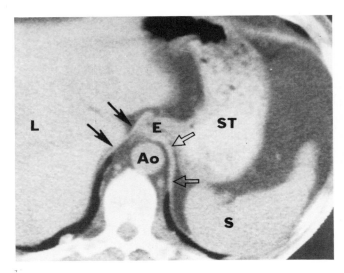

FIG. 1. Gastroesophageal junction. The left crus of the diaphragm (open arrows) remains close to the aorta (Ao), but the right crus (black arrows) is positioned more anteriorly to admit the esophagus (E). This crural separation forms the esophageal hiatus. L, liver; S, spleen; ST, stomach.

lymph toward nodes near the celiac trunk. They are frequently enlarged in patients with abdominal involvement with lymphoma (see Fig. 24a, Chapter 10). Whereas the left gastric vessels are frequently seen in individuals with abundant intraabdominal fat, normal lymph nodes are not routinely observed.

A small bare area of the stomach is present posteriorly, where the cardia comes into intimate contact with the left crus of the diaphragm. Held in a relatively fixed position at the esophageal hiatus, the gastric wall

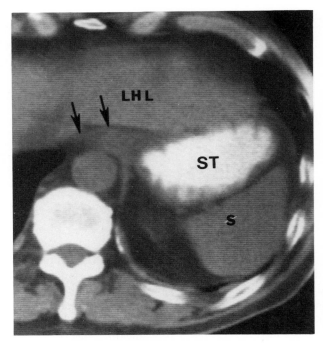

FIG. 2. Gastroesophageal junction in a patient with a large left hepatic lobe (LHL). Note that the right diaphragmatic crus (arrows) extends to the left of the midline. S, spleen; ST, stomach.

in this region courses parallel to the transverse scanning plane. Because of this, the gastric wall may appear to be abnormally thick in this region (11) (Fig. 5). Lateral to the bare area, the posterior aspect of the stomach forms the roof of the superior recess of the omental bursa (lesser peritoneal sac). At the same

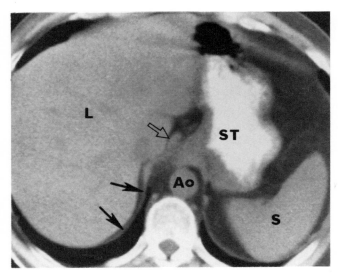

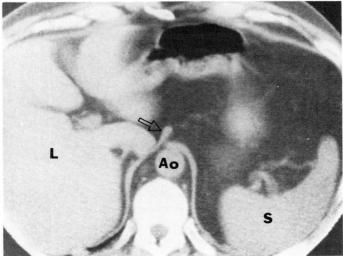

FIG. 3. Anterior protrusion of the right diaphragmatic crus. **Left:** CT scan through the gastroesophageal junction. The somewhat bulbous medial portion of the right diaphragmatic crus (open arrow) is projected into the fat-containing gastrohepatic ligament, and simulates lymph node enlargement. Serial scans documented its continuity with more lateral portions of the right diaphragmatic crus (black arrows). **Right:** CT scan 2 cm inferior to the gastroesophageal junction. The most medial aspect of the right crus (open arrow) is directed anteriorly and protrudes into the region of the gastrohepatic ligament. Its continuity with the remainder of the right diaphragmatic crus is established. L, liver; ST, stomach; Ao, aorta; S, spleen.

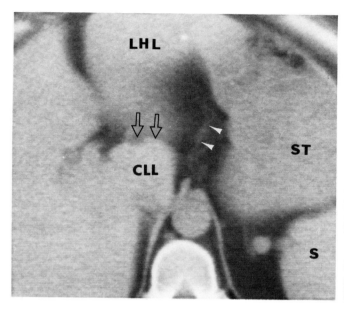

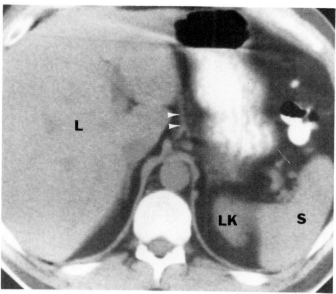

FIG. 4. The region of the gastrohepatic ligament. **Left:** This fat-containing peritoneal reflection extends between the medial aspect of the stomach (ST) and the fissure for the ligamentum venosum (open arrows), which is posterior to the lateral segment of the left hepatic lobe (LHL) and anterior to the caudate lobe (CLL). The left gastric vessels contained within its leaves are seen as ill-defined strands of soft tissue attenuation (arrowheads). **Right:** In another patient, the left gastric artery (arrowheads) is sagitally directed and easily identified. L, liver; S, spleen; LK, left kidney.

level, the peritoneum of the greater peritoneal cavity surrounds the diaphragmatic surface of the spleen to form the perisplenic space (Fig. 6). Between these two spaces, the nonperitonealized medial aspect of the

spleen, lying in the gastrosplenic ligament, makes close contact with the posterior aspect of the stomach. In patients with sufficient omental fat, the short gastric vessels within the gastrosplenic ligament can be observed (Fig. 7). The left gastroepiploic artery, another

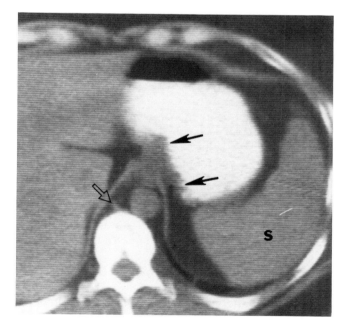

FIG. 5. There is apparent thickening of the medial portion of the gastric wall (black arrows) at a level immediately inferior to the gastroesophageal junction because in this area the stomach wall is parallel to the scanning plane; this normal finding should not be confused with a pathologically thickened gastric wall. Note the normal azygous vein in the retrocrural space (open arrow). S, spleen.

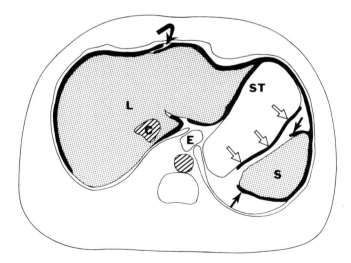

FIG. 6. Schematic diagram of the peritoneal spaces at the level of the gastroesophageal junction. The posterior margin of the stomach forms the roof of the superior recess of the lesser sac (open arrows); the perisplenic space (small black arrows) is continuous with the greater peritoneal space. Between these two peritoneal spaces lies the gastrosplenic ligament, in which the left gastroepiploic vessels and short gastric vessels are found. The discontinuity in the greater peritoneal space on the anterior surface of the liver is caused by the falciform ligament (curved arrow). L, liver; C, inferior vena cava; E, esophagus; S, spleen; ST, stomach.

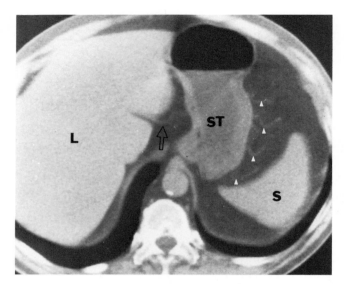

FIG. 7. Scan immediately inferior to the gastroesophageal junction demonstrates multiple serpentine short gastric vessels (white arrowheads), within the gastrosplenic ligament. A small vessel (open arrow) entering the fissure for the ligamentum venosum is an accessory left hepatic artery. L, liver; S, spleen; ST, stomach.

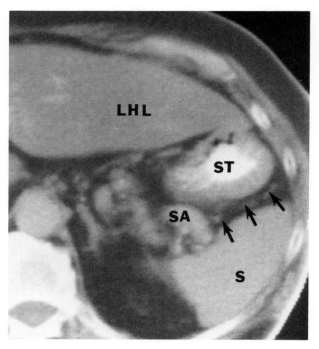

FIG. 8. Scan through the splenic hilus demonstrates the left gastroepiploic artery (arrows), arising from the splenic artery (SA) and coursing along the posterolateral surface of the stomach (ST). This patient has an unusually large left hepatic lobe (LHL). S, spleen.

branch of the splenic artery, may sometimes be seen coursing anteriorly along the greater curvature of the stomach at this level (Fig. 8).

In the area of the gastroesophageal junction, the crura of the diaphragm course roughly parallel to the vertebral bodies. Laterally, the crura are separated from the vertebral bodies by varying amounts of lung and pleura. Centrally, the space anterior to the vertebral body and posterior to the left and right diaphragmatic crus is the retrocrural region (Fig. 9). This contains the aorta, azygous and hemiazygous veins, thoracic duct, and a few lymph nodes. In most patients, the azygous and hemiazygous veins may be seen in cross-section as soft tissue densities 3 to 6 mm in size (3). Occasionally, irregular streaks with muscle attenuation can be seen extending obliquely from the diaphragm toward the ribs and costal cartilages (Fig. 10). They are more often seen on scans taken during suspended inspiration, and probably represent the costal attachments of the diaphragm.

Scans at this level typically demonstrate the dome of the liver. These portions of the right and left hepatic lobes are relatively far from the porta hepatis. Accordingly, the visible structures of the portal triad, including branches of the portal veins, are relatively small. In contrast, the hepatic veins are relatively large and may be seen draining into the inferior vena cava (Fig. 11). The inferior vena cava, immediately posterior to the caudate lobe of the liver in this area, is well anterior to the aorta as it courses toward the right atrium.

In many subjects, a triangular- or spindle-shaped fat

collection may be seen immediately anterior to the left hepatic lobe. This fat, which is extraperitoneal in origin and lies within the root of the falciform ligament, often causes the anterior surface of the left lobe to become quite flat. It may be contiguous with fat within the greater omentum or within the fissure for the ligamentum teres (Fig. 12); sufficient fat may be present to outline the falciform ligament.

The diaphragmatic and gastric surfaces of the spleen are observed on scans at this level in most individuals. The splenic hilus is more likely to be observed at slightly caudal levels. Between the stomach and the spleen is the superior recess of the lesser sac, which is not directly continuous with the perisplenic peritoneal space. The peritoneal spaces at this level (Fig. 6) are, of course, potential spaces and will not be observed by CT unless distended by a pathologic process.

AREA II: SPLENIC HILUS

The hilus of the spleen lies at the junction of two peritoneal ligaments (Fig. 13). The superior, or gastrosplenic, ligament lies between the perisplenic space and the superior recess of the lesser sac and transmits the short gastric and gastroepiploic vessels. A more inferior one, the splenorenal ligament, lies between the perisplenic space and the portion of the lesser sac

9a,b

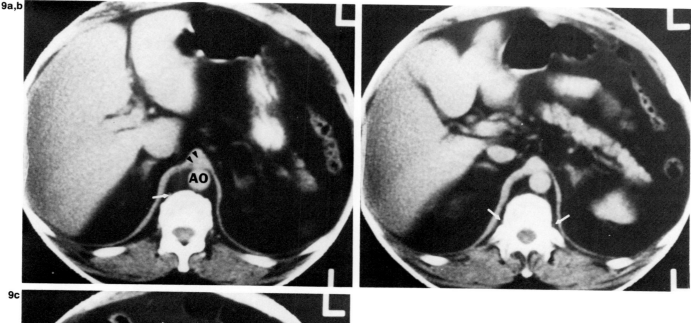

9c

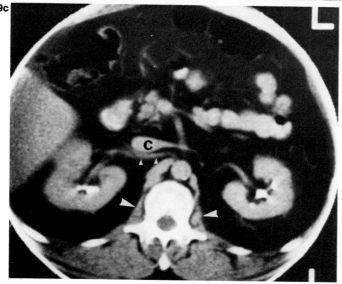

FIG. 9. Retrocrural anatomy. **a:** CT scan 2 cm caudal to the gastroesophageal junction. There is some thickening of the medial portions of the right and left crura, which are slightly separated by fat (arrowheads). A small circular density anterior to the vertebral body on the right (white arrow) represents the azygous vein. AO, aorta. **b:** Scan 2 cm caudad. There is no longer separation of the right and left crura. The fat-containing space posterior to the crura and immediately lateral to the aorta contains the azygous and hemiazygous veins, the thoracic duct, and a few lymph nodes. More posteriorly, the paired ascending lumbar veins (white arrows) course just anterior to the transverse processes. **c:** Scan 4 cm inferiorly. The right and left crura are apposed to the anterior surface of the vertebral body, thus further reducing the amount of retrocrural fat. The psoas muscles (large arrowheads) are well formed at this level. Note the origin and course of the right renal artery (small arrowheads) passing posterior to the inferior vena cava (C).

anterior to the kidney and contains the splenic artery and vein and the tail of the pancreas (Fig. 14). The vascular anatomy in the region of the splenic hilus is somewhat variable. In young patients, the splenic artery predictably lies slightly anterior and cephalic to the splenic vein; but in older individuals, the splenic artery may become markedly tortuous and thus is highly variable in position. In these subjects, it is often calcified, making its identification somewhat easier. The tail of the pancreas is almost always the most anterior structure in the splenic hilus but, in occasional individuals, a small portion of the tail may curl posterior to the splenic artery and vein (13). Rarely, the entire pancreas may be imaged on this section; more commonly, only the tail and a portion of the body will be present. The splenic vein characteristically runs a straight course just posterior to the body of the pan-

creas. The fat plane that is present between the splenic vein and the pancreatic body occasionally may resemble a dilated pancreatic duct (Fig. 15). Its fatty attenuation value and its characteristic position on the posterior aspect of the pancreas should allow its differentiation from a pathologically dilated pancreatic duct (18).

The section containing the splenic hilus also very commonly contains the superior portions of the medial and lateral limbs of the left adrenal gland. The adrenal is within the perirenal fat posterior to the splenic vein, separated from it by the anterior renal fascia (6). Occasionally, a tortuous splenic artery may lie very close to the adrenal and thus simulate enlargement of the gland.

Immediately anterior to the tip of the pancreatic tail at the level of the splenic hilus, the left colic flexure is typically seen (Fig. 16). Anatomically, this represents

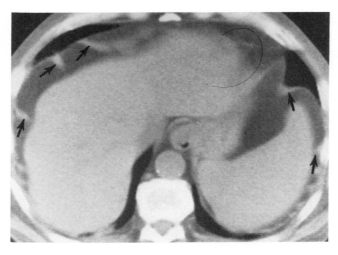

FIG. 10. The folds in the diaphragm (arrows) at its costal attachments are well seen at the level of the gastroesophageal junction. Such prominent folds are probably only observed in suspended inspiration.

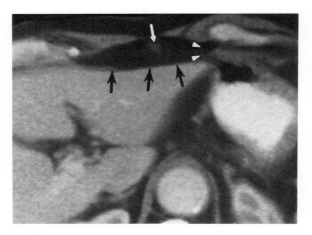

FIG. 12. A triangular- or spindle-shaped collection of extraperitoneal fat is commonly present directly anterior to the left lobe of the liver (black arrows). This fat is extraperitoneal, although it may be contiguous with fat within the greater omentum (white arrowheads). The tip of the xyphoid process was partially contained within the plane of this transverse section and accounts for the central density (white arrow).

the most cephalic portion of the transverse colon, which is still suspended by the transverse mesocolon; actual fusion of the descending colon with the posterior body wall occurs immediately caudal to the tip of the spleen. The body of the stomach, with its characteristic rugal pattern, may be identified just medial to the splenic flexure. Between the stomach and pancreas on sec-

tions at or slightly inferior to the splenic hilum is the duodeno-jejunal flexure, supported by the ligament of Treitz. This flexure is a particularly important anatomic structure, because, if it is collapsed or not opacified with oral contrast material, it may easily be mistaken for a mass or collection within the lesser peritoneal space.

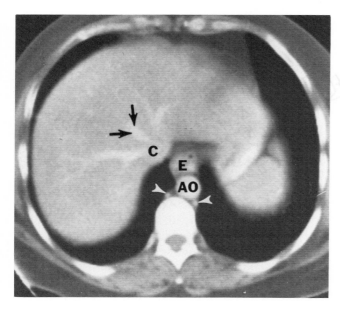

FIG. 11. Contrast-enhanced CT scan through the gastroesophageal junction. The three major hepatic venous trunks converge on the inferior vena cava (C). The middle hepatic vein (arrows) parallels the interlobar fissure. The right and left hepatic veins run in the intersegmental fissures. Note the contrast-enhanced azygous and hemiazygous veins (arrowheads). E, esophagus; AO, aorta.

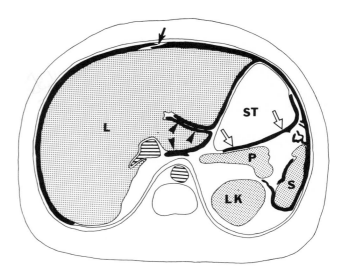

FIG. 13. Schematic diagram of the peritoneal spaces at the level of the splenic hilus. Medially, the lesser peritoneal sac (black arrowheads), which surrounds the caudate lobe, is separated from the greater peritoneal cavity by the gastrohepatic ligament, which here inserts deeply into the fissure for the ligamentum venosum. Laterally, the superior recess of the lesser sac (open arrows) lies anterior to portions of the body and tail of the pancreas. The falciform ligament is again present on the anterior surface of the liver (black arrow). L, liver; LK, left kidney; P, pancreas; S, spleen; ST, stomach.

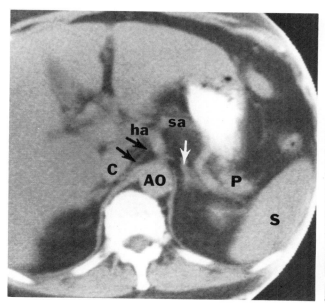

FIG. 14. The splenic hilus. **Left:** At the level of the bifurcation of the celiac trunk, the tortuous splenic artery (sa) can be identified anterolateral to the left adrenal (white arrow) and posteromedial to the tail of the pancreas (P). Note the origin of the right inferior phrenic artery directly from the celiac trunk (black arrows).

Right: Scan 2 cm caudal shows a comparatively straight splenic vein (sv) as it courses directly posterior to the body and tail of the pancreas (P). Note the proximity of the anterior surface of the upper pole of the left kidney (LK) to the splenic vein. S, spleen; C, inferior vena cava; ha, hepatic artery; AO, aorta.

AREA III: PORTA HEPATIS

The porta hepatis is a region on the visceral surface of the liver just anterior to the caudate lobe that transmits the portal vein, the hepatic artery, and the hepatic duct as well as branches of the celiac neural plexus (Fig. 17). The cephalocaudal extent of the porta hepa-

tis is 3 to 4 cm. Two fissures join the porta hepatis and the orientation of these fissures helps establish the exact level of the section. On sections obtained through the most cephalic portions of the porta hepatis (Fig. 18), the inferior margin of the fissure for the ligamentum venosum can be seen coursing in a coronal plane.

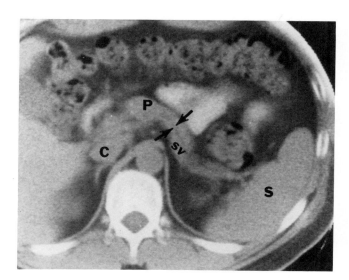

FIG. 15. The splenic hilus. A fat plane (arrows) normally separates the splenic vein (sv) from the body and tail of the pancreas (P). The characteristic posterior position and low attenuation of this fat plane should prevent its being confused with a pancreatic duct. C, inferior vena cava; S, spleen.

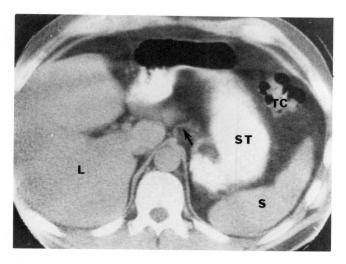

FIG. 16. CT scan slightly cephalic to the splenic hilus. The distal transverse colon (TC) characteristically occupies a position lateral to the stomach (ST) and anterior to the tip of the spleen (S). On more caudal sections, the transverse colon will course posteriorly and join the descending colon in the retroperitoneum caudal to the tip of the spleen. The black arrow points to the left gastric artery. L, liver.

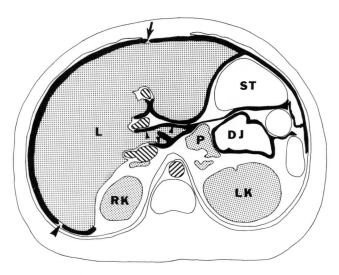

FIG. 17. Schematic diagram of the peritoneal relationships at the level of the porta hepatis. The lesser peritoneal sac (small arrowheads) extends well into the porta hepatis, essentially surrounding the small caudate process. It is at this level that communication between the greater and lesser peritoneal cavities occurs by way of the foramen of Winslow. The right triangular ligament (large black arrowhead) and falciform ligament (black arrow) are also shown. ST, stomach; L, liver; P, pancreas; DJ, duodenojejunal flexure; RK, right kidney; LK, left kidney.

The caudate lobe of the liver lies between this fissure and the inferior vena cava. There is often no fat plane between the anterior surface of the vena cava and the posterior aspect of the caudate lobe, but the two can be distinguished because the inferior vena cava is of

slightly lower attenuation value than the normal caudate lobe. The sagittally directed fissure for the ligamentum teres is seen at this level and continues inferomedial toward the umbilicus. It is sometimes filled with fat, and the obliterated umbilical vein contained therein may then be easily seen (Fig. 19). Fat within this fissure may be continuous with the fat collection in the root of the falciform ligament, anterior to the lateral segment of the left lobe of the liver. Inasmuch as the fissure for the ligamentum teres does not completely separate the lateral segment of the left lobe of the liver from the quadrate lobe, there is a continuity of the hepatic tissue anteriorly on more cephalic sections. Scans at this level include the right and left portal veins and branches of the right and left hepatic arteries. When biliary structures can be identified high in the porta hepatis, they are segments of the right and left hepatic ducts; more caudally, at the level of the portal vein, the common hepatic duct may be visible (Fig. 20).

Scans through the lower aspect of the porta hepatis (approximately 2 cm caudally) demonstrate important differences in portal anatomy (Fig. 21). The caudate lobe of the liver is much smaller (the finger-like inferior extension of the caudate lobe is called the caudate process), and there is a fat plane lying between the inferior vena cava and the unbranched portal vein. The epiploic foramen (of Winslow), which connects the lesser peritoneal space with the greater peritoneal cavity, is present at this level. Anterior to the portal vein, within

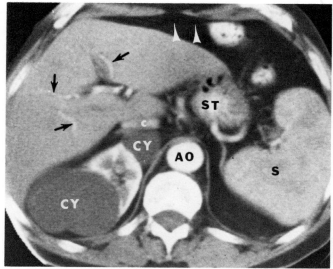

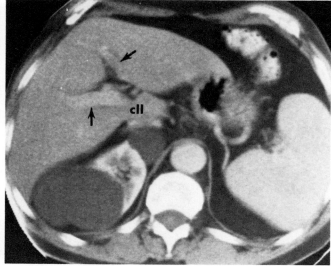

FIG. 18. CT scans through the upper portion of the porta hepatis. **Left:** Fifteen seconds after injection of intravenous contrast material, branches of the left and right hepatic arteries (black arrows) are evident. The fat contained in the greater omentum is more vascular than the fat in the root of the falciform ligament; the line of demarcation (white arrowheads) between these two fat collections represents the peritoneal reflection. The right kidney contains two large simple cysts (CY). **Right:** Thirty seconds later, the right and left portal veins (arrows) have opacified, and are considerably larger than the hepatic arteries. The caudate lobe (cll) divides the portal vein from the inferior vena cava (here displaced anteriorly because of the right renal cyst). c, inferior vena cava; AO, aorta; ST, stomach; S, spleen.

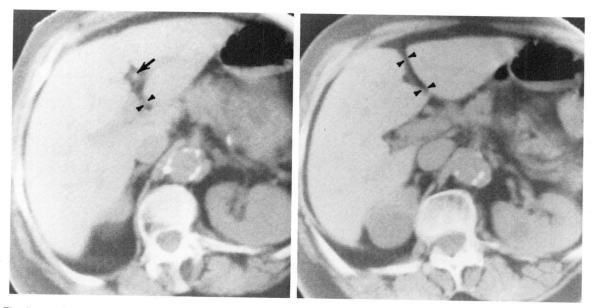

FIG. 19. The fissure for the ligamentum teres. **Left:** The sagitally oriented deep portion of the fissure of ligamentum teres (arrowheads) joins the superior portion of the porta hepatis. The obliterated umbilical vein (arrow) is outlined by plentiful fat contained within the fissure. **Right:** Two centimeters inferiorly, the fissure for the ligamentum teres (arrowheads) forms a complete division between the lateral segment of the left hepatic lobe and the remainder of the liver.

the hepatoduodenal ligament, the proper hepatic artery can be seen. The normal common hepatic duct, which usually cannot be identified without contrast material, lies on the anterior surface of the portal vein lateral to the hepatic artery (Fig. 22). The cystic duct termination is quite variable, and thus absolute differentiation of the common hepatic duct from the common bile duct is not possible on CT. On the right of the porta hepatis at this level two notches are usually displayed (Fig. 23): the anterior notch is important because it points in the plane of the true interlobar fissure and thus delimits the lateral margin of the quadrate lobe. On scans obtained 2 to 4 cm caudally, the long

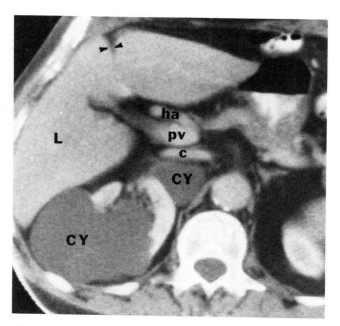

FIG. 21. Lower portion of the porta hepatis. A postcontrast scan (same patient as in Fig. 18) shows the fissure for the ligamentum teres (arrowheads) indenting the anterior surface of the liver. The opacified portal vein (pv) lies in close proximity to the inferior vena cava (c) posteriorly and the proper hepatic artery (ha) anteriorly. The portal vein and hepatic artery occupy the hepatoduodenal ligament. L, liver; CY, renal cysts.

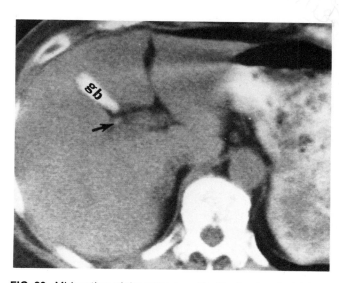

FIG. 20. Midportion of the porta hepatis. Contrast material from a previous cholecystogram remains within the biliary structures. The upper portion of the neck of the gallbladder (gb) as well as a portion of the common hepatic duct (arrow) are opacified.

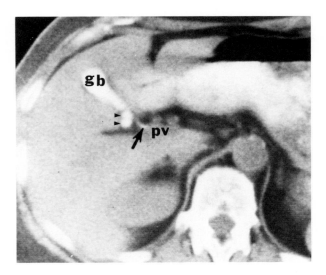

FIG. 22. Caudal portion of the porta hepatis. Residual contrast material from a previous cholecystogram opacifies the fundus and the neck (arrowheads) of the gallbladder (gb). A portion of the common hepatic duct (large arrow) is present, lateral to the peripheral calcified hepatic arteries and anterior to the portal vein (pv).

to the portal vein, a replaced right hepatic artery will most often be seen between the portal vein and the inferior vena cava. Occasionally, an accessory left hepatic artery, arising as a branch of the left gastric artery, may be seen entering the fissure for the ligamentum venosum (Fig. 7).

Scans obtained through the level of the porta hepatis nearly always include the right adrenal gland, occupying a position within the renal fascia immediately posterior to the inferior vena cava. The lateral limb of the adrenal may be intimately apposed to the posteromedial surface of the right lobe of the liver, and it may be difficult to see in asthenic individuals. The body of the stomach occupies an anterior position in this area; its exact position depends on the size and shape of the lateral segment of the left hepatic lobe. Most frequently, the left lobe becomes progressively thinner as one proceeds caudad and the gastric body and antrum, which lie on its posterior surface, thus become progressively more anterior.

AREA IV: GALLBLADDER FOSSA

The gallbladder fossa in most individuals is a notch of variable depth on the anterior aspect of the visceral surface of the liver. The fossa for the gallbladder lies 2 to 4 cm caudal to the porta hepatis and is in the plane of the true interlobar fissure, which can be located by identifying the fat-containing anterior notch to the right of the portal vein at the porta hepatis (5). Cranially, the neck and cystic duct are the most posterome-

axis of the gallbladder will nearly always be present in the same oblique orientation as the interlobar fissure.

Variations in vascular supply to the liver are relatively common. For example, CT may demonstrate a replaced right hepatic artery arising from the superior mesenteric artery or directly from the aorta (16) (Fig. 24). Whereas the normal hepatic artery curves anterior

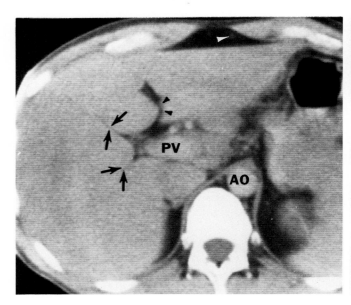

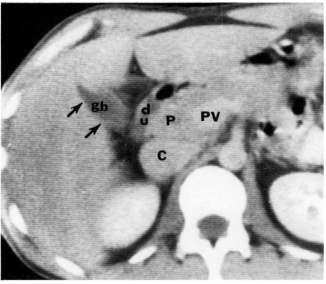

FIG. 23. Hepatic fissural anatomy. **Left:** At the level of the mid-portion of the porta hepatis, lateral to the fissure for the ligamentum teres (arrowheads), the portal fat outlines two distinct notches (arrows). The anterior notch points in the direction of the true interlobar fissure, thus delimiting the surface of the quadrate lobe. The posterior notch points to the intralobar fissure of the right lobe, separating the anterior and posterior segments. The white arrowhead points to the superior epigastric vein. **Right:** Four centimeters caudal, the neck of the gallbladder (gb), which is immediately lateral to the duodenum (du), lies in the same plane as the interlobar fissure (arrows). PV, portal vein; AO, aorta; P, pancreas; C, inferior vena cava.

24a,b

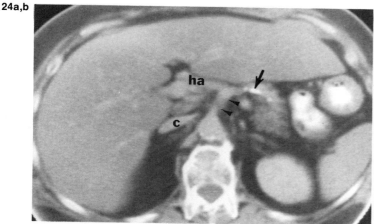
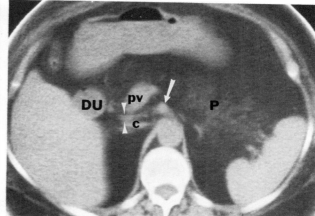

24c

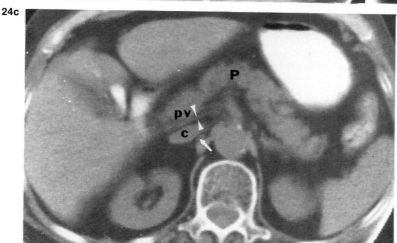

FIG. 24. Vascular anatomy of the upper abdomen. **a:** Normal celiac trunk. Contrast-enhanced CT scan shows the celiac trunk (arrowheads), a proximal portion of the common hepatic artery (ha), and a calcified splenic artery (arrow). **b:** In a patient with diffuse fatty replacement of the pancreas, the vascular structures are easily visible. An accessory right hepatic artery (arrowheads) arises from the superior mesenteric artery (arrow) and passes between the portal vein (pv) and the inferior vena cava (c). **c:** Accessory right hepatic artery (arrowheads) arising directly from the aorta and extending between the inferior vena cava (c) and the portal vein (pv). A portion of the right inferior phrenic artery (arrow) is also visible. P, pancreas; DU, duodenum.

dial structures; scans obtained sequentially in a caudal direction will show the fundus appearing anterolaterally (Fig. 25). In some patients, the gallbladder may be ectopic in position (Fig. 26); rarely, the gallbladder is entirely intrahepatic. The junction of the cystic duct with the common hepatic duct occurs anterior to the portal vein within the hepatoduodenal ligament in the majority of individuals. However, the exact level of this junction is quite variable and is rarely if ever seen on CT. The descending duodenum is immediately medial to the neck of the gallbladder.

As the postbulbar duodenum extends directly posteriorly, it passes lateral to the head of the pancreas and medial to the gallbladder, arriving at a position just anterior to the right renal vein or renal pelvis (Fig. 27). The relationship of the hepatic flexure of the colon to the gallbladder is complex. In most patients, the ascending colon lies lateral to the duodenum and posteromedial to the gallbladder; in successively cephalad slices, it takes a position anteromedial to the gallbladder fossa (Fig. 28). In some patients, however, particularly those with large inferior extension to the left

hepatic lobe, the hepatic flexure may cross completely inferior to the gallbladder fossa (Fig. 29). After cholecystectomy, the descending duodenum or the right colic flexure may occupy the space previously held by the gallbladder (Fig. 30). At the level of the gallbladder fossa, the peritoneal cavity extends between the anterolateral margin of the kidney and the opposed liver to form the hepatorenal fossa (Morrison's pouch). This posterior recess is frequently one of the first sites to be involved in peritoneal fluid collections (Fig. 31). Occasionally, however, the hepatic flexure of the colon may occupy this space. Distinction from a pathologic fluid collection may require additional scans, including the use of rectally administered contrast material or decubitus positioning (Fig. 32). The right colic flexure and proximal transverse colon are mobile structures and can occupy any portion of the greater peritoneal cavity surrounding the liver. Portions of the proximal transverse colon can be interposed between the anterior surface of the liver and the anterior body wall (Fig. 33). Less commonly, the proximal transverse colon may occupy the peritoneal space adjacent to the left

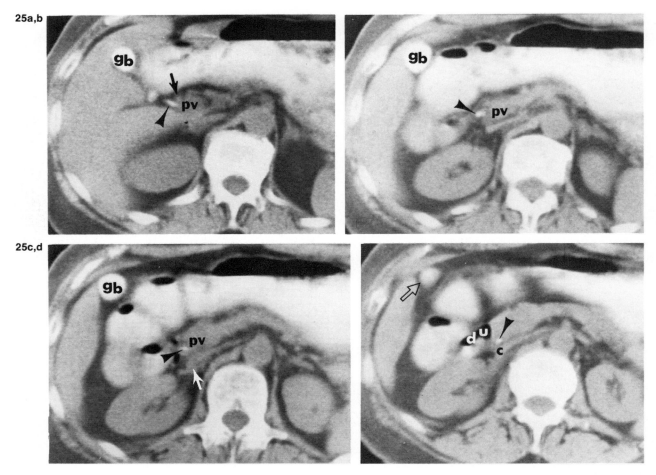

FIG. 25. Serial 1 cm caudal sections starting just below the neck of the gallbladder. **a:** A portion of the gallbladder (gb) is opacified due to previous cholecystographic examination. Several structures are imaged that lie in the cephalic portion of the hepatoduodenal ligament. Contrast-opacified common bile duct (arrowhead) is the most lateral and lies on the anterolateral surface of the portal vein (pv). The round structure immediately medial to the common bile duct is a portion of the proper hepatic artery (arrow). **b:** The common bile duct (arrowhead) has moved posteriorly with respect to the portal vein (pv) and now lies on its lateral aspect. **c:** The gallbladder (gb) now lies more anterior and lateral, and the common duct (arrowhead) is posterior to the portal vein (pv) and lies in the posterolateral margin of the head of the pancreas. Note its proximity to the confluence of the right renal vein and the inferior vena cava (white arrow). **d:** The fundus of the gallbladder (open arrow) is now imaged in its characteristic anterolateral position. At this level, the portal vein blends imperceptibly with the neck and head of the pancreas and cannot be differentiated without administration of intravenous contrast material. The common bile duct (arrowhead) lies on the posterolateral/surface of the head of the pancreas immediately medial to the duodenum (du). This section is obtained close to the level of the ampulla Vater. Note again the proximity of the common bile duct and the pancreas with the inferior vena cava (c).

lobe of the liver where it may mimic a pathologic collection within the lesser peritoneal space (Fig. 34).

AREA V: PANCREATIC HEAD

In most patients, the level of the head of the pancreas is in the same plane as the junction of the left renal vein with the inferior vena cava (7). The head and uncinate process of the pancreas have a great many important and complex relationships (19). Administration of oral, and at times intravenous, contrast material is invaluable in precisely defining anatomic structures in this region.

Directly posterior to the head of the pancreas is the inferior vena cava (Fig. 35). In most normal individuals, there is a well-defined retroperitoneal fat plane that separates the pancreatic head from the inferior vena cava. Within the most posterolateral aspect of the pancreatic head lies the water density common bile duct. Since it is small, and not greatly different from pancreatic parenchyma in attenuation, it is rarely seen on unenhanced scans through the pancreas. However, when intravenous contrast medium is administered, the attenuation difference between the enhanced pancreatic parenchyma and the unenhanced common bile duct permits visualization of the normal bile duct in the majority of patients. Immediately posterior to the body and neck of the pancreas is the splenic vein, which

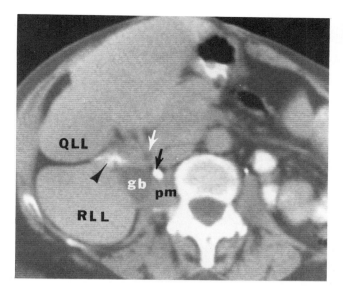

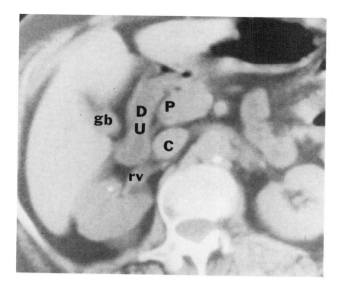

FIG. 26. Unusual anomaly in gallbladder position. The gall-bladder (gb) lies immediately lateral to the right psoas muscle (pm) and posterior to the duodenum (arrowhead). The common bile duct (white arrow) is in its characteristic position on the posterolateral surface of the pancreatic head. The right kidney, visible on more cephalic scans, was almost completely surrounded by hepatic tissue, so that the right ureter (black arrow), lying on the anterior surface of the psoas muscle, passes unusually close to the gallbladder. QLL, quadrate lobe of the liver; RLL, right lobe of the liver.

FIG. 27. The second portion of the duodenum (DU) passes posteriorly, medial to the neck of the gallbladder (gb), and lateral to the pancreatic head (P) and inferior vena cava (C). In this patient, the most posterior portion of the descending duodenum lies immediately anterior to the right renal vein (rv).

unites with the superior mesenteric vein to form the portal vein. In most patients there is no fat plane between the pancreatic neck and the origin of the portal vein (Fig. 36). Thus, when pancreatic masses are suspected in this region, it is particularly important to administer intravenous contrast medium to distinguish between a large portal vein and a pancreatic mass. A fat plane is present between the splenic vein and the body of the pancreas, which may resemble a dilated pancreatic duct; the normal pancreatic duct can be detected in an occasional patient if narrow collimation scans are obtained (1) (Fig. 37).

Posterior to the body of the pancreas, adjacent to the diaphragmatic crura on either side of the midline, lie the nerve fibers of the celiac ganglion, a large neural plexus (Fig. 38). The involvement of these nerve fibers, which are intimately related to the posterior surface of the pancreas, accounts for the back pain that so often accompanies pancreatic carcinoma.

Two to 3 cm inferior to the main portal vein there is

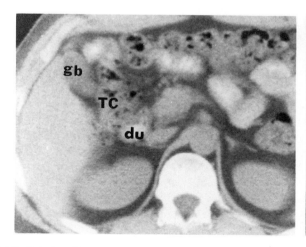

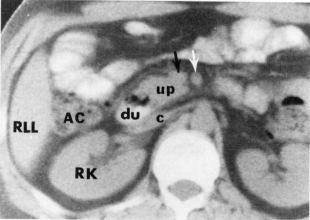

FIG. 28. Relationships of the right colic flexure. Left: The right colic flexure of the transverse colon (TC) lies between the fundus of the gallbladder (gb) and the duodenum (du). Right: The ascending colon is fixed in the anterior pararenal space anterior to the right kidney (RK) and medial to the right lobe of the liver (RLL). The black arrow points to the superior mesenteric vein; the white arrow points to the superior mesenteric artery. du, duodenum; up, uncinate process of the pancreas; c, inferior vena cava.

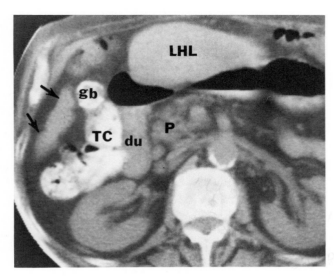

FIG. 29. Relationships of the right colic flexure in a patient with a large left hepatic lobe. CT scan through the fundus of the gallbladder. In this patient, the right colic flexure is oriented so that the transverse colon (TC) courses anteriorly immediately adjacent to the gallbladder fundus (gb). Note calcification in the wall of the gallbladder in this individual. The wavy appearance of the margin of the liver (black arrows) and the relative enlargement of the left hepatic lobe (LHL) were due to cirrhosis. du, duodenum; P, pancreas.

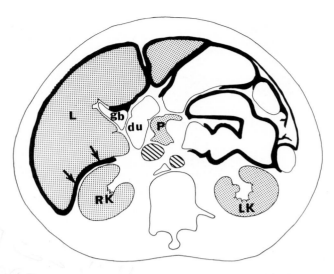

FIG. 31. Schematic diagram of the peritoneal spaces at the level of the gallbladder fossa. A long medial recess posterior to the right hepatic lobe (arrows) and anterolateral to the right kidney (RK) is the hepatorenal fossa (Morrison's pouch). L, liver; gb, gallbladder; du, duodenum; P, pancreas; LK, left kidney.

a posterior extension of pancreatic parenchyma (the uncinate process) whose wedge-shaped appearance is characteristic (Fig. 39). The superior mesenteric vein at this level, just proximal to its junction with the splenic vein, runs on the anterior surface of the uncinate process just to the right of the superior mesenteric artery. A well-defined fat plane between the superior mesenteric artery and the pancreatic body is com-

monly observed; its absence in all but the leanest patients suggests infiltration of the retropancreatic space by a pathologic process, usually pancreatic carcinoma.

This area also contains a portion of the ampullary segment of the common bile duct. Laterally, the pancreatic head is bordered by the descending duodenum. On occasion, the longitudinal fold of the duodenum may be identified and this aids in identifying the exact level of the major duodenal papilla (of Vater). Anteriorly, the pancreatic neck and body are related to either the posterior aspect of the stomach or the left hepatic

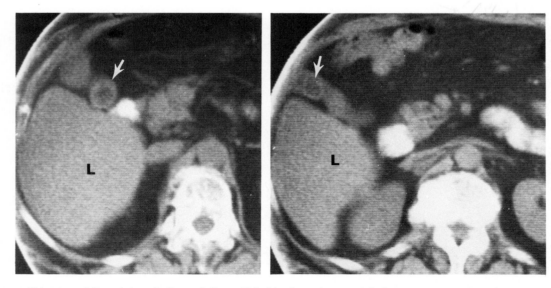

FIG. 30. Sequential scans at 2-cm intervals through the gallbladder fossa in a postcholecystectomy patient demonstrate the anterior portion of the right colic flexure (white arrow) occupying the gallbladder fossa. Particularly on the more caudal scan (right), if the prior surgical history were not known, cholelithiasis would be suspected. L, liver.

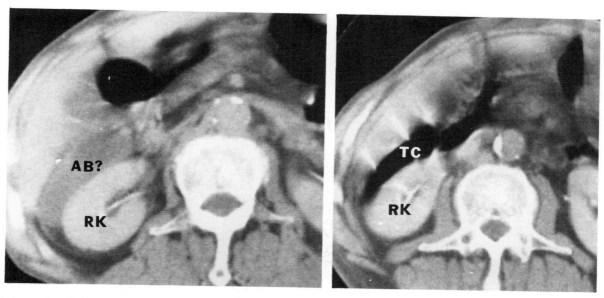

FIG. 32. Normal variation: the right colon within Morrison's pouch. **Left:** CT scan through the gallbladder fossa in a patient with a suspected postoperative abscess shows a near-water density collection (AB?) present within the hepatorenal fossa. **Right:** Repeat scan at the same level, with the patient in the left lateral decubitus position, shows intraluminal colonic gas displacing the fluid within the proximal transverse colon (TC). RK, right kidney.

lobe. Administration of intravenous contrast medium frequently identifies the gastroduodenal artery in cross-section on the anterolateral surface of the pancreas at the level of the portal vein (Fig. 40).

AREA VI: RENAL HILUS

The renal hila (Fig. 41) are at approximately the level of the first lumbar vertebra. The right hilus is

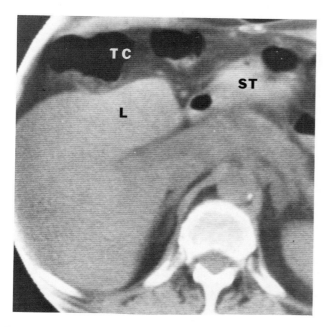

FIG. 33. Transverse colon (TC) interposed between the liver (L) and the anterior abdominal wall. ST, stomach.

generally at the same level as the left or 1 to 2 cm caudal to it. Each renal vein exits the hilus anterior to the renal arteries, although polar arteries may enter the renal parenchyma anterior to the renal vein. The left renal vein crosses between the superior mesenteric artery and the aorta 1 to 2 cm cephalic to the transverse duodenum. Particularly when the superior mesenteric artery lies relatively close to the aorta, the left renal vein may appear pinched and peripherally dilated; this sausage-like appearance should not be confused with renal vein thrombosis (Fig. 35b). Anomalies of venous drainage, including retroaortic or circumaortic left renal veins, are easily demonstrated by CT. The right renal artery passes posterior to the vena cava to enter the right renal hilus. Either artery may bifurcate before reaching the hilus and present a Y-shaped appearance within the sinus fat.

At the level of the renal hilus, the anterolateral aspect of the left kidney is related to the descending colon, which lies in the anterior pararenal space (Fig. 42). Loops of proximal jejunum are generally present immediately anterior to the left renal vein as it courses medially toward the aorta. The left renal vein then passes anterior to the anterior surface of the aorta, posterior to the superior mesenteric artery, and a portion of the uncinate process of the pancreas before entering the inferior vena cava. Similarly, the anterolateral aspect of the right kidney near the hilus is usually in direct apposition to the ascending colon or duodenum, whereas the right renal vein passes directly posterior to the descending duodenum. The right renal vein often runs an oblique craniomedial course toward

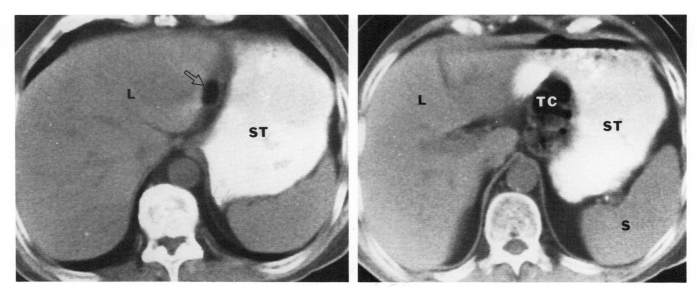

FIG. 34. Transverse colon medial to the left lobe of the liver. **Left:** Unusual air collection (open arrow) between the medial wall of the stomach (ST) and the lateral aspect of the left hepatic lobe (L). **Right:** Two centimeters caudal, air and fecal material are present within the lumen of the transverse colon (TC). Surgical exploration was performed for another cause; no abnormality was present in this area. L, liver; ST, stomach; S, spleen.

35a,b

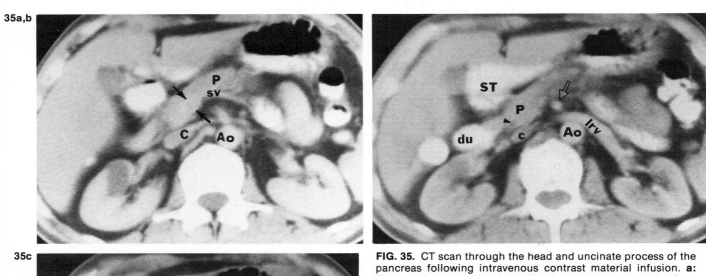

35c

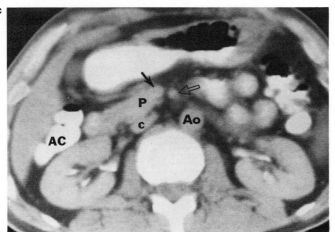

FIG. 35. CT scan through the head and uncinate process of the pancreas following intravenous contrast material infusion. **a:** The splenic vein (sv) lies immediately posterior to the body of the pancreas (P), joining the superior mesenteric vein (black arrows) behind the neck of the pancreas. No fat plane exists between the portal vein and the neck of the pancreas. **b:** Two centimeters caudal, the antrum of the stomach (ST) and the duodenum (du) lie lateral to the pancreatic head (P). The water density common bile duct (arrowhead) can be identified on the posterolateral surface of the head of the pancreas. The left renal vein (lrv) passes between the aorta (Ao) and the superior mesenteric artery (open arrow). Note that the caliber of the left renal vein to the left of the aorta is approximately three times the caliber of the vein to the right of the aorta. This normal finding is probably due to physiologic flattening of the left renal vein by compression between the aorta and superior mesenteric artery. **c:** Two centimeters caudal, the uncinate process of the pancreas (P) lies posterior to the superior mesenteric vein (black arrow) and immediately anterior to the inferior vena cava (c). AC, ascending colon; Ao, aorta.

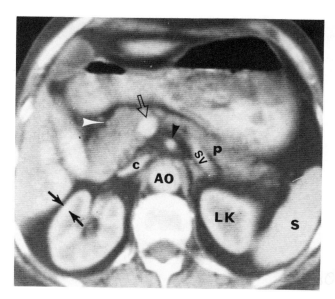

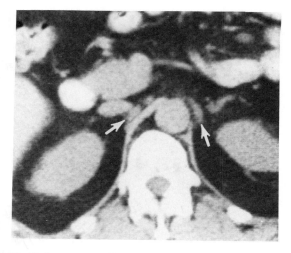

FIG. 36. Scan 30 sec after the administration of contrast medium demonstrates a fat plane between the splenic vein (sv) and the pancreatic tail (p); no fat plane is present between the superior mesenteric vein (open arrow) and the pancreas. The superior mesenteric artery (black arrowhead) is surrounded by retroperitoneal fat. The renal corticomedullary junction (black arrows) is well displayed. The white arrowhead points to the gastroduodenal artery. c, inferior vena cava; AO, aorta; LK, left kidney; S, spleen.

FIG. 38. Celiac ganglia. The neural fibers of the celiac ganglia lie between the right crus of the diaphragm and the inferior vena cava on the right and near the surface of the aorta on the left (white arrows).

the inferior vena cava; thus it is not seen in its entirety on a single scan in most individuals. On successively inferior scans, the descending colon remains on the anterolateral aspect of the renal fascia until well below the lower pole of the left kidney. The right colon, however, occupies a more medial position as scans approach the cecum.

At the level of the kidneys, the retroperitoneum is divided into three spaces: the anterior pararenal, the perirenal, and the posterior pararenal (10) (Fig. 43). Both kidneys are surrounded by an envelope of adipose tissue (perirenal fat). The extent of this fat deposit is limited by the renal fascia, the anterior portion of which is called Gerota's fascia. This fascia may be detected in some normal individuals, particularly on sections through the level of the renal hilus, where the renal fascia is perpendicular to the scanning plane (14) (Fig. 42). Thickening of the anterior portion of the fascia may occur in inflammatory diseases originating in the kidneys or in the pancreas, as well as in neoplastic processes affecting the retroperitoneum. The distribution of fat within the perirenal space differs consid-

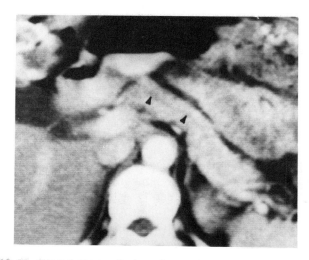

FIG. 37. Normal pancreatic duct. Scan following intravenous contrast enhancement demonstrates a normal pancreatic duct (arrowheads) in the body and tail.

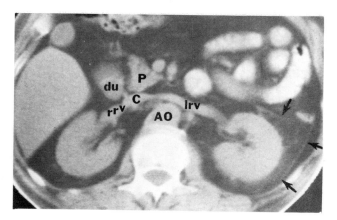

FIG. 39. Scan through the confluence of the renal veins (rrv, lrv) with the inferior vena cava (C). The wedge-shaped uncinate process (P) is well seen, as are the anterior and posterior renal fascia (black arrows) outlining the perirenal space. AO, aorta; du, duodenum.

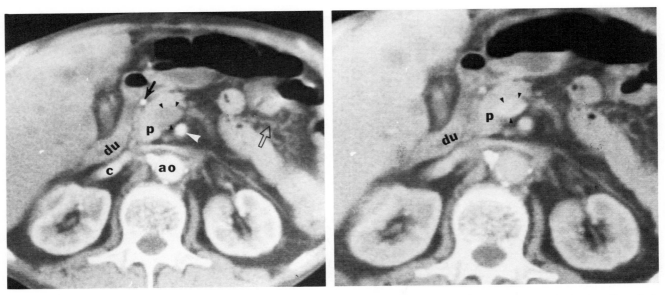

FIG. 40. Vascular anatomy of the region of the head of the pancreas. **Left:** Scan through the neck of the pancreas 15 sec after a bolus injection of contrast medium. The gastroduodenal artery (black arrow) on the anterolateral aspect of the pancreas (p) is well opacified. There is enhancement of pancreatic parenchyma but contrast is not yet present within the superior mesenteric vein (black arrowheads). White arrowhead indicates the superior mesenteric artery; open arrow indicates a branch of the superior mesenteric artery within the jejunal mesentery. **Right:** Fifteen seconds later, contrast medium has now opacified the superior mesenteric vein (arrowheads). du, duodenum; p, pancreas.

erably from individual to individual but, in general, the largest quantity of fat is deposited laterally and slightly posterior to the lower pole of either kidney.

The anterior renal (Gerota's) fascia delimits the posterior border of the anterior pararenal space, which contains the pancreas, duodenum, and both the ascending and descending colon. This space is also continuous with the root of the transverse mesocolon and the root of the mesentery. Lateral to the kidneys, the anterior and posterior renal fascia fuse to form the lateroconal fascia, which separates the perirenal fat from the flank fat. The latter, which forms the familiar

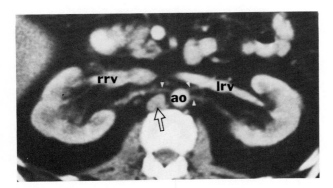

FIG. 41. Contrast-enhanced scan through the renal hila. A single right renal artery and two left renal arteries are indicated by arrowheads. The normal renal veins (rrv, lrv) are larger and more anterior than the renal arteries. Note the prominent inferior portion of the right diaphragmatic crus (open arrow), which should not be confused with an enlarged lymph node. ao, aorta.

flank stripe seen on plain radiography, is continuous with the posterior pararenal space. The posterior pararenal space contains no retroperitoneal organs. Although in most patients it extends as far medially as the psoas muscles, in others it may extend medially only as far as the quadratus lumborum muscles. Medially, the anterior and posterior renal fascia do not form a well-defined anatomic boundary, but fuse with the adventitia of the aorta and inferior vena cava (17). This fusion effectively separates the two perirenal spaces from each other, although cases of communication of the two perirenal spaces across the midline have been reported (19).

Medial to both kidneys and separated from them by the perirenal fat lie the triangular shaped upper sections of the psoas muscles, which attach to anterior portions of vertebral bodies and intervertebral discs. At this level, also, the most inferior slips of the right crus of the diaphragm attach to the anterior surfaces of the L-1 or L-2 vertebral bodies. The wedge-shaped appearance of the crus should not be mistaken for a pathologic process such as an enlarged lymph node (2). Sequential scans obtained immediately above the area will demonstrate its continuity with the remainder of the right crus of the diaphragm. Another potential pitfall is the psoas minor muscle and tendon, present in about 40% of the population and likely to be hypertrophied in young athletic individuals, which appear as a bulge of soft tissue attenuation on the anterior surface of the upper psoas muscle (Fig. 44).

42a,b

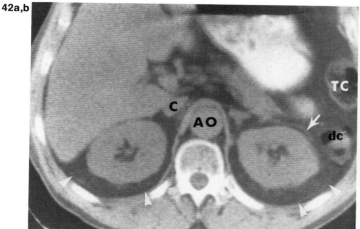
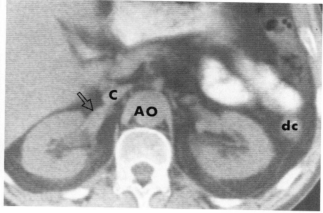

42c

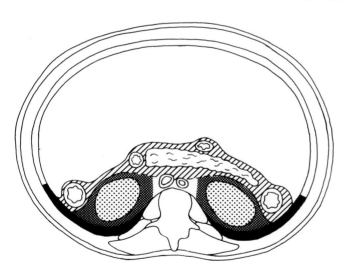

FIG. 42. The renal fascia and perirenal spaces. **a:** Scan 2 cm cephalic to the renal hila. The anterior renal fascia (white arrow) is easily seen on the left. The posterior renal fascia (white arrowheads) is bilaterally well imaged. Both the distal transverse colon (TC) and proximal descending colon (dc) are imaged on this scan. **b:** Scan at the renal hila. The largest accumulation of perirenal fat in this patient, as in most, is posteromedial and slightly caudal to the hila. Open arrow points to a portion of the right renal vein. **c:** Two centimeters caudal to the renal hila, the proximal ureters (black arrows) are within the perirenal space at this level. Note that the most medial extension of the posterior pararenal space (white arrowheads) is lateral to the psoas and quadratus lumborum muscles. The full extent of the left renal vein is well seen at this level (open arrow). dc, descending colon; C, inferior vena cava; AO, aorta; TC, transverse colon.

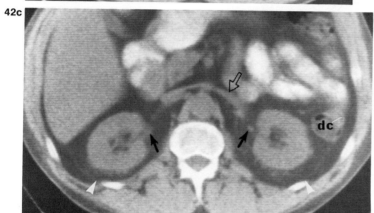

FIG. 43. Schematic diagram of the perirenal and pararenal spaces. The posterior pararenal space (solid black), which contains no retroperitoneal organs, has a variable medial extent and is anteriorly continuous with the flank stripe. The anterior pararenal space (lined) contains the ascending and descending colon, the duodenum, and the pancreas. The perirenal space (cross-hatched) contains a variable quantity of fat, the adrenal gland, the kidney, and proximal ureter. Its medial boundary is not well defined; the renal fascia tends to fuse with the adventitia of the aorta and inferior vena cava. (Modified from Love et al., ref. 10.)

AREA VII: MESENTERY AND SMALL BOWEL

Between the level of the renal hila and the aortic bifurcation, sections of the abdomen display the small bowel and mesentery centrally, with portions of the ascending colon and cecum on the right and descending colon on the left.

On the most cephalic section in this area (Fig. 45), the superior mesenteric artery and vein are evident as side-by-side circular structures of blood density coursing anterior to the transverse duodenum. The origin of the inferior mesenteric artery can be identified at or slightly caudal to the level of the horizontal (third) and ascending (fourth) portions of the duodenum. Jejunal and ileal mesenteric vessels can be noted but not precisely identified within the mesentery (Fig. 46). On occasion, the blood vessels may be traced to the wall of the bowel, thus identifying the mesenteric and antimesenteric surfaces of a single loop. Considerable fat may be present in the root of the mesentery at this level, causing apparent widening of the duodenal loop on routine barium studies.

The psoas muscles originate on the lateral surface of the vertebral bodies and intervertebral discs beginning at the level of the renal hilus and are somewhat more

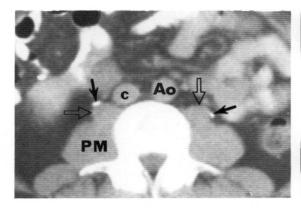

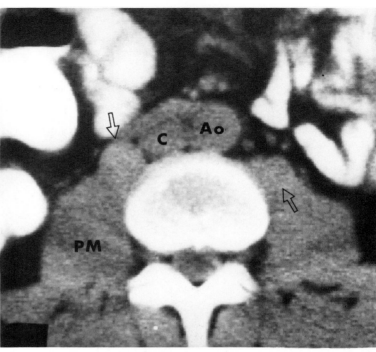

FIG. 44. Psoas minor muscles. **Left:** Scan at level of the L3 vertebral body shows bilateral, slightly asymmetric soft tissue densities (open arrows), due to well-formed psoas minor muscles, anterior to the psoas major muscles (PM). Note the relationship of the ureters (black arrows) to these muscles. c, inferior vena cava; Ao, aorta. **Right:** Another patient with unusually prominent and slightly asymmetric psoas minor muscles (open arrows). PM, right psoas major muscle; C, inferior vena cava; Ao, aorta.

prominent at the level of the horizontal duodenum. On subsequent caudal sections, the muscles become symmetrically broader but maintain their orientation to the adjacent vertebral bodies and intervertebral discs (Fig. 47). Posteromedially, adjacent to the vertebral body, are the tendinous arches of the psoas muscles, which transmit the spinal nerves and ascending lumbar vein (Fig. 48). The ureters lie just anterior to the psoas muscles. On scans obtained near the pelviureteric junction, they are on the lateral aspect of the psoas but migrate medially on more caudal scans. The

tiny gonadal artery and larger gonadal vein accompany the ureter on the anterior surface of the psoas muscles on sections obtained between the origin of the inferior mesenteric artery and the aortic bifurcation. The veins cannot be identified on the CT scan in most normal individuals. Occasionally, enlargement of one or both gonadal veins permits easy identification (Fig. 49).

As is well known from lymphangiography, the region between the aortic bifurcation and the renal hila contains a rich plexus of periaortic and pericaval lymph vessels and nodes. Normal lymph nodes are

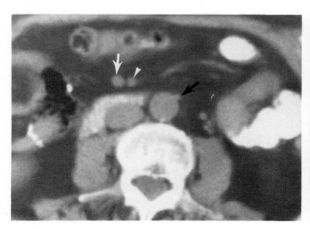

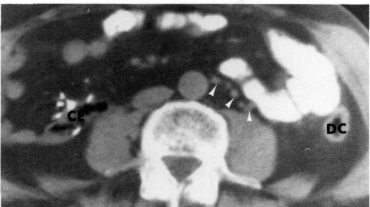

FIG. 45. Normal anatomic structures at the level of the third portion of the duodenum. **Left:** The superior mesenteric vein (white arrow) and artery (white arrowhead) are easily identified, as is the origin of the inferior mesenteric artery (black arrow). **Right:** Two centimeters caudal, the left colic branches of the inferior mesenteric artery (white arrowheads) are seen. The descending colon (DC) remains laterally placed, whereas the cecum (CE) lies somewhat more medial just lateral to the psoas major muscle.

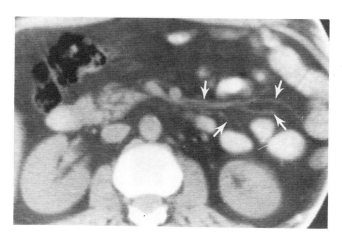

FIG. 46. Tributaries of the superior mesenteric vein (white arrows) drain segments of the jejunum, thus identifying the root of the small bowel mesentery.

less than 1.5 cm in cross-sectional diameter and they lie in any position directly related to the aorta or inferior vena cava. Since a plethora of small vascular structures is present in this region, normal lymph nodes may not be identified with certainty unless a previous lymphangiogram has been performed (Fig.

50). However, there is no normal structure in the immediate vicinity of the inferior vena cava or aorta, which exceeds 1.5 cm in diameter. Thus, if a structure larger than 1.5 cm with an attenuation near soft tissue is seen in this region, lymphadenopathy can be confidently suggested.

On the most caudal sections of the mesentery and small bowel, the cecum and ileocecal valve may be demonstrated. At this level or slightly lower, an indentation is seen in the posteromedial surface of each psoas muscle, well outlined by retroperitoneal fat in most patients. This contains the nerves of the lumbar plexus, which will give rise to the femoral and obturator nerves; in addition, the lumbar arteries and the ascending lumbar vein may be observed (Fig. 51).

AREA VIII: AORTIC-CAVAL BIFURCATION

The aorta bifurcates into the right and left common iliac arteries 1 to 2 cm cephalic to the bifurcation of the inferior vena cava. As the right common iliac artery passes across the midline, it pursues a course directly anterior to the inferior vena cava (Fig. 52). It is often possible in older individuals to identify the common iliac artery and its major branches by the presence of

47a,b

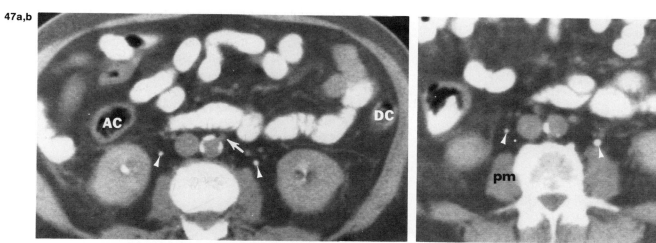

47c

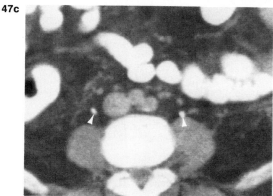

FIG. 47. The inferior mesenteric artery. **a:** Scan at the origin of the inferior mesenteric artery (white arrow). The ureters (arrowheads) exit the perirenal space to lie near the anterolateral surface of the psoas muscles. The ascending colon (AC) lies considerably more medial than the descending colon (DC). Small bowel containing contrast material lies lateral to the ascending colon, a normal variation. **b:** Two centimeters caudal, the ureters (arrowheads) have migrated somewhat medially. The psoas muscles (pm) are slightly wider than on the previous scan. **c:** Two centimeters more caudal, the contour of the psoas muscles is now almost circular. The perirenal space is present at this level, caudal to the lower pole of the kidney, posteromedial to the ascending and descending colon. A variable amount of fat is contained within these spaces. The ureters (white arrowheads) maintain their anteromedial relationship to the psoas muscles.

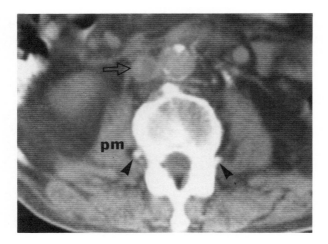

FIG. 48. Ascending lumbar veins. Contrast-enhanced CT scan in a patient with inferior vena cava thrombosis. Partially recanalized lumen of the inferior vena cava can be seen laterally (open arrow). Medial and posterior to the psoas muscles (pm) lie the paired ascending lumbar veins (black arrowheads), larger than normal because of the caval obstruction, which here serve as collateral pathways for blood return from the lower extremities.

intimal calcification. On slightly lower sections, the left common iliac vein passes from right to left posterior to the right common iliac artery. At this level, a portion of the superior aspect of the sacroiliac joint is usually seen. As an external landmark, the depression in the anterior surface of the body wall formed by the umbilicus is often visible at this level.

AREA IX: PELVIC INLET

Male

On this and on all other pelvic sections there is a variety of changes in the musculoskeletal structures supporting the pelvic viscera (9). The level of each section is most easily identified by the appearance of the pelvic bones, and thus the anatomic discussion of each section will begin with a brief description of the musculoskeletal structures.

On sections through the lower aspect of the sacroiliac joint (Fig. 53), the sacrum slants rather abruptly posteriorly, greatly increasing the distance between it

49a,b

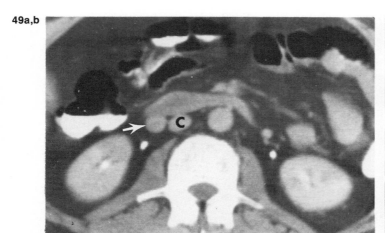

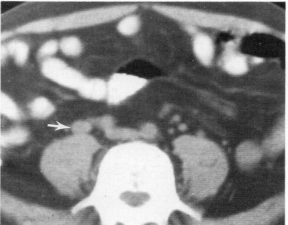

49c

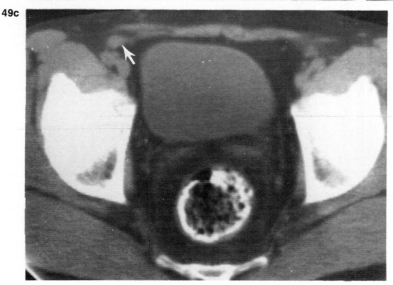

FIG. 49. Normal course of the gonadal vessels illustrated in a patient with an enlarged gonadal vein. **a:** Scan at the level of the third portion of the duodenum shows a soft tissue density (arrow), an enlarged right gonadal vein, to the right of the inferior vena cava (C). Note the relationship of this vein with the right ureter. **b:** Four centimeters caudal, the gonadal vein (arrow) lies on the anterior surface of the psoas muscle, paralleling the course of the ureter. **c:** Scan through the inguinal canal shows the gonadal vein (arrow) passing anteriorly into the spermatic cord.

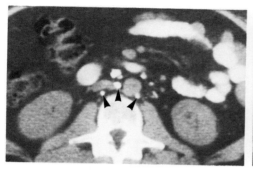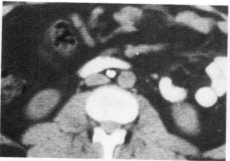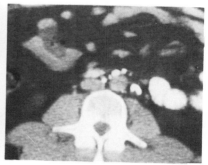

FIG. 50. Normal lymph nodes opacified by a previous lymphangiogram. **Left:** Immediately caudal to the renal hila, lymph nodes (black arrowheads) are seen surrounding the inferior vena cava and aorta. **Center and Right:** Serial caudal scans obtained at 2-cm intervals demonstrate variability in number and distribution of normal lymph nodes.

and the psoas muscle. On this section, the iliacus muscle is well formed, and the fat plane between the iliacus and the psoas is considerably smaller than on more cephalic sections; on more caudal sections, these muscles merge and become indistinguishable. There is an oblique fat-containing cleft on the anterolateral surface of the psoas muscle on this and on subsequent caudal sections. This represents the psoas tendon and is anterior and medial to the course of the femoral nerve. On the medial aspect of the psoas muscle, the common iliac artery lies somewhat anterior to the common iliac vein. At this level, it is occasionally possible to see the origin of the internal iliac (hypogastric) artery curving posteriorly medial to the common iliac vein (Fig. 54). The course of the internal iliac artery is quite variable; its firm identification may be aided by the administration of intravenous contrast medium. The lumbosacral nerve trunk may frequently be identified just lateral to the body of the sacrum. It is a structure with attenuation value intermediate between fat and soft tissue. The remainder of the midportion of the pelvic inlet is

occupied by loops of small bowel; laterally the cecum and descending colon are observed.

On slightly lower sections, the pyriformis muscles are observed extending obliquely between the body of the sacrum through the greater sciatic foramen. On the anterolateral surface of this muscle rests the internal iliac artery and vein (Fig. 55). Indentations for sacral nerves are observed on the anterior surface of this muscle. The sigmoid colon is frequently observed on this scan, passing in a sinuous fashion posteriorly from a position anteromedial to the iliacus muscle. It finally takes up a position very close to the midline immediately anterior to the body of the sacrum, where it reenters the retroperitoneum and becomes the rectum. A rich plexus of arteries and veins surrounds the rectum at all levels.

At this area, there is usually a clear division of the major arteries in the pelvis into three geographical groups (Fig. 56). Anteriorly, the external iliac artery and vein are related to the medial aspect of the iliopsoas muscle. Posteriorly, on the anterolateral surface of the pyriformis muscles, lie the internal iliac artery and vein. Between them, related to the medial aspect of the obturator internus muscle, are the obturator artery and vein, the ureter, and the periureteral vessels. This relationship continues throughout the more caudal scans of the pelvis. The inferior epigastric vessels, posterior to the rectus abdominis, are seen infrequently, whereas the superficial epigastric veins are more commonly observed in cross-section within the subcutaneous tissue of the anterior abdominal wall (Fig. 57).

Female

With minor exceptions, musculoskeletal landmarks described for the male pelvic inlet are identical in females at the level of the pelvic brim. The anteroposterior dimension of the pelvis in women is larger than the side-to-side dimension. In female subjects, fat

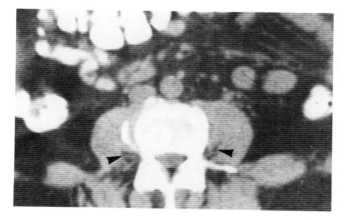

FIG. 51. A fat-containing cleft (arrowheads) is present on the posteromedial aspect of the psoas muscle, containing nerve fibers of the lumbar plexus as well as the ascending lumbar veins. These fibers will form the femoral and obturator nerves.

52a,b

52c,d

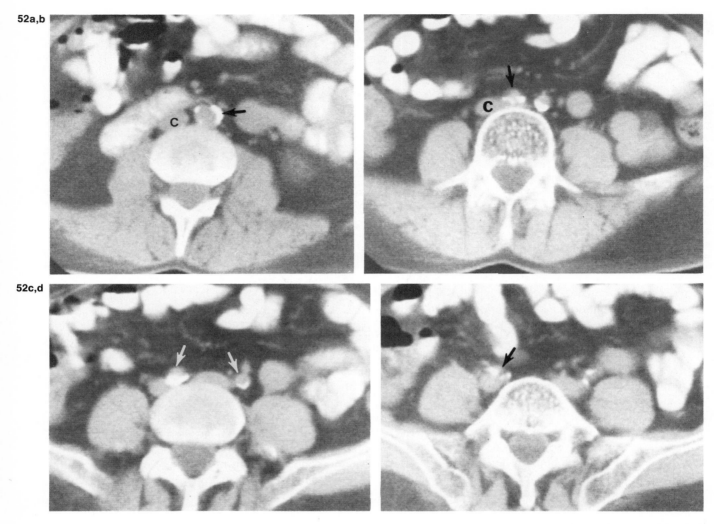

FIG. 52. Normal anatomy of the aortic and caval bifurcations. **a:** Scan through the transverse duodenum shows peripheral calcification (arrow) within the aorta just proximal to its bifurcation. The inferior vena cava (C) is slightly flattened anteriorly by the duodenum. **b:** Two centimeters caudal, the right common iliac artery (arrow) passes just anterior to the inferior vena cava (C). The peripherally calcified iliac arteries are much smaller in di- ameter than the aorta. **c:** Two centimeters caudal, the inferior vena cava has divided into the right and left common iliac veins, which maintain a position to the right and posterior to the iliac arteries (white arrows). **d:** Two centimeters caudal, the iliac arteries (arrow) have taken a position almost directly anterior to the iliac veins.

is usually deposited in the subcutaneous tissues, whereas in men, fat accumulation is predominantly deep to the transversalis fascia. No other appreciable differences are present at this level.

AREA X: ACETABULAR ROOF

Male

On this section, the ilium is a flask-shaped structure whose long axis is directed anterolaterally. On cephalic sections, the iliac wing extended posteriorly to the sacral ala; here, its posterior extent is 5 to 6 cm anterior to the body of the sacrum. The pyriformis muscle, well seen at this level, fills in the intervening space (the greater sciatic foramen) (Fig. 58). On the posteromedial aspect of the ilium, a small part of the obturator internus muscle is seen; the iliopsoas muscles have coursed somewhat more anterior and lateral. The rectus abdominis muscles form the greater portion of the anterior body wall.

Unless medically contraindicated, all patients receiving CT studies of the pelvis are examined with distended urinary bladders. Contrast medium may also be instilled to opacify the urine within the bladder. For this reason, the bladder dome is almost always visible at the level of the acetabular roof. At this level, the bladder occupies a relatively anterior position in the pelvis. The dorsal aspect of the bladder is rarely posterior to the posterior border of the obturator internus

53a,b

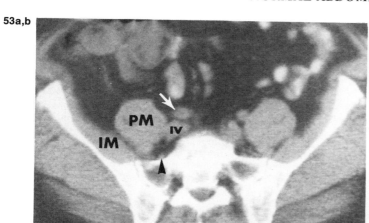

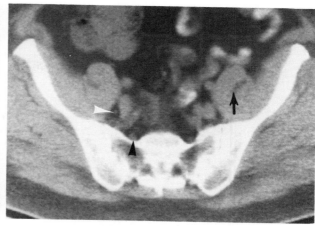

53c

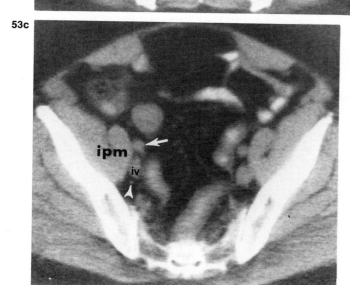

FIG. 53. Serial scans through the pelvic inlet in a normal male. **a:** The surface of the body of S1 lies anterior to the dorsal aspect of the psoas muscles (PM). On this section, the right common iliac artery (white arrow) and vein (iv) lie just medial to the psoas muscle. The iliac muscle (IM) is separated from the psoas by the fat plane. The lumbosacral trunk (arrowhead) lies just lateral to the sacral body. **b:** One centimeter caudal, the sacral body lies posterior to the dorsal surfaces of the psoas muscle. The fat plane between the iliacus and the psoas muscles is no longer present. Fat is present within the psoas tendon (black arrow), which at this level is just anterior to the femoral nerve. The obturator nerve (white arrowhead) and lumbosacral trunk (black arrowhead) are prominent in this subject. **c:** One centimeter caudal, the distance between the sacrum and the iliopsoas (ipm) is greatly increased, but the relative positions of the iliopsoas muscle and the external iliac artery (white arrow), vein (iv), and obturator nerve (white arrowhead) are unchanged.

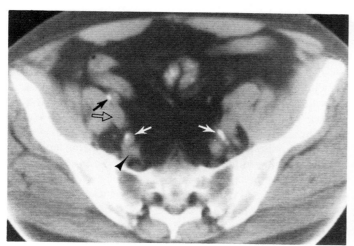

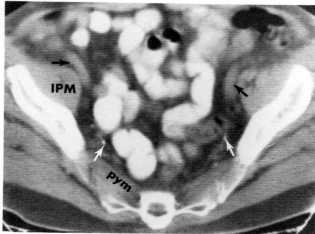

FIG. 54. Normal internal iliac artery. **Left:** In this subject the internal iliac arteries (white arrows) are calcified and their course medial and posterior to the external iliac vein (open arrow) is thus easily followed. They are accompanied by the larger internal iliac veins (black arrowhead). Black arrow points to the external iliac artery. **Right:** Two centimeters caudal, the internal iliac arteries (white arrows) have passed posterolaterally to lie on the ventral surface of the pyriformis muscle (pym). On the same section, the external iliac arteries (black arrows) curve anterolaterally to lie adjacent to the iliopsoas muscle (IPM).

55a

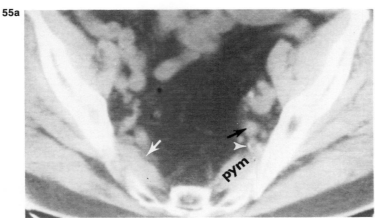

FIG. 55. Normal relationships of the pyriformis muscle. **a:** Section through the pelvic inlet shows that the internal iliac artery (white arrowhead) and vein (black arrow) lie on the anterolateral surface of the pyriformis muscle (pym). An indentation in the right pyriformis muscle (white arrow) contains a sacral nerve. **b:** One centimeter caudal, the pyriformis muscle (pym) extends from the anterior margin of the sacrum to the posterior surface of the ilium. At this level, the sigmoid colon, identified by the presence of numerous diverticula, passes posteromedially toward the rectum. **c:** One centimeter caudal, the pyriformis muscle (pym) exits the pelvis through the greater sciatic foramen. It is accompanied on its anterolateral surface by the sciatic nerve.

55b,c

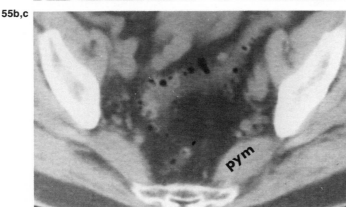
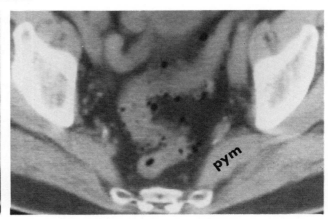

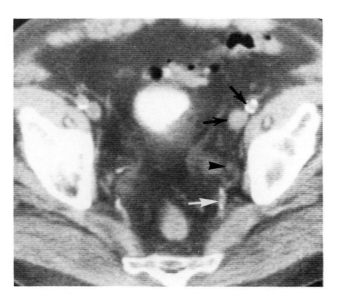

FIG. 56. Division of major pelvic vessels. Three groups of vessels are displayed. An anterior division, medial to the iliopsoas muscle, is the external iliac artery and vein (black arrows). These exit the pelvis below the inguinal ligament. A posterior division, the internal iliac artery and vein (white arrow), lie on the pyriformis muscle. Branches of these vessels exit through the greater sciatic foramen. A middle division (black arrowhead), comprising the obturator branch of the internal iliac artery and tiny periureteral vessels, lies just medial to the obturator internus muscle. The obturator vessels exit through the obturator canal.

muscle. Directly posterior to the bladder, encased in retroperitoneal fat, is the rectum, accompanied by small branches of the superior rectal (hemorrhoidal) arteries and veins. A few loops of distal ileum may be present on the right, anterior to the dome of the bladder. On occasion, these loops may indent the lateral aspect of the bladder wall and suggest a pathologic process. The ureters are visible on the posterolateral aspect of the bladder and continue this relationship caudally to the uretero-vesicle junction.

There is usually sufficient perivesicle fat to separate the urinary bladder from the pelvic side wall. The attenuation value of urine varies with its specific gravity; that is, the higher the specific gravity, the higher the attenuation value. In a well-hydrated patient, the density of urine approaches that of water. The bladder wall can be distinguished from its lumen on the noncontrast scans and measures approximately 1 to 2 mm in thickness when the bladder is adequately distended.

Anteriorly, the spermatic cord is present on this section superficial to the deep inguinal ring and lateral to the rectus abdominis muscles (8) (Fig. 59). Internal to the deep inguinal ring, the ductus deferens can be seen passing directly posterior just medial to the external iliac artery and vein en route to the medial aspect of the prostate (Fig. 60). On this section, the

57a,b

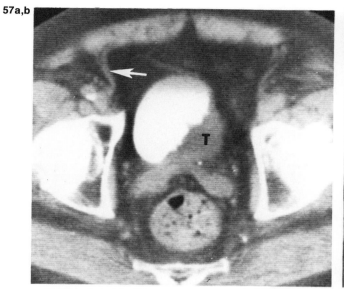

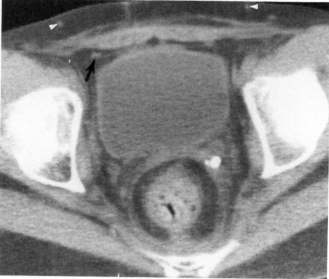

57c

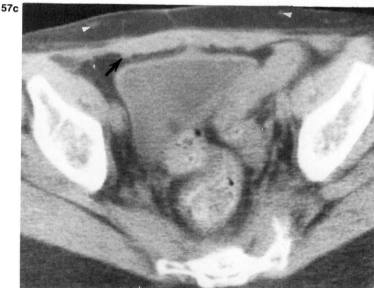

FIG. 57. Inferior epigastric vessels. **a:** The inferior epigastric vein (arrow) drains into the external iliac vein and arcs medial to the deep inguinal ring. The left lateral wall of the bladder in this patient is infiltrated with a large transitional cell carcinoma (T). **b:** In a different patient, the inferior epigastric artery (arrow) is noted posterior to the undersurface of the rectus abdominis muscle. **c:** Two centimeters above b, the vessels enter the rectus sheath and blend with the soft tissue density of the muscle itself. Arrowheads point to the superficial epigastric veins.

pyriformis muscle lies on the posterior aspect of the ilium, having passed through the greater sciatic foramen. On the anteromedial aspect of the pyriformis muscle lies the sciatic nerve, which likewise exits the pelvis through the greater sciatic foramen. On occasion, the inferior gluteal vessels may be seen lying on the anterior surface of the gluteus maximus muscle.

On somewhat more caudal sections, the thin coccygeus muscle crosses anterior to the pyriformis muscle. The internal pudendal and the inferior gluteal vessels may be seen in the narrow space between them. The seminal vesicles (Fig. 61) are positioned immediately posterior to the bladder above the uretero-vesicle junction. These bilateral, lobulated sacs, consisting of irregular pouches, measure approximately 5 cm in length and converge in the midline with the ductus

deferens forming the ejaculatory duct. The seminal vesicles usually can be seen on pelvic CT scans obtained at 1-cm intervals, appearing as a pair of oval-shaped structures of soft tissue attenuation value. A short segment of the ductus deferens often can be seen as a linear structure oriented in the anterioposterior direction lateral to the seminal vesicle; they may be traced anteriorly toward the deep inguinal ring. With the patient supine, the seminal vesicles are clearly separated from the posterior bladder wall by adipose tissue in all but the leanest patients. With the patient prone, the fat plane between the seminal vesicles and the bladder is flattened and the normal seminal vesicle angle is obliterated. The seminal vesicles are quite variable in size; in general, older patients have smaller seminal vesicles than younger patients.

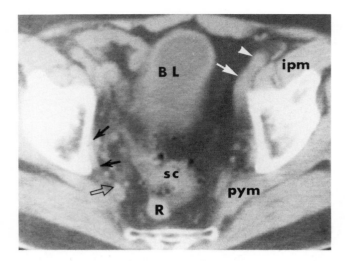

FIG. 58. Normal anatomy at the level of the acetabular roof. The iliopsoas muscle (ipm) has taken a position anterior to the supraacetabular portion of the ilium. Retaining their position anteromedial to the iliopsoas are the external iliac artery (white arrowhead) and vein (white arrow). The pyriformis muscle (pym) has exited the pelvis and will subsequently insert on the greater trochantor of the femur. Branches of the internal iliac vessels (open arrow) lie close to its medial surface. The obturator internus muscle (black arrows) is present at this level; the ureter and obturator vessels lie medial to it. BL, bladder; sc, sigmoid colon; R, rectum.

On occasion the obliterated umbilical artery (medial umbilical ligament) may be seen crossing the ligamentum teres or ductus deferns coursing anteromedially toward the umbilicus (Fig. 62). In an occasional patient, a thin linear midline structure is present at the same level, which represents the urachus (median umbilical ligament).

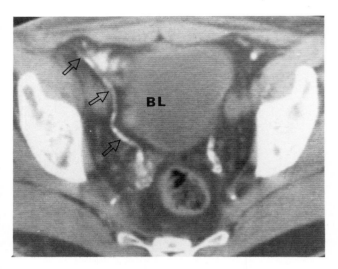

FIG. 60. Ductus deferens. CT scan in a patient with a calcified ductus deferens at the level of the internal inguinal ring demonstrates the vas as a linear structure (open arrows) passing posteriorly just medial to the external iliac artery and vein. More posteriorly, it arcs medially toward its attachment to the medial aspect of the prostate. BL, bladder.

Female

Again, because subjects are examined with a bladder distended at least moderately, the uterus is displaced somewhat cranially and the fundus is usually seen at this level (Fig. 63). The adult postpubertal uterus measures about 7 cm in length, 5 cm in width, and 3 cm in anteroposterior diameter. Although its size is highly variable, the uterus is usually slightly larger in multiparous women. The normal uterus has a uniform soft tissue density. Not uncommonly, the ligamentum

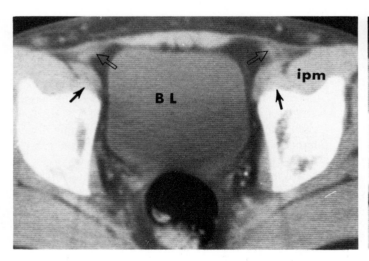

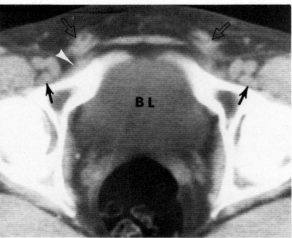

FIG. 59. Normal anatomy of the inguinal canals. **Left:** Scan through the level of the deep inguinal ring. The soft tissue density lateral and deep to the internal oblique muscle represents the spermatic cord (open arrows). It is not infrequent for an undescended testis to be found at this level. Black arrows point to iliopsoas tendon; BL, bladder; ipm, iliopsoas muscle. **Right:** Two centimeters caudal, the spermatic cord (open arrows) has exited the deep inguinal ring and lies within the inguinal canal, immediately anterior to the pectineus muscle (white arrowhead). Note the more medial position of the spermatic cord compared to left scan. Black arrows point to the psoas tendon; BL, bladder.

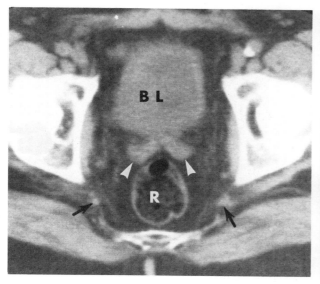 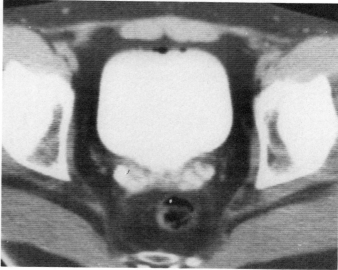

FIG. 61. Seminal vesicle anatomy. **Left:** The seminal vesicles (white arrowheads) are paired, oval structures oriented at approximately 30° to the base of the bladder (BL). There is, therefore, a wedge of perivesicular fat between the vesicles and the bladder. Obliteration of this fat plane would suggest infiltration by a pathologic process. At this level, the gas- and feces-filled rectum (R) is immediately posterior to the seminal vesicles. Caudally, the median lobe of the prostate is related to the central portions of the seminal vesicles. Black arrows point to the inferior gluteal vessels. **Right:** This subject has residual contrast medium from a prior seminal vesiculogram. The convoluted nature of the seminal vesicles is easily appreciated.

teres (round ligament) of the uterus, occupying an analogous anatomic position to the ductus deferens in males, may be seen coursing posteriorly from the inguinal canal to insert on the lateral border of the uterine fundus. Immediately cephalic to this insertion is the ovarian ligament, which is usually not seen on CT scans, but is close to the medial pole of the ovary (Fig. 64). The ovary most commonly lies just lateral and somewhat posterior to the uterine fundus immediately cephalic to the insertion of the ligamentum teres. However, it is quite mobile and need not be present in its expected location.

Sections obtained more caudally demonstrate the rich plexus of vessels (including the uterine, vesical, and vaginal arteries and veins) within the parametrium. The broad ligament itself, which encloses these vessels, is only occasionally seen (Fig. 65).

In both men and women, there is a rich plexus of lymphatic vessels and nodes surrounding the external iliac vessels. Lateral and anterior to the external iliac artery lies the lateral chain; posterior and medial to the external iliac vein is the medial chain; an intermediate or middle chain lies between the two. In normal subjects, it is difficult to distinguish lymph nodes from small vascular structures reliably unless a previous lymphangiogram has been performed.

AREA XI: SYMPHYSIS PUBIS

Male

On sections through the symphysis pubis, the head, neck, and greater trochanter of the femur are normally well imaged (Fig. 66). Posteromedially, the acetabular portion of the ischium is present. There is a separation between the pubis and the ischium at this level, which

FIG. 62. Medial and median umbilical ligaments. Obliquely to the vas deferens (black arrows), the superior vesicle branch of the internal iliac artery (white arrowheads) passes medially toward the posterior aspect of the rectus abdominis muscle. Its most anterior extension is the obliterated umbilical artery (medial umbilical ligament). The midline soft tissue density (open arrow) represents the urachus (median umbilical ligament). sc, sigmoid colon; R, rectum.

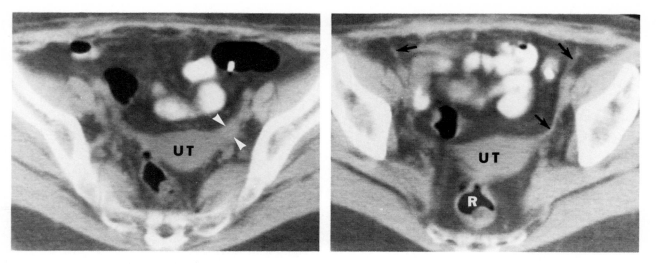

FIG. 63. Normal round ligaments. **Left:** Scan through the uterine fundus (UT) demonstrates the left ovary (white arrowheads) within the ovarian fossa. **Right:** One centimeter caudal, both round ligaments (black arrows), which have the same course as the vas deferens in males, are evident. R, rectum.

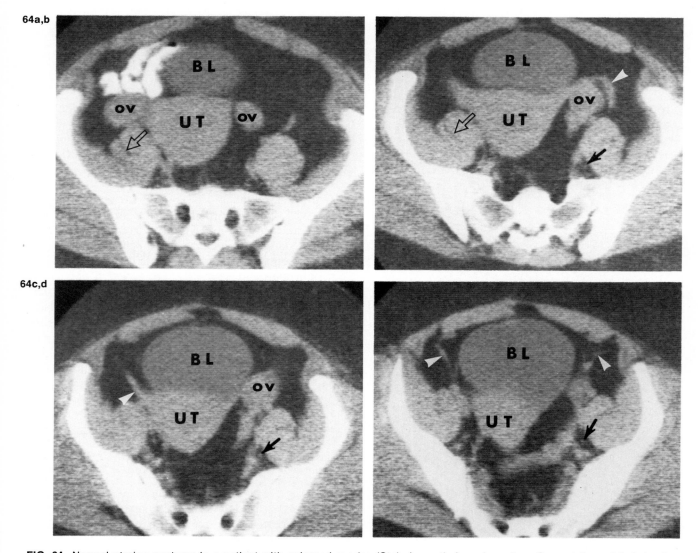

64a,b

64c,d

FIG. 64. Normal uterine anatomy in a patient with enlarged ovaries (Stein-Leventhal syndrome). **a:** Scan at the pelvic brim demonstrates both ovaries (ov) adjacent to the uterine fundus (UT). The dome of the urine-distended bladder (BL) is seen anteriorly. **b:** One centimeter caudal, a segment of the left fallopian tube (arrowhead) is present. **c:** One centimeter caudal, the right round ligament (arrowhead) is imaged near its junction with the uterus. **d:** One centimeter caudal, the anterior segment of both round ligaments (arrowheads) is present. BL, bladder; UT, uterus; ov, ovary; black arrow, obturator nerve; open arrow, psoas tendon.

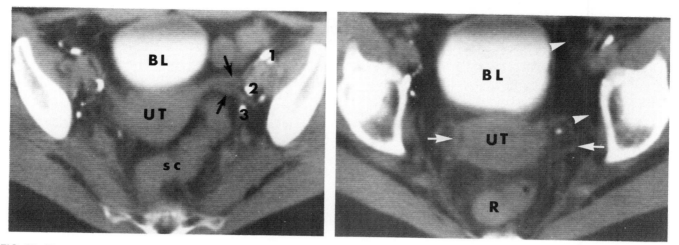

FIG. 65. The broad ligament and normal pelvic lymph nodes. **Left:** Scan in a woman following a normal lymphangiogram shows three chains of external iliac nodes: a lateral chain (1), anterior to the external iliac artery; a middle chain (2), posterior to the external iliac vein; and a medial chain (3), the obturator group, lying near the obturator vessels and nerve. A portion of the left broad ligament (black arrows) is unusually well seen. **Right:** Two centimeters caudal, the periuterine vessels (white arrows) lie lateral to the uterus (UT). White arrowheads point to the left medial umbilical ligament. BL, bladder; UT, uterus; R, rectum; sc, sigmoid colon.

66a,b

66c,d

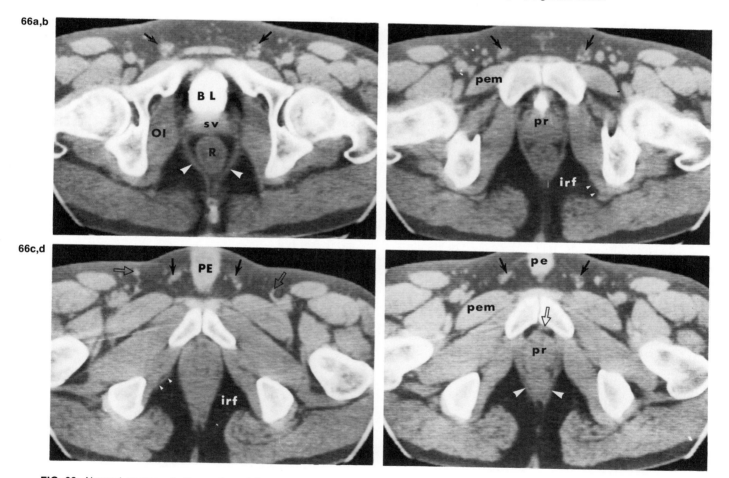

FIG. 66. Normal anatomy in the region of the symphis pubis. **a:** Anteriorly, the spermatic cords (black arrows) lie anterior to the pectineus muscle, lateral to the rectus abdominis muscle. The iliopsoas muscle and tendon lie posterolateral to the femoral artery and vein. The fibers of the obturator internus muscle (OI) form the medial border of the obturator canal, containing the obturator nerve, artery, and vein. The urinary bladder (BL), opacified with contrast medium, occupies the anterior part of the pelvic cavity. Posteriorly, the seminal vesicles are present (sv) anterior to the rectum (R). On this section, the rectum is surrounded by fibers of the levator ani muscle (white arrowheads). **b:** One centimeter caudal, the prostate (pr) is visible, but is somewhat difficult to separate from the base of the bladder. On this section, the pudendal vessels and nerves course through the posterolateral portion of the ischiorectal fossa within the pudendal canal (white arrowheads). Black arrows point to the spermatic cords; pem, pectineous muscle; irf, ischiorectal fossa. **c:** One centimeter caudal, the fat plane separating the prostate and the rectum is not visible. The proximal portion of the penile shaft (PE) is now imaged. Note the progressively medial position of the spermatic cord as more caudal scans are obtained. Open arrows point to the saphenous veins. White arrowheads, pudendal canal. **d:** One centimeter caudal, a fat-containing space posterior to the symphysis pubis, in which lies the dorsal vein of the penis or the prostatic plexus, is imaged. On this section, the fibers of the levator ani (white arrowheads) are seen separate from the rectum. pe, penis; black arrows point to the spermatic cords.

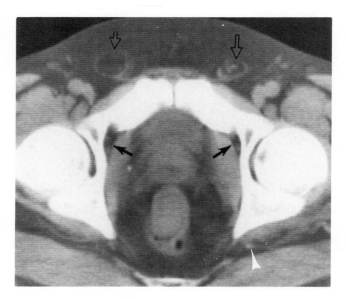

FIG. 67. The spermatic cords (open arrows) lie on the anterior aspect of the pectineus muscle at the level of the symphysis pubis and enclose variable amounts of fat. The obturator vessels are clearly seen within the obturator canals (black arrows). A white arrowhead points to the inferior gluteal vessels.

represents the obturator foramen. Immediately anterior to the symphysis, the tendon of the rectus abdominis muscle and the pyramidalis muscle can be seen. Anterolaterally lie the pectineus muscles. The obturator internus muscle attaches to the posterolateral aspect of the pubis; just medial to its attachments lie the fibers of the levator ani, which encircle the bladder, prostate, and rectum. The iliopsoas has taken a position anterior to the femoral neck. On its anterolateral margin is the sartorius muscle; this normal structure should not be confused with an enlarged inguinal node.

Sections at this level pass through the prostate and bladder base, as well as through the rectum near the anal verge. The prostate appears as a round mass of soft tissue attenuation on transverse CT scans (22). It lies caudal to the bladder. The periurethral glands and the true prostatic capsule cannot be seen as separate structures. There is usually a fat plane between the prostate and the rectum on more cephalic scans; however, this fatty layer becomes much smaller on caudal scans and it may not be possible to distinguish the prostate from the rectum at all levels. The size of the prostate increases equally in all dimensions with advancing age. Central punctate calcifications may also be seen with increasing incidence in older individuals, reaching a maximum of 60% in patients over 60 years of age. The spermatic cord, having passed through the superficial inguinal ring, is more medial than on previous cephalic sections and lies in the notch between the medial border of the pectineous muscle and the lateral border of the rectus abdominis muscle (Fig. 67). Occasionally, the fibrous sheath of the cord may be seen, enclosing variable amounts of fat. Between the iliopsoas and pectineus muscles lie the femoral artery, vein, and nerve, as well as inguinal lymph nodes. The origin of the deep femoral artery may occasionally be seen. A triangular space is formed by the posterolateral border of the pubis, the anteromedial border of the ischium and the lateral border of the obturator internus muscle; in this triangle (the obturator canal), the obturator nerve, artery, and vein are routinely identified. On the medial surface of the obturator internus muscle posteriorly is the trapezoid-shaped, fat-filled ischiorectal fossa, bound medially by the levator ani muscle. Along the lateral and posterior margins of the ischiorectal fossa lies the pudendal canal, which contains the internal pudendal artery and vein. The levator ani forms

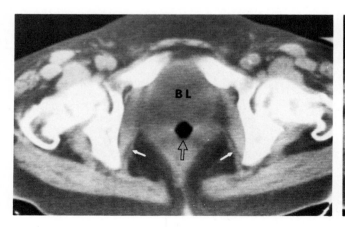

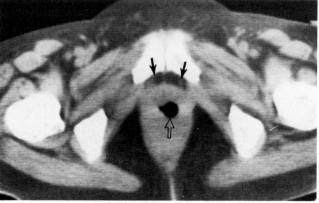

FIG. 68. Normal female symphysis pubis. **Left:** A tampon has been positioned to outline the vagina. The tip of the tampon (open arrow) lies against the cervix. The bladder base (BL) is easily visible anteriorly. The fascial planes of the pudendal canal (white arrows) are seen on the lateral aspect of the ischiorectal fossi adjacent to the obturator internus muscles. **Right:** Two centimeters caudal, the tampon (open arrow) outlines the vaginal vault. The anus lies posteriorly; the urethra, not visible without catheterization, fuses with the anterior vaginal wall. The dorsal veins of the clitoris and the vaginal veins (arrows) reside within the fat-containing retropubic space.

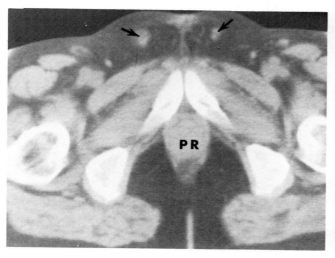 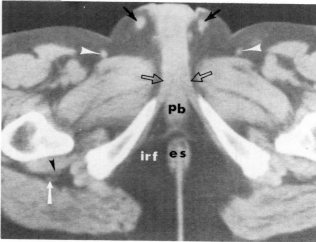

FIG. 69. Male perineum. **Left:** Scan through the lower portion of the symphysis pubis shows the spermatic cords (black arrows) lying medially within the scrotum at this level. The prostate (PR) is present immediately posterior to the symphysis. **Right:** Two centimeters caudal, the paired ischiocavernosus muscles (open arrows) at the base of the penis are demonstrated. Spermatic cords (black arrows) are present within the scrotum. Laterally, the greater saphenous vein (white arrowhead) lies on the anterior surface of the adductor longus muscle. Posteriorly lies the ischiorectal fossa (irf). Lateral to the ischial tuberosity and anterior to the gluteus maximus muscle lies the inferior gluteal artery (white arrow), which accompanies the sciatic nerve (black arrowhead). es, external sphincter; pb, penile bulb.

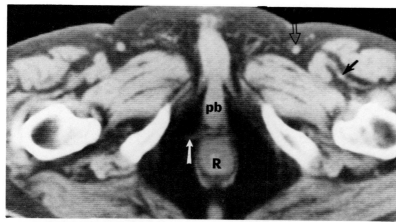
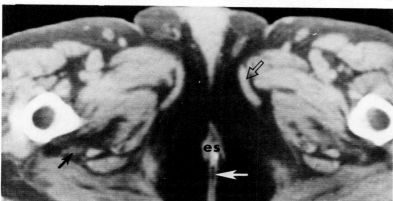

FIG. 70. Normal male perineal anatomy. **Above:** Scan 2 cm below the symphysis pubis. The saphenous vein (open arrow) lies in the subcutaneous tissue medial to the femoral vein. The lateral femoral circumflex artery exits the femoral artery at this level. The penile shaft and penile bulb (pb) are also present. White arrow points to the superficial transverse perineal muscle. R, rectum. **Below:** Two centimeters caudal, the gracilis muscle (open arrow) attaches to the ischiopubic ramus. The natal cleft (white arrow) leads to the external sphincter(es). Black arrow points to the sciatic nerve.

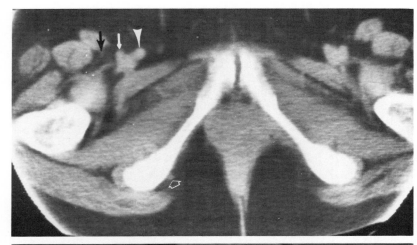

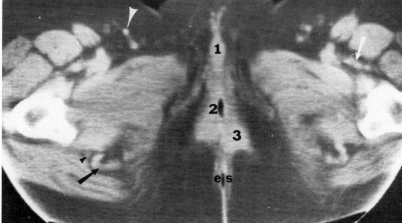

FIG. 71. Normal female perineal anatomy. **Above:** Scan through the lower part of the symphysis pubis shows the femoral nerve (black arrow), artery (white arrow), and vein (white arrowhead) in the femoral canal. Open arrow points to a pudendal vessel. **Below:** Two centimeters caudal, a portion of the bulb of the clitoris (1) is displayed. The urethra fuses with the tissue on the anterior aspect of the vagina (2). Immediately posterior to the vaginal canal are prominent vestibular glands (3). White arrowhead points to the great saphenous vein; white arrow points to the lateral femoral circumflex artery. The black arrow points to the hamstring tendon; the black arrowhead points to the sciatic nerve. es, external anal sphincter.

a sling containing the rectum, prostate, and bladder base. A distinct fat plane is usually present on cephalic scans between the rectum and the prostate, but the prostate may be difficult to distinguish from the bladder. The inferior gluteal artery and vein may also be seen lying on the anterior surface of the gluteus maximus at this level.

Female

On this section, the bladder base and rectum are separated by the inferior aspect of the cervix or, more caudally, by the superior aspect of the vagina (Fig. 68). To define the extent of the vagina, a tampon is routinely positioned in all female patients in whom the pelvis is the primary area of interest. Although the urethra is present at this level, it is not normally seen; its path may be evident if a urethral catheter has been placed.

AREA XII: PERINEUM

Male

Scans obtained inferior to the symphysis pubis (Fig. 69) display perineal anatomy (21). The ischiopubic

rami form an inverted V symmetrically about the midline. Lateral to the rami are the adductor muscles of the thigh and the obturator externus. Anterior to the ischiopubic rami lie the slender ischiocavernosus muscles, which encircle the crura of the corpora cavernosum. The spermatic cords approach the midline as they pass caudally into the scrotum. The pectineus muscle now supports the femoral artery and vein. The medial femoral circumflex artery may be seen passing posteriorly between the pectineus and iliopsoas muscles. The lateral femoral circumflex artery can often be seen passing laterally between the rectus femoris and iliopsoas muscle. The great saphenous vein lies in the subcutaneous fat lateral to the spermatic cord and anterior to the femoral vessels. In a fatty triangle lateral to the ischial tuberosity bordered by the quadratus femoris anteriorly, the gluteus maximus posteriorly, and the ischial tuberosity medially, the inferior gluteal vessels can easily be identified. The sciatic nerve (Fig. 70) can be distinguished as a bulge on the posterior surface of the quadratus femoris muscle.

Female

On this section, the urethra has fused with the anterior wall of the vagina. These two structures and the rectum are surrounded by the paired levator ani muscles. Posteriorly, the external anal sphincter may occasionally be seen. The crura of the clitoris extend anteriorly. Perineal tributaries of the greater saphenous vein are prominent on these sections (Fig. 71). The bulb of the vaginal vestibule, containing the glands of Bartholin, may be especially prominent on these sections.

REFERENCES

1. Berland LL, Lawson TL, Foley WD, Geenen JE, Stewart ET: CT of the normal and abnormal pancreatic duct: Correlation with pancreatic ductography. *Radiology* 141:715–724, 1981
2. Callen PW, Filly RA, Korobkin M: CT evaluation of the diaphragmatic crura. *Radiololgy* 126:413–416, 1978
3. Callen PW, Korobkin M, Isherwood I: CT evaluation of the retrocrural prevertebral space. *AJR* 129:907–910, 1977
4. Halber MD, Daffner RH, Thompson WM: CT of the esophagus. I. Normal appearance. *AJR* 133:1047–1050, 1979
5. Havilla TR, Reich NE, Haaga JR, Seidelmann FE, Cooperman AM, Alfidi RJ: CT of the gallbladder. *AJR* 130:1059–1067, 1978
6. Karstaedt N, Sagel SS, Stanley RJ, Melson GL, Levitt RG: CT of the adrenal gland. *Radiology* 129:723–730, 1978
7. Kuhns LR, Borlaza GS, Seigel R, Cho KJ: Localization of the head of the pancreas using the junction of the left renal vein and the inferior vena cava. *J Comput Assist Tomogr* 2:170–172, 1978
8. Lee JKT, McClennan BL, Stanley RJ, Sagel SS: Utility of CT in the localization of the undescended testis. *Radiology* 135:121–125, 1980
9. Levitt RG, Sagel SS, Stanley RJ, Evens RG: CT of the pelvis. *Semin Roentgenol* 73:193–200, 1978
10. Love L, Meyers MA, Churchill RJ, Reynes CJ, Moncada R, Gibson D: CT of extraperitoneal spaces. *AJR* 136:781–789, 1981
11. Marks WM, Callen PW, Moss AA: Gastroesophageal region source of confusion on CT. *AJR* 136:359–362, 1981
12. Meyers MA: *Dynamic Radiology of the Abdomen*. Berlin, Springer-Verlag, 1976
13. Neumann CH, Hessel SJ: CT of the pancreatic tail. *AJR* 135:741–745, 1980
14. Parienty RA, Pradel J, Picard JD, Ducellier R, Lubrano JM, Smolarski N: Visibility and thickening of the renal fascia on CT. *Radiology* 139:119–124, 1981
15. Petasnick JP: Normal anatomy as seen on the abdominal computed tomogram. *CRC Crit Rev Diagn Imaging* 10:291–323, 1978
16. Ralls PW, Quinn MF, Rogers W, Halls J: Sonographic anatomy of the hepatic artery. *AJR* 136:1059–1063, 1981
17. Sandler CM, Jackson H, Kaminsky RI: Right perirenal hematoma secondary to a leaking abdominal aortic aneurysm. *J Comput Assist Tomogr* 5:264–266, 1981
18. Seidelmann FE, Cohen WN, Bryan PJ: CT demonstration of the splenic vein—pancreatic relationship: The pseudo-dilated pancreatic duct. *AJR* 129:17–21, 1977
19. Somogyi J, Cohen WN, Omar MM, Makhuli Z: Communication of right and left perirenal spaces demonstrated by CT. *J Comput Assist Tomogr* 3:270–273, 1979
20. Stanley RJ, Sagel SS, Levitt RG: CT evaluation of the pancreas. *Radiology* 124:715–722, 1977
21. Tisnado J, Amendola MA, Walsh JW, Jordan RL, Turner MA, Krempa J: CT of the perineum. *AJR* 136:475–481, 1981
22. VanEngelshoven JMA, Kreel L: CT of the prostate. *J Comput Assist Tomogr* 3:45–51, 1979
23. Whalen J: *Radiology of the Abdomen: Anatomic Basis*. Philadelphia, Lea and Febiger, 1976

Chapter 7

Liver and Biliary Tract

Robert J. Stanley

Since 1975, computed body tomography (CT) and gray scale ultrasonography (US) have made major contributions to the evaluation of the liver. In many clinical settings, these noninvasive methods provide information that previously could be obtained only by invasive studies, such as angiography or percutaneous transhepatic cholangiography. Experience in numerous centers has established that both imaging methods are highly accurate in diagnosing hepatic disease (69, 115–117).

In this chapter, the application of CT to the assessment of focal and diffuse liver disease, as well as the evaluation of the biliary tree, will be discussed and illustrated.

TECHNIQUE

Contiguous, serial transverse images, usually with 10-mm collimation, are obtained at 1-cm intervals when the liver is the primary organ of interest and at 2-cm intervals when it is being surveyed as a more incidental part of an abdominal examination. After processing, all scans should be reviewed on the video console, varying the window width and level to optimize detection of lesions whose attenuation value (density) differs minimally from the surrounding normal liver; additionally, the density of the liver should be compared with the other visualized organs. The adequacy of the study is determined, while concomitantly ascertaining the need for additional measures, such as the administration of intravenous contrast medium or the obtaining of more thinly collimated sections.

Either an intravenous bolus (50–100 ml) or a rapid infusion (150 ml of a 60% solution or 300 ml of a 30% solution) of a standard urographic contrast agent, usually a diatrizoate or iothalamate, is used. With the availability of rapid (2–5 sec) scanners, an increasing number of investigators have used the combination of rapid bolus injections of renal contrast agents and timed sequential scans to determine different and

sometimes characteristic enhancement patterns of focal hepatic lesions. In many cases, the enhancement properties of primary or secondary hepatic neoplasms during the first pass of the contrast agent through the liver are markedly different than after contrast material has reached a state of relative equilibrium between the intra- and extravascular spaces.

NORMAL ANATOMY

Gross Morphology

A more detailed section on the anatomy of the liver and surrounding structures will be found in Chapter 6. Important general considerations of hepatic morphology and their clinical relevance will be presented here. The largest intraabdominal organ, the liver occupies the right and midportions of the upper abdomen (Fig. 1). Considerable individual variation exists in the normal size and shape. The right lobe is often larger than the left (Fig. 2), which may be congenitally quite small. The cephalic and right margins are convex, whereas the inferior or visceral surface generally is concave. The inferior or caudal extent of the right lobe usually assumes a more anterior position, being indented posteriorly by the contents of the right renal fossa. Reidel's lobe, generally found in women, is an infrequently encountered caudal bulbous extension of the right lobe. It is recognized by observing consecutive inferior tapering of the right lobe, followed by bulbous widening on more caudad scans near the level of the umbilicus. The left lobe, which is especially inconsistent in size and shape, extends across the midline to varying degrees, even as far as the left lateral, upper abdominal wall. Thinning of the left lobe, which sometimes measures only 1.5 cm from front to back, is not infrequent and causes difficulty in the interpretation of radionuclide images (115). Correlating the CT scan findings with RN images often can obviate further investigation of suspected focal defects due to this developmental variant.

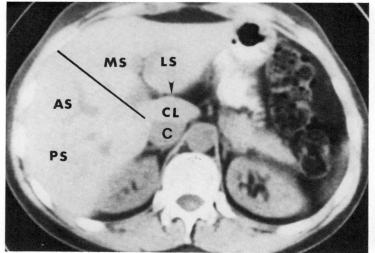
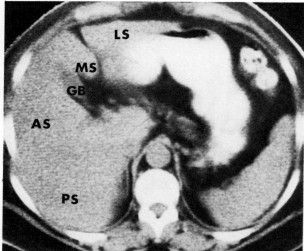

FIG. 1. Normal hepatic anatomy. **Left:** The right and left hepatic lobes divide along a vertical plane that intercepts the sulcus of the inferior vena cava (C) posteromedially and the bed of the gallbladder along the inferior (visceral) surface of the liver. The line indicates the approximate location of this plane. The actual fissure is rarely seen on CT. The left lobe is divided into the medial (MS) and lateral (LS) segments by the fissure of the ligamentum teres; the right lobe is divided into anterior (AS) and posterior (PS) segments. The caudate lobe (CL) lies between the inferior vena cava and the fissure of the ligamentum venosum (arrowhead). **Right:** At a more caudad level in a different patient, the medial (MS) and lateral (LS) segments of the left lobe are more clearly defined. The position of the gallbladder (GB) demarcates the location of the interlobar fissure. The medial segment is also referred to as the quadrate lobe.

Segmental Anatomy

Classically, the liver has been considered to be divided into right and left lobes by a plane extending from the falciform ligament anteriorly through the left sagittal fossa and the ligamentum venosum. However, investigations using injected corrosion casts have shown that the hepatic lobes are usually separated by a main lobar fissure that, on the visceral surface of the liver, corresponds approximately to a line extending through the fossa of the gallbladder caudally and the fossa (or sulcus) for the inferior vena cava posteriorly (75) (Fig. 1). Although this fissure passes through the fossa of the gallbladder, no indication of its presence is seen on the visceral hepatic surface, making it difficult to determine its exact location on images at some levels.

Each lobe is subdivided by a segmental fissure into two segments. The right intersegmental fissure, rarely apparent on a CT image, divides the right lobe into anterior and posterior segments. The left lobe is divided into medial and lateral segments by the left intersegmental fissure (fissure of the ligamentum teres), which corresponds to what classically was described as the division between right and left lobes (Fig. 3). The lateral segment of the left lobe thus matches to the

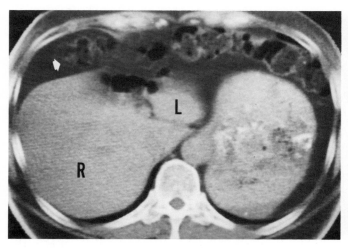
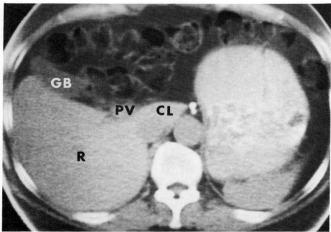

FIG. 2. In this patient with colonic interposition (arrow), the left lobe (L) is diminutive compared with the right (R). The gallbladder (GB) indicates the location of the plane dividing the two lobes. PV, portal vein; CL, caudate lobe.

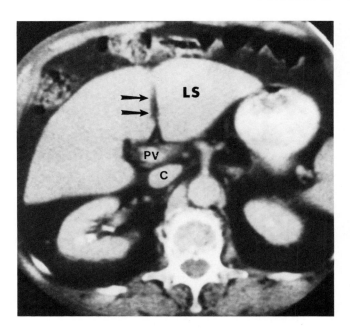

FIG. 3. By classic topographic anatomy criteria, the "left lobe" lies to the left of the fissure of the ligamentum teres (arrows). In modern anatomic nomenclature, the classic "left lobe" actually represents the lateral segment (LS) of the left lobe, here quite prominent. At this level, the portal vein (PV) and inferior vena cava (C) are adjacent to each other; caudally, these two vascular structures diverge.

classic "left lobe," whereas the medial segment conforms to the quadrate lobe. The caudal and anterior portions of the left intersegmental fissure are continuous with the falciform ligament, an extrahepatic remnant of the fetal ventral mesentery. Fibro-fatty tissue within the fissure of the ligamentum teres frequently produces a prominent low density cleft on CT scans. The ligamentum teres, the obliterated umbilical vein, courses in the ventral margin of the falciform ligament and enters this intersegmental fissure to join the left portal vein. It is usually seen on end when sufficient fibro-fatty tissue is present and may be quite prominent when serving as a collateral venous pathway in portal hypertension. Although not readily appreciated with CT, segmental branches of the portal vein, bile ducts, and hepatic arteries course within each hepatic segment and do not cross the segmental or lobar fissures. The major hepatic veins run within fissures between lobes and segments.

The caudate lobe should be considered a structure separate from the left and right lobes. It is a posterior portion of the liver, the bulk of which is located cephalad to the bifurcation of the main portal vein. It is bounded posteriorly by the fossa of the inferior vena cava and anteriorly by the fissure of the ligamentum venosum. Separating the caudate lobe from the anteriorly located lateral segment of the left lobe, the fissure of the ligamentum venosum is frequently seen in both longitudinal and transverse sonograms as a

strong specular reflection, but only rarely is it seen on CT scans (91). Occasionally, a thin tongue of the caudate lobe, the caudate process, may project caudally between the main portal vein and the inferior vena cava. Arterial and portal venous branches from both right and left lobes supply the caudate lobe. In addition, veins from the caudate lobe empty directly into the inferior vena cava. This separate anatomical status of the caudate lobe may account for the relative sparing of this portion of the liver in certain diffuse parenchymal diseases (44).

Gallbladder

The gallbladder, seen in cross-section as an oval or elliptical near-water density structure, normally lies in a fossa on the inferior surface of the liver, just inferolateral to the quadrate lobe, in the plane that divides the right and left hepatic lobes (Figs. 1 and 2). Gallbladders with an intrahepatic or unusual ectopic position have been localized precisely with CT (Fig. 4). Occasionally, the normal gallbladder will extend beyond the inferior margin of the liver, appearing as an isolated near-water density structure, surrounded by perivisceral fat, adjacent to the right colic flexure and lateral to the second portion of the duodenum. When the normal gallbladder is profiled in this manner, a thin wall (1–2 mm) can be perceived.

Portal and Hepatic Venous Systems

In most patients with a normal liver, there is sufficient inherent density difference between the flowing blood within the portal and hepatic venous systems and the surrounding hepatic parenchyma to provide the definition of these vascular structures on a CT scan in their more central locations within the liver. This inherent density difference of blood and hepatic parenchyma can be accentuated by a reduction in the attenuation value of the blood (e.g., in anemia) or an increase in the attenuation value of the liver parenchyma (e.g., hemochromatosis). The density differential may be reversed by the intravenous administration of a urographic contrast agent, increasing the attenuation value of the blood compared to the liver (Fig. 5), or in the presence of diffuse fatty infiltration of the liver where the normal blood vessels stand out as structures of relatively greater density, even without the aid of an intravenous contrast agent (Fig. 6).

The main portal vein, originating at the junction of the splenic and superior mesenteric vein, extends cephalad in its extrahepatic course, toward the right, and slightly posterior within the hepatoduodenal ligament. It closely approaches or actually contacts the inferior vena cava, which lies posterior to it, at or near the porta hepatis, a deep transverse fissure coursing

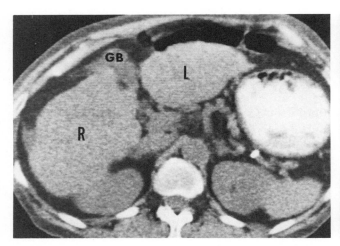
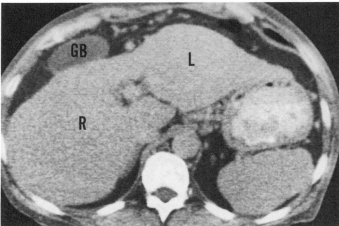

FIG. 4. Left: The separation of the right (R) and left (L) hepatic lobes is prominently shown in this cirrhotic patient. The neck of the gallbladder (GB) indicates the plane of the interlobar fissure. **Right:** The body of the gallbladder (GB) lies in an unusual, ectopic location on the anterior surface of the right lobe.

between the fissure of the ligamentum teres and the cephalad end of the gallbladder fossa (Fig. 3). Within the porta hepatis, the main portal vein divides into a more caudad posterior right portal vein and a more cephalad and anterior left portal vein. Hepatic veins are less frequently visualized by CT than are the portal veins. The confluence of the hepatic veins with the inferior vena cava is sometimes obscured on CT scans by artifacts due to cardiac motion. However, this problem is greatly reduced when sub-5 sec rotary motion CT scanners are used (Figs. 5 and 6). Depending on the plane of the CT image, both portal and hepatic veins appear as round, linear, and branching structures having the density of flowing blood. Portal veins may be reliably distinguished from hepatic veins on CT by carefully tracing their course on serial scans. Portal veins enlarge as they approach the porta hepatis, whereas hepatic veins increase in diameter as they ap-

proach the diaphragm and their junction with the inferior vena cava.

Arterial and Biliary Systems

Hepatic arteries and bile ducts course contiguous to the portal veins. The extrahepatic portions of these systems are seen relatively frequently in high quality CT scans. Within the hepatoduodenal ligament, the hepatic artery is located anterior and medial to the main portal vein, whereas the common hepatic duct is anterior and lateral to the main portal vein. In approximately one-fourth of cases, an aberrant right hepatic artery will arise separately from either the celiac axis or the superior mesenteric artery. It is recognized on CT as a vascular structure, passing between the inferior vena cava and the portal vein in the majority of cases, entering the medial surface of the right lobe of

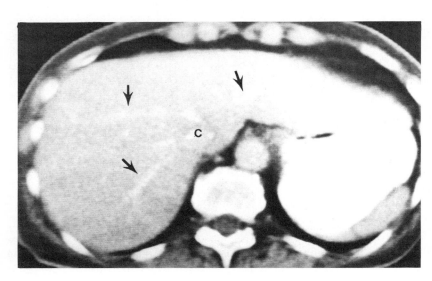

FIG. 5. During a rapid intravenous infusion of contrast medium, the hepatic veins (arrows), close to their confluence with the inferior vena cava (C), appear dense with respect to the hepatic parenchyma.

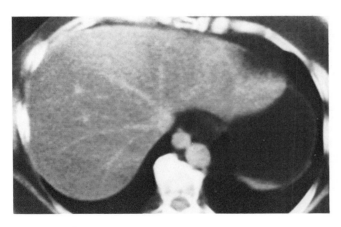

FIG. 6. The hepatic veins appear dense, not due to enhancement from intravenous contrast medium, but because the surrounding hepatic parenchyma is of unusually low density due to diffuse fatty infiltration.

the liver (67,88). A minority of aberrant right hepatic arteries will pass anterior to the portal vein.

The caudal end of the common bile duct lies within the head of the pancreas, medial to the second portion of the duodenum. Demonstration of the normal intrahepatic portions of these structures peripheral to the central or hilar area is unusual. Occasionally small tubular structures are identified adjacent to the right portal vein or left portal vein, but it is usually difficult to identify with certainty whether they are arteries or bile ducts. Even when enhanced with biliary contrast agents, only the more central portions of the right and left hepatic ducts are seen as discrete structures. However, in approximately one-third of patients with a normal biliary tree, the common hepatic duct or common bile duct can be seen on end as a water-density structure, varying in diameter from 3 to 6 mm (35). The likelihood of demonstrating the common bile duct is increased by producing enhancement of surrounding pancreatic parenchyma and vascular structures with the use of an intravenous renal contrast agent (Fig. 7). Narrow collimation (5-mm sections) also may be helpful.

Hepatic Parenchyma

The normal unenhanced hepatic parenchyma has a density slightly higher than other upper abdominal organs (pancreas, kidneys, spleen). Although the range of attenuation values is somewhat variable among normal livers—40 to 80 Hounsfield units (HU)—in the individual patient the range is narrower, resulting in a relatively homogenous parenchymal appearance, except for the slightly lower density branching vascular structures. Following the intravenous administration of iodinated contrast media, the liver parenchyma will increase in attenuation value in a dose-related fashion,

often as high as 120 to 140 HU. Although the larger vascular structures within the liver are usually visible either prior to the intravenous administration of a urographic contrast agent or immediately after the injection of a bolus, they become less visible or even isodense with the surrounding liver parenchyma during the subsequent equilibrium phase of the injected contrast agent. For this reason, intravenous contrast agents commonly are employed when one is attempting to differentiate branches of a slightly dilated intrahepatic biliary tree, which will not enhance, from smaller branches of the vascular system (Fig. 8).

Image Degradation and Artifacts

An important principle in all CT interpretations is that the densities recorded in a CT reconstruction represent the attenuation of X-rays by all of the tissues within the volume of the CT slice. Unless a structure occupies the entire thickness (Z axis) of a slice, the displayed densities of that structure also will include contributions from underlying and overlying material within the slice (116). This partial volume averaging concept relates the size of the structure or lesion compared with the thickness of the scanning slice. Improvements in both spatial and contrast resolution can be achieved by reducing the thickness of the slice from

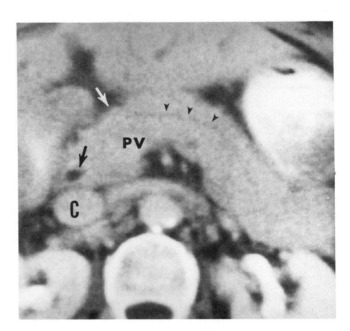

FIG. 7. Detail view of CT scan obtained during infusion of intravenous contrast media shows the normal caliber distal common bile duct (black arrow) as it enters the head of the pancreas. The neck of the pancreas (white arrow), usually the thinnest portion of the pancreas in the anteroposterior dimension, lies anterior to the slightly enhanced portal vein (PV). A normal caliber main pancreatic duct (arrowheads) is visible in the body and tail. Five millimeter collimation was used in this study. C, inferior vena cava.

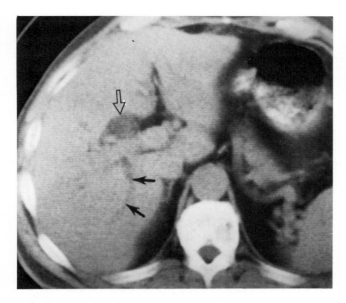

FIG. 8. Although a moderately dilated common hepatic duct (open arrow) could be seen precontrast in this patient with biliary obstruction due to pancreatitis, the mildly dilated intrahepatic tributaries (solid arrows) were only visible on postcontrast images.

the usual 10 to 5 mm or less by thinner collimation. This generally will result in closer agreement between the densities displayed and the true attenuation values of the structures being studied. A trade-off related to narrow collimation is the fact that the image may appear very grainy due to increased statistical noise (a photon deficient scan), especially if the part of the body being studied is large (e.g., abdomen of an obese patient).

With slower scanners (18 sec or longer), respiratory motion can seriously degrade the diagnostic quality of the image and result in gross artifacts. Suspension of breathing during the scan is essential in producing a technically superior CT examination of the liver. Small focal intrahepatic lesions and mildly dilated bile ducts can be obscured on the CT image if breath holding is not maintained. A low density, benign hepatic cyst could appear to have a higher density more characteristic of an abscess or neoplasm owing to partial volume averaging produced by respiratory motion. Near the dome of the liver, cardiac pulsations may produce additional artifacts even with suspended respirations. The introduction of circular motion, multidetector equipment capable of scanning times of less than 5 sec, now in use in our department, has substantially diminished the effect of these biologic motion factors.

PATHOLOGY

Diseases of the Hepatic Parenchyma

Neoplasms

There are no CT criteria to distinguish, absolutely, primary from secondary or benign from malignant he-

patic neoplasms, with probably one exception. With the development of "CT angiography" techniques, cavernous hemangiomas, the most common benign liver tumor, may have a characteristic pattern of enhancement (10,56,60).

In addition, as experience with bolus technique and sequential scanning increases, patterns of enhancement are being recognized in both malignant and other benign hepatic tumors that help in their differentiation (4,54,73,97).

Primary malignant neoplasms.

Hepatocellular carcinoma (hepatoma) is the commonest primary malignant tumor of the liver in adults. It has a high association with cirrhosis. Certain CT features favoring the diagnosis of hepatoma over metastatic neoplasm include a solitary or few in number large lesion(s), an attenuation value very close to normal parenchyma, a tendency to alter the contour by projecting beyond the surface of the liver, and dense, diffuse, nonuniform enhancement following bolus administration of intravenous contrast medium, which quickly diminishes to uniform enhancement similar to the enhancement of normal parenchyma (54,57,68) (Figs. 9–11). Fairly uniform enhancement may be noted if only an infusion of contrast material is used. Morphologic changes of cirrhosis, some of which are readily identified on CT (44), in association with one or a few large, focal lesions, should suggest the strong possibility of hepatocellular carcinoma, complicating the patient's diffuse liver disease.

Involvement of the portal vein by direct invasion of a hepatoma is a recognized complication of this tumor. Tumor thrombus within the branches of the portal vein and hepatic artery-portal vein shunting have been frequently recognized angiographically and at autopsy. Gross involvement of the portal vein usually constitutes a contraindication for attempted surgical resection. Several reports have described the CT appearance of this complication (37,52,125). Both before and after intravenous contrast medium administration, the thrombus within the portal vein appears as relatively low density material within the vein compared with blood in the aorta or vena cava. The portal vein may be enlarged in diameter and, following a bolus of intravenous contrast medium, transient dense enhancement of the wall of the vein may occur. Additionally, there may be associated diminished density of the entire lobe or segment supplied by the branch of the portal vein; this attenuation difference may be accentuated on scans obtained after intravenous contrast medium administration (87) (Fig. 12). A somewhat similar appearance of patchy enhancement has been described in cases of the Budd-Chiari syndrome, involving the lobe or segment drained by the affected hepatic vein (100).

9a,b

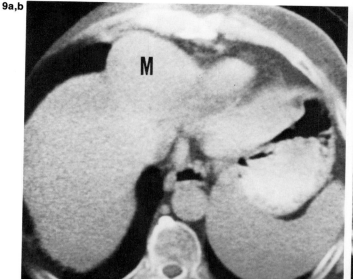

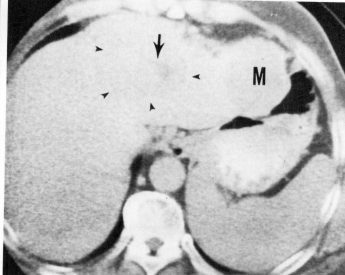

9c

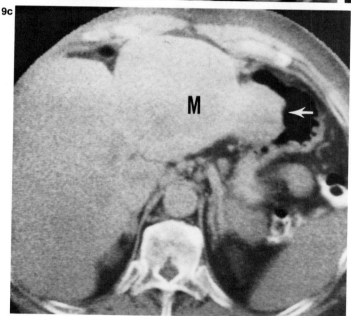

FIG. 9. Hepatoma. **a:** A focal bulge in the contour of the anterior surface of the liver dome is the only indication of the presence of an isodense hepatoma (M), at this level. **b:** Three centimeters caudad, the nearly isodense tumor (arrowheads) contains a small focus of necrosis (arrow). A second lower density mass (M) projects from the lateral aspect of the lateral segment. **c:** Four centimeters caudad to level (b), the large isodense mass (M) prominently distorts the configuration of the lateral segment of the left lobe; the second, smaller lesion (white arrow) distorts the lumen of the stomach.

Computed tomography can be valuable in the preoperative assessment of primary liver tumors because of its ability to define precisely the extent of involvement of a lobe or segment by the tumor. Improvements in surgical technique permit a more aggressive approach to these lesions, and subtotal hepatectomies will be attempted if a remaining segment can be shown to be free of tumor. In this regard, CT and angiography appear complementary, since CT is best at defining the segments of the left lobe, whereas angiography is weakest in this area. Yet, knowledge of the precise anatomy and possible involvement of the hepatic artery divisions, a requirement for the hepatic surgeon, is best supplied by selective arteriography. Such an application has been emphasized in children with hepatoblastomas (66).

Metastatic neoplasms.

On CT, most metastases are less dense than normal liver and are relatively well marginated (Fig. 13). Some, however, are poorly circumscribed and gradually change in density from near normal parenchyma peripherally to a low value centrally due to necrosis (Figs. 14–16). Rarely, metastases may be more dense than the liver due either to diffuse calcification or fresh hemorrhage, or because of fatty infiltration of the surrounding hepatic parenchyma (Fig. 17). Cystic metastases, closely simulating benign cysts (9,31), and necrotic tumors resembling abscesses have been seen in metastatic leiomyosarcoma, colon carcinoma, melanoma, and carcinoid (89,126). A peculiar, scalloped appearance to the surface of the liver, suggesting cap-

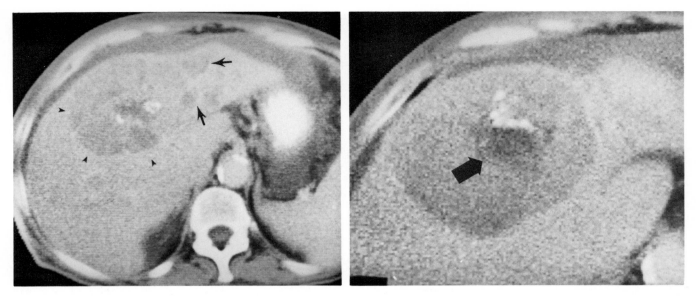

FIG. 10. Hepatoma with central calcification. **Left:** A large mass (arrowheads), slightly lower in density than the surrounding normal hepatic parenchyma, arises in the area of the medial segment of the left lobe; discrete calcifications lie on the periphery of a central zone of necrosis. Satellite nodules (arrows) are visible in the lateral segment, as well as ascites. **Right:** Detail view of primary tumor shows a central area of necrosis (arrow) and foci of calcification on the perimeter of the necrotic zone.

11a,b

11c,d

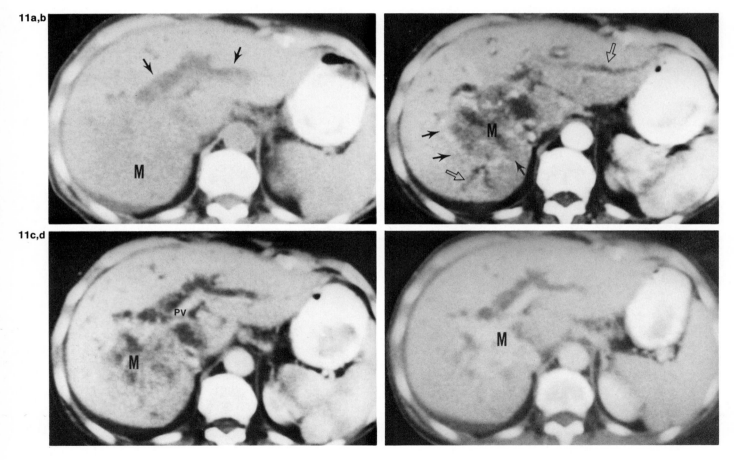

FIG. 11. Hepatoma producing biliary obstruction. **a:** A poorly defined area of diminished density in the posterior aspect of the right lobe (M) suggests the presence of a mass lesion. Dilated intrahepatic bile ducts (arrows) are seen. **b:** During the arterial phase of a postbolus injection scan sequence, the hypervascular rim (solid arrows) of the centrally located hepatoma (M) is defined. More peripheral segments of the dilated intrahepatic biliary tree (open arrows) can be seen postcontrast. **c:** Later in the scanning sequence, the portal vein (PV) is well shown poste-rior to the dilated left hepatic duct. The tumor (M) margins are less well defined as the rest of the lesion begins to enhance, following the transient hypervascular phase. **d:** Eight seconds later, the central portion of the tumor (M) now reaches its maximum level of enhancement and the perimeter of the tumor has become isodense with the surrounding hepatic parenchyma. This cycle of enhancement is completed in a period of time, generally less than 30 sec, much shorter than would be seen with a cavernous hemangioma.

12a,b

12c,d

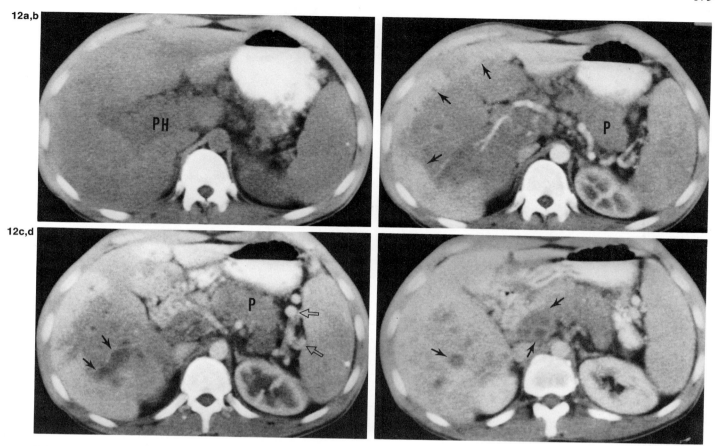

FIG. 12. Portal vein thrombosis by tumor. **a:** The area of the porta hepatis (PH) is widened on this precontrast scan. **b:** Following a bolus injection of contrast media, only the peripheral one-third of the liver (arrows) initially enhances during the arterial phase, a phenomenon not readily explained. The body and tail of the pancreas (P) appear unusually prominent. **c:** Six seconds later, patchy enhancement of the hepatic parenchyma persists. The nonenhancing branch of the tumor-filled right portal vein (arrows) now is visible. Tributaries of a dilated proximal splenic venous system (open arrows) reflect the distal obstruction. The enlarged appearance of the pancreas (P) is partially accounted for by a distended splenic vein filled with tumor thrombus just posterior to the pancreas. **d:** Sixteen seconds later, nonenhancing areas near the neck of the pancreas and within the liver (arrows) represent more of the thrombosed portal venous system. At operation an extensive, undifferentiated retroperitoneal tumor was found with extension directly into the entire portal venous system.

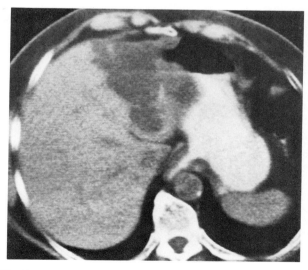

FIG. 13. Metastatic breast carcinoma. High in the dome of the left lobe, sharply defined, low density areas represent largely necrotic metastatic carcinoma.

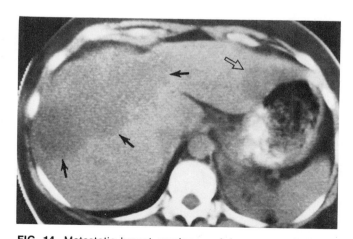

FIG. 14. Metastatic breast carcinoma. A large area of slightly diminished density (solid arrows) occupies the anterior half of the right lobe and extends into the medial segment of the left lobe. A second smaller focus of metastatic tumor (open arrow) lies beneath the capsule of the left lateral segment. The boundaries of the lower density areas do not always indicate the actual margins of the tumor, which in some cases may be considerably smaller.

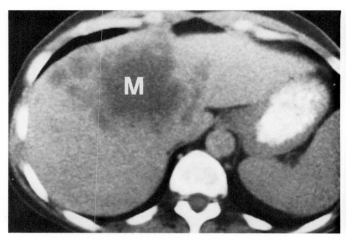
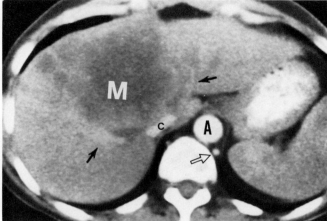

FIG. 15. Metastatic carcinoma of the pancreas. **Left:** A large low density metastasis (M) with surrounding satellite nodules occupies an area close to the interlobar fissure. **Right:** During the portal phase of a postbolus injection study, the faintly enhanced branches of the portal vein (solid arrows) are splayed apart by the central mass (M). Prominent filling of the hemiazygous vein (open arrow) may reflect some relative compression of the inferior vena cava (C) by the tumor. A, aorta.

sular or subcapsular cystic implants, has been seen in metastatic ovarian carcinoma and in pseudomyxoma peritonei (109).

Metastatic tumors with punctate or amorphous calcification in an area of diminished density are occasionally seen, most often due to mucin-producing metastatic colon carcinoma (13) (Fig. 18). This appearance may also be seen with metastatic pseudomucinous cystadenocarcinoma of the ovary, adenocarcinoma of the stomach, islet cell carcinoma of the pancreas, and, rarely, adenocarcinoma of the kidney and breast or melanoma (33).

Some metastases may be isodense with the normal liver parenchyma before or after intravenous contrast enhancement. The exact incidence of this occurrence

is uncertain, since most of the data thus far reported relate to older translate-rotate scanners and contrast medium infusion technique. In a 1979 study evaluating the effect of an infusion of intravenous contrast medium on the detectability of liver neoplasms, the majority of metastases (58%) were equally well demonstrated before and after the contrast medium (82). In 16%, the lesions were better defined before contrast medium and in 13% the abnormalities were diagnostically visible only before contrast medium. In a small percentage of cases, 3%, lesions were diagnostically visible only after contrast medium. Correlation between tumor histology and the degree of contrast enhancement, which is a function of both intravascular

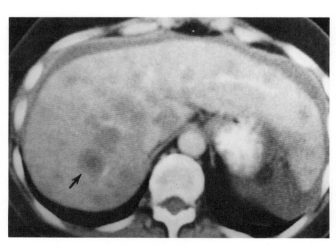

FIG. 16. Metastatic cystadenocarcinoma of the ovary. Multiple small metastases of varying diameter are present in both lobes. The smallest lesions are nearly isodense on this postcontrast scan. A central zone of lower density tissue, probably reflecting necrosis, can be seen in one of the larger metastases in the right lobe (arrow).

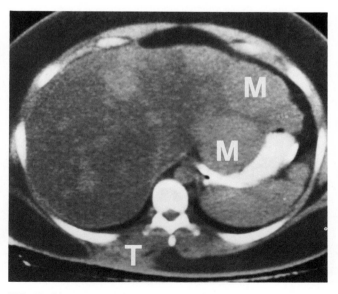

FIG. 17. Metastatic melanoma. Large (M) and small metastases stand out against a lower density background of diffuse fatty infiltration. The persistent primary tumor (T) lies to the right of the midline.

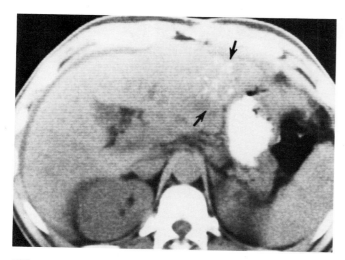

FIG. 18. A cluster of calcific densities (arrows) identifies the center of a metastasis from a mucin-producing carcinoma of the colon. In comparison to the discrete foci of calcification sometimes seen in hepatomas, the calcification in the metastases of mucin-producing tumors is often amorphous and diffuse.

and extravascular contrast medium distribution, was poor with the infusion technique.

However, it has been shown that the enhancement characteristics of metastatic tumors can be significantly altered if a large bolus of contrast medium is injected directly into the hepatic artery via an indwelling arterial catheter (97). Lesions that only minimally enhanced by the slow infusion technique were shown to be positively enhanced and very visible on the CT image, as one would have anticipated from prior experience with selective hepatic angiography. This hypervascular phase of contrast enhancement was shown to be of short duration and the subsequent pattern of enhancement, after several systemic circulations of the

contrast agent, was quite variable and approximated the spectrum seen when the infusion technique was used.

Subsequent investigations using rapid CT scanners (2–5 sec), a bolus injection of 50 to 100 ml of standard urographic contrast agent, and timed sequential scans, starting shortly after completion of the injection and repeated every 10 to 30 sec (so-called CT angiography), have clearly shown the vascular structures of the liver and contrast enhancement properties of primary and metastatic tumors similar to the findings of the direct hepatic artery injection study cited above (4, 21,73) (Figs. 11,19–21). Tumor vascularity, arteriovenous shunting, and variable patterns of enhancement could be seen. In those tumors with positive enhancement compared to the surrounding hepatic parenchyma, some remained positively enhanced on only the initial scan, reflecting hepatic arterial flow alone, whereas others persisted in a state of positive enhancement for a prolonged period of time, a pattern characteristic of cavernous hemangiomas. A pattern of early, transient, peripheral enhancement was commonly seen in low-density, centrally necrotic metastases, which would have appeared not to enhance if only delayed, postcontrast equilibrium scans were evaluated.

As a generality, those factors that would favor the diagnosis of metastatic neoplasm on CT include multiplicity, tumors of variable size, a near-isodense periphery with a gradual decrease in attenuation value as the center is approached, a nodular margin, diffuse, punctate, or amorphous calcification, and peripheral enhancement on postinfusion scans or transient, dense rim enhancement following bolus technique (4,54) (Figs. 23 and 24).

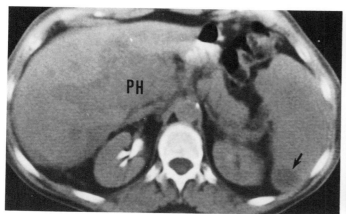

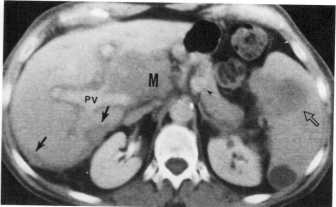

FIG. 19. Metastatic ovarian carcinoma to the liver and spleen. **Left:** The extent of the hepatic metastases is unclear on this scan; the area of the porta hepatis (PH) appears expanded. A single definite low density lesion is apparent in the spleen (arrow). The scan was obtained several hours after an excretory urogram, accounting for contrast material in the right kidney. **Right:** Immediately following a bolus injection of contrast mate-

rial, the margins of the dominant hepatic metastasis (M), occupying primarily the porta hepatis, are more clearly defined. Smaller, subcapsular metastases (solid arrows) are confirmed. A second, previously isodense metastasis in the spleen (open arrow) can now be appreciated. The splenic vein (arrowhead), seen end-on, and the portal vein (PV) are well enhanced by the rapid passage of contrast medium.

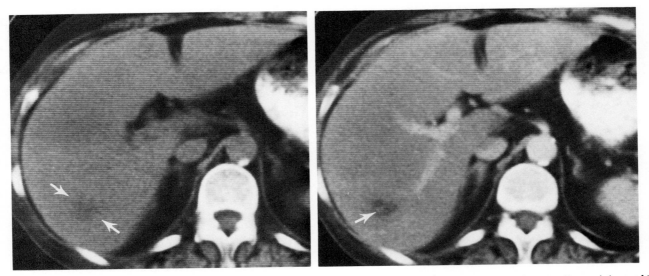

FIG. 20. Metastatic lung cancer. **Left:** Although the center of this single metastasis to the right lobe is easily seen, the periphery of the lesion blends imperceptibly into the surrounding parenchyma. **Right:** Following intravenous contrast medium, the lesion is more sharply defined. An enhancing nodule (arrow) appears to be in the center of an otherwise non-enhancing, low-density zone, a finding not infrequently encountered with metastatic tumors.

Hepatic involvement with lymphoma is recognized in over 50% of cases at autopsy, but is detected with difficulty clinically. Computed tomography has not been shown to be more sensitive than radionuclide imaging (RI) in this regard (129). Recent investigations with a new colloid-based hepatic contrast agent, however, suggest that the CT detection of hepatic and splenic involvement with lymphoma will be greatly improved by this agent, Ethiodized Oil Emulsion (EOE-13) (2,121–123).

When lymphoma is detected with CT, the single or multiple low-density areas of involvement resemble other primary or metastatic tumors. Hepatosplenomegaly may also be present but is a nonspecific finding. The major advantage of CT over RI in the staging of subdiaphragmatic lymphoma relates to its capability of demonstrating the entire retroperitoneal and intraperitoneal compartments in the search for lymph node and extranodal (visceral) involvement.

Benign neoplasms.

A variety of benign neoplasms, including hemangiomas, adenomas, hamartomas, and focal nodular

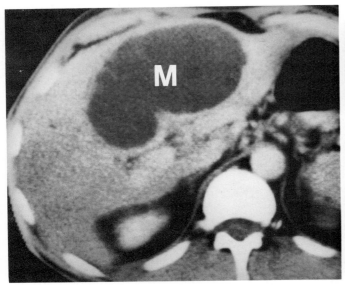

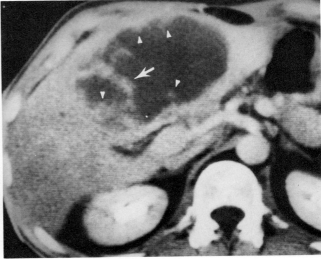

FIG. 21. Low-density, "cystic" appearing hepatoma postradiation therapy. **Left:** At this level, the bilobed, uniformly low-density (near-water value) mass (M) simulates a hepatic cyst. **Right:** Two centimeters caudad, enhancing mural nodules (arrowheads) and septations (arrow) indicate the active, neoplastic nature of this hepatoma. The significance of the overall low attenuation value of this tumor related to prior radiation therapy is not known, since a pretreatment CT scan was not obtained.

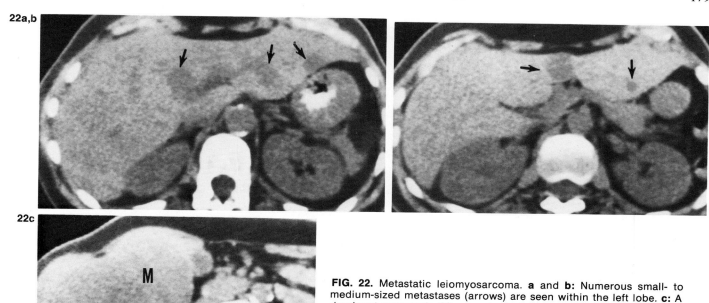

FIG. 22. Metastatic leiomyosarcoma. **a** and **b:** Numerous small- to medium-sized metastases (arrows) are seen within the left lobe. **c:** A dominant metastasis (M) arises in the inferior portion of the right lobe. Such multiplicity and variation in size are typical of metastatic liver disease.

hyperplasia (FNH), have been shown with CT (7, 10,56,60,99,115,116). To date, with the exception of cavernous hemangiomas and certain "classic" presentations of hepatic adenoma and FNH, no reliable characteristics for consistently distinguishing these benign tumors from each other or from more commonly demonstrated malignant neoplasms have emerged. However, the increasing use of "CT angiography" techniques has resulted in some clarification of

the enhancement patterns of these tumors. As with selective hepatic angiography, most adenomas and areas of FNH (Fig. 24) show transient positive enhancement reflecting their hepatic arterial flow during a CT study employing sequential scans following bolus administration of intravenous contrast medium.

It is of clinical importance to distinguish between a hepatic adenoma, which has a high association with the use of oral contraceptives, and FNH, which does

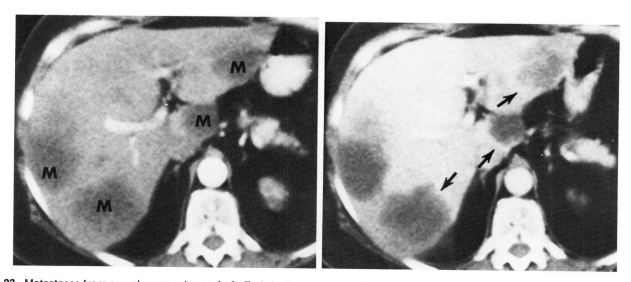

FIG. 23. Metastases from an unknown primary. **Left:** Early in the sequence of a postbolus study, the margins of multiple metastases (M) are still poorly defined. **Right:** Fifteen seconds later, transient, faint rim enhancement (arrows) of these more sharply defined metastatic nodules can be appreciated against the background of enhancing hepatic parenchyma. A narrow window setting would improve the detectability of this transient phenomenon.

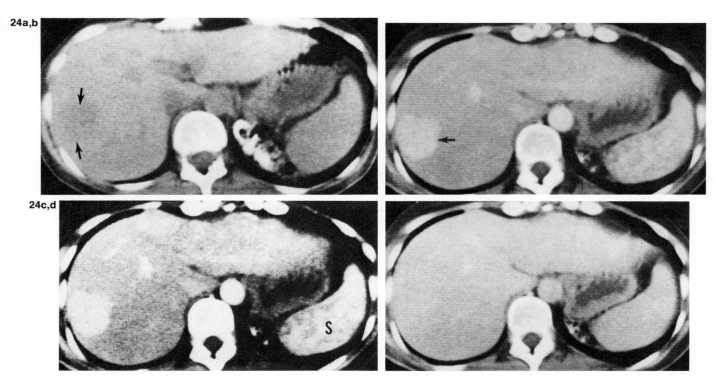

FIG. 24. Focal nodular hyperplasia (FNH). **a:** On the precontrast scan, the nearly isodense focal defect (arrows) is barely perceptible. **b** and **c:** Standard and narrow window setting images of the lesion, early in a postbolus contrast medium study, show the dense, homogeneous, transient enhancement of this vascular, benign lesion (arrow). The level of the scan was not through the center of the tumor and therefore did not show the central, non-enhancing stellate scar characteristic of FNH and present in this lesion when examined pathologically. Note the typical, nonuniform early enhancement pattern of the spleen (S). **d:** At the same level as (b) and (c) and 30 sec later in the sequence, the lesion is now isodense with the surrounding hepatic parenchyma and virtually imperceptible. This enhancement pattern is very similar to that which would be seen with a hepatic adenoma. Without evidence of a fresh intratumoral hemorrhage, common with adenomas, the two lesions would be difficult to differentiate. This lesion would not have been detectable if the early scan after the bolus injection of contrast material had not been obtained or probably if the rapid infusion technique had been used.

not. Spontaneous hemorrhage, sometimes of life threatening proportions, is a relatively common feature of adenomas (3). Young women with adenomas frequently present with the acute onset of pain associated with the bleeding episode, and emergency surgery may be necessary. If a CT examination of such a patient shows a well-defined, nearly isodense mass with a central area of increased density on precontrast medium scans, which uniformly and transiently densely enhances (except for the central area of non-enhancing hemorrhage), the diagnosis is almost certainly hepatic adenoma. If the bleeding episode is chronologically remote, the central area of the tumor will appear of low density, reflecting either an evolving hematoma or central cellular necrosis. Additional diagnostic studies should be unnecessary except for preoperative angiographic mapping of arterial anatomy if resection is planned.

One reported adenoma was shown on CT to be surrounded by a narrow band of tissue with density slightly lower than water, which pathologically was shown to consist of a zone of hepatocytes containing large fat vacuoles (3). Since such cells are not seen in

FNH, the authors suggested that the finding may be unique to benign adenomas. Adenomas have been reported to regress following withdrawal of oral contraceptives; such spontaneous regression of a biopsy-proven adenoma under these clinical circumstances has been shown with CT (95).

Focal nodular hyperplasia is usually discovered incidently; the male to female ratio of this tumor occurrence is 1 to 4 and there is no definite association with the use of oral contraceptives (99). Spontaneous hemorrhage is a rare occurrence. This benign tumor is composed of normal hepatocytes and Kupffer cells, thus allowing for variable degrees of uptake of radiocolloids, ranging from a focus of photon deficiency to an area of increased activity compared with the surrounding parenchyma (7,18,99). A characteristic gross morphologic feature of FNH is the presence of a central, stellate, fibrous scar with peripherally radiating septae. This central scar is usually large enough to be imaged with CT if bolus technique and state-of-the-art CT equipment are used (7). Thus, if a moderate to large-sized, nearly isodense mass is seen on precontrast scans, which transiently and diffusely enhances, except for a central stellate area, the diagnosis is almost certainly FNH. Despite optimal CT technique, the central scar may not be imaged in all cases of FNH, and the tumor will appear identical to a hepatic adenoma that has not yet undergone central hemorrhage or necrosis. Subsequent demonstration of radiocolloid uptake in the area of the tumor, however, will ensure the correct diagnosis. Since the majority of these tumors have a very benign, silent clinical course, nothing further needs to be done diagnostically or therapeutically.

Cavernous hemangiomas are the most commonly occurring benign liver tumors. They have a male-female occurrence ratio similar to FNH, 1:4.5, and quite different from the ratio in hepatomas, which is approximately 8:1 (10,56,60). On precontrast CT scans they usually appear as well-defined circular or oval areas of low density, most frequently located in the posterior aspect of the right hepatic lobe. Isolated foci of calcification have been reported and the tumors may be multiple. Thus, on the precontrast scans, they cannot be readily differentiated from metastatic tumors or hepatomas. However, on postcontrast

scans, the sequential enhancement properties of cavernous hemangiomas may be sufficiently characteristic to warrant a presumptive diagnosis of that lesion on the CT study alone (10,56,60) (Figs. 25–27). The initial precontrast scans show a homogeneous circumscribed area having reduced attenuation values compared to the surrounding normal liver parenchyma. Serial scans following a bolus of intravenous contrast medium usually demonstrate early peripheral enhancement, whereas the attenuation values of the central portion of the lesion remain low. Sequential scans over a period of minutes show, in the larger lesions, a centripetally advancing border of enhancement as the central area of low density becomes progressively smaller. Although the overall level of enhancement gradually diminishes, it remains positive with respect to the surrounding parenchyma for relatively prolonged periods (5 to 10 min). In the smaller lesions (1–2 cm in diameter), the early enhancement usually involves the entire tumor and prolongation of enhancement is not as prominent a feature as in the larger hemangiomas.

Although it is accepted that selective angiography

25a,b

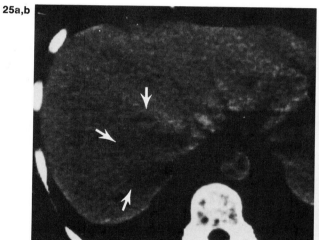
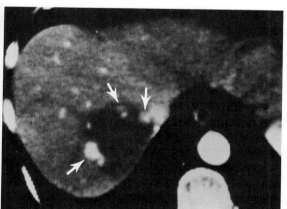

25c

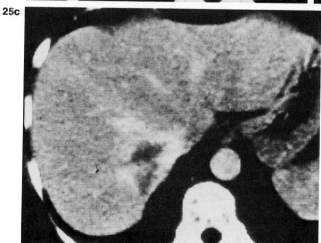

FIG. 25. Cavernous hemangioma. **a:** Its detectability improved by a narrow window setting, this nearly isodense cavernous hemangioma (arrows) is located in the posterior aspect of the right lobe near the dome. This location, i.e., posterior aspect of the right lobe, is a very common site for cavernous hemangiomas. The incidental discovery of a lesion in this location, especially in an asymptomatic woman, should suggest the high probability of this benign tumor. **b:** Early in the vascular phase of a bolus technique study, prominent collections (arrows) of contrast medium appear on the perimeter of the otherwise initially nonenhancing lesions. **c:** At 2 min into the sequence, the prominent, discrete peripheral collections of contrast media have diffused in a centripetal fashion, slowly producing a prolonged positive enhancement of the center of this tumor, composed of interconnecting venous lakes, which could still be detected at five minutes. (Case courtesy of Dr. Bruce Vest, Alton, Illinois.)

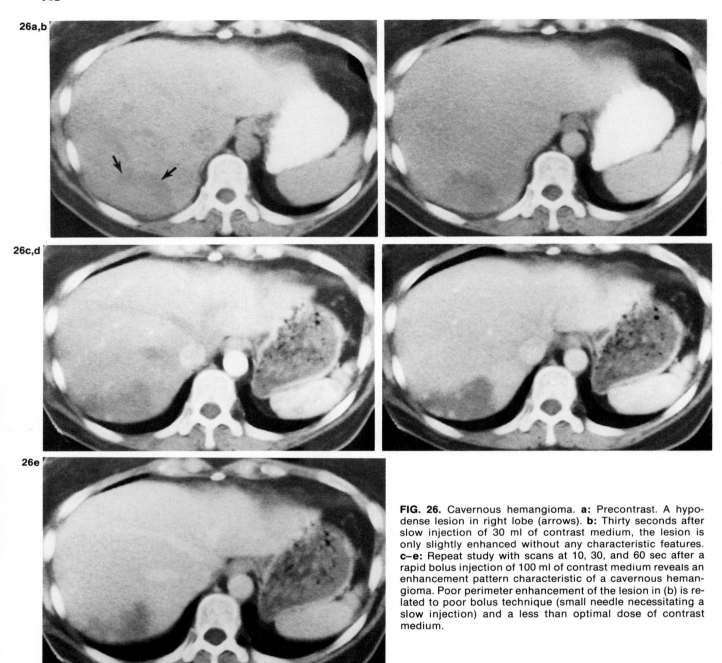

FIG. 26. Cavernous hemangioma. **a:** Precontrast. A hypodense lesion in right lobe (arrows). **b:** Thirty seconds after slow injection of 30 ml of contrast medium, the lesion is only slightly enhanced without any characteristic features. **c–e:** Repeat study with scans at 10, 30, and 60 sec after a rapid bolus injection of 100 ml of contrast medium reveals an enhancement pattern characteristic of a cavernous hemangioma. Poor perimeter enhancement of the lesion in (b) is related to poor bolus technique (small needle necessitating a slow injection) and a less than optimal dose of contrast medium.

provides the most accurate diagnosis of this tumor, short of biopsy, we believe that the increasing use of "CT angiography" technique in the assessment of unexpected, solitary (or few) focal lesions of the liver will show this pattern of enhancement to be characteristic in nearly all but the smallest cavernous hemangiomas, and will obviate angiographic confirmation in the majority of these patients. The more invasive techniques can then be limited to the equivocal lesions. A

technical consideration related to equivocal lesions is our own observation that some cavernous hemangiomas will fail to show the characteristic enhancement pattern after a bolus of 25 to 50 ml of a standard urographic contrast agent is injected, but, on a subsequent repeat examination using a larger bolus (75–100 ml), will show the typical features of the tumor. In addition, if the tumor is large and very peripheral, its major blood supply may enter the tumor

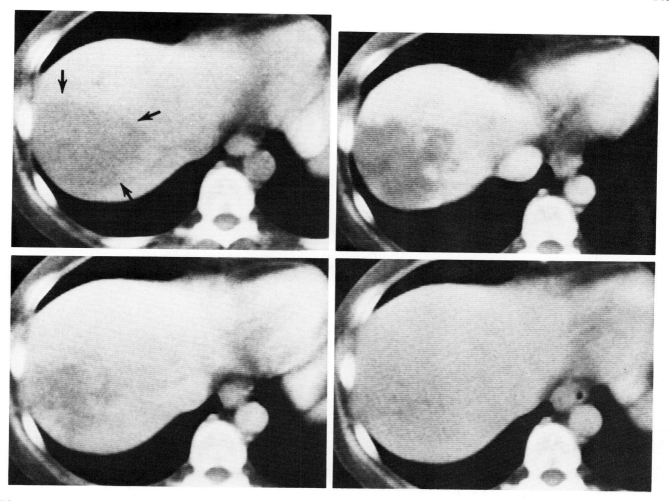

FIG. 27. Cavernous hemangioma high in the dome of the right lobe (arrows). Postcontrast scans at 0, 30, 120, and 240 sec. A similar pattern of perimeter enhancement, gradual centripetal advance of the contrast medium, and virtual isodensity, except at the center, is shown in this sequence following a 75-ml bolus. Experience with cases such as Fig. 26 and this one have led to our use of larger volumes of contrast medium (100–125 ml) administered through a large bore needle (16 gauge) or intravenous catheter. Case confirmed by selective angiography.

from only a single sector, in which case the advancing border of enhancement will cross the tumor from the near to the far side rather than centripetally (Fig. 28).

Cysts

Hepatic cysts occur in congenital and acquired forms. Congenital lesions are more frequent than the acquired types, which can be secondary to inflammation, trauma, or parasitic disease. Benign cysts, frequently solitary, are not uncommon and are a frequent cause of an unexpected focal lesion detected on a radionuclide liver study (69). Multiple hepatic cysts usually are seen with polycystic renal disease but may occur without renal lesions.

On CT scans, benign hepatic cysts are sharply defined, homogeneous areas of near-water density (0–20

HU), which do not enhance with intravenous contrast agent (115,116) (Fig. 29). However, if a small cyst does not occupy the entire thickness of a CT slice, its density will be averaged with adjacent tissue (partial volume averaging), causing an erroneously high value (Fig. 30). Generally, the CT appearance of a cyst is so characteristic that no further evaluation is indicated unless the clinical history suggests the possibility of a cystic neoplasm or abscess. Included in the differential of entities that have the potential to mimic a benign hepatic cyst on CT are a variety of cystic neoplasms, both the rare primary benign biliary cystadenoma and metastatic leiomyosarcoma, colon carcinoma, melanoma and carcinoid, certain stages of hydatid disease, old intrahepatic hematomas, and pseudocysts within the liver substance secondary to pancreatitis (9,31,36) (Fig. 31). A visibly thick wall, diffuse or focal in ex-

28a,b

28c,d

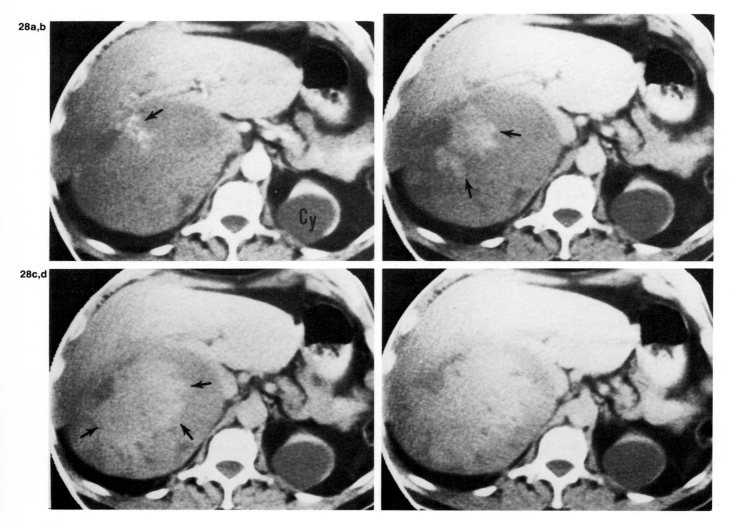

FIG. 28. Large cavernous hemangioma with atypical enhancement pattern. Scan sequence 30, 60, 120, and 240 sec postbolus injection of 100 ml of contrast medium. **a:** The blood supply to this huge tumor arises from a single location (arrow) at its point of origin from the posterior surface of the right lobe. Cy, incidental renal cyst. **b–d:** The advancing border of contrast medium expands as it crosses from the near to the far side of the tumor (arrows). At 240 sec, nearly the entire tumor has become enhanced.

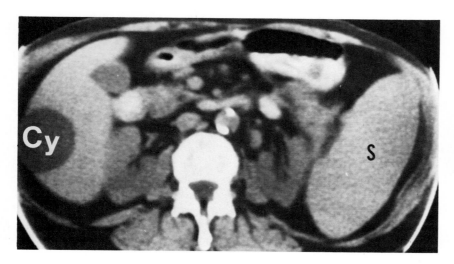

FIG. 29. Benign hepatic cyst. An incidentally found sharply defined, water density, homogeneous mass (Cy) in the lateral aspect of the right lobe was subsequently proven to be a benign cyst. Splenomegaly (S) is related to the patient's known lymphoma.

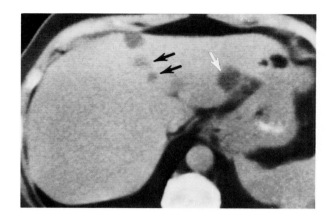

FIG. 30. A spectrum of densities is shown here, related to the size of these multiple benign hepatic cysts. The smaller cysts (black arrows) have an attenuation value midway between water and normal hepatic parenchyma, primarily reflecting volume averaging and resulting in falsely high values. The largest cyst (white arrow), which occupies the full thickness of the slice, measures correctly near the attenuation value of water.

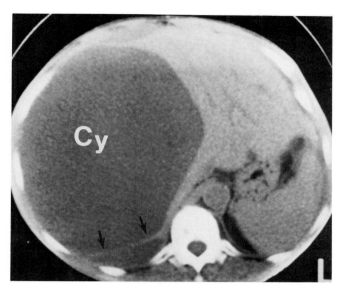

FIG. 31. This huge, benign hepatic cyst (Cy), with septation posteriorly (arrows), was drained of several liters of clear fluid at operation. Based on the CT findings alone, this lesion could not be distinguished from a biliary cystadenoma, or a variety of other cystic lesions, all of which would require at least needle aspiration for further clarification.

tent, mural nodules, septations, or nonhomogeneous fluid content, or enhancement of the wall on postcontrast CT images should alert one to the possibility that something other than a benign cyst is present. Percutaneous needle aspiration may then be indicated for further clarification. Ultrasound has also been shown to be very useful in the evaluation of cystic liver lesions (31,36,98); it is particularly good for defining wall thickness, mural nodules, and septations.

Abscess

Abscesses are the most frequent inflammatory masses, although, occasionally, solid inflammatory lesions without frank pus formation will be identified. In our

experience, the majority occur in the posterior portion of the right lobe for reasons not firmly established but thought to be due to the pattern of portal venous flow (62).

Computed tomography shows most abscesses as sharply defined homogeneous areas whose density is usually greater than a benign cyst but lower than a solid neoplasm (20–30 HU) (Fig. 32). Overlap, however, does occur between low-density abscesses and benign cysts, as well as between high-density abscess-

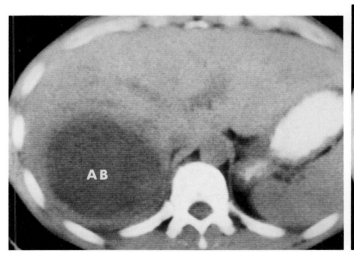
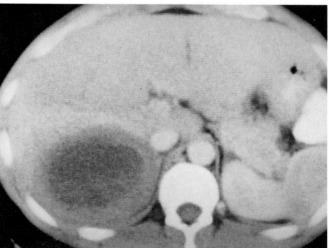

FIG. 32. Amebic abscess. **Left:** A large, well-defined low-density mass (25 HU) (AB) is shown in the posterior aspect of the right lobe, a very common location for solitary abscesses. The patient's history and clinical course were suggestive of an amebic abscess. **Right:** Following a rapid infusion of contrast medium, a ''halo'' effect is obtained as the perimeter of the abscess appears to enhance slightly compared to the nonenhancing center, consisting of ''anchovy paste'' debris. Operatively drained.

es and low-density neoplasms with centers of necrosis or liquefaction (9,115). Identification of gas within a low density hepatic mass, which when present is highly suggestive of an abscess, is helpful in differentiating it from some other lesion. However, the occurrence of gas within a hepatic abscess unrelated to recent surgery or trauma is uncommon compared with abscesses elsewhere in the body.

If linear or branching collections of gas are noted within the liver of a patient who has recently had hepatic artery embolization, either as part of the procedure of infusing chemotherapeutic agents or as specific treatment to deprive primary or metastatic liver tumors of their arterial blood supply, one should not automatically conclude that the gas arises from gas-forming organisms in an abscess. The bland nature of these gas collections has been emphasized. It has been suggested that the gas is inadvertently injected during the embolization procedure or is related either to gas trapped within the embolic particles or to oxygen release produced from some form of anaerobic metabolism (15,74).

Being avascular, abscess cavities do not enhance after intravenous contrast medium administration, but a rim of tissue around the cavity may become more dense than the normal liver (Fig. 32). This "rim sign" is not specific; the same finding may be seen associated with a necrotic neoplasm. When the diagnosis of hepatic abscess is not certain from either the clinical history or the CT findings, percutaneous needle aspiration of the lesion can help resolve the question (42).

Immunosuppressed patients may present with fever, hepatomegaly, and multiple, small abscesses due to unusual organisms such as fungi (22). These patients present special management problems, since the size

and multiplicity of the abscesses make drainage by surgical or catheter techniques difficult or impossible, and the response to antibiotic therapy is slow at best (Fig. 33).

In humans, the liver is the most frequently involved organ in hydatid disease. The CT and US findings in cysts of *Echinococcus granulosis* are distinctly different from those caused by *Echinococcus alveolaris* (38,40,106). Cysts due to *E. granulosis* may be unilocular, but usually are multiocular, with distinct internal daughter cysts (Fig. 34). They are typically sharply delineated from the surrounding normal liver by a well-defined dense wall; the density of the central cyst fluid varies from 0 to 30 HU. Crescent- or ring-shaped calcifications are present in the walls in about 60% of cases. The lesions due to *E. alveolaris,* in comparison, have an indistinct margin, lack a well-defined wall and internal structure, and may be confused with a necrotic neoplasm both radiologically and clinically (Fig. 35). Small nodular calcifications occur in about 80% of lesions.

Diffuse Liver Disease

As a rule, CT is of less value in assessing diffuse parenchymal disease than in the evaluation of focal lesions. The CT appearance of diffuse parenchymal disease is quite variable, depending on the etiology of the disease and the severity of involvement. Acute hepatitis, for example, will not produce any change in the density or contour of the liver, although, if actual liver volume is measured, varying degrees of hepatomegaly may be present. In contradistinction, the late stages of posthepatitic cirrhosis are usually quite apparent on CT, based on marked alterations in

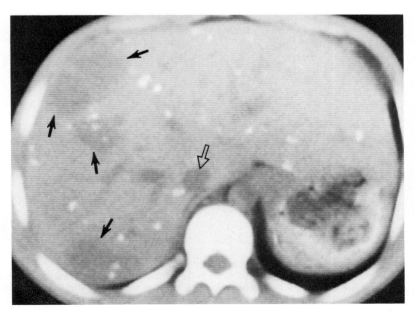

FIG. 33. Multiple areas of calcification reflect prior healed inflammatory granulomatous disease (histoplasmosis) within the liver of this young immunosuppressed patient. Numerous zones of decreased density (black arrows) at this level and throughout the liver on other scans represent multiple, active abscesses, the management of which presents special problems. Other circular and linear, low-density structures in this scan represent the inferior vena cava (open arrow) and intrahepatic vessels.

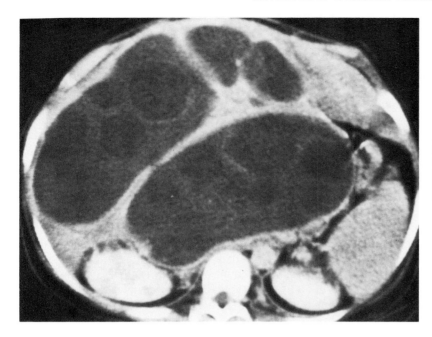

FIG. 34. Classic appearance of hydatid disease within the liver due to *E. granulosis.* Daughter cysts of slightly lower density are visible within the parent cysts. (Case courtesy of Dr. M. A. Rudwan, Ibn Sina Hospital, Kuwait.)

the contour of the liver, as well as segmental areas of atrophy or regeneration (44). In addition, liver diseases that cause substantial modification in the density (attenuation value) of the hepatic parenchyma will be readily detected on a CT study. Ultrasound has also been found to be sensitive in detecting parenchymal alterations in alcoholic liver disease ranging from fatty infiltration to advanced stages of fibrosis, although, like CT, its overall clinical value in this diffuse parenchymal disease is not as well established as in the assessment of focal disease (118).

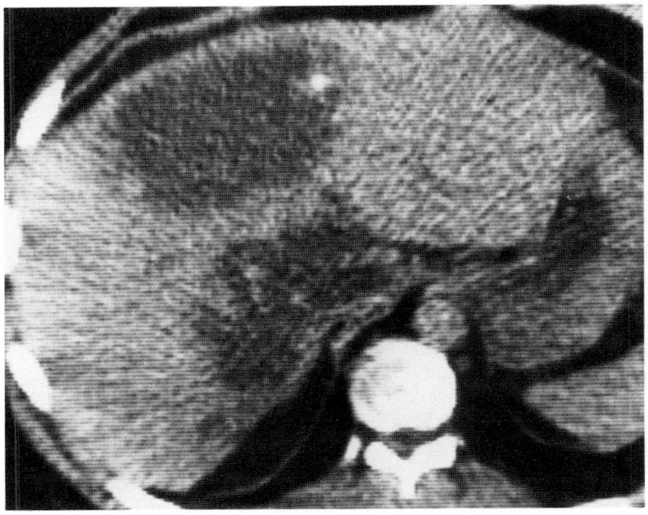

Fatty infiltration, whether at an early stage of cirrhosis or in a variety of other disorders, including diabetes mellitus, cystic fibrosis, or malnourishment for whatever reason, results in a decrease in hepatic density (27,69) (Fig. 36). Mild degrees of change may be subtle and not appreciated unless liver density is carefully compared to that of other abdominal organs such as the spleen. Although the attenuation values of the normal liver and spleen may vary widely from person to person, in a given subject the values will be concordant, with the liver on the average being 6 to 12 HU greater than the spleen (96). Reversal of this relationship is the earliest CT indication of fatty infiltra-

FIG. 35. Homogeneous, low density lesions of *E. alveolaris* are indistinguishable from a wide variety of focal hepatic lesions ranging from abscesses to primary and metastatic tumors. Note the focus of calcification in the wall of the anterior lesion, a common finding in this disease. (Case courtesy of Dr. Maurice Coyle, Providence Hospital, Anchorage, Alaska.)

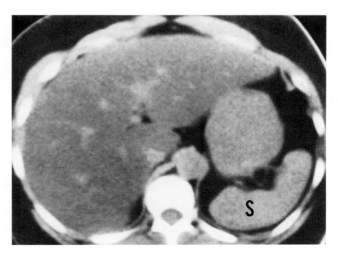

FIG. 36. In this noncontrast-enhanced scan, the hepatic vasculature appears dense against the background of diffuse fatty infiltration. Note the higher density of the spleen (S) compared with the liver.

tion of the liver. A relatively linear relationship between the amount of fat deposited and the attenuation value appears to exist. With more advanced changes, the hepatic parenchyma becomes clearly less dense than intrahepatic vessels and, in severe cases, the parenchymal density may even be less than water (0 HU) and in the negative attenuation value range.

In most instances, fatty infiltration is diffuse and uniform, but nonuniform, focal distribution can occur (85,87,107). These areas of focal fatty infiltration are usually lobar or segmental in distribution (Fig. 37) and can appear and disappear quite rapidly, related to a patient's changing nutritional status. A strong clue to the presence of focal fatty infiltration is that the course of the hepatic vessels (hepatic artery/portal vein) is undistorted through the area of involvement. Radionuclide imaging of the liver will show these areas of involvement to have relatively less uptake of the radiocolloid than surrounding uninvolved hepatic parenchyma. Thus, the findings may lead to the false conclusion that a focal mass lesion is present. Even on CT, this patchy or irregular fat distribution can resemble neoplastic changes. Whenever focal fatty infiltration is suspected, and the CT findings are not conclu-

sive, CT-directed needle biopsy of the liver can be used to resolve this diagnostic dilemma (42).

Hemochromatosis (Fig. 38), either primary or secondary to such conditions as beta-thalassemia or hemosiderosis, causes a generalized increase in liver density (28,70,76,101). Liver densities between 86 and 132 HU have been reported in patients having clinical evidence of iron overloading (76). In children, glycogen storage disease as well as iron overload can cause increased liver density and hepatomegaly (101). However, low attenuation values due to fatty infiltration also occur in glycogen storage disease. In most circumstances, the clinical diagnosis would be known and CT would not be used to establish the primary diagnosis.

In early cirrhosis, the liver sometimes may be enlarged, smooth, and uniformly infiltrated with fat. Advanced forms typically are characterized by lobar or segmental atrophy and gross nodular irregularity of the surface and overall contour of the liver related to the presence of regenerating nodules and interposed fibrotic bands. Usually, the parenchyma has normal density. Frequently, ascites, splenomegaly, and dilated collateral veins may be seen (25,90).

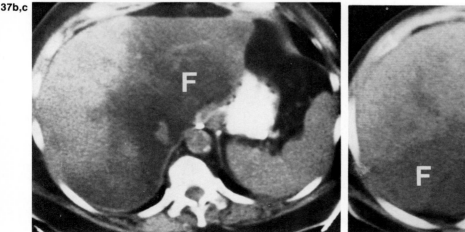
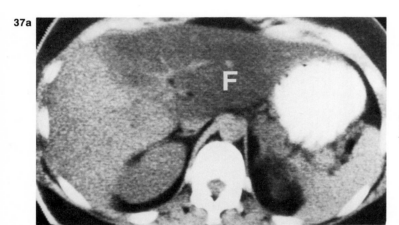
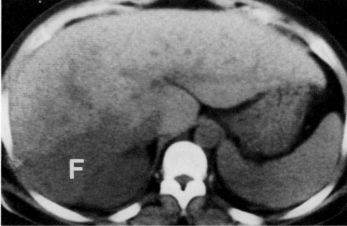

FIG. 37. Three separate cases of focal fatty infiltration (F) are illustrated here. In **a** and **b** the distribution is primarily lobar, whereas in **c** only the posterior segment of the right lobe is affected by the process (biopsy proven).

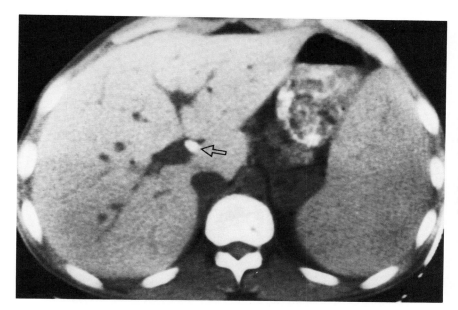

FIG. 38. The marked contrast between the hepatic parenchyma and the hepatic vasculature is related to the high attenuation value (90 HU) of the parenchyma secondary to hemochromatosis. A densely mineralized node (arrow) is present medial to the portal vein. The spleen can also show unusually high density in this disease of abnormal iron absorption and deposition.

Collateral veins appear as a lobulated mass or a cluster of discrete, round (end-on) or tubular structures in the typical locations for the varices in portal hypertension. On precontrast scans they will have the same density as the blood in the aorta or vena cava and, following the intravenous infusion of contrast medium, will enhance to a similar degree (25) (Fig. 39). Regenerating nodules, which may appear as focal lesions on a radionuclide liver-spleen scan, in our experience are most often isodense with the liver. Intravenous contrast medium should be administered, however, to minimize the risk of missing a precontrast medium isodense hepatoma. Regenerating nodules usually enhance in a fashion identical to the surrounding hepatic parenchyma, although lower density exceptions to this rule have, on occasion, been encountered.

It has been recognized that enlargement of the caudate and left lobes is a frequent finding in advanced cirrhosis (Fig. 40). The ratio between the transverse width of the caudate lobe and the right lobe has been found to be the most reliable indicator in differentiating normal from cirrhotic livers (44). The mean value of this ratio for normal livers was 0.37 ± 0.16 and the mean for cirrhotic livers was 0.83 ± 0.20. None of the normal livers had a value greater than 0.55, and only one cirrhotic liver was less than 0.60. Using this criterion, cirrhotic livers could be differentiated from noncirrhotic livers with a sensitivity of 84%, a specificity of 100%, and an accuracy of 94%. However, a recent case report of a patient with the Budd-Chiari syndrome described a similar abnormal ratio of 0.94, without histologic evidence of cirrhosis (19). This suggests that the specificity may only approach 100%.

Trauma

Computed tomography has not been widely used to evaluate acute hepatic trauma. Limited experience shows that a hematoma may be accurately localized to either the perihepatic or intrahepatic area (16,30,32) (Fig. 41). Subcapsular collections are lenticular in configuration, compressing liver parenchyma away from the capsule, whereas central collections are of variable outline but usually round or oval. The density of a fresh hematoma may be as high as 70 to 80 HU and can appear denser than the liver parenchyma. Over a period of days and weeks, the density of the hematoma will decrease due to the breakdown of blood products and the influx of fluid, during which time it may briefly appear isodense with the liver parenchyma. As the clot retracts and lyses, the old hematoma will stabilize at a density comparable to serum (approximately 25 HU). Occasionally, a fluid-fluid interface will be visible within an intrahepatic hematoma produced by dependent layering of cellular debris (Fig. 42).

With the use of bolus technique and rapid, sequential scanning, detection of an intrahepatic pseudoaneurysm, which developed a month or more after blunt trauma and surgical treatment, has been possible (34). Similarly, a postliver biopsy arteriovenous fistula located by CT has been reported (8). On precontrast CT scan, the fistula or pseudoaneurysm may appear as an isolated focal, low-density area in the periphery of the liver or as a local enlargement of one of the major vascular structures closer to the hilum. Following a bolus of contrast medium and rapid sequential scanning, the enhancement pattern of the

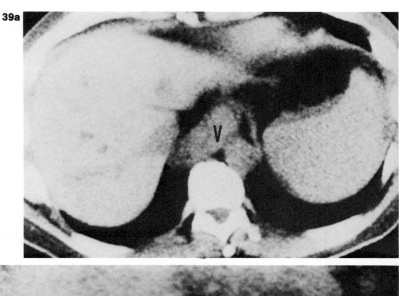

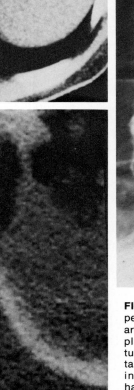

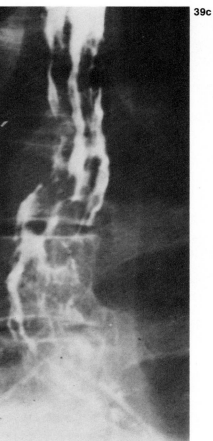

FIG. 39. Esophageal varices in portal hypertension. **a:** A mass (V) is present in the area of the esophageal hiatus. Possible explanations include hiatus hernia, primary tumor of the esophagus, and varices. **b:** Detail view of the same area following a rapid infusion of contrast medium shows enhancement, equal to the blood in the aorta, of numerous contiguous rounded structures (veins seen end-on) characteristic of esophageal varices. **c:** Detail view of distal esophagus from a barium swallow confirms the diagnosis of prominent esophageal varices.

lesion will coincide with that of the aorta at the same level in its density and time of appearance (Fig. 43). Opacification of the portal vein will occur several seconds later. Depending on the level of the lesion in the liver with respect to its venous drainage, one may or may not see early enhancement of the inferior vena cava, well ahead of the normal arteriovenous circulation time. In addition, diffuse hepatic artery-hepatic vein shunting can be seen in hereditary hemorrhagic telangiectasia. On CT, enlarged hepatic arteries and veins, as well as postcontrast evidence of shunting, has been reported (50).

Radiation Injury to the Liver

Radiation injury to the liver is detectable with CT (59,65). In patients studied within days to several months following the completion of radiation therapy, a sharply defined area of low attenuation value with relatively straight borders has been shown, corresponding to the radiation port. Follow-up CT scans with intervals ranging from 10 weeks to 14 months after the initial study showed partial or complete resolution of the abnormal area. The low attenuation shown by CT in the radiated areas reflects the his-

40a,b

40c,d

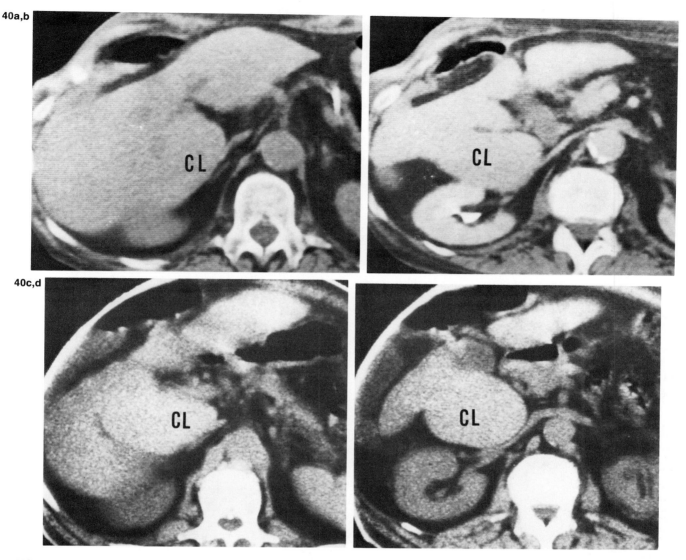

FIG. 40. Caudate lobe hyperplasia in cirrhosis. **a** and **b:** The caudate lobe (CL) is increased in size, out of proportion to the other lobes, in this patient with alcoholic cirrhosis. **c** and **d:** More advanced atrophy of the right and left lobes accentuates the disparity in size between the caudate lobe (CL) and the rest of the liver in another patient with advanced cirrhosis.

tologic combination of evolving hemorrhage and fatty change. The unusual, straight configuration of its border on CT, cutting across normal anatomical boundaries, such as intralobar fissures, is the key feature that distinguishes this lesion from metastatic tumors or focal fatty infiltration, unrelated to radiation.

Miscellaneous

Investigational CT contrast agents.

The development of new contrast agents that are specifically concentrated in the liver parenchyma holds promise for increasing the accuracy of CT. Results have been reported in animal studies using lipoid-based contrast material (2,122), high atomic number particulate contrast agents involving members of the lanthanide series of elements and silver iodide (48, 108), and an iodinated starch suspension (26). However, to date there are only a few reports of clinical trials in which a lipoid-based contrast agent has been used (2,121,123).

This lipoid-based agent, EOE-13, appears to improve the detection of neoplastic deposits in both the liver and spleen significantly by markedly enhancing normal hepatic and splenic parenchyma while not producing any enhancement of the neoplastic tissue. If its clinical safety can be documented by continuing investigative studies, its use may play a major role not only in the detection of hepatic metastases but espe-

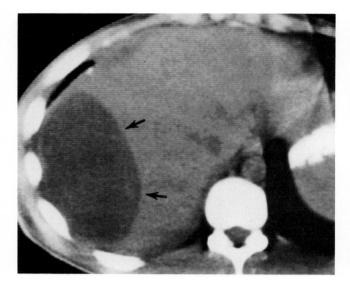

FIG. 41. This low-density, lenticular collection of fluid (arrows) is an evolving 2-week-old subcapsular hematoma. A fresh intrahepatic hematoma could appear hyper- or isodense with the adjacent hepatic parenchyma.

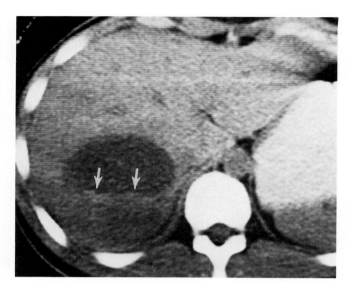

FIG. 42. Posttraumatic intrahepatic hematoma of 1-week duration. A fluid-fluid level (arrows) is present produced by dependent layering of cellular debris. This interface could be shifted by change in the patient's position.

cially in the staging of lymphoma, because the demonstration of hepatic and splenic involvement is a crucial factor in planning treatment. At present, the detection of hepatic and splenic involvement with lymphoma by radionuclide, US, and CT examinations is relatively insensitive (129). This inability to stage these organs accurately, noninvasively in lymphoma (especially Hodgkin's disease) frequently necessitates splenectomy and open liver biopsy.

Measurement of liver volume and tumor volume.

The volume of the liver and spleen, as well as other organs in the abdomen, can be accurately measured with CT (49,81). In a study in which the volume of the liver, spleen, and kidneys of dogs was measured with CT, an estimate within ±5% of the true organ volume, as determined by water displacement, was obtained (81). Other investigators concluded that the ability to

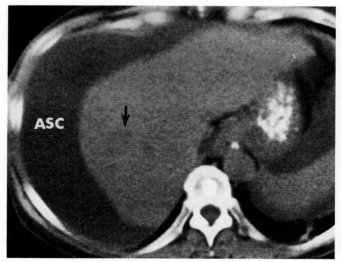

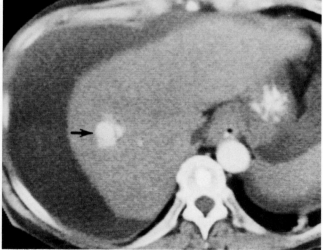

FIG. 43. Postbiopsy arteriovenous fistula. **Left:** In this patient with biopsy-proven cirrhosis and marked ascites (ASC), a barely perceptible focal defect (arrow) is present in the right lobe, in the general area of a biopsy performed several weeks earlier. **Right:** During the early arterial phase of a bolus technique scanning sequence, the enhancement of the lesion (arrow) is simultaneous and nearly equal in density to the blood in the aorta. At a more cephalad level (not shown), prompt filling of a hepatic vein confirmed that this was an AV fistula secondary to biopsy.

measure liver volume accurately had two clinical applications, i.e., as a unit of reference in quantitative hepatic function tests and as an index of the progress of liver disease (49).

Ultrasound has been used to measure hepatic tumor size in response to therapy. The lesions could be judged to be improved, worsened, or unchanged by US, correlating well with other imaging methods and clinical course (14). With a somewhat different approach, total tumor volume compared to total liver volume has been measured with CT (79). A software program involving a two-component system was used where CT attenuation values for normal liver parenchyma were chosen. Those values falling lower than this range were considered tumor tissue. This method of computing total volume of normal parenchyma and a separate volume of tumor tissue worked best when discrete foci of tumor were present, rather than diffuse involvement. These investigators concluded that quantitative CT techniques allowed for rapid, reproducible measurements of liver parenchyma and tumor volume, and that small changes in organ volume may be accompanied by substantial changes in tumor volume.

Diseases of the Biliary Tract

By the appropriate utilization of a variety of laboratory tests of liver function, combined with the pertinent historical and physical findings, the clinician is able to predict the correct etiology in the majority of patients presenting with clinical or biochemical evidence of jaundice. Despite that high predictive ability, there is nevertheless a growing trend to make use of the noninvasive imaging capability of US and CT to confirm or alter the clinical impression rapidly. In addition to demonstrating the presence or absence of morphologic changes that would be indicative of obstructive jaundice (extrahepatic cholestasis), both CT and US can show the precise level and, in many cases, the actual cause of obstruction (11,39,41,46,64, 78,92–94,104,110,111,128).

Methodology

When clinical or chemical evidence of an elevated serum bilirubin is present, or when obstruction of the biliary tree is suspected solely on the basis of an elevated alkaline phosphatase, several precontrast CT scans through the liver should be obtained to exclude diffuse fatty infiltration or extensive and obvious metastatic tumor involvement of the liver as the underlying cause of the clinical or chemical abnormality. Although oral contrast medium is routinely administered for CT examinations of the abdomen, it may be initially withheld if a common duct stone causing biliary obstruction is strongly suspected based on the clinical presentation. Dense contrast in the lumen of the duodenum and, more specifically, within the lumen of a duodenal diverticulum, which commonly live very close to the course of the distal common bile duct, can cause problems in the detection of opaque stones.

With the exception of occasionally being able to define the main right and left hepatic ducts, the normal caliber intrahepatic biliary tree is not visible except when densely enhanced by the presence of an iodinated biliary contrast agent or if air is present within normal caliber bile ducts. Usually, scans after intravenous urographic contrast medium administration are necessary to detect minimal dilatation of the intrahepatic biliary tree confidently. Enhancement of the hepatic parenchyma and vasculature causes the nonenhancing branches of the biliary tree to become more visible (Fig. 44).

Scanning during a rapid infusion of intravenous renal contrast medium also greatly assists in the evaluation of the extrahepatic portion of the biliary tree. The intravenous contrast medium enhances the contiguous vascular structures and the pancreatic parenchyma, causing the normal or dilated common duct to be much more detectable in its cross-sectional, end-on appearance (Figs. 7 and 45). Starting at the level of the junction of the left and right hepatic ducts, sequential scans of the common duct at 1-cm or less intervals, using 5- or 10-mm collimation, should be obtained, continuing caudally through the head of the pancreas until the level of the third-fourth duodenum is confidently reached.

The normal caliber extrahepatic common duct, ranging in diameter from 2 to 6 mm, can be identified in approximately one-third of patients on intravenous contrast-enhanced scans depending on the collimation used and quality of the CT scanner (35). This ability to demonstrate the normal caliber duct may be improved when thin collimation (5 mm) is used. By proceeding in this sequential fashion, one can measure the length of the dilated common duct proximal to the point of obstruction and predict whether the junctional, suprapancreatic, intrapancreatic, or ampullary portion of the duct is the site of the obstructing lesion (11,92,93) (Fig. 46).

Biliary Obstruction

The CT diagnosis of biliary obstruction is based on the demonstration of dilated intrahepatic or extrahepatic bile ducts. Dilated intrahepatic bile ducts will be apparent as linear, branching, or circular structures of near-water density, enlarging as they approach the junction of the left and right hepatic ducts in the porta hepatis (Figs. 46–48).

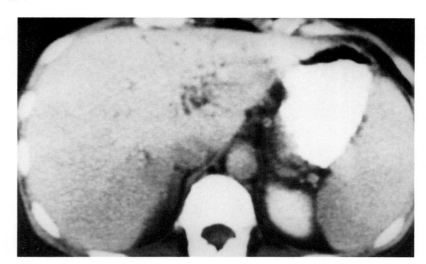

FIG. 44. Sclerosing cholangitis. The minimally dilated, tortuous, and irregular ducts within the left lobe could only be adequately appreciated on this postcontrast scan. This pattern of clustered, focally ectatic ducts is not seen in simple biliary obstruction. (From Koehler and Stanley, ref. 64, with permission of the publisher.)

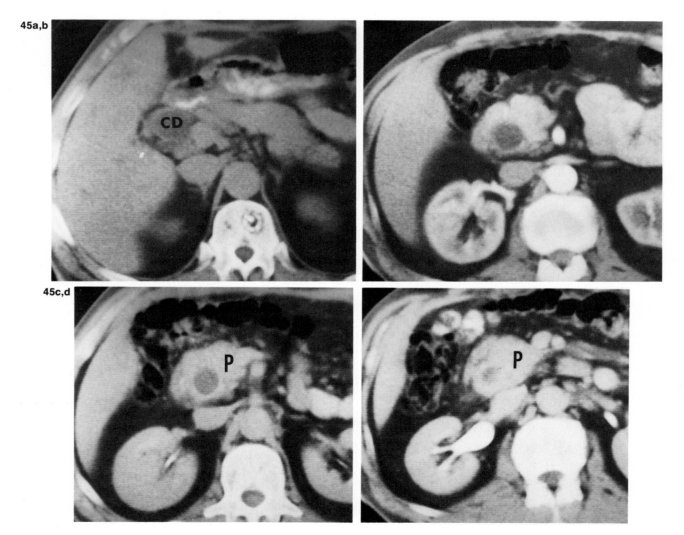

FIG. 45. Mild jaundice and a history of chronic pancreatitis. Sequential scans at 2-cm intervals, starting at the suprapancreatic level oɩ the common duct (CD), shows a gradual tapering of the common duct as it traverses a moderately enlarged pancreatic head (P). The final point of narrowing occurred at the level of the ampulla, 1 cm below the level shown in (d). By enhancing the surrounding pancreatic parenchyma with a bolus of intravenous contrast medium (scan b), the non-enhancing, dilated duct becomes much more visible. (From Koehler and Stanley, ref. 64, with permission of the publisher.)

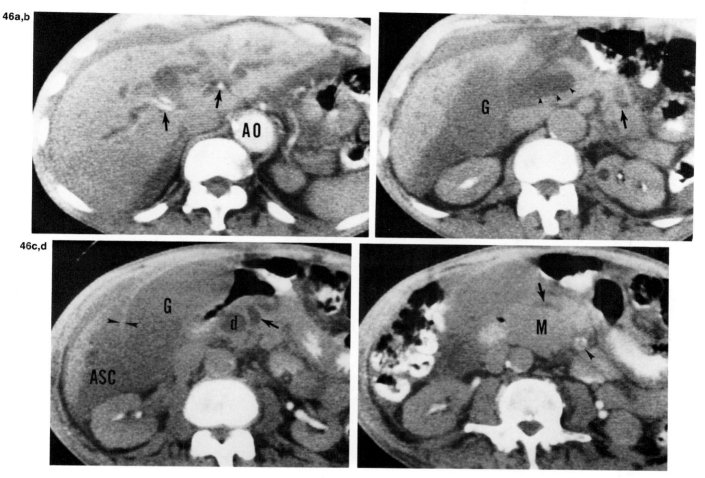

46a,b

46c,d

FIG. 46. Biliary obstruction due to a locally extensive carcinoma of the head of the pancreas. **a:** At the level of the liver, gross intrahepatic biliary dilatation is seen. Dense enhancement of the aorta (AO) and branches of the hepatic artery (arrows) is obtained with bolus technique. Ascites is noted anterior to the liver. **b:** A prominent horizontal portion of the dilated common duct (arrowheads) is shown at this level. A segment of the dilated main pancreatic duct (arrow) is also seen. G, gallbladder. **c:** Two centimeters caudad to (b), the medially positioned continuation of the common bile duct (d) is still visible, just to the right of the dilated main pancreatic duct (arrow). A markedly distended gallbladder (G) reflects the low level of the obstruction; the adjacent ascitic fluid (ASC) helps to delineate the thinned wall of the gallbladder (arrowheads). **d:** Two centimeters caudad to (c), the lumen of the bile duct is obliterated by a large mass (M) in the head of the pancreas, which displaces the superior mesenteric artery (arrowhead) to the left. A portion of the dilated pancreatic duct system is still visible (arrow).

Segmental dilatation of only a portion of the intrahepatic biliary tree, with the remainder of the intra- and extrahepatic biliary trees appearing normal, can be demonstrated with CT (6,119) (Fig. 49). In these patients, the serum bilirubin level may be normal, and the clue to biliary tract disease may be an elevated serum alkaline phosphatase.

The extrahepatic bile duct is considered unequivocally dilated if it is 9 mm or more in diameter (11, 41,45,83,105,128). Ducts of 7 or 8 mm diameter are of borderline size and raise the suspicion of obstruction. Those less than 7 mm are considered normal in caliber. These size criteria should apply equally to postcholecystectomy patients. A recent study has shown that there is no consistent increase in the caliber of the common bile duct following cholecys-

tectomy (83). If the duct is normal in caliber prior to cholecystectomy and measures larger subsequently, some element of obstruction should be suspected.

Unfortunately, there is not always a direct relationship between the caliber of the biliary tree and the presence or absence of clinically significant obstruction. In patients with significant dilatation of the biliary tree in whom the obstruction is later relieved surgically or by spontaneous passage of a calculus, the bile duct may remain somewhat more dilated than normal for the remainder of the patient's life. In such patients, the CT findings can falsely suggest the presence of biliary obstruction. In patients with little or no clinical or biochemical evidence for biliary obstruction in whom CT shows a dilated bile duct but no tumor, calculus, or other obstructing lesion, one must be skeptical about

47a,b

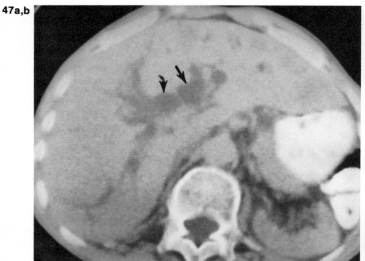

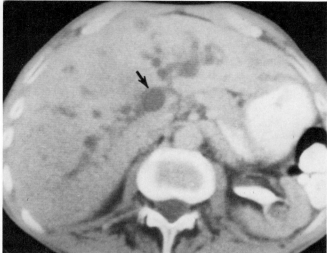

47c

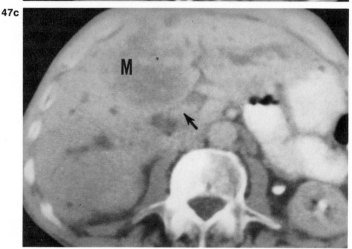

FIG. 47. Cholangiocarcinoma with obstruction of the common hepatic duct and metastasis to the liver. **a:** The left and right hepatic ducts (arrows) and their tributaries are grossly dilated. **b:** At the level of the proximal common hepatic duct (arrow), the diameter of the duct measures 18 mm. **c:** Two centimeters caudad the lumen of the common hepatic duct is obliterated and, in its expected location, only a small soft-tissue density (arrow) is present. A large metastatic lesion (M) replaces and enlarges the medial segment of the left lobe. The study confirms the presence and level of biliary obstruction and strongly suggests the cause and stage of the malignant process based on the CT findings alone. (From Koehler and Stanley, ref. 64, with permission of the publisher.)

the presence of obstruction. In this situation, percutaneous cholangiography can be used to determine how readily bile passes from the dilated bile duct into the duodenum and whether a stricture is present in the distal common bile duct. Radionuclide imaging using imidodiacetic acid derivatives, i.e., Technetium-HIDA, may provide similar functional evaluation.

Isolated dilatation of the extrahepatic bile ducts, without intrahepatic biliary duct dilatation, has been well documented in patients with proven biliary obstruction (11,93,110,128) (Fig. 50). Also, a normal caliber bile duct can be present with a surgically correctible cause of jaundice. Intermittently obstructing calculi and subtle strictures of the extrahepatic ducts may be present when overall duct caliber is normal. When the clinical course, including liver function tests, suggests the possibility of an intermittent or low-grade obstruction, while the CT or US examinations demonstrate a "normal" caliber duct, cholangiography by the intravenous, percutaneous, or en-

doscopic route may be necessary to provide more precise anatomic details.

Evidence of main pancreatic duct dilatation would help to localize the level of obstruction to the pancreatic or ampullary segment (Fig. 51). By careful attention to the appearance of the transition point from dilated to narrowed (or obliterated), one can make further predictions concerning the nature of the obstruction. For example, an abrupt transition from dilated to obliterated would be most characteristic of neoplasm (Figs. 46 and 47), whereas a gradual continuous tapering of the common duct into and through the pancreatic segment would be far more characteristic of narrowing due to chronic pancreatitis (Fig. 45). In such an instance, one would carefully evaluate the pancreas and peripancreatic areas for additional signs of pancreatitis.

Biliary obstruction due to lymphoma can be diagnosed based on the extensive involvement of nodes in the area of the porta hepatis, associated with involve-

48a,b

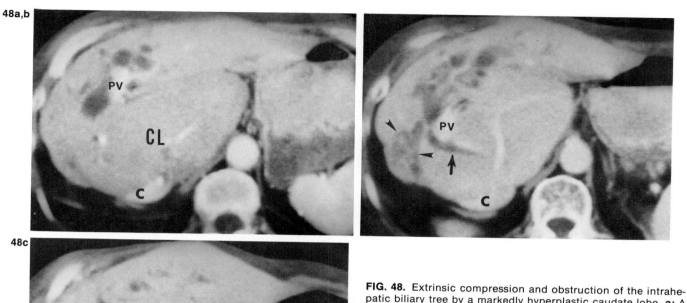

48c

FIG. 48. Extrinsic compression and obstruction of the intrahepatic biliary tree by a markedly hyperplastic caudate lobe. **a:** A huge caudate lobe (CL) displaces the inferior vena cava (C) posteriorly and the portal vein (PV) anterolaterally, while causing intrahepatic biliary dilatation by compression of the common hepatic duct. **b:** At the level of the porta hepatis dilated ducts from the atrophied right lobe (arrowheads), more normal-sized left lobe, and huge caudate lobe (arrow) converge anterolateral to the portal vein (PV). C, inferior vena cava. **c:** At the point of extrinsic compression, the common hepatic duct (arrow) appears slit-like. At the same level, the portal vein (PV) and vena cava (C) appear more dilated, reflecting the relative impairment of flow through these vessels at this point by the caudate lobe (CL).

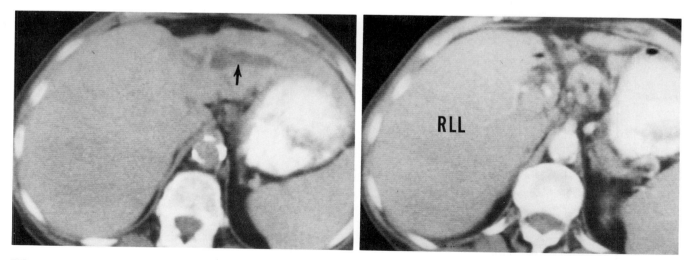

FIG. 49. Left: Isolated dilatation of the left hepatic duct system (arrow) in this patient was associated with atrophy of the left hepatic lobe secondary to a vascular injury, rather than actual obstruction of the ducts. **Right:** At the level of the porta hepatis, the hypertrophied right lobe (RLL) displaces the hilus of the liver to the left.

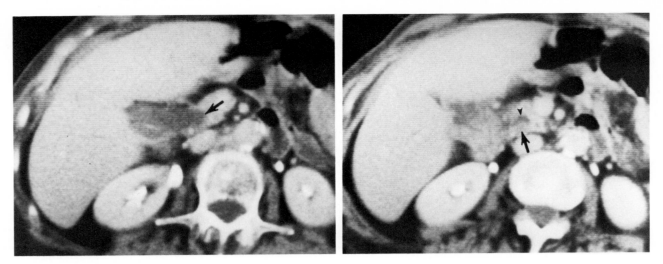

FIG. 50. Left: No detectable intrahepatic biliary dilatation was present in this patient with a mildly dilated (10 mm), obliquely oriented common duct (arrow) at the point where it enters the head of the pancreas. **Right:** Two centimeters caudad, a tissue-density calculus (arrow) nearly fills the lumen of the distal common bile duct, leaving a crescent of bile (arrowhead) as a clue to the presence of this intraluminal filling defect. This "crescent sign" should be carefully sought when common duct stones are suspected and an obvious calcified stone is not initially detected. (From Koehler and Stanley, ref. 64, with permission of the publisher.)

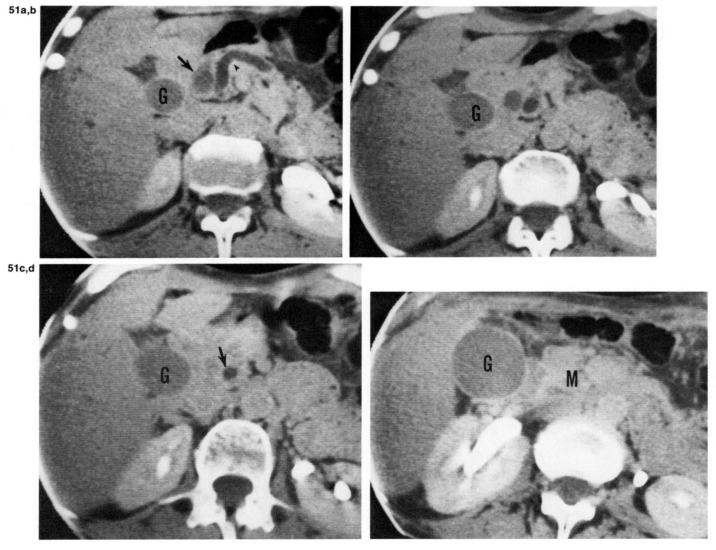

FIG. 51. Five-millimeter collimated scans at four descending levels in a patient with ductal obstruction by pancreatic carcinoma. **a:** Both the common bile duct (arrow), seen in cross-section, and the main pancreatic duct (arrowhead), seen longitudinally, are dilated above the tumor. **b:** Both dilated ducts, running parallel, are now seen in cross-section. **c:** At the level of tumor, the bile duct is obliterated while the pancreatic duct (arrow) is still patent. **d:** Two centimeters lower, both ducts are obliterated. A poorly defined mass (M) is present. Note the loss of the retropancreatic fat planes due to tumor infiltration. G, gallbladder. (From Koehler and Stanley, ref. 64, with permission of the publisher.)

ment of other nodal groups including the paraaortic, paracaval, mesenteric, celiac axis, and splenic groups as well as involvement of other organs, e.g., spleen, kidneys, and gastrointestinal tract (Fig. 52).

Since carcinoma of the head of the pancreas, producing biliary obstruction, frequently has already metastasized to the liver at the time of initial presentation, CT will often not only establish the level and cause of obstruction but also show the metastases in the liver or peripancreatic nodes, in essence staging the tumor (Fig. 53).

Despite the above-described pitfalls, CT has proven to be useful and accurate in establishing a diagnosis of biliary obstruction. In one study, obstruction was correctly identified in 45 (96%) of the 47 patients later proven to have obstructive jaundice (11). But a 2-cm common bile duct was incorrectly thought to indicate

obstruction in one patient in whom percutaneous cholangiography subsequently showed that bile passed freely from the dilated duct through the ampulla of Vater into the duodenum. Computed tomography was quite sensitive in detecting gallstones and obstructing stones within the common duct (Figs. 50,54–56). Computed tomography has also been shown to be accurate in detecting intrahepatic ductal calculi (53) (Fig. 57).

In another study in which 67 jaundiced patients were analyzed, the precise level of obstruction was determined in 65, and the cause of obstruction was correctly determined in 57 cases based on the CT findings alone (92,93). In another 6 cases, the patient's history was essential for the final diagnosis, although the level of obstruction could be correctly determined. The authors found that: (a) marked dilatation of the intrahe-

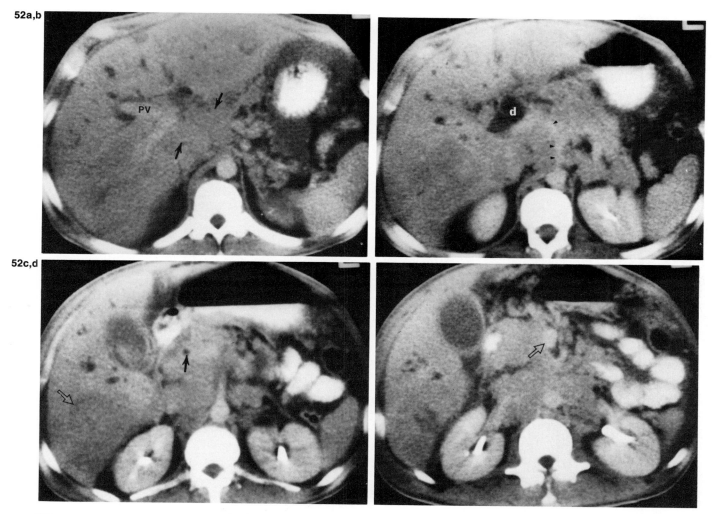

52a,b

52c,d

FIG. 52. Biliary obstruction due to lymphoma. **a:** The enhanced portal vein (PV) is profiled, anteriorly by moderately dilated intrahepatic bile ducts. Enlarged nodes (arrows) fill the medial aspect of the porta hepatis. **b:** A grossly dilated common hepatic duct (d) is seen at this level. Confluent, enlarged nodes surround the celiac axis and its branches (arrowheads). **c:** Abrupt change in the caliber of the common duct (arrow) local- izes the level of obstruction to the proximal common hepatic duct. The paraaortic and paracaval areas are filled with enlarged nodes and lymphomatous involvement of the posterior right lobe of the liver also is noted (open arrow). **d:** The superior mesenteric vein (open arrow) is displaced anteriorly by the nodel masses in the paraaortic, paracaval, and mesenteric areas. The findings in the case are typical of biliary obstruction due to lymphoma.

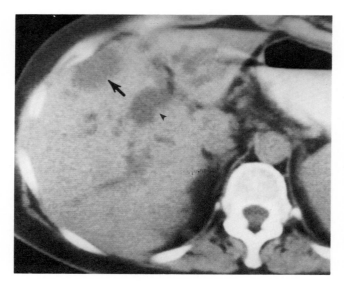

FIG. 53. In this patient with obstruction of the biliary tree by a small ampullary carcinoma, the stage of the disease is indicated by the presence of a metastasis (arrow) to the subcapsular area of the liver. Note the difference in attenuation value between the metastatic lesion and the bile within the dilated duct (arrowhead) at the level of the junction.

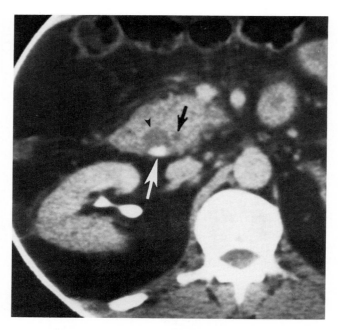

FIG. 55. In this patient with intermittent pain and fluctuating levels of serum bilirubin, moderate dilatation of the common bile duct (arrowhead) and slight dilatation of the pancreatic duct (black arrow), shown here at the level of the uncinate process of the pancreas, were due to impaction of a small calcium bilirubinate stone in the ampulla. Several other stones (white arrow) are seen layered in a dependent position just proximal to the point of obstruction. Although they may not be visible on a radiograph, most of the stones found within the gallbladder and biliary tree will contain sufficient calcium to be seen on CT.

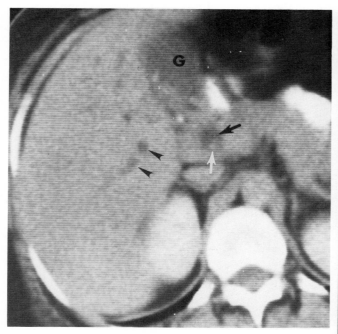

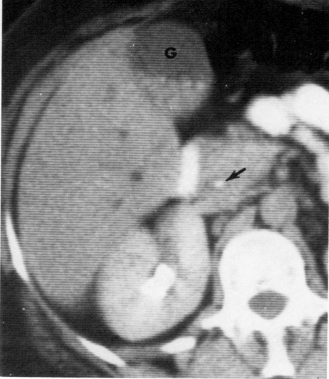

FIG. 54. Cholelithiasis and choledocholithiasis. **Left:** Minimal intrahepatic (arrowheads) and moderate (12 mm) extrahepatic (black arrow) biliary dilatation is shown at the level of the head of the pancreas. A common duct stone (white arrow) is visible within the lumen. G, gallbladder. **Right:** Multiple stones are present within the gallbladder (G). A small stone is shown impacted within the ampulla (arrow).

56a,b

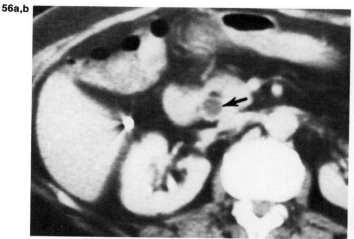
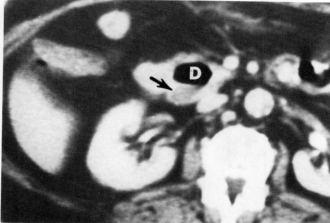

56c

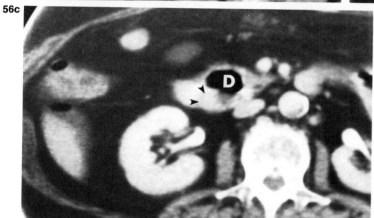

FIG. 56. Noncalcified common duct stone. **a:** A moderately dilated distal common bile duct (arrow) is present at this level. A dense metal clip, to the right, is from a prior cholecystectomy. **b:** A gas-filled duodenal diverticulum (D) lies immediately anterior to the distal bile duct (arrow), seen here turning obliquely toward the duodenal lumen. Oral contrast material within a duodenal diverticulum is a potential source of confusion in the diagnosis of common duct stones. If strongly suspected, oral contrast material should be initially withheld. **c:** Retrospectively, an almost imperceptible non-opaque, near-tissue density stone (arrowheads) is seen impacted in the ampulla, bulging into the duodenal lumen. D, diverticulum.

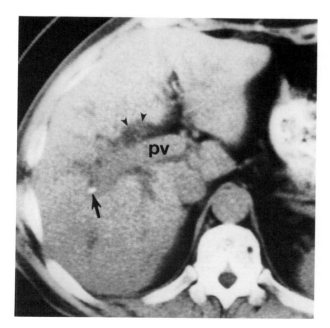

FIG. 57. In this patient with distal duct obstruction due to stones, several intrahepatic ductal stones were encountered, one of which is shown here (arrow). Arrowheads, dilated hepatic duct; PV, portal vein.

patic biliary tree had a very high association with malignancy, (b) associated dilatation of the main pancreatic duct was most often due to an obstructing lesion at the intrapancreatic or ampullary level, and (c) of 17 cases with obstructing ductal calculi, the calculi were clearly visible in 14. In addition, they claimed that a prominent horizontal configuration to the dilated suprapancreatic segment of the common duct was most often associated with obstruction by cancer of the pancreas.

However, we and others (11,58) have not found such a high association between a transverse-oriented segment of the common duct and obstruction by cancer of the pancreas. Obstruction due to choledocholithiasis occurred with a frequency similar to malignant obstruction in this subset of patients.

By careful attention to all factors, presuming the availability of sub-5 sec scanners with high spatial and contrast resolution, one should be able to exclude the normal, unobstructed biliary tracts and to specify the level and cause of obstruction in almost all patients with biliary obstruction who are evaluated with CT. The adequacy of the diagnostic information provided

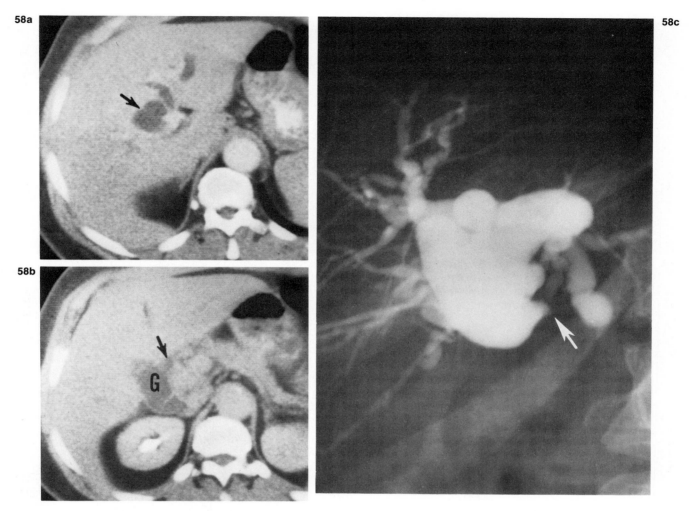

FIG. 58. Cholangiocarcinoma of proximal common hepatic duct. **a:** At the level of the junction of the right and left hepatic ducts (arrow), prominent intrahepatic dilatation is seen. **b:** Three centimeters caudad, a normal caliber common hepatic duct (arrow) is visible just anterior to the gallbladder (G). Between the level shown in (a) and this level, the lumen of the common duct was obliterated but no appreciable soft tissue mass could be seen. **c:** Percutaneous transhepatic cholangiogram shows the point of obstruction (arrow) to be at the level of the proximal common hepatic duct, as indicated on the CT scan. A small cholangiocarcinoma was found at operation.

by CT usually should obviate additional preoperative invasive diagnostic techniques such as percutaneous transhepatic cholangiography (PTC) or endoscopic retrograde cholangiography. Exceptions to this involve patients who require interventional procedures to decompress the biliary tree either as definitive treatment or in preparation for subsequent operation, or to provide access to the site of a primary biliary tumor for intraductal irradiation (51,84). In these cases, the PTC serves as the initial step of a catheterization procedure. Another exception in which PTC may follow a diagnostic CT study is in the patient with a high obstruction near or involving the junction of the right and left hepatic ducts (Fig. 58). If surgical decompression is planned, knowledge of the precise location and extent of the ductal obstruction can be best provided by PTC. Even in this group of patients, however, the information provided by CT assists in the

selection of candidates as well as in the planning of the interventional procedure itself. The precise segmental location of the most dilated ducts can be shown with CT, thereby eliminating possible prolongation of the procedure in a complex case.

Gallbladder Disease

It is unlikely that CT will ever become a primary radiologic method of evaluating suspected gallbladder disease. Oral cholecystography, US, and, more recently, RI accomplish this task quite satisfactorily. In rare situations, when both conventional radiography and US fail to provide a definitive diagnosis, CT can then be used as a reasonable alternative.

Computed tomography may reveal unsuspected cholelithiasis during studies performed for other reasons. Gallstones and bile duct calculi not visible by

59a,b

59c,d

59e,f

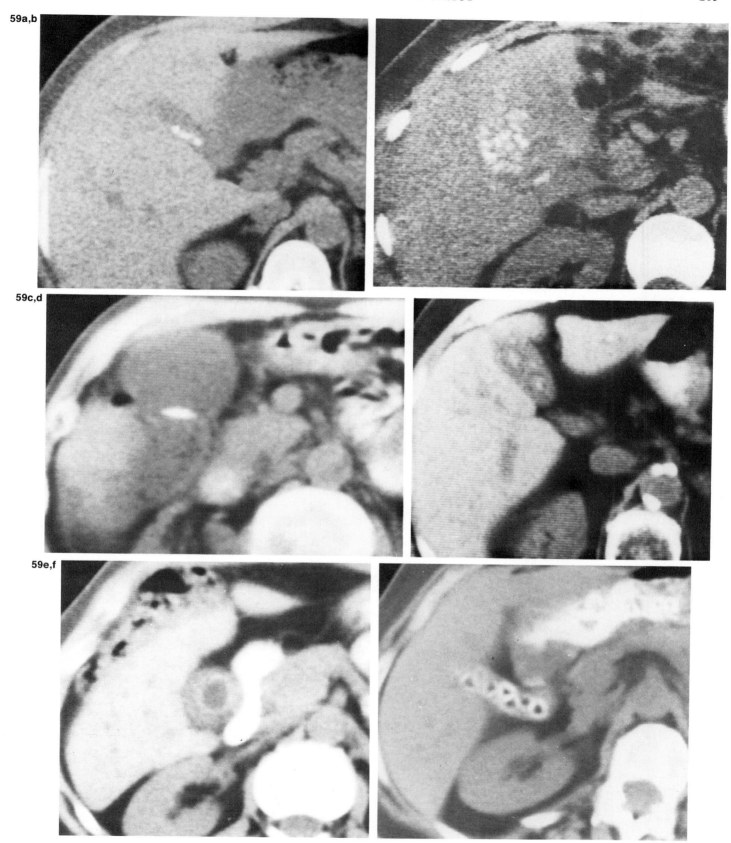

FIG. 59. a–f. Variety of calcium bilirubinate (a–c) and mixed (d–f) gallstones as shown by CT. (From Koehler and Stanley, ref. 64, with permission of the publisher.)

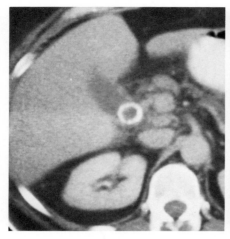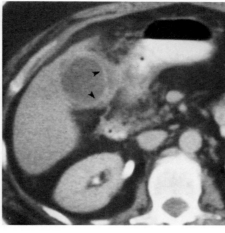

FIG. 60. Cholelithiasis with cholecystitis. **Left:** Mixed composition calculus in the neck of the gallbadder. **Right:** The gallbladder wall (arrowheads) is uniformly thickened. Also note the increased density of the pericholecystic fat, medially, reflecting the inflammatory process.

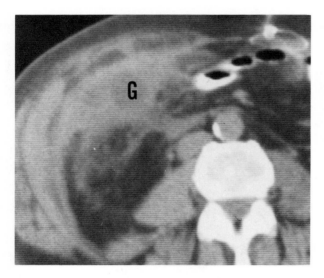

FIG. 61. In this acutely ill patient, the gallbladder (G) is surrounded by higher density tissue, obscuring the outer surface of the gallbladder wall. The appearance is characteristic of a pericholecystic abscess, spreading anteriorly and laterally. Operatively proven. (From Koehler and Stanley, ref. 64, with permission of the publisher.)

conventional radiographic plain film technique can be detected by CT (11,47,53,92,120) (Fig. 59). Calcium bilirubinate and most mixed stones contain sufficient calcium to be seen on a CT scan (64,80,114). Pure cholesterol stones with an attenuation value lower than bile, which is near-water density, are more difficult to define with CT, but can sometimes be recognized as filling defects within the bile (114). Evidence of cholecystitis, either acute or chronic, may be diagnosed by observing uniform thickening or calcification of the gallbladder wall (47,120) (Figs. 60 and 61). Using rapid CT scanners, which have high spatial resolution and contrast sensitivity, the wall of the gallbladder can be identified and evaluated with greater precision than with the slower CT scanners.

The CT and US findings in gallbladder carcinoma have been reported and are quite similar (55,103,127). The CT findings can be classified into three main categories: massive, thickened wall, and intraluminal. Common CT abnormalities encountered were a focal low-density area in the liver adjacent to the gallbladder, mass in the region of the gallbladder, gallstones, biliary tract obstruction (usually high in the common hepatic duct or at the junction of the right and left hepatic ducts), gallbladder wall thickening, intraluminal mass in the gallbladder, liver metastases, and enlarged regional lymph nodes (55,127) (Fig. 62). Gallbladder wall thickening due to carcinoma is usually focal or discontinuous, but occasional cases exhibit uniform thickening, which can mimic the appearance of cholecystitis. CT abnormalities can be particularly difficult to interpret in patients who have both gallbladder wall thickening due to chronic cholecystitis and metastatic liver disease from some other source.

In a series of 27 patients with gallbladder carcinoma, 20 patients were correctly diagnosed as gallbladder cancer by CT (55). In retrospect, 4 other patients had definite CT findings of this disease. In only 3 patients were CT findings equivocal or misleading.

Cystic Disease of the Biliary Tree

Choledochal cyst.

Although experience with the CT evaluation of congenital or developmental anomalies of the biliary tree is limited, the clarity with which rapid, rotary CT scanners can image the normal and abnormal bile ducts indicates a strong potential capability for noninvasive imaging in this category of disease.

Choledochal cysts of the Alonso-Lej Type 1 have been clearly defined with CT and US (5,43,86). In this entity both intra- and extrahepatic cystic dilatation can be present. The intrahepatic dilatation is limited to the central portion of the left and right main hepatic ducts,

62a,b

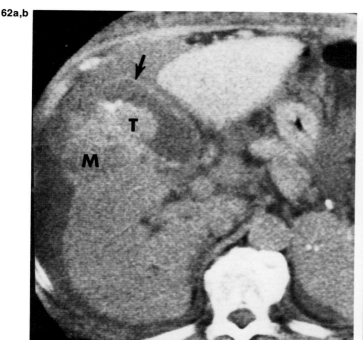

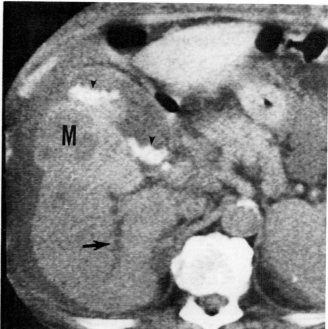

62c

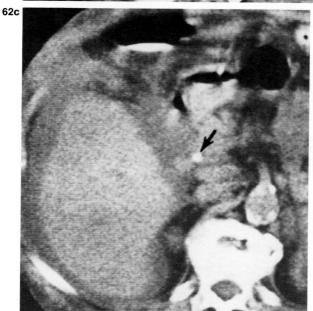

FIG. 62. Carcinoma of the gallbladder and obstruction by choledocholithiasis. **a:** An oval mass (T) arises from the wall of the gallbladder (arrow), which is profiled by ascitic fluid. Direct extension of the tumor into the adjacent hepatic parenchyma (M) is present, producing an inhomogeneous mass that bulges the surface contour. **b:** Numerous small, dense stones (arrowheads) are present within the gallbladder. A dilated tributary of the right hepatic duct (arrow) indicates biliary obstruction. M, hepatic metastasis. **c:** The actual cause of obstruction was an impacted calculus (arrow) in the distal common bile duct. When carcinoma of the gallbladder is associated with biliary obstruction and jaundice, the cause usually is direct extention of the tumor into the bile duct. (From Koehler and Stanley, ref. 64, with permission of the publisher.)

in contrast to the more generalized involvement of the intrahepatic biliary tree in acquired obstruction, where gradually decreasing dilatation extends into the periphery (Fig. 63).

When only extrahepatic dilatation is present, the diameter of the dilated segment is usually out of proportion to the remainder of the biliary tree and the transition point from dilated to normal is usually abrupt (5). Jaundice may be present in uncomplicated choledochal cysts without an accompanying pattern of obstructive dilatation of the intrahepatic ducts. If a known or

suspected choledochal cyst appears to have a superimposed pattern of obstructive dilatation of the intrahepatic ducts, a secondary complication, such as tumor, should be sought, especially in view of the association of malignancy with this anomaly.

In some cases, one cannot be certain that the cystic mass is in communication with the biliary tree. The use of intravenous meglumine iodipamide (Cholegrafin®) may help resolve this question by showing enhancement of the cystic fluid on CT scans obtained 30 to 60 min after infusion (86).

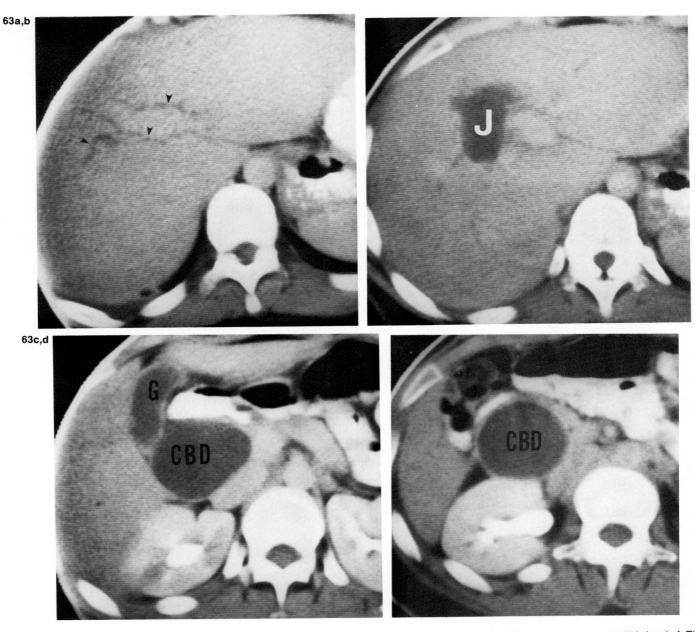

FIG. 63. Choledochal cyst—Alonso-Lej Type I. **a:** Minimally dilated ducts (arrowheads) are present in the middle zone of the liver. **b:** An abrupt transition to markedly dilated ducts, close to the level of the junction (J), is seen; this would be most unusual for simple obstruction. **c:** A normal size gallbladder (G) and a grossly dilated common bile duct (CBD), measuring approximately 6 cm in maximum diameter, are present at this level. **d:** The distal common duct (CBD), in its intrapancreatic course, remains markedly dilated. The duct tapered rapidly below this point, to a normal caliber at the ampulla. The findings in this case are diagnostic of a choledochal cyst. (From Koehler and Stanley, ref. 64, with permission of the publisher.)

Caroli's disease.

Congenital cystic dilatation of the intrahepatic bile ducts, first described by Caroli in 1958, is a rare condition thought to be inherited as an autosomal recessive trait (24). The disease has been classified into two groups: (a) a pure form, unassociated with cirrhosis and portal hypertension and having a high incidence of cholangitis and calculus formation and (b) a type associated with congenital hepatic fibrosis in which the predominant clinical features are those of portal hypertension (23). In the latter type, complications of bile stasis may be latent or occur late in the patient's course.

Imaging findings in Caroli's disease have been previously reported with both US and CT examinations (12,61,77,113,117). On CT scans, multiple low-density branching tubular structures, characteristic of dilated bile ducts communicating with focal areas of increased ectasia, are present (Fig. 64). As with the choledochal

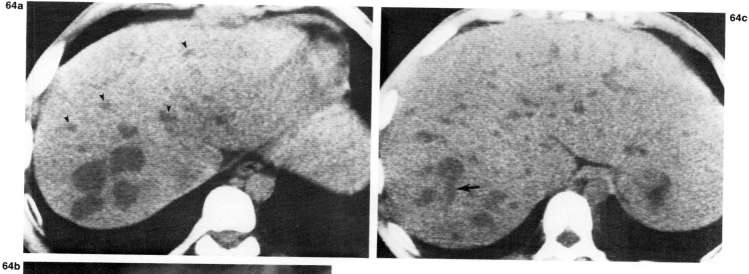

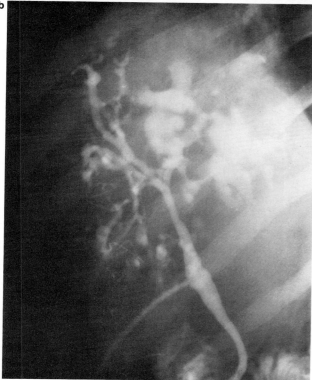

FIG. 64. Caroli's disease. **a:** A cluster of low-density, cystic-appearing areas is noted in the posterior aspect of the dome of the liver. Numerous smaller, low-density areas lie anteriorly (arrowheads). **b:** Two centimeters caudad, several of the cystic areas appear to communicate with more tubular structures (arrow), suggesting that the cystic areas are focally ectatic portions of the biliary tree. **c:** T-tube cholangiogram demonstrates focal cystic dilatation of intrahepatic portions of the biliary tree in the areas shown by the CT scan. (From Koehler and Stanley, ref. 64, with permission of the publisher.)

cyst, intravenous meglumine iodipamide may be of use in confirming communication of the cystic spaces with the biliary tree, if this relationship is not readily apparent (113).

The discovery of hepatic bile duct cysts on a CT examination in a patient with polyarteritis nodosa prompted one group of investigators to study its possible etiology in an animal model (29). They found that bile duct cysts could be produced in monkeys by injecting silicone particles to occlude the peripheral hepatic artery. They postulated that occlusion of small peripheral hepatic arteries led to ischemic infarction and bile duct epithelial necrosis. The bile duct cysts

were formed as a result of bile extravasation. The pathologic appearance of these cysts was identical to that in Caroli's disease, the cysts communicating with the biliary tree in both diseases. The clinical significance of this observation remains to be clarified.

Correlative Studies

The availability of sub-5 sec CT scanners with narrow collimation capability has greatly improved our ability to detect small, subtle lesions within the liver without interference from biologic motion. Modern gray scale and real time US has paralleled CT with its advances in technology and operator experience.

How CT and US compare with RI in the detection of focal liver disease is not yet clearly established. Numerous studies have attempted to determine the relative merits of the various imaging methods, considered both alone and in combination (17,20,63,71, 72,102,112,124). However, these studies have been flawed for a variety of reasons, including unequal quality of the imaging systems being compared, retrospective analysis, incompletely proven cases, and lack of adequate statistical analysis.

One prospective study evaluating metastatic colon and breast cancer to the liver, using state-of-the-art CT and US technology compared with RI, has been reported (1). Considering overall accuracy, sensitivity and specificity, CT consistently outperformed the other two imaging methods, although the differences were not marked. Despite the superiority of CT, Alderson et al. (1) still consider RI a reasonable primary screening method. Although we currently share that opinion, continuing improvement in CT technology, permitting a larger number of patients to be rapidly evaluated, may alter that concept.

Several studies of jaundiced patients have compared the accuracy of CT and US in determining whether or not obstructive jaundice was present (11,39,78). Although CT and US were essentially equal in the ability to detect the presence or absence of biliary obstruction (90–95%), CT was superior to US in determining both the level and cause of obstruction (11,78).

RECOMMENDATIONS FOR USE OF US, CT, AND RI

Considering the findings of comparative studies and our own experience, the following conclusions and recommendations for the use of US, CT, and RI are suggested.

In the patient suspected of having a focal lesion(s) in the liver, RI is the screening procedure of choice because of its ease and rapidity of performance, low cost, and sensitivity, which is at least equal to that of US or CT. However, in the continuing evaluation of oncology patients, where the liver is only one of several organs and areas of interest in the abdomen, CT may be the most efficacious imaging method. Both CT and US have the additional advantage over RI of providing important information about other upper abdominal structures (e.g., metastatic involvement of lymph nodes and the adrenal glands) in addition to hepatic and splenic imaging. In this regard, CT is superior to US in many cases, since CT is less organ directed than US. Any one of the three methods may occasionally demonstrate lesions not shown by the other two. When clinical features strongly suggest a hepatic abnormality and RI is negative, either US or CT may be helpful.

If a focal process is identified by RI or if the RI is equivocal, either US or CT may accurately further characterize the lesion or define an anatomical variant explaining the RI findings. Whether US or CT is the optimal procedure to use depends on a number of factors including body habitus, the location of the lesion, technical quality, and interpreter experience. The ability to suspend respiration, which was often difficult for many patients when 18-sec or slower scanners were in use, is no longer a major problem with CT scanners having a scanning time of 2 to 5 sec.

Radionuclide imaging presently is more sensitive (although of uncertain clinical significance) in the detection of hepatocellular disease than CT or US. Computed tomography appears to be the most accurate method for identifying fatty infiltration. Also, pre- and postintravenous contrast medium CT has, in our experience, proven to be the most reliable method of differentiating regenerating nodules from concommitant neoplasm.

Computed tomography and US have comparable sensitivity in detecting the presence of biliary obstruction but CT appears to be somewhat more accurate in defining the level and underlying etiology. Because of its nonionizing nature and lower cost, we employ US as the screening procedure for evaluating most patients suspected of having obstructive biliary tract disease. When the intra- and extrahepatic ducts are well seen sonographically and are normal in caliber, no further radiologic evaluation is needed in most patients. Computed tomography plays a major role in those patients in whom (a) sonographic abnormalities indicate ductal dilatation but do not clearly establish the level and etiology of the obstruction, (b) sonographic findings are equivocal, or (c) there is strong clinical suspicion of biliary obstruction despite apparent normal findings on sonography. In patients who are obese and in those with prior biliary-enteric bypass procedures, one can anticipate the likelihood of an unsatisfactory sonographic examination and in these patients CT is the optimal procedure. We currently reserve PTC or endoscopic retrograde cholangiography for patients in whom both CT and US are equivocal or unsatisfactory, or for patients in whom a fluoroscopically guided biliary drainage procedure is planned. In selected patients with ductal obstruction high in the porta hepatis, we also employ PTC to help the surgeon decide whether or not to attempt a surgical biliary-enteric bypass procedure.

In the evaluation of gallbladder disease, CT can play an important role in the detection and staging of carcinoma of the gallbladder; it has been shown to be very useful in evaluating patients with this often difficult diagnostic problem. It has an ancillary role in the study of cholecystitis, pericholecystic inflammatory disease, and calculous gallbladder disease but one should be familiar with the appearance of these conditions since they are commonly encountered in patients studied for other reasons.

REFERENCES

1. Alderson PO, Adams DF, McNeil BJ, et al.: A prospective study of computed tomography, ultrasound and nuclear imaging of the liver in patients with breast or colon cancer. *J Nucl Med* 22:P35, 1981
2. Alfidi RJ, Laval-Jeantet M: A promising contrast agent for computed tomography of the liver and spleen. *Radiology* 121:491, 1976
3. Angres G, Carter JB, Velasco JM: Unusual ring in liver cell adenoma. *AJR* 135:172–174, 1980
4. Araki T, Itai Y, Furui S, Tasaka A: Dynamic CT densitometry of hepatic tumors. *AJR* 135:1037–1043, 1980
5. Araki T, Itai Y, Tasaka A: CT of choledochal cyst. *AJR* 135:729–734, 1980
6. Araki T, Itai Y, Tasaka A: Computed tomography of localized dilatation of the intrahepatic bile ducts. *Radiology* 141:733–736, 1981
7. Atkinson GO Jr, Kodroff M, Sones PJ, Gay BB Jr: Focal nodular hyperplasia of the liver in children: A report of three new cases. *Radiology* 137:171–174, 1980
8. Axel L, Moss AA, Berninger W: Dynamic computed tomography demonstration of hepatic arteriovenous fistula. *J Comput Assist Tomogr* 5:95–98, 1981
9. Barnes PA, Thomas JL, Bernardino ML, et al.: Pitfalls in the diagnosis of hepatic cysts by CT. *Radiology* 141:129–134, 1981
10. Barnett PH, Zerhouni EA, White RI, Siegelman SS: Computed tomography in the diagnosis of cavernous hemangioma of the liver. *AJR* 134:439, 1980
11. Baron RL, Stanley RJ, Lee JKT, Koehler RE, Melson GL, Balfe DM, Weyman PJ: Prospective comparison of the evaluation of biliary obstruction with computed tomography and ultrasound. *Radiology* (in press)
12. Bass EM, Funston MR, Shaff MI: Caroli's disease: An ultrasonic diagnosis. *Br J Radiol* 50:366–369, 1977
13. Bernardino ME: Computed tomography of calcified liver metastasis. *J Comput Assist Tomogr* 3:32–35, 1979
14. Bernardino ME, Green B: Ultrasonographic evaluation of chemotherapeutic response in hepatic metastases. *Radiology* 133:437–441, 1979
15. Bernardino ML, Chung VP, Wallace S, Thomas JL, Soo C-S: Therapeutically infarcted tumors: CT findings. *AJR* 136:527–530, 1981
16. Bhatt GM, Jason RS, Delany HM, Rudavsky AZ: Hepatic hematoma: Percutaneous drainage. *AJR* 135:1287–1288, 1980
17. Biello DR, Levitt RG, Siegel BA, Sagel SS, Stanley RJ: Computed tomography and radionuclide imaging of the liver. A comparative evaluation. *Radiology* 127:159–163, 1978
18. Biersack HJ, Thelen M, Torres JF, Lackner K, Winkler CG: Focal nodular hyperplasia of the liver as established by 99mTc sulfur colloid and HIDA scintigraphy. *Radiology* 137:187–190, 1980
19. Blickman JG, McArdle CR: Budd-Chiari syndrome. *J Comput Assist Tomogr* 5:409–410, 1981
20. Bryan PJ, Dinn WM, Grossman ZD, Wistow BW, McAfee JG, Kieffer SA: Correlation of computed tomography, gray scale ultrasonography and radionuclide imaging of the liver in detecting space-occupying process. *Radiology* 124:387–393, 1977
21. Burgener FA, Hamlin DJ: Contrast enhancement in abdominal CT: Bolus vs infusion. *AJR* 137:351–358, 1981
22. Callen PW, Filly RA, Marcus FS: Ultrasonography and computed tomography in the evaluation of hepatic microabscesses in the immunosuppressed patient. *Radiology* 136:433–434, 1980
23. Caroli J: Diseases of intrahepatic bile ducts. *Isr J Med Sci* 4:21–35, 1968
24. Caroli J, Soupalt R, Kossakowski J, Placker L, Pavadowska: La dilatation polykystique congenitale des voies biliaries intrahepatiques. Essai de classification. *Sem Hop Paris* 34:488–495, 1958
25. Clark KE, Foley WD, Lawson TL, Berland LL, Maddison FE: CT evaluation of esophageal and upper abdominal varices. *J Comput Assist Tomogr* 4:510–515, 1980
26. Cohen Z, Seltzer SE, Davis MA, Hanson RN: Iodinated starch particles: new contrast material for computed tomography of the liver. *J Comput Assist Tomogr* 5:843–846, 1981
27. Cunningham DG, Churchill RJ, Reynes CJ: Computed tomography in the evaluation of liver disease in cystic fibrosis patients. *J Comput Assist Tomogr* 4:151–154, 1980
28. Doppman JL, Cornblath M, Dwyer AJ, Adams AJ, Girton ME, Sidbury J: Computerized tomography of the liver and kidneys in glycogen storage disease. *J Comput Assist Tomogr* 6:67–71, 1982
29. Doppman JL, Dunnick NR, Girton M, Fauci AS, Popovsky MA: Bile duct cysts secondary to liver infarcts: Report of a case and experimental procedure by small vessel hepatic artery occlusion. *Radiology* 130:1–5, 1979
30. Druy EM, Rubin BE: Computed tomography in the evaluation of abdominal trauma. *J Comput Assist Tomogr* 3:40–44, 1979
31. Federle MP, Filly RA, Moss AA: Cystic hepatic neoplasms: Complementary roles of CT and sonography. *AJR* 136:345–348, 1981
32. Federle MP, Goldberg HI, Kaiser JA, Moss AA, Jeffrey RB, Mall JC: Evaluation of abdominal trauma by computed tomography. *Radiology* 138:637–644, 1981
33. Federle MP, Jeffrey RB, Minagi H: Calcified liver metastasis from renal cell carcinoma. *J Comput Assist Tomogr* 5:771–772, 1981
34. Foley WD, Berland LL, Lawson TL, Maddison FE: Computed tomography in the demonstration of hepatic pseudoaneurysm with hemobilia. *J Comput Assist Tomogr* 4:863–865, 1980
35. Foley WD, Wilson CR, Quiroz FA, Lawson TL: Demonstration of the normal extrahepatic biliary tract with computed tomography. *J Comput Assist Tomogr* 4:48–52, 1980
36. Forrest ME, Cho KJ, Shields JJ, Wicks JD, Silver TM, McCormick TL: Biliary cystadenomas: Sonographic-angiographic-pathologic correlations. *AJR* 135:723–727, 1980
37. Freeny PC: Portal vein tumor thrombus: Demonstration by computed tomographic arteriography. *J Comput Assist Tomogr* 4:263–264, 1980
38. Gharbi HA, Hassine W, Brauner MW, Dupuch K: Ultrasound examination of the hydatic liver. *Radiology* 139:459–463, 1981
39. Goldberg HI, Filly RA, Korobkin M, Moss AA, Kressel HY, Callen PW: Capability of CT body scanning and ultrasonography to demonstrate the status of the biliary ductal system in patients with jaundice. *Radiology* 129:731–737, 1978
40. Gonzalez LR, Marcos J, Illanas M, Hernandez-Mora M, Pena S, Picouto JP, Cienfuegof JA, Alvarez JIR: Radiologic aspects of hepatic echinococcosis. *Radiology* 130:21–27, 1979
41. Graham MF, Cooperberg PL, Cohen MM, Burhenne HJ: Ultrasonographic screening of the common hepatic duct in symptomatic patients after cholecystectomy. *Radiology* 138:137–139, 1981
42. Haaga JR, Vanek J: Computed tomographic guided liver biopsy using the Menghini needle. *Radiology* 133:405–408, 1979
43. Han BK, Babcock DS, Gelfand MH: Choledochal cyst with bile duct dilatation: sonography and 99mTc IDA cholescintigraphy. *AJR* 136:1075–1079, 1981
44. Harbin WP, Robert NJ, Ferrucci JT: Diagnosis of cirrhosis based on regional changes in hepatic morphology. *Radiology* 135:273–283, 1980
45. Haubek A, Pedersen JH, Burcharth F, Gammelgaard J, Hancke S, Willumsen L: Dynamic sonography in the evaluation of jaundice. *AJR* 136:1071–1074, 1981
46. Havrilla TR, Haaga JR, Alfidi RJ, Reich NE: Computed tomography and obstructive biliary disease. *AJR* 128:765–768, 1977
47. Havrilla TR, Reich NE, Haaga JR, Seidelmann SE, Cooper-

man AM, Alfidi, RJ: Computed tomography of the gall-bladder. *AJR* 130:1059–1067, 1978

48. Havron A, Davis MA, Seltzer SE, Paskins-Hurlburt AJ, Hessel SJ: Heavy metal particulate contrast materials for computed tomography of the liver. *J Comput Assist Tomogr* 4:642–648, 1980

49. Henderson JM, Heymsfield SB, Horowitz J, Kutner MH: Measurement of liver and spleen volume by computed tomography. *Radiology* 141:525–527, 1981

50. Henderson JM, Liechty EJ, Jahnke RW: Liver involvement in hereditary hemorrhagic telangiectasia. *J Comput Assist Tomogr* 5:773–776, 1981

51. Herskovic A, Heaston D, Engler MJ, Fishburn RI, Jones RS, Noell KT: Irradiation of biliary carcinoma. *Radiology* 139:219–222, 1981

52. Itai Y, Araki T, Furui S, Tasaka A, Atomi Y, Kuroda A: CT of hepatoma: Effects of portal vein obstruction. *AJR* 136:349–353, 1981

53. Itai Y, Araki T, Furui S, et al.: Computed tomography and ultrasound in the diagnosis of intrahepatic calculi. *Radiology* 136:399–405, 1980

54. Itai Y, Araki T, Furui S, Tasaka A: Differential diagnosis of hepatic masses on computed tomography, with particular reference to hepatocellular carcinoma. *J Comput Assist Tomogr* 5:834–842, 1981

55. Itai Y, Araki T, Yoshikawa K. Furui S, Yashiro N, Tasaka A: Computed tomography of gallbladder carcinoma. *Radiology* 137:713–718, 1980

56. Itai Y, Furui S, Araki T, Yashiro N, Tasaka A: Computed tomography of cavernous hemangioma of the liver. *Radiology* 137:149–155, 1980

57. Itai Y, Nishikawa J, Tasaka A: Computed tomography in the evaluation of hepatocellular carcinoma. *Radiology* 131:165–170, 1979

58. Jacobson JB, Brodey PA: The transverse common duct. *AJR* 136:91–95, 1981

59. Jeffrey RB, Moss AA, Quivey JM, Federle MP, Wara WM: CT of radiation-induced hepatic injury. *AJR* 135:445–448, 1980

60. Johnson CM, Sheedy PF, Stanson AW, Stephens DH, Hattery RR, Adson MA: Computed tomography and angiography of cavernous hemangiomas of the liver. *Radiology* 138:115–121, 1981

61. Kaiser JA, Mall JC, Salmen BJ, Parker JJ: Diagnosis of Caroli disease by computed tomography. Report of two cases. *Radiology* 132:661–664, 1979

62. Kinney TD, Ferrebee JW: Hepatic abscess: Factors determining its localization. *Arch Pathol* 45:41, 1948

63. Knopf DR, Torres WE, Fajman WJ, Sones PJ: Liver lesions: Comparative accuracy of scintigraphy and computed tomography. *AJR* 138:623–627, 1982

64. Koehler RE, Stanley RJ: Computed tomography. In: *Diagnostic and Interventional Radiology of the Gallbladder and Bile Ducts*, ed. by RN Berk, JT Ferrucci, and GR Leopold, Philadelphia, Saunders, 1982

65. Kolbenstvedt A, Kjolseth I, Klepp O, Kolmannskog F: Postirradiation changes of the liver demonstrated by computed tomography. *Radiology* 135:391, 1980

66. Korobkin M, Kirks DR, Sullivan DC, Mills SR, Bowie JD: Computed tomography of primary liver tumors in children. *Radiology* 139:431–435, 1981

67. Kuhns LR, Borlaza G: Normal roentgen variant: Aberrant right hepatic artery on computed tomography. *Radiology* 135:392, 1980

68. Kunstlinger F, Federle MP, Moss AA, Marks W: Computed tomography of hepatocellular carcinoma. *AJR* 134:431–437, 1980

69. Levitt RG, Sagel SS, Stanley RJ, Jost RG: Accuracy of computed tomography of the liver and biliary tract. *Radiology* 124:123–128, 1977

70. Long JA, Doppman JL, Nienhus AW, Mills SR: Computed tomographic analysis of beta-thalassemic syndromes with hemochromatosis: Pathologic findings with clinical and laboratory correlations. *J Comput Assist Tomogr* 4:159–165, 1980

71. MacCarty RL, Stephens DH, Hattery RR, Sheedy PF: Hepatic imaging by computed tomography. A comparison with ⁹⁹ᵐTc-sulfur coloid ultrasonography and angiography. *Radiol Clin North Am* 17:137–156, 1979

72. MacCarty RL, Wahner WH, Stephens DH, Sheedy PF, Hattery RR: Retrospective comparison of radionuclide scans and computed tomography of the liver and pancreas. *AJR* 129:23–28, 1977

73. Marchal GJ, Baert AL, Wilms GE: CT of noncystic liver lesions: Bolus enhancement. *AJR* 135:57–65, 1980

74. Marks WM, Filly RA: Computed tomographic demonstration of intraarterial air following hepatic artery ligation. *Radiology* 132:665–666, 1979

75. Michels NA: Newer anatomy of the liver and its variant blood supply and collateral circulation. *Am J Surg* 112:337–347, 1966

76. Mills SR, Doppman JL, Neinhus AW: Computed tomography in the diagnosis of disorders of excessive iron storage of the liver. *J Comput Assist Tomogr* 1:101–104, 1977

77. Mittelstaedt CA, Volberg FM, Fischer GJ, McCartney WH: Caroli's disease: Sonographic findings. *AJR* 134:585–587, 1980

78. Morris AI, Fawcitt RA, Wood R, Forbes WSC, Isherwood I, Marsh MN: Computed tomography, ultrasound and cholestatic jaundice. *Gut* 19:685–688, 1978

79. Moss AA, Cann CE, Friedman MA, Marcus FS, Resser KJ, Berninger W: Volumetric CT analysis of hepatic tumors. *J Comput Assist Tomogr* 5:714–718, 1981

80. Moss AA, Filly RA, Way LW: In vitro investigation of gallstones with computed tomography. *J Comput Assist Tomogr* 4:827–831, 1980

81. Moss AA, Friedman MA, Brito AC: Determination of liver, kidney, and spleen volumes by computed tomography: An experimental study in dogs. *J Comput Assist Tomogr* 5:12–14, 1981

82. Moss AA, Schrumpf J, Schnyder P, Korobkin M, Shimshak RR: Computed tomography of focal hepatic lesions: A blind clinical evaluation of the effect of contrast enhancement. *Radiology* 131:427–430, 1979

83. Mueller RO, Ferrucci JT, Simeone JF, Wittenberg J, vanSonnenberg E, Polansky A, Isler RJ: Postcholecystectomy bile duct dilatation: Myth or reality? *AJR* 136:355–358, 1981

84. Mueller RP, Harbin WP, Ferrucci JT, Wittenberg J, vanSonnenberg E: Fine-needle transhepatic cholangiography: Reflections after 450 cases. *AJR* 136:85–90, 1981

85. Mulhern CB, Arger PH, Coleman BG, Stein GN: Nonuniform attenuation in computed tomography study of the cirrhotic liver. *Radiology* 132:399–402, 1979

86. Nakata H, Nobe T, Takahashi M, Maeda T, Koga M: Choledochal cyst. *J Comput Assist Tomogr* 5:99–101, 1981

87. Nishikawa J, Itai Y, Tasaka A: Lobar attenuation difference of the liver on computed tomography. *Radiology* 141:725–728, 1981

88. Noon MA, Young SW: Aberrant right hepatic artery: A normal variant demonstrated by computed tomography. *J Comput Assist Tomogr* 5:411–412, 1981

89. Noon MA, Young SW, Castellino RA: Leiomyosarcoma metastatic to the liver: CT appearance. *J Comput Assist Tomogr* 4:527–530, 1980

90. Park SC, Glanz S, Gordon DH, Johnson M: Computed tomography and angiography in the Cruveilhier-Baumgarten syndrome. *J Comput Assist Tomogr* 5:19–21, 1981

91. Parulekar SG: Ligaments and fissures of the liver: Sonographic anatomy. *Radiology* 130:409–411, 1979

92. Pedrosa CS, Casanova R, Lezana AH, Fernandez MC: CT in obstructive jaundice, Part II: The cause of obstruction. *Radiology* 139:635–646, 1981

93. Pedrosa CS, Casanova R, Lezana AH, Rodriguez R: CT in obstructive jaundice. Part I: The level of obstruction. *Radiology* 139:627–634, 1981

94. Pedrosa CS, Casanova R, Rodriguez R: CT cholangiography: Multiplanar reconstruction in obstructive jaundice. *J Comput Assist Tomogr* 5:503–508, 1981

95. Penkava RR, Rothenberg J: Spontaneous resolution of oral-contraceptive-associated liver tumor. *J Comput Assist Tomogr* 5:102–103, 1981

96. Piekarski J, Goldberg HI, Royal SA, Axel L, Moss AA: Difference between liver and spleen CT numbers in the normal adult: Its usefulness in predicting the presence of diffuse liver disease. *Radiology* 137:727−729, 1980

97. Prando A, Wallace S, Bernardino ME, Lindell MN, Jr.: Computed tomographic arteriography of the liver. *Radiology* 130:697−701, 1979

98. Roemer CE, Ferrucci JT, Mueller PR, Simeone JF, vanSonnenberg E, Wittenberg J: Hepatic cysts: Diagnosis and therapy by sonographic needle aspiration. *AJR* 136:1065−1070, 1981

99. Rogers JV, Mack LA, Freeny PC, Johnson ML, Sones PJ: Hepatic focal nodular hyperplasia: angiography, CT, sonography, and scintigraphy. *AJR* 137:983−990, 1981

100. Rossi P, Sposito M, Simonetti G, Sposato S, Cusumano G: CT diagnosis of Budd-Chiari syndrome. *J Comput Assist Tomogr* 5:366−369, 1981

101. Royal SA, Beiderman BA, Goldberg HI, Koerper M, Chaler MN: Detection and estimation of iron, glycogen and fat in liver of children with hepatomegaly using CT. *Pediatr Res* 13:408, 1979

102. Rubinson HW, Isikoff MB, Hill MC: Diagnostic imaging of hepatic abscesses: A retrospective analysis. *AJR* 135:735−740, 1980

103. Ruiz R, Teyssou H, Fernandez N, Carrez JP, Gortchakoff M, Manteau G, Ter-Davtian PM, Tessier JP: Ultrasonic diagnosis of primary carcinoma of the gallbladder: A review of 16 cases. *J Clin Ultrasound* 8:489−495, 1980

104. Sample WF, Sarti DA, Goldstein LI, Weiner M, Kadell BM: Gray-scale ultrasonography of the jaundiced patient. *Radiology* 128:719−725, 1978

105. Sauerbrei EE, Cooperberg PL, Gordon P, Li D, Cohen MM, Burhenne HJ: The discrepancy between radiographic and sonographic bile-duct measurements. *Radiology* 137:751−755, 1980

106. Scherer U, Weinzierl M, Sturm R, Schildberg F-W, Zrenner M, Lissner J: Computed tomography in hydatid disease of the liver. A report of 13 cases. *J Comput Assist Tomogr* 2:612−617, 1978

107. Scott WW, Sanders RC, Siegelman SS: Irregular fatty infiltration of the liver: diagnostic dilemmas. *AJR* 135:67−71, 1980

108. Seltzer SE, Adams DF, Davis MA, Hessel SJ, Havron A, Judy PF, Paskins-Hurlburt AJ, Hollenberg NK: Hepatic contrast agents for computed tomography: High atomic number particulate material. *J Comput Assist Tomogr* 5:370−374, 1981

109. Seshul MB, Coulam CM: Pseudomyxoma peritonei: Computed tomography and sonography. *AJR* 136:803−806, 1981

110. Shanser JD, Korobkin M, Goldberg HI, Rohlfing BM: Computed tomographic diagnosis of obstructive jaundice in the absence of intrahepatic ductal dilatation. *AJR* 131:389−392, 1979

111. Shimizu H, Ida M, Takayama S, Seki T, Yoneda M, Nakaya S, Yanagi T, Bando B, Sato H, Uchiyama M, Okumura T, Miura S, Fujisawa M: The diagnostic accuracy of computed tomography in obstructive biliary disease: A comparative evaluation with direct cholangiography. *Radiology* 138:411−416, 1981

112. Snow JH, Goldstein HM, Wallace S: Comparison of scintigraphy, sonography and computed tomography in the evaluation of hepatic neoplasms. *AJR* 132:915−918, 1979

113. Sorensen KW, Glazer GM, Francis IR: Diagnosis of cystic ectasia of intrahepatic bile ducts by computed tomography. *J Comput Assist Tomogr* 6:486−489, 1982

114. Stanley RJ, Sagel SS: Computed tomography of the liver and biliary tract. In: *Radiology of the Gallbladder and Bile Ducts,* ed. by RN Berk and AR Clemett, Philadelphia, Saunders, 1977, p 352

115. Stanley RJ, Sagel SS, Levitt RG: Computed tomography of the liver. *Radiol Clin North Am* 15:331−348, 1977

116. Stephens DH, Sheedy PF, Hattery RR, MacCarty RL: Computed tomography of the liver. *AJR* 128:579−590, 1977

117. Taylor KJW, Carpenter DA, Hill CR, McCready VR: Gray scale ultrasound imaging. The anatomy and pathology of the liver. *Radiology* 119:415−423, 1976

118. Taylor KJW, Gorelick FS, Rosenfield AT, Riely CA: Ultrasonography of alcoholic liver disease with histological correlation. *Radiology* 141:157−161, 1981

119. Thomas JL, Bernardino ME: Segmental biliary obstruction: Its detection and significance. *J Comput Assist Tomogr* 4:155−158, 1980

120. Toombs BD, Sandler CM, Conoley PM: Computed tomography of the nonvisualizing gallbladder. *J Comput Assist Tomogr* 5:164−168, 1981

121. Vermess M, Bernardino ME, Doppman JL, Fisher RI, Thomas JL, Velasquez WS, Fuller LM, Russo A: Use of intravenous liposoluble contrast material for the examination of the liver and spleen in lymphoma. *J Comput Assist Tomogr* 5:709−713, 1981

122. Vermess M, Chatterji DC, Doppman JL, Grimes G, Adamson RH: Development and experimental evaluation of contrast medium for computed tomographic examination of the liver and spleen. *J Comput Assist Tomogr* 3:25−31, 1979

123. Vermess M, Doppman JL, Sugarbaker P, Fisher RI, Chatterji DC, Luetzeler J, Grimes G, Girton M, Adamson RH: Clinical trials with a new intravenous liposoluble contrast material for computed tomography of the liver and spleen. *Radiology* 137:217−222, 1980

124. Vicary FR, Shirly I: Ultrasound and hepatic metastases. *Br J Radiol* 51:596−598, 1978

125. Vigo M, DeFaveri D, Biondetti PR, Benedetti L: CT demonstration of portal and superior mesenteric vein thrombosis in hepatocellular carcinoma. *J Comput Assist Tomogr* 4:627−629, 1980

126. Wooten WB, Bernardino ML, Goldstein HM: Computed tomography of necrotic metastases. *AJR* 131:839−842, 1978

127. Yeh HC: Ultrasonography and computed tomography of carcinoma of the gallbladder. *Radiology* 133:167−173, 1979

128. Zeman RK, Dorfman GS, Burrell MI, Stein S, Berg GR, Gold JA: Disparate dilatation of the intrahepatic and extrahepatic bile ducts in surgical jaundice. *Radiology* 138:129−136, 1981

129. Zornoza J, Ginaldi S: Computed tomography in hepatic lymphoma. *Radiology* 138:405−410, 1981

Chapter 8

Pancreas

Matthew A. Mauro and Robert J. Stanley

Prior to the advent of the current cross-sectional imaging methods, radiographic evaluation of pancreatic abnormalities consisted of plain radiographs, gastrointestinal barium examinations, and the more invasive techniques such as angiography, endoscopic retrograde cholangiopancreatography (ERCP), and percutaneous transhepatic cholangiography (PTC). Although plain abdominal radiographs may show a focal ileus in acute pancreatitis, extraluminal air in pancreatic abscess, or calcifications in chronic pancreatitis, and barium studies may demonstrate displacement or distortion of adjoining stomach and duodenum, these studies are insensitive and nonspecific. More invasive techniques have improved accuracy; however, they also have associated morbidity and still do not directly image the gland. Computed tomography and ultrasonography (US) offer the unique ability to image the pancreas and adjacent structures directly, allowing visualization of the primary pancreatic abnormality rather than an indirect manifestation of the disease.

NORMAL ANATOMY

There is considerable variation in the orientation, shape, and size of the pancreas. Appreciation of the myriad of normal forms that the pancreas can assume is necessary for both proper conduct and correct interpretation of CT examinations. Despite the retroperitoneal location of the pancreas, the organ is located predominantly anterior to the midcoronal plane of the body. An oblique orientation of the pancreas across the upper abdomen is most often seen with the tail lying several centimeters cephalad to the head. Transverse and U-shaped orientations, where the body is slightly cephalad and anterior to the head and tail, are not uncommon. When the pancreas is relatively horizontal, three to four contiguous 1-cm-thick images usually encompass the entire gland (Fig. 1).

Form

Assessment of pancreatic size is important because both neoplastic and inflammatory processes com-

monly alter the size of the gland. However, the many variations of size and shape, some of which may simulate a focal mass, make it difficult to determine whether or not the gland is enlarged. With current sub-5-second scanners, measurements of the pancreas remain variable; the head averages approximately 2.0 cm and the body and tail approximately 1.2 cm when measured perpendicular to the long axis of the gland on the cross-sectional view (14). Such values are comparable to those previously reported with US. With aging, the pancreas normally decreases in size and may show fatty replacement; therefore, any measurements must be correlated with the patient's age (21,53). However, due to the variability in size, a focal contour change is a more reliable indicator of pancreatic pathology than any measurement. The pancreas gradually tapers from head to tail except at the neck where there is a normal narrowing due to the dorsal crossing of the portal vein (Fig. 1).

The surface of the pancreas is smooth or lobulated. The lobulated appearance is due to fatty septae and is being seen more often with sub-5-second scanners (Fig. 2) (67). Fatty replacement of the pancreas is a common degenerative process seen in the elderly (Figs. 3 and 4). Pancreatic ductal dilatation can also occur with aging, with ductal diameters reported to increase 8% per decade after the fifth decade (38). The term *fatty infiltration* is preferred in obese patients where the process is not pathologic and is reversible. Severe fatty replacement may be associated with a compromise of pancreatic function and may be seen as a late sequela to chronic pancreatitis (53).

Anatomic Relationships

The splenic vein serves as one of the major CT landmarks for the body and tail of the pancreas. It lies on the dorsal surface of the body and tail of the pancreas caudal to the splenic artery. A fat plane often separates the splenic vein from pancreas and should not be mistaken for a dilated pancreatic duct (Fig. 4). In difficult cases where the substance of the pancreas cannot be easily distinguished from the splenic vein, intravenous contrast material administration aids dis-

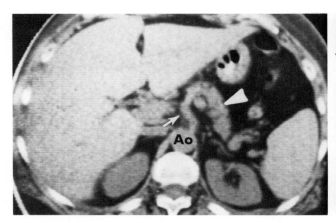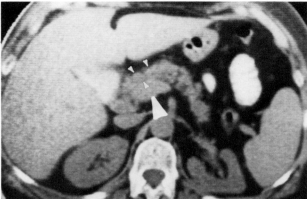

FIG. 1. Normal pancreas. **Left:** The celiac axis (arrow) can be seen emerging from the aorta (Ao). The splenic vein is seen end on in this patient as it courses dorsal to the pancreas (large arrowhead). **Right:** One centimeter inferiorly, normal narrowing of the neck of the pancreas (small arrowheads) is demonstrated due to dorsal crossing of the portal vein (large arrowhead).

tinction by opacifying the vein (Fig. 5). The left adrenal gland lies posterior to the splenic vein and the pancreas at the junction of the body and tail.

The tail of the pancreas extends to the splenic hilus, entering the splenorenal ligament and becoming intraperitoneal for a short distance. Although generally located anterior to the splenic vein, the tail may rarely curve posterior to the splenic vein. In almost all normal patients, the tail is located anterior or anterolateral to the left kidney (Fig. 6), but rarely lies adjacent to the aorta and anteromedial to the kidney simulating a mass (50). In patients with an absent (surgical or congenital) or small left kidney, the tail will

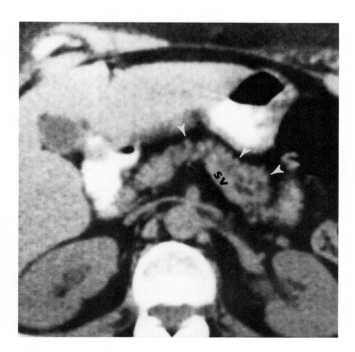

FIG. 2. Normal pancreas. Lobulated pancreatic surface (arrowheads) due to fatty septae. sv, splenic vein.

often be displaced posteromedially adjacent to the spine, occupying the empty renal fossa (10).

The body of the pancreas arches over the superior mesenteric artery and aorta, separated by a distinct fat plane (Fig. 2). The superior mesenteric vein runs parallel to and to the right of the superior mesenteric artery and is usually larger in diameter (Fig. 7). The superior mesenteric vein joins the splenic vein forming the portal vein just dorsal to the neck of the pancreas. Intravenous contrast material often is needed to distinguish the superior mesenteric and portal veins from the pancreas.

The head of the pancreas lies medial to the second portion of the duodenum, to the right and caudal to the portal vein, and just anterior to the inferior vena cava. The uncinate process, a structure of variable prominence, is a hook-like inferior extension of the head that is lateral to the superior mesenteric vein and curves posteriorly under it at the level of the renal veins (Figs. 7 and 8). The normal sized common bile duct measuring 3 to 6 mm in diameter can be seen in cross-section at the lateral aspect of the head as a circular, near water-density structure (Fig. 6), especially in scans performed after intravenous contrast enhancement (25). It is unusual to see the normal pancreatic duct with routine 1-cm collimation. However, with 5-mm collimation, small field of view, and intravenous contrast material administration, the normal duct can be seen in almost 70% of patients and measures up to 5 mm in the head and 2 mm in the body and tail (5). The normal duct is usually seen either in cross-section within the head medial to the common bile duct or as a tubular structure within the body and tail, but only very rarely in its entirety. A normal appearing pancreatic duct on CT does not exclude mild ductal dilatation (5,8).

The pancreas lies in the anterior pararenal space and is related to the second segment of the duodenum

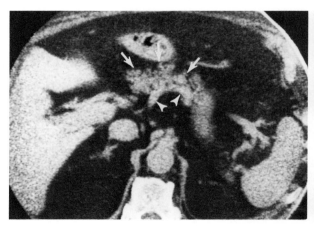
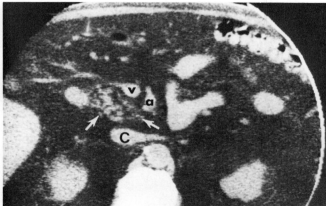

FIG. 3. Fatty infiltration of the pancreas. Pancreatic lobules are seen amid the fat in this extremely obese patient. **Left:** Level through body of pancreas (arrows). Arrowheads indicate splenic vein. **Right:** Level of uncinate process (arrows). C, inferior vena cava; v, superior mesenteric vein; a, superior mesenteric artery.

along the lateral surface of the head, and the third and fourth segments of the duodenum along the inferior surface of the body and tail. The stomach is anterior to the pancreas and separated from it by the lesser sac, a potential space. The peritoneal leaves of the transverse mesocolon, which form the inferior boundary of the lesser sac, fuse as they come off the entire ventral surface of the pancreas.

The retroperitoneal fat is the tissue most responsible for defining the pancreas on CT scans. When fat is lacking, contiguous organs can blend imperceptibly with the pancreas. Fortunately, the structures most likely to present a problem (adjacent gastrointestinal viscera and blood vessels) can be opacified with contrast material. Nonopacified loops of bowel contig-

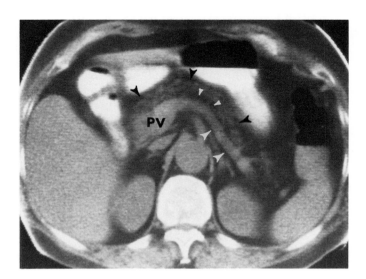

FIG. 4. Normal splenic vein (large white arrowheads) coursing along the dorsal surface of the body and tail of the pancreas (black arrowheads). The pancreatic lobules are well projected by extensive fatty infiltration. Note fat plane (small white arrowheads) separating the splenic vein and pancreas. PV, portal vein.

uous with the body and tail of the pancreas can simulate a pancreatic tumor. Adequate volumes of oral contrast medium must be used to avoid misinterpreting such pseudotumors (Fig. 9). Tortuous splenic arteries and veins also can simulate a mass lesion. Bolus technique will usually resolve this potential source of error (Fig. 10).

PATHOLOGIC CONDITIONS

Neoplasia

Adenocarcinoma

Adenocarcinoma represents 95% of the primary malignant tumors of the pancreas (4). The major CT finding is a focal soft tissue mass altering the contour of the gland (Figs. 11 and 12) (57). The density of the mass usually is similar to or slightly less than that of the normal organ. Sometimes the difference in density between a pancreatic carcinoma and the normal parenchyma may be accentuated by intravenous contrast media, which generally causes perceptible opacification of the normal pancreas and its vascular bed while leaving the relatively hypovascular tumor unenhanced. Pancreatic adenocarcinoma virtually never calcifies; however, a cancer may arise in a gland containing calcification (62). Since the attenuation value of tumor is similar to that of normal tissue, the lesion usually must alter the contour of the pancreas in order to be detected. Most pancreatic carcinomas at clinical presentation are large enough to be detected by CT. With the improved resolution of newer scanners, more subtle changes may be detectable—such as loss of the lobulated appearance or faint low density areas in a tumor (necrosis or cystic degeneration)—before a gross mass is apparent. Normal pancreatic parenchyma is frequently heterogeneous in its density due to the interdigitation of fat. A focal area of

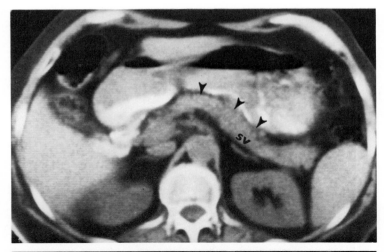

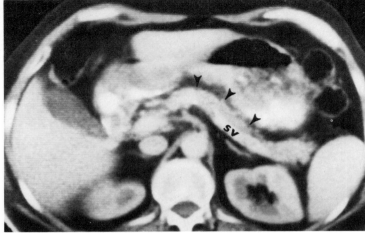

FIG. 5. Above: Differentiation of splenic vein (sv) and substance of the pancreas (arrowheads) is not obvious. **Below:** Following bolus injection of intravenous contrast material, the splenic vein (sv) opacifies and is easily distinguished from pancreas (arrowheads).

homogeneous density, even without apparent mass enlargement, should be viewed with suspicion in the patient with clinical signs or symptoms of pancreatic disease (Fig. 13).

In one large series, 61% of pancreatic cancers occurred in the head, whereas 13% were in the body, 5% in the tail, and 21% diffusely involved the gland (4). Due to the pancreatic head's intimate relationship to the common bile duct and duodenum, carcinomas arising there tend to present earlier. They are, therefore, generally smaller than tumors of the body or tail, but large carcinomas may be present in the head of the pancreas in patients who are not jaundiced. In the absence of a calculus, combined dilatation of the common bile duct and main pancreatic duct strongly suggests the presence of an ampullary or pancreatic head tumor even though the tumor itself may not be recognizable as a discrete mass (Fig. 14). Small neoplasms of the uncinate process can be detected on CT by noting a round or oval shape to the normally slender, hook-like process. Rounded, convex borders to both anterior and posterior surfaces of the uncinate should be considered abnormal (Fig. 15) (40).

Occasionally, the entire gland is infiltrated with tumor and usually appears grossly enlarged and distorted.

A carcinoma of the pancreatic head may produce changes on CT in the body and tail of the pancreas such as a dilated pancreatic duct, pseudocyst (Figs. 16 and 17) or retention cyst, edema, or atrophy (Fig. 12) (34). If the gland is transversely oriented, the obstructed dilated pancreatic duct will appear either as an obvious tubular structure or as a series of adjacent rounded or oval cystic spaces within the substance of the pancreas, the latter occasionally being confused with pseudocysts (Figs. 13 and 14) (33). A dilated pancreatic duct is a sensitive indicator of pancreatic disease, but is not specific for carcinoma and can occur in pancreatitis with or without impacted calculi and in duodenal inflammatory disease (5,28,33). In a patient without a history of pancreatitis, a dilated pancreatic duct should imply a proximal tumor. Occasionally, with malignant obstruction of the pancreatic duct, intraductal pressure will rise to a point causing rupture of small ducts and enzyme release. These patients may have clinical and biochemical evidence of pancreatitis and develop retention cysts,

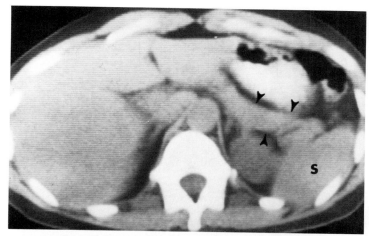

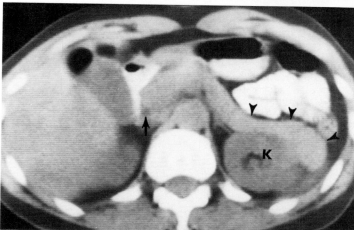

FIG. 6. **Above:** The pancreatic tail (arrowheads) courses toward the hilum of the spleen (S). **Below:** Two centimeters inferiorly, the pancreatic tail (arrowheads) lies in intimate association with the anterolateral surface of the left kidney (K) in this lean patient. A normal common bile duct (arrow) is seen in the lateral portion of the pancreatic head.

pseudocysts, and edema. Such patients with carcinoma presenting as acute pancreatitis are middle to older aged with only a short history of pancreatitis without apparent cause (41). If a neoplasm is suspected as the cause of a dilated main pancreatic duct, but is not apparent on CT, ERCP would be indicated for further evaluation.

Although a focal mass is the primary CT finding of adenocarcinoma of the pancreas, other findings include (a) obliteration of peripancreatic fat planes posteriorly, especially the fat surrounding the superior mesenteric vessels, celiac trunk, and aorta (Figs. 11, 12, and 17), (b) peripancreatic, periaortic, pericaval, and portal lymph node enlargement, and (c) liver metastases (40,67). Neoplastic invasion of the fat surrounding the superior mesenteric artery and celiac trunk may result in a thickened appearance of these vessels on CT (Figs. 18–20) (44). Peripancreatic fat invasion is almost always associated with an obvious mass, especially with tumors of the body and tail. Common bile duct, pancreatic duct, and splenic vein dilatation from obstruction can be seen with carcinoma, but can occur with pancreatitis as well. Due to the rich vascular and lymphatic supply of the

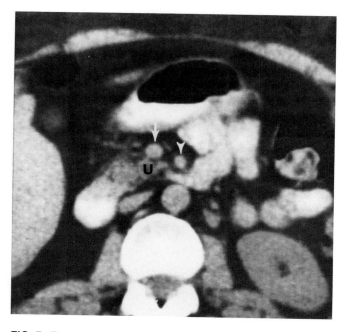

FIG. 7. The superior mesenteric vein (arrow), coursing parallel to and to the right of the superior mesenteric artery (arrowhead), lies immediately anterior to the medial tip of the uncinate process (U).

218

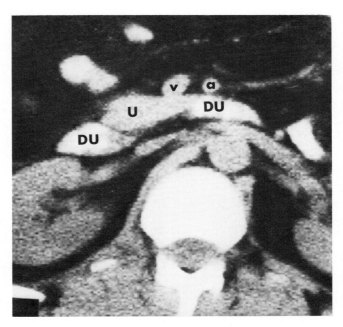

FIG. 8. Uncinate process (U), lateral and posterior to the superior mesenteric vessels, is distinguished from the adjacent duodenum (DU), which is filled with orally administered contrast medium. v, superior mesenteric vein; a, superior mesenteric artery.

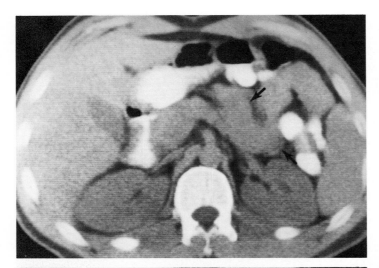

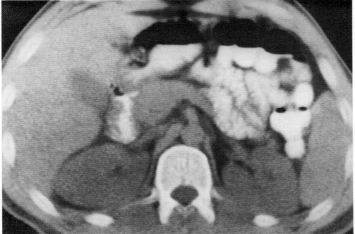

FIG. 9. Pancreatic "pseudotumor." **Above:** A possible soft tissue mass (arrows) is present in the region of the pancreatic tail. Is this a neoplasm or unopacified loops of bowel? **Below:** Scan following additional oral contrast shows the "mass" to be simply proximal jejunum.

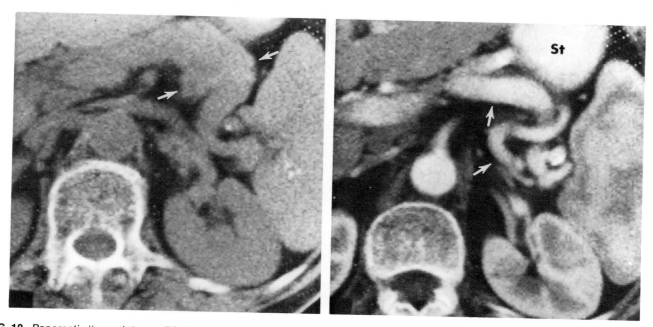

FIG. 10. Pancreatic "pseudotumor." **Left:** Suspicion of a mass lesion (arrows) in the region of the pancreatic tail. **Right:** Scan following intravenous bolus enhancement demonstrates the "mass" to be tortuous splenic vessels (arrows). St, stomach.

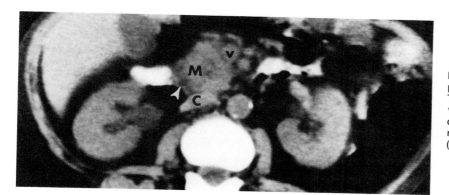

FIG. 11. Carcinoma of the head and uncinate process. A large, irregular mass (M) is present. The fat plane between the pancreas and inferior vena cava (C) and superior mesenteric vein (v) is obliterated, suggesting the possibility of non-resectability. A normal distal common bile duct (arrowhead) can be seen.

FIG. 12. Carcinoma of the pancreatic body. Mass (M) abruptly distorts the contour of the gland and appears to obliterate the fat plane between the pancreas and the superior mesenteric artery at one point (black arrowhead). There is atrophy of the pancreatic tail (white arrowhead).

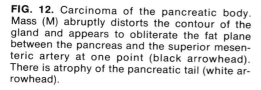

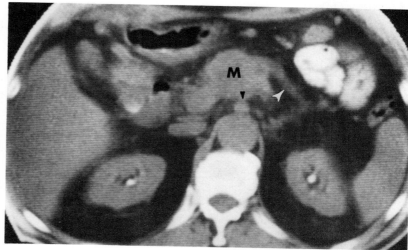

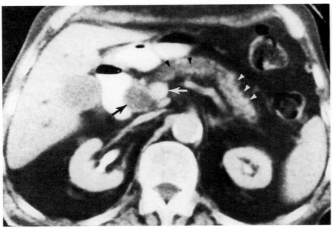
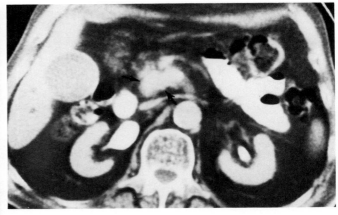

FIG. 13. Small carcinoma of the head of the pancreas producing obstructive jaundice. **Left:** A distal common bile duct (black arrow), 2 cm in diameter, lies lateral to the portal vein (white arrow). Dilatation of the main pancreatic duct (black arrowheads) is also seen. Note the contour of the lobulated pancreatic parenchyma partially infiltrated with fat in the body and tail (white arrowheads). **Right:** The obstructing mass (arrows) arising in the head of the pancreas does not produce obvious enlargement of the gland. However, the homogeneous and slightly higher density of the tumor is distinctly different from the typically lobulated heterogeneous density of the normal pancreatic parenchyma.

pancreas and lack of a capsule, regional metastases tend to occur early (Fig. 21). However, peripancreatic lymph node metastases may be inseparable from the primary pancreatic mass on CT. An adenocarcinoma of the tail may rarely extend posterior to the splenic vein via a superior or inferior route and simulate a left adrenal mass (7). The CT criteria for unresectability include a pancreatic mass with evidence of regional lymph node, hepatic or distant metastases, invasion of contiguous organs, encasement of vascular structures, and high density (hemorrhagic) ascites (Figs. 17–21) (26).

A focal mass alone is not specific for carcinoma and can be seen in acute or chronic pancreatitis (60,67). When focal pancreatitis results in a mass, it is usually in the head. Only when secondary signs of malignancy are present can a confident diagnosis of adenocarcinoma be made. If a focal mass is seen on CT in a patient whose clinical features are more compatible with acute pancreatitis, follow-up scans should be obtained to document its resolution. In equivocal or indeterminate cases, ERCP or direct percutaneous thin needle biopsy can assist in diagnosis. The combined use of CT and ERCP improves diagnostic accuracy compared with either method alone in pancreatic carcinoma (5,24,48). In several centers, CT- or

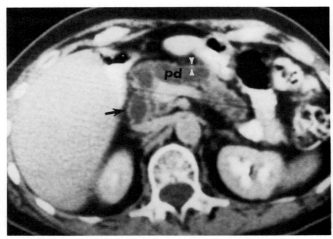
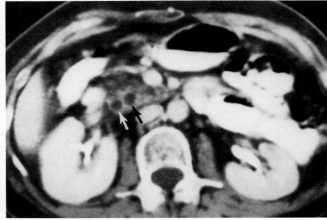

FIG. 14. Ampullary carcinoma producing obstructive jaundice. **Left:** Obstruction of the level of the ampulla produces marked dilatation of the main pancreatic duct (pd) with compression and thinning of the pancreatic parenchyma (arrowheads). A dilated common bile duct (arrow) is also visible. **Right:** Several centimeters caudad, the dilated common bile duct (white arrow) and main pancreatic duct (black arrow) lie side by side, an appearance characteristic of obstruction at the ampullary level.

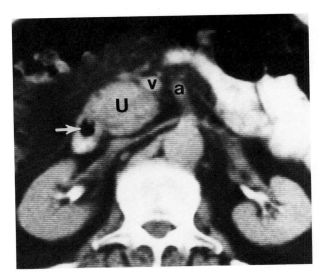

FIG. 15. Carcinoma of the uncinate process. There is rounding of the normal slender hook-like configuration of the uncinate process (U) as it extends posterior to the superior mesenteric vein (v). Convex borders to both the anterior and posterior surfaces of the uncinate process should be considered abnormal. Arrow indicates duodenum. a, superior mesenteric artery.

US-guided percutaneous biopsies in equivocal cases have produced positive results in 85% of patients with carcinoma (22,29,47). The utility of this procedure, however, is strongly dependent on the expertise of the cytopathologist.

Islet Cell Tumors

Islet cell tumors that are hormonally active are most often found to be small at clinical presentation and are frequently not seen on CT. Computed tomography will only show the primary islet cell tumor (especially hypervascular insulinomas opacified with intravenous contrast material) in approximately 30 to 40% of pa-

tients and rarely identifies a tumor not seen on angiography (Fig. 22) (17,18). Although CT is not as reliable as angiography in the evaluation of islet cell tumors, it remains the initial radiologic method in the evaluation because CT is noninvasive and can detect approximately one-third of primary tumors as well as hepatic metastases. Computed tomography has not detected small tumors in ectopic locations (stomach, duodenum, jejunum, splenic hilum) or diffuse pancreatic islet cell hyperplasia. However, metastatic lymphadenopathy from ectopically located tumors may be detected even when the primary tumor is not visible (Fig. 23). Because islet cell tumors can occur as part of a multiple endocrine adenomatosis syndrome, the abdominal CT examination should include a search for tumors of the adrenals. Bilaterally enlarged adrenal glands representing adrenal hyperplasia can also be seen due to an ACTH-secreting islet cell tumor (62). The more sensitive angiographic and venous sampling techniques are reserved for cases with negative CT results.

Malignant islet cell tumors, which tend to be larger when they come to clinical attention, resemble adenocarcinoma, but are more equally distributed throughout the pancreas. They may calcify, appear cystic, and are usually more vascular in comparison to pancreatic adenocarcinoma, a feature that may become evident after intravenous administration of contrast material (17).

Cystic Neoplasms

The relatively rare cystic neoplasms of the pancreas are commonly grouped together, but are composed of two distinct groups that have notable therapeutic and prognostic differences.

The first group is the macrocystic adenoma-adenocarcinoma (cystadenoma-cystadenocarcinoma or mu-

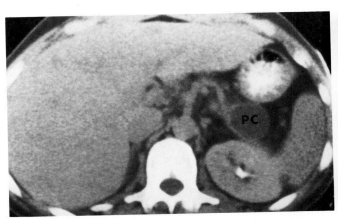

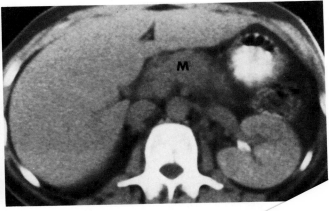

FIG. 16. Pancreatic carcinoma and pseudocyst. **Left:** A pseudocyst (PC) is present in the tail of the pancreas second of the main pancreatic duct. **Right:** The obstructing adenocarcinoma (M) is shown in the body of the pancreas.

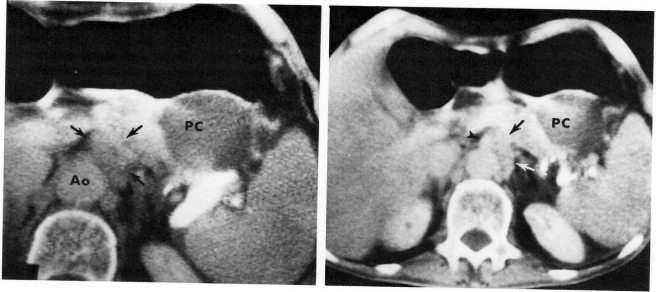

FIG. 17. Carcinoma of the pancreas. **Left:** Scan in the region of the tail of the pancreas shows a prominent low density cystic structure (PC). Note a soft tissue mass (arrows) infiltrating the fat plane between the posterior surface of the pancreas and the left anterolateral wall of the aorta (Ao). (From Weyman et al., ref. 67, with permission.) **Right:** Post-infusion contrast scan demonstrates the left paraaortic mass (arrows) more clearly. This invasive carcinoma involved the wall of the superior mesenteric artery (arrowhead) and obstructed the main pancreatic duct, accounting for the cystic mass (PC) in the tail.

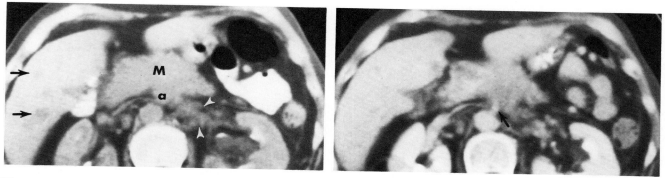

FIG. 18. Carcinoma of the pancreas. **Left:** Scan following intravenous infusion of contrast medium shows a pancreatic mass (M) encasing the superior mesenteric artery (a), obliterating its surrounding fat planes and giving a thickened appearance to the artery. Hepatic metastases (arrows) are also present. There is also tumor extension (arrowheads) toward the left kidney. **Right:** Repeat scan following a bolus injection shows the lumen of the superior mesenteric artery (arrow) encased by surrounding neoplasm near its origin.

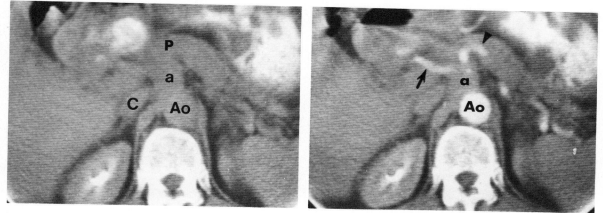

FIG. 19. Carcinoma of the pancreas. **Left:** A thickened celiac axis (a) is present indicating vascular encasement and unresectability. P, pancreas; C, vena cava; Ao, aorta. **Right:** Using an intravenous bolus injection of contrast material, the splenic (arrowhead) and hepatic (arrow) arteries can be seen emerging from the encased celiac artery (a). Ao, aorta.

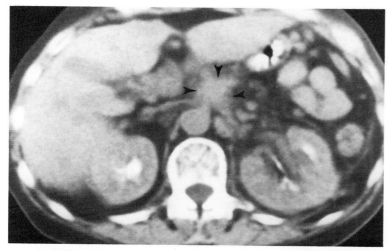

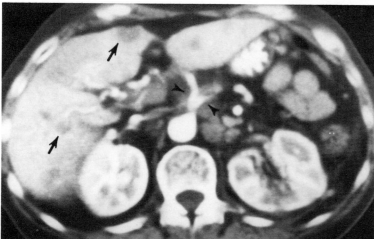

FIG. 20. Pancreatic carcinoma. **Above:** A soft tissue density mass (arrowheads) surrounds the celiac trunk indicating vascular invasion and unresectability. **Below:** Scan following a bolus of intravenous contrast media shows vascular encasement (arrowheads) of the vessels by the surrounding malignant neoplasm. Multiple hepatic metastases (arrows) are also documented.

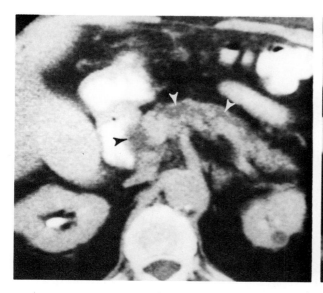

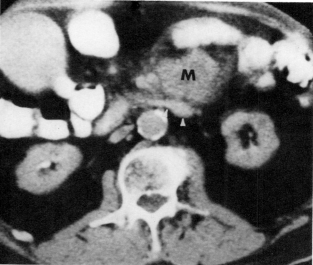

FIG. 21. Pancreatic carcinoma. **Left:** Dilated common bile (black arrowhead) and pancreatic (white arrowheads) ducts are seen, indicating obstruction in the distal common duct region. **Right:** Although the primary pancreatic lesion was not seen, a metastatic mass (M) in lymph nodes in the root of the mesentery, anterior to the left renal vein (arrowheads), was identified indicating a malignant etiology that had spread beyond surgical curability.

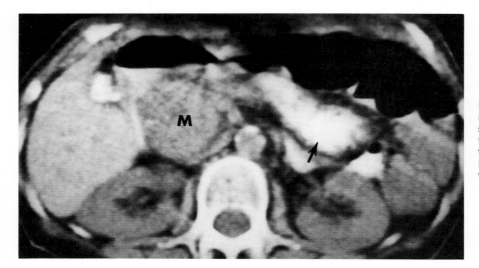

FIG. 22. Gastrinoma. This large mass (M) in the head of the pancreas represented a gastrinoma in a patient with the Zollinger-Ellison syndrome. Note the dilated loops of proximal small bowel (arrow), commonly associated with this disease.

FIG. 23. Ectopic islet cell tumor. A small gastrinoma was found in the proximal jejunum at surgery in this patient with the Zollinger-Ellison syndrome. Although the primary tumor was not identified on CT, regional metastatic lymphadenopathy (N) was seen.

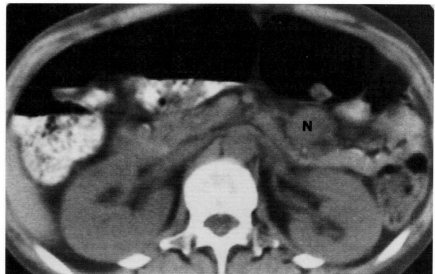

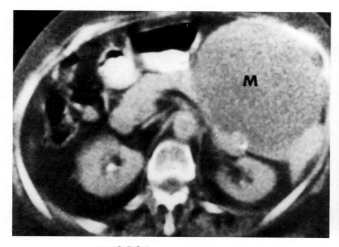
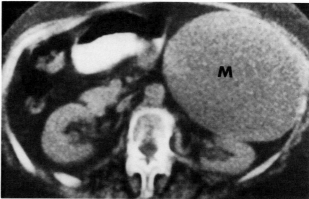

FIG. 24. Macrocystic adenoma of the pancreas. **Left:** A large unilocular cystic mass (M) arises from the pancreatic tail. **Right:** The wall is relatively thin and this neoplasm (M) could not be easily differentiated from a pseudocyst.

cinous cystic neoplasm of the pancreas). These tumors tend to be located in the body or tail and occur predominantly in middle-aged (40- to 60-year-old) women. They are usually large encapsulated tumors, approximately 10 cm in size, composed of multiloculated low density areas greater than 2 cm in size intermixed with stromal elements (septa). The wall of the tumor and the septae occasionally calcify (69). The stromal matrix varies in amount and, when small, the septa cannot be identified on CT. The tumor may then appear unilocular and simulate a pseudocyst (Fig. 24) (9). Pathologically, there is a large amount of cytoplasmic and intracystic mucin present; these lesions are either frankly malignant or have cellular atypia and substantial malignant potential (12).

Microcystic adenoma (glycogen-rich cystadenoma) is the second type of cystic tumor with distinctive CT and pathologic appearances. The microcystic adenoma is a benign tumor with no malignant potential. It predominantly affects a more elderly population (mean age near 70) than the mucinous cystic tumor and occurs without a strong sex predilection (11). The tumor can be found in all parts of the pancreas, but predominates in the head. This neoplasm usually appears well circumscribed with a smooth or nodular contour and consists of numerous cysts, typically ranging from several millimeters to 2 cm in size. There is a characteristic central soft tissue stellate density seen on CT formed by centrifugally radiating bands of connective tissue that frequently calcify in a radial pattern (Fig. 25) (69). Occasionally, a dominant cyst greater than 2 cm is present, making the distinction from a macrocystic adenoma more difficult and at times impossible from CT appearances alone (Fig. 26). Pathologically, however, the cytoplasm is rich in glycogen with little or no mucin, in contradistinction to the mucinous cystic tumor (11).

The major diagnoses to be differentiated from these two groups of cystic neoplasms of the pancreas are focal pancreatitis with calcification or pseudocyst formation or a necrotic adenocarcinoma (52). Patients with focal pancreatitis or an isolated pseudocyst will usually have some clinical history of either pancreatitis or trauma. However, based on the CT findings alone, it is usually impossible to differentiate a thin-walled cystadenoma from a pseudocyst. A necrotic adenocarcinoma characteristically has a thick irregular wall on CT without calcification (36).

Other Neoplastic Lesions

Lymphomatous involvement of the pancreas or peripancreatic nodes is usually part of a systemic disease where retroperitoneal or mesenteric lymphadenopathy is also present. Peripancreatic lymphadenopathy secondary to lymphoma or metastatic disease without other findings on rare occasion may be indistinguishable from a primary pancreatic carcinoma (62,67). However, with lymphomatous involvement of peripancreatic tissue, the pancreas itself usually is displaced anteriorly, and adjacent blood vessels are frequently lifted, displaced, and remain patent (Fig. 27), rather than encased and obliterated as usually occurs with extensive pancreatic carcinoma. Occasionally, the pancreas may be directly infiltrated by lymphomatous tissue and appear diffusely enlarged. Tumors originating from the posterior surface of the left lobe of the liver or other peripancreatic areas can also mimic a primary pancreatic lesion (40).

Inflammation

Acute Pancreatitis

A broad spectrum of inflammatory changes may occur in acute pancreatitis ranging from mild edematous interstitial inflammation to fulminant necrotizing

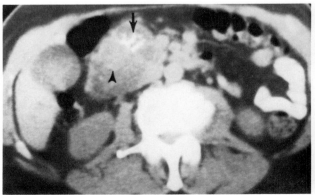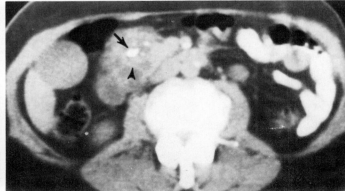

FIG. 25. Microcystic adenoma. Two serial scans at a 1-cm interval show a multicystic tumor in the head of the pancreas with central soft tissue density (arrowheads), cysts varying in size from 5 mm to 2 cm in diameter, and calcifications (arrows) arranged in a radial pattern.

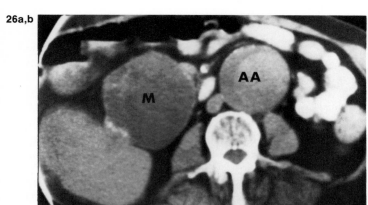

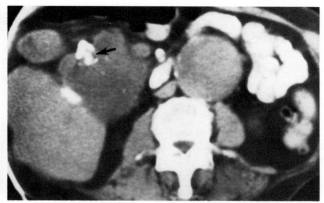

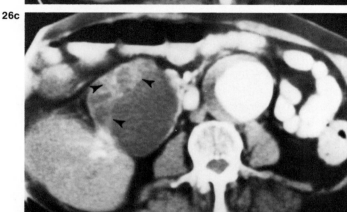

FIG. 26. Microcystic adenoma of the head of the pancreas. **a** and **b:** Scans show a large cystic mass (M) in the head of the pancreas. Calcification within soft tissue septae (arrow) is noted on the anterolateral aspect of the mass. An aortic aneurysm (AA) is present. **c:** Scan at the same level as (a), following bolus injection of intravenous contrast media shows enhancement of the septations (arrowheads), documenting the multicystic nature of the mass; one cyst is dominant.

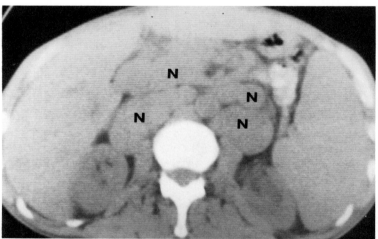

FIG. 27. Peripancreatic lymphoma. **Above:** Multiple nodular masses (N) are present in the peripancreatic region. **Below:** After intravenous bolus enhancement, the splenic, portal, and left renal veins are densely enhanced and the pancreas (arrows) is seen to be anteriorly displaced by the lymph nodes (N) enlarged by lymphoma. Note that the fat plane surrounding the superior mesenteric artery (arrowheads) remains intact, unlike with the usual extensive adenocarcinoma of the pancreas. sv, splenic vein; pv, portal vein; rv, left renal vein.

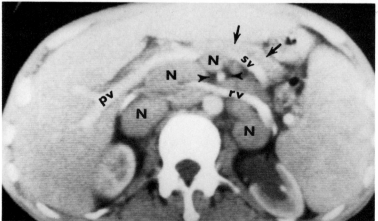

hemorrhagic pancreatitis. Acute pancreatitis may be associated with an exudation of fluid into the interstitium of the pancreas and a subsequent leakage of pancreatic juice with its proteolytic enzymes into the peripancreatic tissues. The pancreas exhibits a wide spectrum of response to this insult. In some patients the inflammatory process results in no more than transient edema of the gland with full recovery. At the other end of the spectrum, the extensive inflammation and tissue destruction are life threatening. Appearances on CT may vary from a normal appearing gland to a diffusely enlarged gland with low and high density areas representing necrosis and hemorrhage, respectively.

Computed tomography shows a normal appearing gland in as many as one-third of patients with acute pancreatitis (60). The abnormal CT findings of acute uncomplicated pancreatitis include (a) diffuse enlargement of the gland, often with decreased attenuation values secondary to edema (Fig. 28), (b) focal enlargement (Fig. 29), and (c) irregular contour with indistinct margins of the gland and increased density of peripancreatic fat planes (Fig. 28) (46, 59,60). Transient focal enlargement of the gland in acute pancreatitis is almost always within the head. Such a focal mass alone cannot easily be distinguished from a malignant neoplasm; follow-up scans can demonstrate resolution of the enlargement (Fig. 30).

The diagnosis of uncomplicated acute pancreatitis is usually readily established by clinical and biochemical means, without resorting to CT. However, CT is quite valuable when the diagnosis has not been firmly established clinically or in the detection and evaluation of suspected complications of acute pancreatitis. Complications include the development of intrapancreatic or peripancreatic fluid collections, a pancreatic and peripancreatic phlegmon, abscess, hemorrhage, and ascites (37,46,59,60).

Pancreatic and extrapancreatic fluid collections result from duct rupture with escape of pancreatic fluid and represent the most common complications seen on CT. When these secretions escape from the pancreas, they are typically located on the anterior or anterolateral surface of the gland, which is covered only by a thin layer of loose connective tissue. When these fluids penetrate this thin tissue layer, they become extrapancreatic and spread beyond the pancreas along fascial planes (Fig. 31). The fluid initially leaks into the immediately adjacent spaces: the lesser sac and the left anterior pararenal space. Most of these collections are not cyst-like, but rather conform somewhat to the shape of the involved space (retroperitoneal or intraperitoneal compartment). An acute pancreatic collection is a distinct entity, different from a pseudocyst that has a well-defined fibrous capsule, has relative permanence, and is usually associated with subacute or chronic pancreatitis. Fluid collections do not have a fibrous capsule, distend an already existing space, and may be transient, often resolving spontaneously (59,66,67).

The lesser sac is a potential space anterior to the pancreas and posterior to the stomach and is separated from the pancreas by only a thin layer of connective tissue and the parietal peritoneum, thereby explaining its common involvement in pancreatitis (Fig. 32). Anterior perforation leads to direct tracking of fluid into the lesser sac. Fluid from the lesser sac rarely enters the greater peritoneal cavity due to closure of the foramen of Winslow. The rare escape of fluid into the greater peritoneal space produces pancreatic ascites. The anterior pararenal space is filled first if the disruption is in the posterior portion of the gland or the tail. Signs of anterior pararenal space involvement are a collection posterior to the pancreas or descending colon, blurring of the lateral margin of the pancreas, obliteration of the splenorenal interface, and irregular

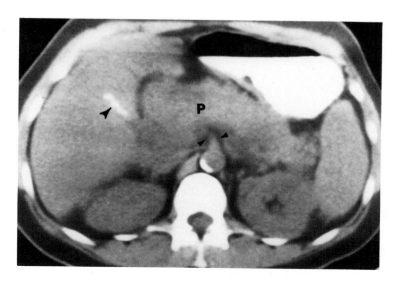

FIG. 28. Acute pancreatitis. Diffuse enlargement and blurring of the margins of the gland (P) are present. Note preservation of fat planes surrounding the superior mesenteric artery (small arrowheads). Gallstones are also seen (large arrowhead).

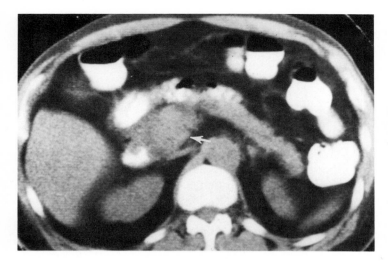

FIG. 29. Focal pancreatitis. The head of the pancreas (arrow), but not the body and tail, is diffusely enlarged. Based on the CT appearance alone, this manifestation of focal pancreatitis cannot be differentiated from a neoplasm.

thickening of the anterior surface of Gerota's fascia (Fig. 33) (15,51,59).

Involvement of the ascending or descending colon in acute pancreatitis can be severe enough to lead to hemorrhage as well as necrosis, perforation, and stricture formation (63). Furthermore, a pancreatic inflammatory mass involving the colon may be difficult to distinguish from colonic malignancy with local spread on CT scans alone. Clues to the neoplastic nature of such a process include the relatively high density of the mass and the normal appearance of the retroperitoneal fat immediately contiguous with the mass (Fig. 34).

Less frequently involved sites of extrapancreatic inflammatory processes include (a) the right anterior pararenal space (Fig. 35), (b) the perirenal space after penetrating Gerota's fascia, (c) the posterior pararenal space (Fig. 36) with spread to the pelvis and upper thigh, (d) the left lobe of the liver via the lesser sac and fissure of the ligamentum venosum (Fig. 37), (e) the spleen, (f) between the crura of the diaphragm into the mediastinum, (g) along the transverse mesocolon to the transverse colon (Fig. 38), and (h) along the root of the small bowel mesentery (Fig. 32) (37,46,59,60). When spread of the inflammatory process extends into the root of the mesentery, the fat plane surrounding the superior mesenteric artery and vein characteristically remains intact, and the vessels remain visible (Figs. 32 and 35). This is in contrast to the findings in pancreatic carcinoma occurring in the same area.

Although spontaneous extrapancreatic escape of pancreatic juice may lead to many undesirable consequences, the drainage of this fluid may exert a salubrious effect by decompressing the inflamed

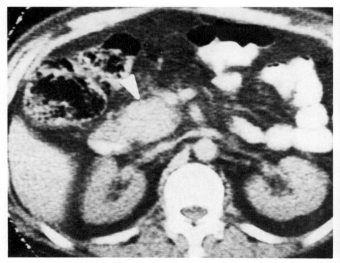
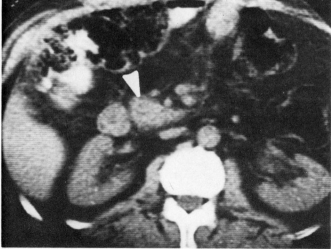

FIG. 30. Acute focal pancreatitis. **Left:** Diffusely enlarged head and uncinate process (arrowhead). The body and tail of the pancreas were normal. **Right:** Six-week follow-up scan at similar level shows resolution of inflammatory process. The uncinate process (arrowhead) has returned to a normal size and shape.

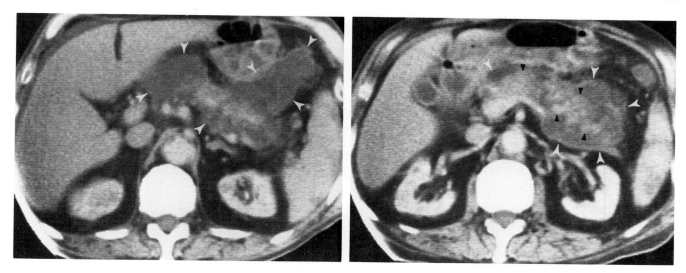

FIG. 31. Fluid collections. **Left:** A fluid collection (arrowheads) is seen extending into the lesser sac. **Right:** On a scan 2-cm caudad, the fluid collection (white arrowheads) surrounds the lobules of pancreatic tissue (black arrowheads). A small amount of ascites is present.

pancreas. Extrapancreatic fluid collections may retain a communication with the pancreatic duct system, and an equilibrium may be established between the secretions absorbed from the collection and those produced by the pancreas. Detection of extrapancreatic inflammatory masses is important because they are often the cause of prolonged symptoms and may become infected with subsequent abscess formation.

A phlegmon is a diffuse spreading edematous inflammation within specified compartments and along tissue planes and is not of drainable consistency (Fig. 38) (46,60,62). A pancreatic phlegmon is, therefore, a mass of inflamed and indurated pancreas and peripancreatic tissue, and on CT will appear as an irregular mass with attenuation values distinctly greater than water. Distinction between phlegmons and fluid collections is sometimes not possible (Fig. 39). The attenuation value alone will not reliably differentiate between the two. Phlegmons may be complicated by suppuration and necrosis leading to a lower density process and may then be termed a fluid collection.

A pancreatic abscess occurs where there is secondary infection of pancreatic or extrapancreatic fluid collections, phlegmons, or of the associated devitalized tissue. The extrapancreatic abscesses spread along fascial planes similar to other extrapancreatic collections (20,45). The attenuation value of an abscess is quite variable, but is generally higher than

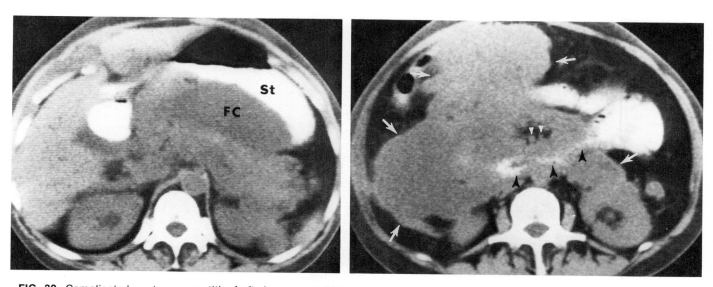

FIG. 32. Complicated acute pancreatitis. **Left:** Lesser sac fluid collection (FC) displacing the stomach (St) anteriorly. **Right:** The massive inflammatory exudate (arrows) dissects the leaves of the mesentery, surrounds the third–fourth duodenum (black arrowheads) and superior mesenteric vascular bundle (white arrowheads), and extends to the area of the cecum and anterior abdominal wall.

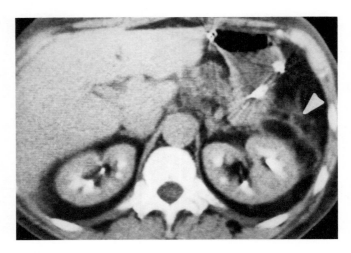

FIG. 33. Acute pancreatitis. One of the earliest CT changes in acute pancreatitis is thickening and blurring of the anterior surface of the perinephric (Gerota's) fascia (arrowhead), reflecting spread of the inflammatory process in the left anterior pararenal space.

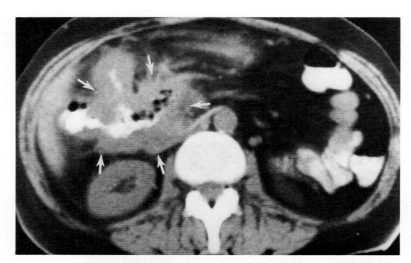

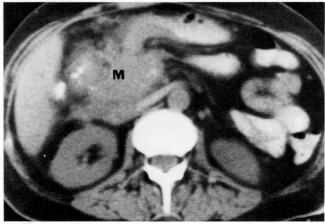

FIG. 34. Colon carcinoma simulating complicated pancreatitis. **Above:** An extensive circumferential soft tissue mass (arrows) is present distorting the hepatic flexure. **Below:** Scan 1 cm cephalad shows the mass (M) involving the region of the pancreatic head. At presentation, this patient had biochemical evidence of pancreatitis and the CT was interpreted as a pancreatic phlegmon involving the colon. After follow-up scans showed no improvement, the presence of a malignancy was suggested. At surgery, a large hepatic flexure carcinoma was present infiltrating the pancreatic bed.

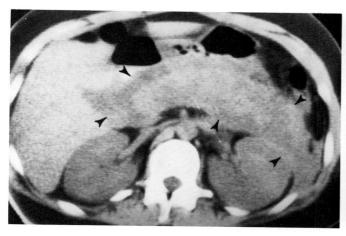
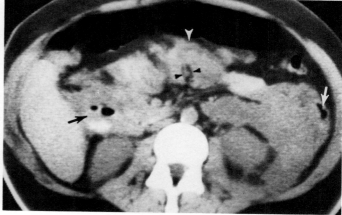

FIG. 35. Extensive pancreatitis. **Left:** Large peripancreatic fluid collection (arrowheads) with extension into left anterior pararenal space. The margins of the pancreas are barely discernible within the inflammatory process. **Right:** Extension of inflammatory process in the left and right anterior pararenal spaces with involvement of the hepatic flexure of the colon (black arrow), descending colon (white arrow), and root of mesentery (white arrowhead). Note preservation of fat planes surrounding mesenteric vessels (black arrowheads).

that of sterile fluid collections or pseudocysts (49). Gas within a collection is the most reliable sign of abscess formation on CT, but is present in only 29 to 64% of cases (20,46,70). More often a pancreatic abscess appears as a poorly defined inhomogeneous mass or fluid collection often with displacement of adjacent structures (Fig. 40) (20,45,67). However, without examination and/or culture of the contents,

often obtainable via needle aspiration under CT or US guidance, an abscess is usually indistinguishable from a sterile fluid collection, phlegmon, or pseudo-cyst on CT (26,45,70). Although extraluminal gas is the most diagnostic CT sign for an abscess, it is not pathognomonic. Inflammatory collections or pseudo-cysts that communicate with the gastrointestinal tract, either spontaneously or surgically, may contain

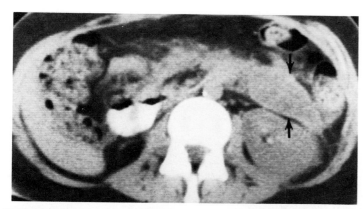

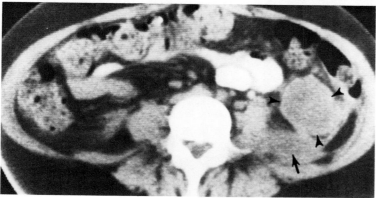

FIG. 36. Above: The anterior pararenal space is distended by extrapancreatic fluid (arrows) lying between the posterior parietal peritoneum and the anterior surface of the perinephric (Gerota's) fascia. **Below:** At a more caudad level, the communication between the anterior (arrowheads) and posterior (arrow) pararenal spaces is shown by the spreading pancreatic effusion.

232

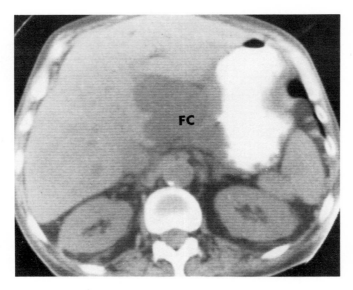

FIG. 37. An extrapancreatic fluid collection (FC) is shown dissecting into the fissure of the ligamentum venosum. Collections reach the liver by first entering the lesser sac and then extending to the right to reach the porta hepatis.

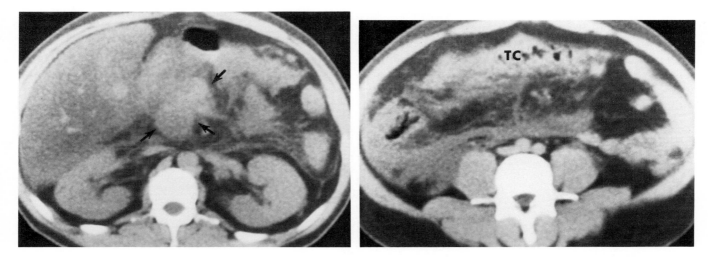

FIG. 38. Pancreatic phlegmon. **Left:** The peripancreatic inflammatory process (arrows) blurs the outline of the pancreatic head and diffusely raises the density of the mesenteric fat (compare with the perinephric fat). Note fatty infiltration of the liver. **Right:** The inflammatory process extends through the transverse mesocolon to involve the transverse colon (TC) directly (compare with Fig. 35).

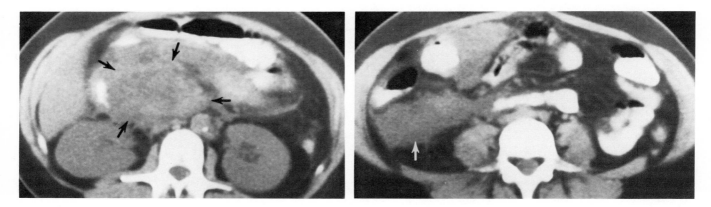

FIG. 39. Extrapancreatic fluid collection versus phlegmon. **Left:** Extrapancreatic inflammatory process (arrows) involving the lesser sac. Note the increased density of peripancreatic fat compared with the fat in the perinephric space reflecting the contiguous inflammatory process. **Right:** The process extends into the right anterior pararenal space (arrow), conforming to the fascial compartment. The soft tissue density of the process suggests that it is not of a consistency that would be easily drained.

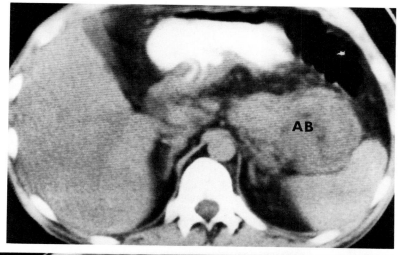

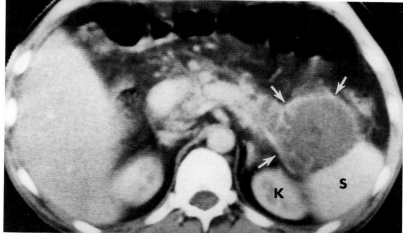

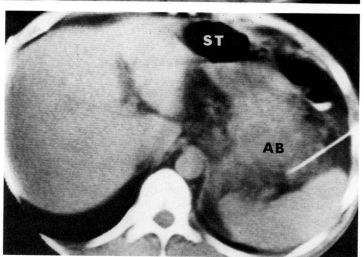

FIG. 40. Pancreatic abscess. **Top:** Inhomogeneous mass (AB) occupying the left anterior pararenal space and lesser sac in a febrile patient with acute pancreatitis. **Center:** A scan after intravenous contrast material administration and 2-cm caudad shows a lower density component to the mass (arrows) arising from the pancreatic tail. S, spleen; K, kidney. **Bottom:** CT-guided thin needle aspiration revealed pus. ST, stomach; AB, inhomogeneous mass.

gas as well as fluid and are not necessarily infected (37,45). Scattered pockets of gas throughout the collection almost always represent an abscess (Fig. 41), whereas a larger collection of gas or a gas-fluid level may be related to bland communication with gut as well as to a real abscess. Clinical correlation is mandatory in this setting.

Acute necrotizing hemorrhagic pancreatitis repre-

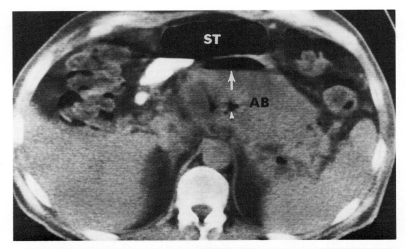

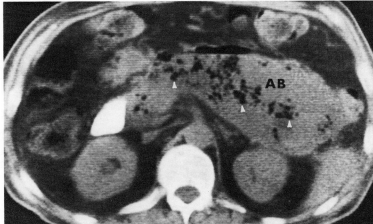

FIG. 41. Pancreatic abscess. **Above:** The stomach (ST) is displaced anteriorly by an infected fluid collection (AB). Note the air fluid level (arrow) and smaller bubbles (arrowhead). **Below:** At the level of the pancreas, gas bubbles (arrowheads) are distributed throughout this large abscess (AB), a grave complication of pancreatitis and an indication for emergency drainage.

sents the most severe form of acute pancreatitis and is reported to have a mortality rate approaching 50% (46). But CT has shown evidence of focal hemorrhage in patients with pancreatitis who are not moribund and who survive without surgery. Thus, some investigators believe that the reported high mortality figures reflect a subset of patients in whom the hemorrhage is massive and tissue destruction is extensive. Acute hemorrhage (less than 1 week) within or around the pancreas appears as a poorly marginated mass with attenuation values equal to or higher than those of normal parenchyma. After a week, the attenuation values of the resolving hematoma begin to approach those of other pancreatic fluid collections (35,60).

Chronic Pancreatitis

Patients with chronic pancreatitis have had recurrent bouts of acute pancreatitis and are usually evaluated during an acute exacerbation or because of complications. The size of the gland may be normal, small, or enlarged. In one reported series, the CT scan was entirely normal in approximately 16% of patients with chronic pancreatitis, presumably mild cases. In advanced cases, an atrophic gland may be seen with or without fatty replacement (21,67). Atrophy is a late sequela of the disease, but it is not specific and can also be seen proximal to an obstructing neoplasm, associated with diabetes mellitus or as part of the aging process. Atrophy limited to the tail or body and tail should alert one to search for an underlying neoplasm. Pancreatic enlargement in chronic pancreatitis may be focal or diffuse and often represents edema in association with an acute exacerbation or fibrosis (Fig. 42). A focal mass from chronic pancreatitis may be indistinguishable from carcinoma and summons the need for either follow-up scans or other diagnostic techniques such as ERCP, percutaneous biopsy, or angiography. Since it is extremely rare for an adenocarcinoma of the pancreas to calcify, a focal mass with evenly distributed calcifications is more likely inflammatory. However, a cancer can arise within a gland already containing calcifications due to chronic pancreatitis.

Additional CT findings in chronic pancreatitis include pancreatic duct dilatation, parenchymal and

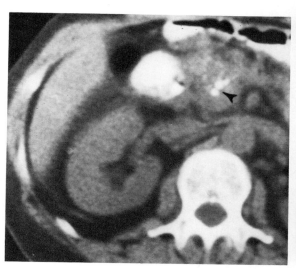 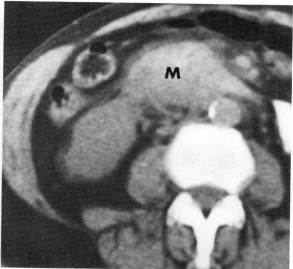

FIG. 42. Chronic pancreatitis. **Left:** Calculi (arrowhead) are present in the course of the main pancreatic duct in the head of the pancreas. **Right:** An inflammatory mass (M) extends inferiorly in the anterior pararenal space displacing the third duodenum (not shown) in a caudad direction.

ductal calcification (Fig. 43), and pseudocyst formation (Figs. 44–46) (21). Uniform enlargement of the pancreatic duct or combined enlargement of both the pancreatic and common bile ducts is nonspecific and can be seen in either chronic pancreatitis or malignant obstruction. A dilated pancreatic duct simply confirms the presence of obstructive pancreatic disease and, when the common bile duct is also dilated, indicates the level of obstruction (23,28,33). Parenchymal and ductal calcification alone or in combination with the other less specific findings is a reliable CT indicator of chronic pancreatitis (Fig. 43)

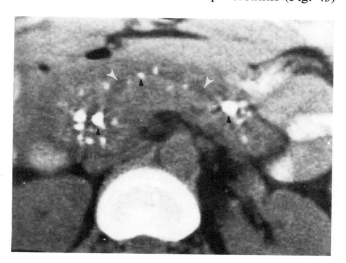

FIG. 43. Chronic pancreatitis. Multiple intraductal calculi (black arrowheads) conform to the course of the mildly dilated main pancreatic duct (white arrowheads) and its major tributaries. The gland appears moderately enlarged. (From Weyman et al., ref. 67, with permission.)

(21). Splenic artery calcifications will occasionally mimic pancreatic calcifications, but careful examination of contiguous scans or the use of intravenous contrast material generally alleviates the confusion.

Pseudocysts are most commonly associated with subacute or chronic pancreatitis. The term *pseudocyst* should be reserved for pancreatic or extrapancreatic fluid collections with a measurably thick fibrous capsule or wall (Figs. 17, 45, and 46). On CT, pseudocysts are readily detected as unilocular or multilocular mass-like lesions with a near water density center and a well-defined wall that occasionally calcifies (Figs. 44–46) (39). There is some variability in the density of pseudocysts, depending on the amount of internal cellular debris and protein composition. A pseudocyst with an unusually high attenuation value should suggest the presence of either superimposed infection or hemorrhage (54). Infected pseudocysts need not have attentuation values much greater than water, and sampling via thin needle aspiration or surgery may be the only way of determining the presence of superimposed infection. Along with hemorrhage and superinfection, another major complication of pseudocyst formation is spontaneous rupture. Pseudocysts may rupture into the peritoneal cavity with the development of ascites, into the extraperitoneal spaces, or into the gastrointestinal tract. As emphasized before, with rupture into the gastrointestinal tract, gas may be seen within the pseudocyst and does not necessarily indicate abscess formation (45,46,65).

Pseudocysts can be mimicked by a cystic or necrotic tumor, a dilated and tortuous pancreatic duct, or an

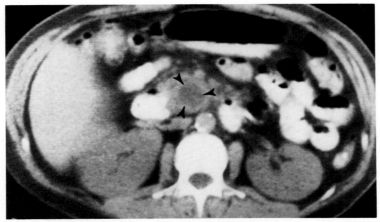

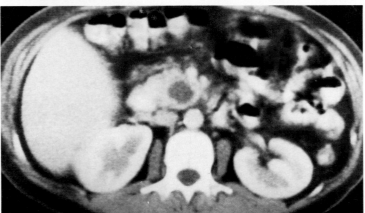

FIG. 44. Pancreatic pseudocyst. **Above:** A low-density area is present in the head of the pancreas (arrowheads). **Below:** Scan following intravenous contrast material administration shows enhancement of the pancreatic parenchyma resulting in better definition of this small pseudocyst in the area of the uncinate process; the cyst was subsequently shown by endoscopic retrograde pancreatography to communicate with the main pancreatic duct.

45a,b

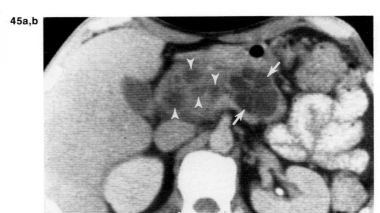
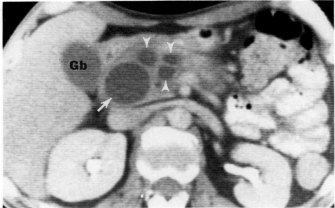

45c

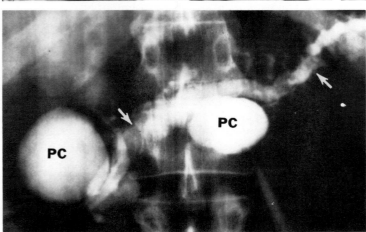

FIG. 45. Multiple pseudocysts in a patient with chronic pancreatitis. **a:** A large septated pseudocyst (arrows) as well as smaller cystic areas (arrowheads) are present in an enlarged pancreatic body. **b:** A scan 2 cm caudad shows several other small pseudocysts (arrowheads) in addition to a large unilocular pseudocyst (arrow) in the head of the pancreas. Gb, gallbladder. **c:** An intraoperative pancreatogram shows an enlarged pancreatic duct (arrows) with contrast filling of the two dominant pseudocysts (PC). The smaller pseudocysts are either not adequately filled with contrast material or are not in free communication with the main pancreatic duct.

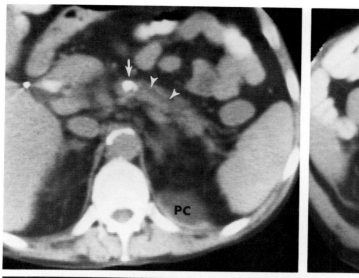

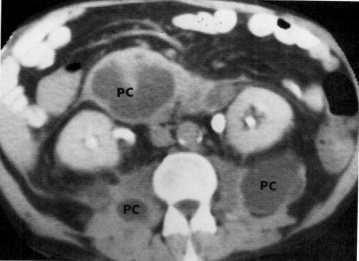

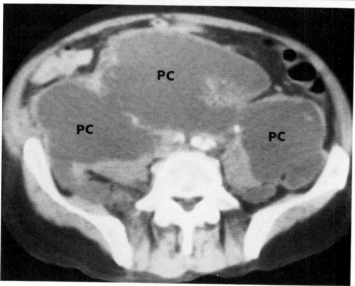

FIG. 46. Extensive pseudocysts (PC) complicating chronic pancreatitis. A sequence of scans shows remarkable ability of pancreatic effusions to dissect into multiple compartments including the posterior pararenal space, the fascial compartments of the psoas muscle, and the root of the mesentery, as well as the more common involvement of the anterior pararenal space. Arrow indicates intraductal calculi; arrowheads, dilated main pancreatic duct. (Case courtesy of G. Wilson and associates, Columbia Regional Hospital, Columbia, Missouri.)

aneurysm or false aneurysm of an adjacent vessel (36). Cystic tumors usually occur in patients without a history of pancreatitis and may show some characteristic CT findings as described previously. Necrotic tumors generally have thick and irregular walls that rarely if ever calcify compared to the discrete, occasionally calcific walls of pseudocysts. Aneurysms or false aneurysms will enhance with bolus intravenous contrast medium administration, easily distinguishing them from pseudocysts. The presence of a pseudocyst is not pathognomonic for pancreatic inflammatory disease and can also be seen proximal to an obstructing carcinoma.

Retention cysts of the pancreas, like pseudocysts, are seen as a result of increased intraductal pressure. As opposed to the fibrous-lined pseudocyst, which not infrequently extends beyond the pancreas, retention cysts are lined with epithelium and remain confined to

the pancreas. Intrapancreatic pseudocyts (Figs. 44 and 45) and retention cysts are indistinguishable on CT (32,62).

Miscellaneous

Trauma

Due to its relatively fixed extraperitoneal location just anterior to the spine, the pancreas is not uncommonly affected in blunt upper abdominal trauma. Either blunt or sharp abdominal trauma may cause pancreatic ductal disruption with subsequent escape of pancreatic enzymes and the potential development of the entire spectrum of acute pancreatitis. Appearances of traumatic pancreatitis on CT are the same as with a nontraumatic etiology (64).

Fatty Replacement of the Pancreas

Fatty replacement of the pancreas can be seen as part of the benign aging process as well as secondary to chronic obstruction of the pancreatic duct. Other entities associated with or predisposing to fatty replacement include chronic pancreatitis (Fig. 47), cystic fibrosis (Fig. 17, Chapter 18), diabetes mellitus, and hepatic disease (53). There is a spectrum of the severity of fatty replacement from only mild involvement to essentially complete fatty replacement, in which case the main pancreatic duct is seen as a tissue density line coursing through the center of the fat replaced gland.

ACCURACY

The overall accuracy of CT in diagnosing pancreatic diseases has ranged from 83 to 94% (31,43,58,61). The sensitivity of CT in pancreatic carcinoma is 88 to 94% compared with 56 to 90% in pancreatitis (19,40). Although fewer than 10% of symptomatic patients with carcinoma have normal CT studies, a normal appearing gland is not infrequently seen in either acute or chronic pancreatitis (62).

Diagnostic accuracy has clearly increased with improvements in scanner technology and in the conduction and interpretation of the studies. False positive interpretations of pancreatic carcinoma have resulted from mistaking intrinsic normal morphology (pancreatic lobulations) or unopacified bowel for neoplasm. In addition, focal pancreatitis, tumors from adjacent regions, or peripancreatic lymphadenopathy due to lymphoma, metastatic carcinoma, or granulomatous disease all can be mistaken for primary pancreatic carcinoma.

Small intrapancreatic lesions that do not alter the gland's contour are usually undetectable and can cause a false negative scan result. Most often in our experience, false negative scans have resulted from interpreter failure to appreciate the abnormality. In patients with pancreatic cancer evaluated with a 3 second scanner, only 83% of patients had a mass discovered prospectively, but in 100% the mass was seen retrospectively (43). Similarly, a pancreatic mass may be falsely classified as indeterminate when the secondary signs of malignant or inflammatory disease, which would allow for a firm diagnosis, are overlooked. It should be recognized that, because of variations in normal and pathologic morphology, some pancreatic CT examinations may be inconclusive. In these cases, information provided by other diagnostic examinations is essential.

CLINICAL APPLICATIONS

Computed tomography is a highly accurate noninvasive method of evaluating pancreatic pathology. Its use is not only in the diagnosis of pancreatic inflammatory or neoplastic disease, but also in the evaluation of the extent of carcinoma or detection of complications of pancreatitis. Because CT can image other upper abdominal structures simultaneously, the detection of unsuspected additional or ancillary abnormalities, which may be responsible for clinical symptoms, will also be possible.

The high sensitivity of CT in carcinoma of the pancreas is in part due to the relatively advanced nature of pancreatic carcinoma at clinical presentation. Although CT is a safe, convenient, highly effective method to diagnose such carcinomas, there is no evidence to indicate that CT has had a noticeably favorable influence on the high rate of mortality associated with this disease. Nevertheless, combining

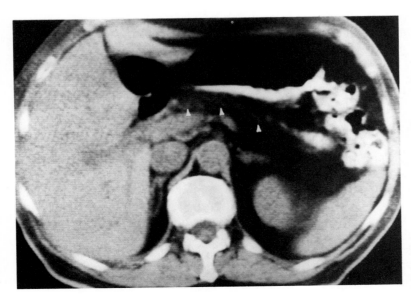

FIG. 47. Pancreatic insufficiency. Linear duct structures, fibrous septae, and a few lobules of tissue (arrowheads) are all that remain of this patient's pancreatic parenchyma, which has been replaced by fat.

CT with percutaneous biopsy and biliary drainage procedures not only expedites the diagnosis but also alters management and may prevent unnecessary laparotomies.

The indeterminate pancreatic mass, that is, a focal soft tissue mass without secondary signs of malignancy or pancreatitis, remains a problem in CT diagnosis. The use of follow-up scans, CT-directed percutaneous thin needle biopsy, ERCP, transhepatic cholangiography, or, rarely, angiography may be necessary.

Computed tomography is unnecessary in patients with a well-established clinical diagnosis of acute or chronic pancreatitis. However, there are no techniques short of laparotomy that are superior to CT in displaying the effects of complicated pancreatitis such as fluid collections, hemorrhage, phlegmons, pseudocysts, or abscesses.

Computed tomography and US are both accurate and sensitive in the evaluation of pancreatic disease (1,2). However, the success rate in delineating the entire pancreas is higher with CT than with US. With sub-5 second scanners, technically adequate examinations can be obtained on nearly every patient (43). Abundant abdominal fat and intestinal gas (commonly present in patients with acute pancreatitis) may preclude total visualization of the pancreas with US in approximately 20% of patients (42,43,55,68). Fat and gas offer no problem for CT (Fig. 48). Furthermore, CT often provides a better topographic display of the pancreas and adjacent structures.

Computed tomography is our preferred method in screening adult patients with suspected pancreatic disease. In cachectic patients with little body fat and patients who are unable or unwilling to suspend respiration, US is a better imaging method. In addition,

the use of sound waves and not ionizing radiation makes US preferable in pregnant women and young children. Because US is significantly less costly than CT, US is the preferred method in situations where multiple follow-up studies are necessary.

Endoscopic retrograde pancreatography is used in patients with a high clinical suspicion of pancreatic disease when the CT scan is normal, equivocal, or technically unsatisfactory. The use of ERCP alone is sensitive and accurate for pancreatic carcinoma, but the combined use of ERCP and CT increases the accuracy in carcinoma detection compared with either technique alone. Endoscopic retrograde pancreatography can also evaluate the periampullary region and biliary tree and obtain pancreatic secretions for cytology (13). However, ERCP is a more invasive technique than CT and is heavily dependent on the technical ability of the endoscopist. Ultrasound- or CT-guided percutaneous thin needle aspiration of the pancreas is useful in equivocal masses and has a low morbidity (3,30). Percutaneous transphepatic cholangiography is extremely valuable in the jaundiced patient when it is necessary to delineate precisely the pathologic biliary anatomy. It also serves as the initial step in percutaneous biliary decompression.

Angiography is infrequently used in our department in the evaluation of pancreatic adenocarcinoma or pancreatitis. It may be used when other techniques (CT, US, ERCP, PTC) are unsatisfactory or equivocal or to evaluate further a tumor judged resectable by CT or US. Selective angiography may detect previously unsuspected vessel encasement and offers a vascular road map to the surgeon. Angiography remains the primary radiographic method in the evaluation of islet cell tumors of the pancreas that are too small to be detected with CT (27,56). Percutaneous transhepatic

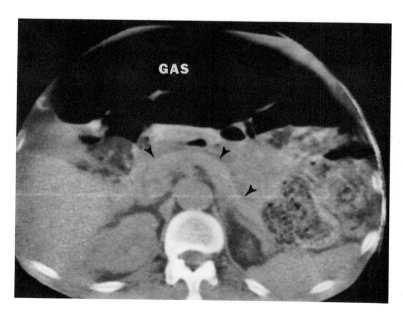

FIG. 48. Patient with a nonvisualized pancreas on ultrasound. CT shows a normal pancreas (arrowheads) and a large amount of intestinal gas accounting for the previous unsuccessful sonographic examination.

pancreatic venous sampling is also helpful in the detection of small functioning islet cell tumors or islet cell hyperplasia, but is not in widespread use (6,16).

REFERENCES

1. Arger PH, Mulhern CB, Bonavita JA, Stauffer DM, Hale J: An analysis of pancreatic sonography in suspected pancreatic disease. *J Clin Ultrasound* 7:91–97, 1979
2. Barkin J, Vining D, Miale A, Gottlieb S, Redlhammer E, Kalser MH: Computerized tomography, diagnostic ultrasound, and radionuclide scanning. *JAMA* 238:2040–2042, 1977
3. Beazley RM: Needle biopsy diagnosis of pancreatic cancer. *Cancer* 47:1685–1687, 1981
4. Beazley RM, Cohn I: Pancreatic cancer. *Ca* 31:346–358, 1981
5. Berland LL, Lawson TL, Foley WD, Geenen JE, Stewart ET: Computed tomography of the normal and abnormal pancreatic duct: Correlation with pancreatic ductography. *Radiology* 141:715–724, 1981
6. Burcharth F, Stage JG, Stadil F, Jensen LI, Fischermann K: Localization of gastrinomas by transphepatic portal catheterization and gastrin assay. *Gastroenterology* 77:444–450, 1979
7. Callen PW, Breiman RS, Korobkin M, De Martini J, Mani JR: Carcinoma of the tail of the pancreas: An unusal CT appearance. *AJR* 133:135–137, 1979
8. Callen PW, London SS, Moss AA: Computed tomographic evaluation of the dilated pancreatic duct. *Radiology* 134:253–255, 1980
9. Carroll B, Sample WF: Pancreatic cystadenocarcinoma: CT body scan and gray scale ultrasound appearance. *AJR* 131:339–341, 1978
10. Charnsangavej C, Elkin M: Displacement of the tail of the pancreas in the absence of the left kidney. *Radiology* 137:156, 1980
11. Compagno J, Oertel JE: Microcystic adenomas of the pancreas (glycogen-rich cystadenomas). *Am J Clin Pathol* 69:289–298, 1978
12. Compagno J, Oertel JE: Mucinous cystic neoplasms of the pancreas with overt and latent malignancy (cystadenocarinoma and cystadenoma). *Am J Clin Pathol* 69:573–580, 1978
13. Cotton PB, Lees WR, Vallon AG, Cottone M, Croker JR, Chapman M: Gray-scale ultrasonography and endoscopic pancreatography in pancreatic diagnosis. *Radiology* 134:453–459, 1980
14. de Graaff CS, Taylor JKW, Simonds BD, Rosenfield AJ: Gray-scale echography of the pancreas. *Radiology* 129:157–161, 1978
15. Dembner AG, Jaffee CC, Simeone J, Walsh J: A new computed tomographic sign of pancreatitis. *AJR* 133:477–479, 1979
16. Doppman JL, Brennan MF, Dunnick NR, Kahn CR, Gorden P: The role of pancreatic venous sampling in the localization of occult insulinomas. *Radiology* 138:557–562, 1981
17. Dunnick NR, Doppman JL, Mills SR, McCarthy DM: Computed tomographic detection of nonbeta pancreatic islet cell tumors. *Radiology* 135:117–120, 1980
18. Dunnick NR, Long JA, Krudy A, Shawker TH, Doppman JL: Localizing insulinomas with combined radiographic methods. *AJR* 135:747–752, 1980
19. Fawcitt RA, Forbes C, Isherwood I: Computed tomography in pancreatic disease. *Br J Radiol* 51:1–4, 1978
20. Federle MP, Jeffrey RB, Crass RA, van Dalsem V: Computed tomography of pancreatic abscesses. *AJR* 136:879–882, 1981
21. Ferrucci JT, Wittenberg J, Black EB, Kirkpatrick RH, Hall DA: Computed body tomography in chronic pancreatitis. *Radiology* 130:175–182, 1979
22. Ferrucci JT, Wittenberg J, Mueller PR, Simeone JF, Harbin WP, Kirkpatrick RH, Taft PD: Diagnosis of abdominal malignancy by radiologic fine-needle aspiration biopsy. *AJR* 134:323–330, 1980
23. Fishman A, Isikoff MB, Barkin JS, Friedland JT: Significance of a dilated pancreatic duct on CT examination. *AJR* 133:225–227, 1979
24. Foley WD, Stewart ET, Lawson TL, Geenan J, Loguidice J,

25. Maher L, Unger GF: Computed tomography, ultrasonography and endoscopic retrograde cholangiopancreatography in the diagnosis of pancreatic disease: A comparative study. *Gastrointest Radiol* 5:29–35, 1980
26. Foley WD, Wilson CR, Quiroz FA, Lawson TL: Demonstration of the normal extrahepatic biliary tract with computed tomography. *J Comput Assist Tomogr* 4:48–52, 1980
27. Freeny PC, Ball TJ: Endoscopic retrograde cholangiopancreatography (ERCP) and percutaneous transhepatic cholangiography (PTC) in the evaluation of suspected pancreatic carcinoma: Diagnostic limitations and contemporary roles. *Cancer* 47:1666–1678, 1981
28. Freeny PC, Ball TJ, Ryan J: Impact of new diagnostic imaging methods on pancreatic angiography. *AJR* 133:619–624, 1979
29. Gold RP, Seaman WB: Computed tomography and the dilated pancreatic duct: an ominous sign. *Gastrointest Radiol* 6:35–38, 1981
30. Goldstein HM, Zornoza J, Wallace S, Anderson JH, Bree RL, Samuels BI, Lukeman J: Percutaneous fine needle aspiration biopsy of pancreatic and other abdominal masses. *Radiology* 123:319–322, 1977
31. Haaga JR, Alfidi RJ: Precise biopsy localization by computed tomography. *Radiology* 118:603–607, 1976
32. Haaga RJ, Alfidi RJ, Havrilla TR, Tubbs R, Gonzalez L, Meaney TF, Corsi MA: Definitive role of CT scanning of the pancreas. *Radiology* 124:723–730, 1977
33. Haubrich WS, Berk JE: Cysts of the pancreas: Medical aspects. In: *Gastroenterology, Vol. 3*, ed. by HL Bockus, Philadelphia, Saunders, 1976, pp 1155–1164
34. Hauser H, Battikha JG, Wettstein P: Computed tomography of the dilated main pancreatic duct. *J Comput Assist Tomogr* 4:53–58, 1980
35. Inamoto K, Yamazaki H, Kuwata K, Okamoto E, Kotoura Y, Ishikawa Y: Computed tomography of carcinoma in the pancreatic head. *Gastrointest Radiol* 6:343–347, 1981
36. Isikoff MB, Hill MC, Silverstein W, Barkin J: The clinical significance of acute pancreatic hemorrhage. *AJR* 136:679–684, 1981
37. Kaplan JO, Isikoff MB, Barkin J, Livingstone AS: Necrotic carcinoma of the pancreas: "The pseudo-pseudocyst." *J Comput Assist Tomogr* 4:166–167, 1980
38. Kolmannskog F, Kolbenstvedt A, Aakhus T: Computed tomography in inflammatory mass lesions following acute pancreatitis. *J Comput Assist Tomogr* 5:169–172, 1981
39. Kreel L, Sandin B: Changes in pancreatic morphology associated with aging. *Gut* 14:962–970, 1973
40. Kressel HY, Margulis AR, Gooding GW, Filly RA, Moss AA, Korobkin M: CT scanning and ultrasound in the evaluation of pancreatic pseudocysts: A preliminary comparison. *Radiology* 126:153–157, 1978
41. Lee JKT, Stanley RJ, Melson GL, Sagel SS: Pancreatic imaging by ultrasound and computed tomography. *Radiol Clin North Am* 16:105–117, 1979
42. Levine E: Carcinoma of the pancreas presenting as acute pancreatitis: CT diagnosis. *Gastrointest Radiol* 6:29–33, 1981
43. Levitt RG, Geisse G, Sagel SS, Stanley RJ, Evens RG, Koehler RE, Jost RG: Complementary use of ultrasound and computed tomography in studies of the pancreas and kidney. *Radiology* 126:149–152, 1978
44. Levitt RG, Stanley RJ, Sagel SS, Lee JKT, Weyman PJ: Computed tomography of the pancreas: 3 second scanning vs 18 second scanning. *J Comput Assist Tomogr* 6:259–267, 1982
45. Megibow AJ, Bosniak MA, Ambos MA, Beranbaum ER: Thickening of the celiac axis and/or superior mesenteric artery: A sign of pancreatic carcinoma on computed tomography. *Radiology* 141:449–453, 1981
46. Mendez G Jr., Isikoff MB: Significance of intrapancreatic gas demonstrated by CT: A review of nine cases. *AJR* 132:59–62, 1979
47. Mendez G, Isikoff MB, Hill MC: CT of acute pancreatitis: Interim assessment. *AJR* 135:463–469, 1980
48. Mitty HA, Efemidis SC, Yeh HC: Impact of fine needle biopsy on management of patients with carcinoma of the pancreas. *AJR* 137:1119–1121, 1981
49. Moss AA, Federle M, Shapiro HA, Ohto M, Goldberg H,

Korobkin M, Clemett A: The combined use of computed tomography and endoscopic retrograde cholangiopancreatography in the assessment of suspected pancreatic neoplasm: A blind clinical evaluation. *Radiology* 134:159–163, 1980

49. Moss AA, Kressel HY: Computed tomography of the pancreas. *Dig Dis* 22:1018–1027, 1977

50. Neumann CH, Hessel SJ: CT of the pancreatic tail. *AJR* 135:741–745, 1980

51. Nicholson RL: Abnormalities of the perinephric fascia and fat in pancreatitis. *Radiology* 139:125–127, 1981

52. Parienty RA, Ducellier R, Lubrano JM, Picard JD, Pradel J, Smolarski N: Cystadenomas of the pancreas: Diagnosis by computed tomography. *J Comput Assist Tomogr* 4:364–367, 1980

53. Patel S, Bellon EM, Haaga J: Fat replacement of the exocrine pancreas. *AJR* 135:843–845, 1980

54. Pistolesi GF, Marzoli GP, Colosso PQ, Pederzoli P, Procacci C: Computed tomography in surgical pancreatic emergencies. *J Comput Assist Tomogr* 2:165–169, 1978

55. Pollock D, Taylor KJW: Ultrasound scanning in patients with clinical suspicion of pancreatic cancer. *Cancer* 47:1662–1665, 1981

56. Rosch J, Keller FS: Pancreatic arteriography, transhepatic pancreatic venography, and pancreatic venous sampling in diagnosis of pancreatic cancer. *Cancer* 47:1679–1684, 1981

57. Sheedy PF, Stephens DH, Hattery RR, MacCarty RL: Computed tomography in the evaluation of patients with suspected carcinoma of the pancreas. *Radiology* 124:731–737, 1977

58. Sheedy PF, Stephens DH, Hattery RR, MacCarty RL, Williamson B: Computed tomography of the pancreas. *Radiol Clin North Am* 15:349, 1977

59. Siegelman SS, Copeland BE, Saba GP, Cameron JL, Sanders RC, Zerhouni EA: CT of fluid collections associated with pancreatitis. *AJR* 134:1121–1132, 1980

60. Silverstein W, Isikoff MB, Hill MC, Barkin J: Diagnostic imaging of acute pancreatitis: Prospective study using CT and sonography. *AJR* 137:497–502, 1981

61. Stanley RJ, Sagel SS, Levitt RG: Computed tomographic evaluation of the pancreas. *Radiology* 124:715–722, 1977

62. Stephens DH, Sheedy PF: Computed tomography (pancreas). In: *Alimentary Tract Radiology, Vol. 3*, ed. by AR Margulis and HJ Burhenne, St. Louis, Mosby, 1979, pp 251–274

63. Strax R, Toombs BD, Rauschkolb EN: Correlation of barium enema and CT in acute pancreatitis. *AJR* 136:1219–1220, 1981

64. Toombs BD, Lester RG, Ben-Menachem Y, Sandler CM: Computed tomography in blunt trauma. *Radiol Clin North Am* 19:17–35, 1981

65. Torres WE, Clements JL, Sones PJ, Knopf DR: Gas in the pancreatic bed without abscess. *AJR* 137:1131–1133, 1981

66. Vick CW, Simeone JF, Ferrucci JT, Wittenberg J, Mueller PR: Pancreatitis-associated fluid collections involving the spleen: sonographic and computed tomographic appearance. *Gastrointest Radiol* 6:247–250, 1981

67. Weyman PJ, Stanley RJ, Levitt RG: Computed tomography in evaluation of the pancreas. *Semin Roentgenol* 16:301–311, 1981

68. Whalen JP: Radiology of the abdomen: Impact of new imaging methods. *AJR* 132:585–618, 1979

69. Wolfman NT, Ramquist NA, Karstaedt N, Hopkins MB: Cystic neoplasms of the pancreas: CT and sonography. *AJR* 138:37–41, 1982

70. Woodard S, Kelvin FM, Rice RP, Thompson WM: Pancreatic abscess: importance of conventional radiology. *AJR* 136:871–878, 1981

Chapter 9

Spleen

Robert E. Koehler

The spleen is an organ that is well demonstrated on CT scans of the abdomen in virtually every patient. The normal spleen appears as a smoothly bordered, oblong or ovoid organ in the left upper abdomen (Fig. 1). The contour of the superior lateral border of the spleen is smooth and convex, conforming to the shape of the adjacent abdominal wall and left hemidiaphragm (Fig. 2). The hilum is usually directed anteromedially and the splenic artery and vein and their branches can be seen entering the spleen in this region. The posteromedial surface of the spleen behind the hilum is often concave where it conforms to the shape of the adjacent left kidney. The medial surface anterior to the hilum is in contact with the stomach and also assumes a shallow concave shape in most patients. Typically, the spleen measures about 12 cm in length, 7 cm in anteroposterior diameter, and 4 cm in thickness (48). It varies so much in position and orientation from one patient to the next that measurements of this sort are rarely made on CT scans in actual practice; however, precise measurements can be made if needed (42). On scans performed without the use of intravenous contrast material, the normal spleen appears homogeneous in density with a CT attenuation number equal to or slightly less than that of the normal liver (41,55). The margins of the spleen are smooth and the parenchyma is sharply demarcated from the adjacent fat.

The splenic vessels are well seen without the benefit of intravenous contrast material in all but the thinnest of individuals. Only occasionally will contrast material need to be given to visualize the splenic artery and vein. The splenic vein follows a fairly straight course toward the splenic hilum (Fig. 1), running transversely along the posterior aspect of the body and tail of the pancreas in most patients. Unlike the splenic vein, the splenic artery is sometimes very tortuous in older patients. On any given CT slice, it may appear as a curvilinear structure or it may wander in and out of the plane of the slice and appear as a series of round densities, each of which represents a cross-sectional image of a portion of the artery. Also in older individuals, it is common to see calcified atheromas within the wall of the splenic artery.

It is sometimes useful to administer urographic

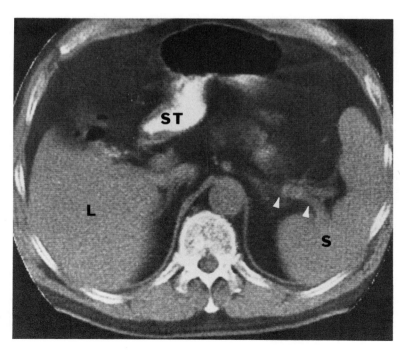

FIG. 1. Normal spleen (S). The lateral border is convex and conforms to the shape of the adjacent body wall. The medial surface is concave and slightly lobulated. The splenic vein (arrowheads) is seen entering the hilum. L, liver; ST, stomach.

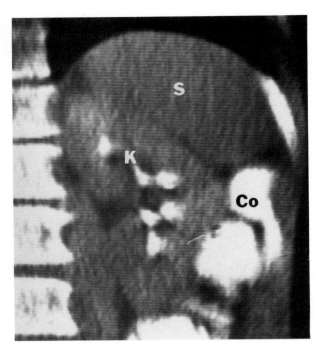

FIG. 2. Direct coronal scan of the normal spleen (S). Note the intimate relationship of the spleen to the kidney (K), and ribs. Co, colon.

contrast material intravenously when examining the spleen by CT. Scans performed immediately after a bolus injection are useful for clarifying the nature of soft tissue densities in the splenic hilar and retropancreatic regions which can mimic abnormalities of the pancreas or left adrenal but which may, in fact, be due to normal splenic vasculature. The splenic artery and vein and their branches undergo dense contrast enhancement after bolus injection and are easily identified on scans of this type (Fig. 3a). Splenic parenchymal opacification also occurs and is sometimes used to improve the detectability of focal mass lesions within the spleen. When the injection is made slowly, over a period of minutes, a uniform increase in the density of the splenic parenchyma results. However, when contrast material is given by rapid intravenous injection, most patients exhibit a heterogeneous pattern of splenic opacification reflecting variable blood flow patterns within different compartments of the spleen (22) (Fig. 3). Only after the passage of a minute or more does the splenic parenchyma return to a uniform, homogeneous appearance. Care must be taken not to misinterpret heterogeneity of splenic density on scans obtained immediately after injection of contrast material as an indication of focal abnormalities.

A promising area currently under investigation is the use of emulsified liposoluble contrast materials, which are taken up by reticuloendothelial cells in the spleen, liver, and other areas (29). Experimental studies in animals (58) and humans (57,59) have demonstrated that the CT attenuation number of the spleen can be increased by as much as 82 Hounsfield units (HU) with the intravenous injection of ethiodized oil emulsion (EOE-13). Nodules of lymphoma and other lesions only a few millimeters in size can be demonstrated in the spleen with this technique.

3a,b

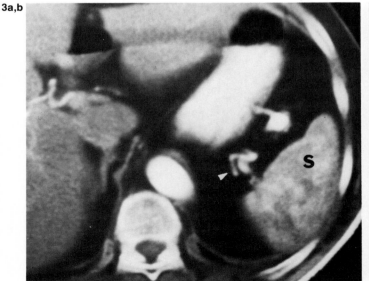 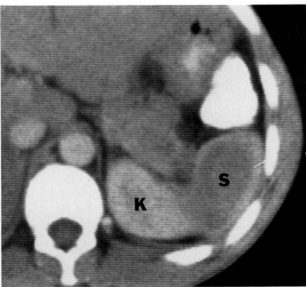

FIG. 3. CT appearance of the normal spleen (S) in two patients immediately after bolus intravenous injection of contrast material. The heterogeneity of parenchymal opacification is transient and the spleen appeared homogeneous on scans obtained 1 min later in both patients. **a:** Patchy pattern of splenic parenchymal enhancement. The aorta and hepatic and splenic arteries (arrowhead) are densely opacified. **b:** Rim-like pattern of parenchymal opacification. K, kidney.

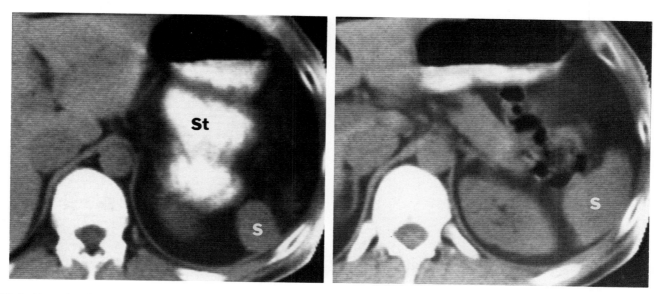

FIG. 4. Normal variation in splenic position. The spleen (S) is partially inverted with its hilum directed medially and superiorly. **Left:** Scan high in the abdomen shows the upper pole as a small rounded density. St, stomach. **Right:** The spleen appears more usual in shape on a scan 2 cm lower in the abdomen.

NORMAL VARIANTS AND CONGENITAL ANOMALIES

The size, shape, and position of the normal spleen can vary considerably from one individual to another (Figs. 4 and 5). Commonly there is a bulge or lobule of splenic tissue that extends medially from the visceral surface of the spleen to lie anterior to the upper pole of the left kidney (23,34,48) (Fig. 6). This can simulate the appearance of a left renal or adrenal mass on intravenous urography but is usually identifiable without difficulty by CT. Clefts between adjacent lobulations can be sharp and are occasionally as deep as 2 or 3 cm (Fig. 7). Liposoluble contrast material has been used to separate renal and splenic parenchyma visually on CT in patients in whom this interpretive problem is encountered (60). Occasionally, a lobule of splenic tissue can lie partially behind the left kidney and displace it anteriorly.

The spleen is sufficiently soft and pliable in texture that left upper abdominal masses or organ enlargement can cause considerable displacement and deformity in its shape. When this happens, the spleen conforms to the shape of the adjacent mass and the resulting

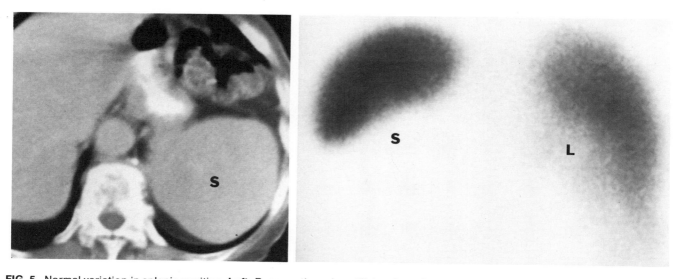

FIG. 5. Normal variation in splenic position. **Left:** Because the spleen (S) is oriented transversely high under the left hemidiaphragm, it appears round and larger than normal. The cranio caudal extent was only 4 cm. **Right:** Posterior view from radionuclide scan confirms the normal appearance and transverse orientation. L, liver.

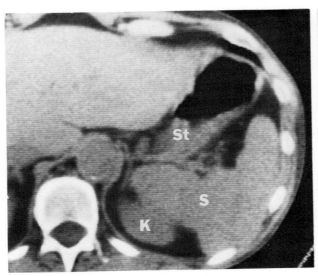
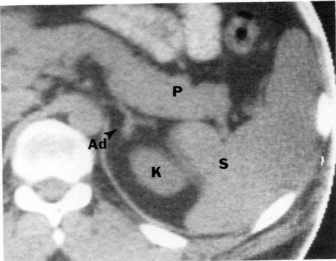

FIG. 6. Normal splenic lobulation. **Left:** Prominent lobule of splenic tissue extending medially between the stomach (St) and left kidney (K). **Right:** Medial lobulation of the spleen (S). Note the intimate relationship between this portion of the spleen and the adjacent kidney, adrenal (Ad), and pancreatic tail (P).

deformity can be quite striking (Fig. 8). Likewise, changes in the position of the spleen occur when adjacent organs are surgically removed (Figs. 9a and b). This is particularly true in patients who have undergone left nephrectomy, in which case the spleen can occupy the left renal fossa (Fig. 9c). Occasionally, there is sufficient laxity in the ligamentous attachments of the spleen that it lies in an unusual position in the absence of an abdominal mass or previous operation. The upside-down spleen (11,63) is a variant in which the splenic hilum is directed superiorly toward the medial or, occasionally, the lateral portion of the left hemidiaphragm.

The "wandering" spleen is another congenital variant that sometimes causes diagnostic difficulties (25,30). In this condition, there is striking laxity of the suspensory splenic ligaments, which permits the spleen to move about in the abdomen and to simulate the presence of a mid or lower abdominal neoplasm. The CT findings consist of an abdominal mass of appropriate size and the absence of a splenic shadow in the normal location (Fig. 10). It may be possible to

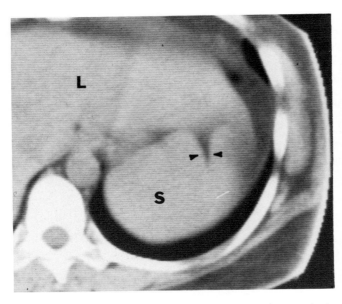

FIG. 7. Prominent cleft (arrowheads) between adjacent splenic lobulations. This anatomic variant can simulate an abnormality on radionuclide scan, especially in patients with suspected splenic trauma. L, liver; S, spleen.

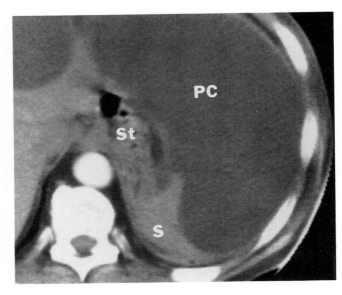

FIG. 8. Marked alteration in splenic shape and position due to compression by an adjacent pancreatic pseudocyst (PC). At operation the spleen (S) was compressed but otherwise unaffected by the adjacent inflammatory process. St, stomach.

9a,b

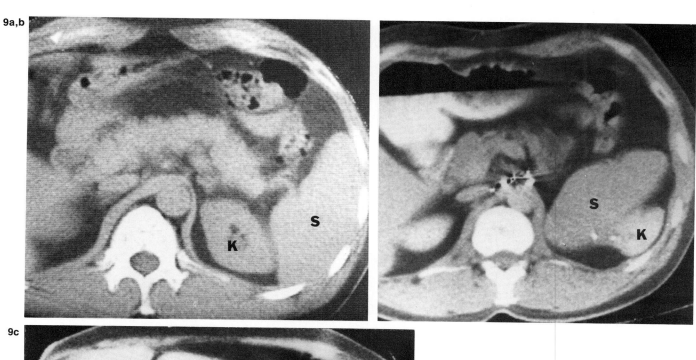

9c

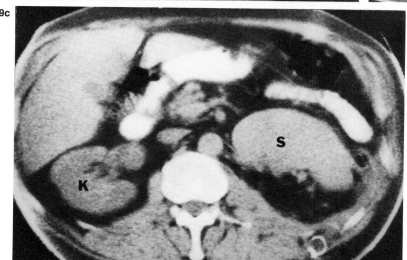

FIG. 9. Altered splenic position after left upper abdominal operation. **a:** Preoperative scan shows spleen (S) to be in normal position. **b:** Postoperative intravenous urogram showed lateral displacement of the left kidney (K) but CT shows that this is due to shift in relative positions of spleen and kidney. **c:** In another patient, scan after left nephrectomy shows that spleen has shifted into position formerly occupied by the left kidney. Splenic hilum is now directed posterosuperiorly.

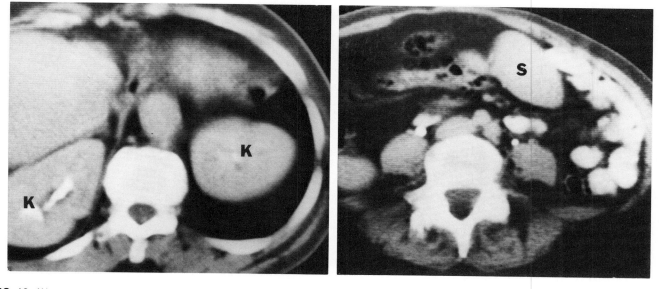

FIG. 10. Wandering spleen. **Left:** No splenic shadow is seen in the left upper abdomen. K, kidney. **Right:** The spleen (S) is seen in the lower mid abdomen and mimics the appearance of an abdominal tumor.

recognize the characteristic shape of the spleen; and the density and pattern of enhancement after bolus injection of intravenous contrast material may lend additional support to the diagnosis. When there is uncertainty as to whether the mass truly represents an ectopically located spleen, scanning after administration of EOE-13 or radionuclide imaging with ⁹⁹ᵐTc-sulfur colloid may resolve the dilemma. The condition is usually one of little clinical significance but in an occasional patient the wandering spleen undergoes torsion with compromise of its vascular supply (31,54).

Accessory spleens occur in 10 to 30% of individuals (4,15) and are a common finding on CT. They probably arise as a result of the failure of fusion of some of the multiple buds of splenic tissue in the dorsal mesogastrium during embryonic life. They occur most commonly near the hilum of the spleen but are sometimes found in its suspensory ligaments or in the tail of the pancreas. Rarely, they occur in the wall of the stomach or intestine, in the greater omentum or mesentery, or even in the pelvis or scrotum (64). They vary from microscopic deposits that are not visible on CT to nodules that are of soft tissue density and 2 or 3 cm in diameter (Fig. 11). In most patients they represent an incidental finding of no clinical significance.

Occasionally, it is important to identify the presence of accessory splenic tissue, particularly when it is confused with a mass of another type. For instance, an accessory spleen can mimic the findings of a pancreatic, left adrenal, or other retroperitoneal mass on intravenous urography (10,56). When there is uncertainty as to whether a nodule seen on CT represents an accessory spleen, one can compare the CT attenuation number of the structure in question

with that of the spleen before and after intravenous injection of urographic or emulsified (EOE-13) contrast material because accessory splenic tissue tends to exhibit the same pattern of contrast enhancement as does the spleen itself (22,48).

Another situation in which it can be important to identify accessory splenic tissue is in patients with splenic pathology (Fig. 12) or who have previously undergone splenectomy. In this situation, accessory spleens may hypertrophy and reach a size of 5 cm or more (4,33). Identification is particularly important in patients in whom the splenectomy was initially performed for a hematologic disorder resulting in hypersplenism. In these people, the growth of accessory splenic tissue may lead to a return of splenic hyperactivity with resultant relapse.

Polysplenia is a rare combination of congenital anomalies characterized by multiple aberrant right-sided splenic nodules, central or left-sided liver, absence of the gallbladder, cardiac anomalies, incomplete development of the inferior vena cava, and anomalies of other organs. When this condition is present, CT can demonstrate the nodules of splenic tissue in the right upper abdomen, the altered shape of the liver, and other features of the syndrome (13).

PATHOLOGIC CONDITIONS

Splenomegaly

Enlargement of the spleen is detectable by a variety of means including physical examination, and CT is rarely necessary to document the presence of splen-

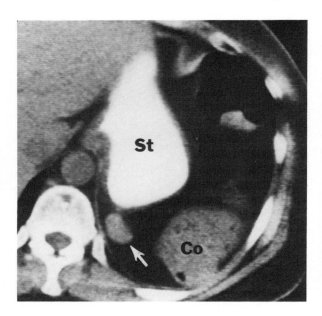

FIG. 11. Small accessory spleen (arrow) in a patient with prior splenectomy. Co, colon; St, stomach.

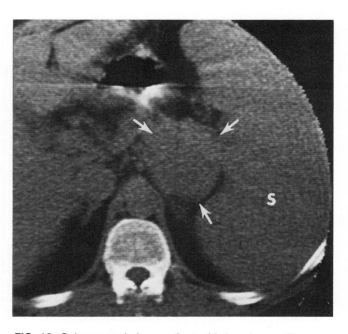

FIG. 12. Splenomegaly in a patient with lymphoma. The mass (arrows) in the splenic hilar region represents an enlarged accessory spleen (S) that was also affected by the tumor.

omegaly. However, confusion sometimes arises as to whether a mass felt in the left upper abdomen truly represents an enlarged spleen. In such cases, CT can provide a definite answer as to whether the spleen is enlarged or whether there is a separate abdominal mass (6). Methods have been described for accurately estimating the volume of the spleen from cross-sectional images (35). An accuracy of ±5% has been reported (42) in determining splenic volume in experimental animals by tracing the area of the spleen on contiguous scans at 1 cm intervals and using a computer program to add the volume of each slice. In actual practice, most experienced radiologists judge the volume of the spleen as normal or enlarged on a more subjective basis using certain visual clues. A craniocaudal span exceeding 14 cm should suggest the presence of splenomegaly. When the spleen is enlarged, the concavity of the visceral surface is often lost as the spleen assumes a more globular shape (Fig. 13). When splenomegaly is present, there are often CT findings that suggest the etiology of the splenic enlargement. Tumor, abscess, or cyst can be appreciated within the spleen. Associated abdominal lymph node enlargement can suggest the presence of lymphoma. Cirrhotic patients with splenomegaly on the basis of portal hypertension often show characteristic alterations in the size and shape of the liver and prominence of the venous structures in the splenic hilum and gastrohepatic ligament (Fig. 14). There is an increase in the CT attenuation number of the spleen in some patients with hemochromatosis of either the primary or secondary type (39).

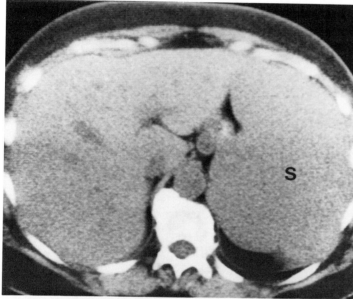

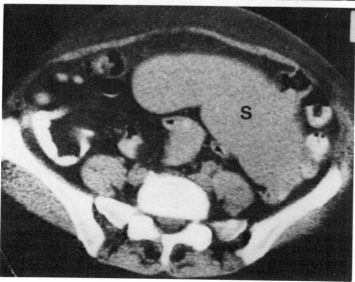

FIG. 13. Splenomegaly in a patient with chronic lymphocytic leukemia. **Above:** The spleen (S) is globular in shape and its medial border is predominantly convex. **Below:** The lower pole of the spleen extends into the pelvis.

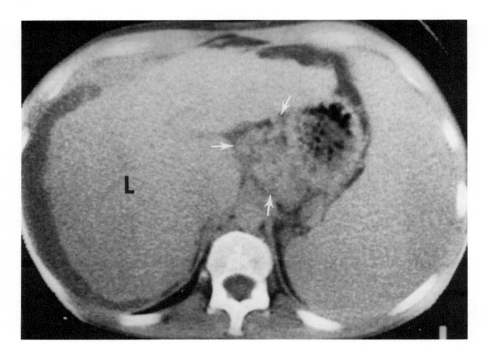

FIG. 14. Splenomegaly in a patient with cirrhosis and portal hypertension. The small nodular liver (L) and varices (arrows) in the gastrohepatic ligament indicate portal hypertension as the cause for splenic enlargement.

Neoplasms

The spleen is often affected in patients with lymphoma of both the Hodgkin's and non-Hodgkin's types. The sensitivity for detecting splenic involvement with CT in patients with lymphoma has been reported to be 50 to 90% (1,7,20,28,49). When there is homogeneous lymphomatous infiltration of the spleen without enlargement, the CT appearance can be normal. More commonly, however, splenomegaly is evident either with or without focal low density nodules in the parenchyma (Figs. 15 and 16). Some

observers have found that as many as half of the patients who have CT abnormalities indicating splenic involvement show focal low density lesions (20,28), whereas others find focal lesions to be infrequent (9). Splenic abnormalities are seen most often in scans of patients with lymphoma of the diffuse histiocytic type (19,51) and somewhat less commonly in patients with Hodgkin's disease. This is particularly true of focal low density nodules in the spleen, which are rarely

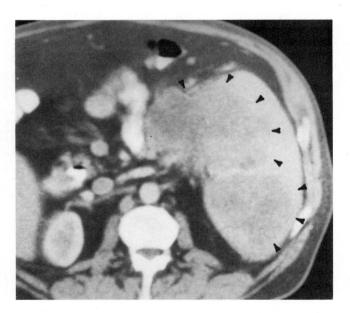

FIG. 16. Complex low density masses (arrowheads) in the spleen, one of which appeared to extend into the adjacent tail of the pancreas. At operation, there were multiple foci of lymphoma in the spleen, splenic hilum, and pancreas.

FIG. 15. Splenomegaly in a patient with diffuse histiocytic lymphoma. A focal low density lesion (arrowheads) is also noted.

demonstrated by CT in patients with lymphoma other than the diffuse histiocytic type (37).

In patients with non-Hodgkin's lymphoma, the finding of splenomegaly indicates a high probability of splenic involvement by the tumor. In patients with Hodgkin's disease, however, as many as one-third of those with splenomegaly are found not to have splenic involvement at the time of splenectomy (28).

In some series an even more common cause of focal low density nodules in the spleen is metastatic disease in patients with carcinoma or sarcoma originating in other areas (19,48) (Figs. 17a and b). Malignant melanoma is often the tumor of origin (Fig. 17c) but metastases can also arise from tumors of the lung, breast, and a variety of other organs. Typical CT findings consist of one or more nodules that are 10 to 20 HU lower in density than the surrounding splenic

tissue. Metastatic nodules containing areas of necrosis and liquifaction can exhibit irregularly shaped regions within them that approach water density (Fig. 17d). Splenic enlargement may or may not be present.

Primary tumors of the spleen are rare and are usually sarcomas arising from cells of vascular origin. To date there is little experience to indicate the spectrum of CT appearances to be expected with primary splenic tumors (Fig. 18). Rare benign tumors such as cystic hamartoma (8) and lymphangiomatosis are occasionally encountered.

Inflammatory Disease

Scattered punctate calcifications in the spleen are commonly encountered on CT and indicate the presence of healed granulomata (Fig. 19). In most pa-

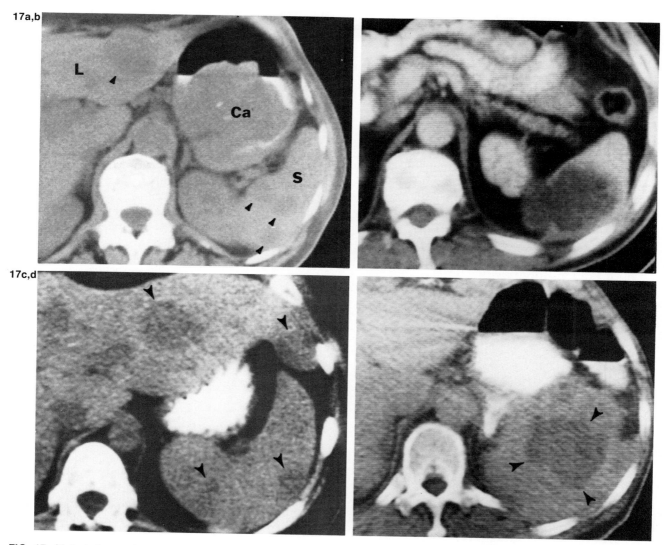

FIG. 17. Metastatic carcinoma to the spleen. **a:** Large gastric adenocarcinoma (Ca) with metastatic nodules (arrowheads) in the liver (L) and spleen (S). The nodules are only slightly lower in density than the normal parenchyma. **b:** Low density focus of metastatic bronchogenic carcinoma in the spleen on a contrast enhanced scan. **c:** Metastatic deposits (arrowheads) in the liver and spleen in a patient with malignant melanoma. **d:** Irregular low density area (arrowheads) in a large nodule of metastatic carcinoma in the spleen indicates central necrosis and liquifaction.

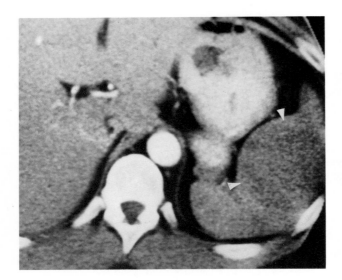

FIG. 18. Spherical low density splenic mass (arrowheads) in a patient with a primary sarcoma of the spleen.

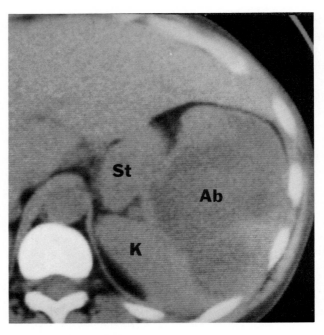

FIG. 20. Splenic abscess (Ab) in a patient with fever and alcoholic withdrawal. The spleen is enlarged and the abscess appears as a lobulated, low density region within it. K, kidney; St, stomach.

tients in the midwestern United States, these are presumed to be due to prior histoplasmosis. Tuberculous infection can also cause calcified splenic granulomata. Large, thin-rimmed, concentrically laminated calcifications have been described in splenic granulomata due to brucellosis (2).

Computed tomography can be important in the detection of splenic abscess. This serious disease carries a 60% mortality rate, partially because it is often not diagnosed until the time of operation or autopsy (26). The CT appearance of abscesses in the spleen is similar to that of abscesses in other areas (19,43) (Fig. 20). Typically there is a focal lesion with a density lower than that of the surrounding splenic tissue. The CT attenuation number of the abscess

depends on the nature of its contents and can vary from 20 to 40 HU or more. The abscess is usually well circumscribed and is often spherical or slightly lobulated in shape. It may contain gas or there may be layering of material of different densities within the cavity. The rim of the abscess is often isodense with the surrounding spleen but may enhance when iodinated contrast material is injected intravenously.

Splenic abnormalities of an inflammatory nature can also be seen in patients with pancreatitis. Fluid may collect around the spleen, particularly laterally (Fig. 8) (62). Pseudocysts can arise in the tail of the pancreas or adjacent splenic hilum (45) and can extend beneath the splenic capsule or even into the spleen itself. Like abscesses, pancreatic pseudocysts have low density material within them and the cyst wall may enhance after administration of contrast material.

Cysts

Three types of cysts are known to occur in the spleen and, unless the spleen is removed and examined histologically, it is usually not possible to distinguish one type from another. Most splenic cysts, particularly those encountered in older individuals, are posttraumatic in origin and are thought to represent the final stage in the evolution of a splenic hematoma. Histologically, they do not contain an epithelial lining and they are probably best referred to as pseudocysts. They may or may not calcify. Like other types of splenic

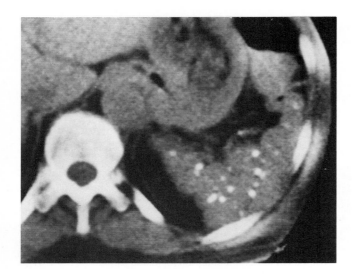

FIG. 19. Multiple calcified splenic granulomata presumed due to histoplasmosis.

cysts, they are sharply demarcated from the adjacent splenic parenchyma and contain fluid of a density similar to or slightly above that of water (Fig. 21). Echinococcal cysts are rare, even in patients with known echinococcal disease elsewhere in the body. They are well circumscribed, spherical lesions that tend to enlarge the spleen and commonly contain extensive calcification within their wall. Epidermoid cysts are congenital in origin (12,27). They are also spherical, sharply circumscribed, water density lesions and they show no central or rim enhancement when intravenous contrast material is given. The wall of an epidermoid cyst will occasionally calcify (16), but this does not usually occur.

Trauma

Computed tomography has proven to be quite useful for detecting splenic injury in patients with blunt abdominal trauma (5,14,17,18,32,40,50). Injury to the spleen can take the form of subcapsular hematoma, laceration, or, less commonly, intrasplenic hematoma. Subcapsular hematomas appear as crescentic collections of fluid that flatten or indent the lateral margin of the spleen (Figs. 22 and 23). When the hematoma has been present for only 1 to 2 days, its density may be equal to or even greater than that of the splenic parenchyma. Over the next 10 days the density of the fluid within the hematoma gradually decreases (36), becoming less than that of the spleen. Injection of intravenous contrast material improves the detectability of fresh subcapsular hematomas and may be essential for detection of those which are isodense.

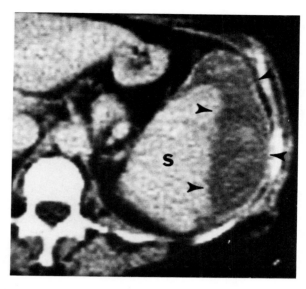

FIG. 22. Traumatic subcapsular hematoma. The low density hematoma (arrowheads) is sharply demarcated from the adjacent spleen (S) in this postcontrast scan. (Case courtesy of Dr. Melvyn Korobkin.)

Splenic lacerations may occur with or without accompanying subcapsular hematoma. CT findings include splenic enlargement, an irregular cleft or defect in the splenic border, and the presence of free blood in the peritoneal cavity (3,18) (Fig. 24).

Conservative surgical management of splenic trauma is becoming more prevalent as the increased risk of serious infection is being recognized in patients who have previously undergone splenectomy. Some centers are now performing splenorrhaphy, suturing of

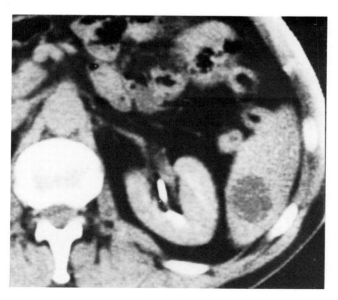

FIG. 21. Splenic cyst. The lesion is round, sharply circumscribed, and of low density. At cholecystectomy, the spleen felt normal and was not removed. The cyst is presumed to be on a posttraumatic basis.

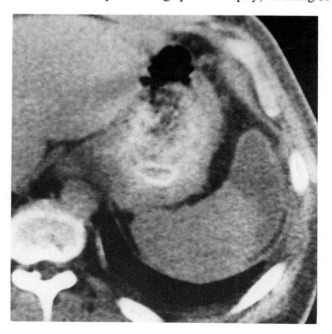

FIG. 23. Spontaneous subcapsular splenic hematoma in a patient without abdominal trauma.

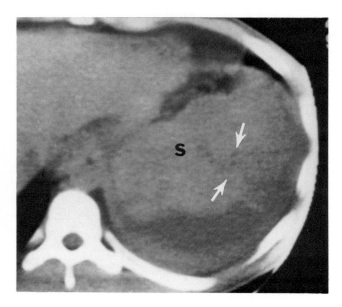

FIG. 24. Splenic laceration. The spleen (S) is enlarged, irregular in shape, and contains a low density defect in its lateral margin (arrows). A collection of blood surrounds the posterior and lateral aspects of the spleen.

splenic lacerations without removing the spleen, and CT has been found to be useful in the postoperative evaluation of these patients (21). In those who are doing well postoperatively, the spleen appears essentially normal after splenorrhaphy. Subcapsular hematoma and perisplenic fluid collections can, of course, be recognized if they are present. In some centers, radiopaque Teflon felt plegets are laid over the laceration to aid in keeping the sutures in place. These plegets appear as focal areas of radioopacity on the splenic capsule, which have a density of 85 to 100 HU (24).

It has been found that physiologic splenic activity can develop again in as many as half of patients undergoing splenectomy for trauma (46). This can be due either to growth of an accessory spleen not removed at the time of operation or to seeding of the peritoneal cavity with viable splenic tissue at the time of the initial trauma or subsequent operation, a condition sometimes known as splenosis. Computed tomography can be used to detect these foci of splenic tissue in the abdomen, particularly when liposoluble contrast material is used (61), and it can be helpful in determining that an apparent abdominal mass represents splenosis or an accessory spleen rather than a neoplasm.

Miscellaneous Conditions

A focal low density region in the spleen can indicate the presence of a splenic infarct (19,48) (Fig. 25). The

defect may be wedge-shaped, with its base at the splenic capsule and its apex toward the hilum. Gas bubbles have been seen scattered throughout a large, nonsuppurative splenic infarct caused by transcatheter embolization of the splenic arterial bed (38).

Patients with sickle cell anemia usually undergo repeated episodes of splenic infarction that eventually result in a small spleen containing diffuse microscopic deposits of calcium and iron. Computed tomography has been helpful in establishing that the finding on bone scan of a focal area of uptake of ^{99m}Tc-diphosphonate in the left upper abdomen was due to uptake in the spleen rather than in a focus of osteomyelitis in the overlying rib (47).

CLINICAL APPLICATIONS

Computed tomography can serve many useful purposes and answer many questions in patients with known or suspected splenic disease. Normal splenic lobulations, clefts between adjacent lobulations, and positional anomalies may present confusing appearances on radionuclide liver spleen images, making interpretation difficult. This is especially true in patients in whom splenic trauma is suspected (53). When clarification is needed of an abnormality suspected on the basis of radionuclide imaging, CT constitutes an excellent means of clarifying the true size, shape, position, and physical integrity of a spleen.

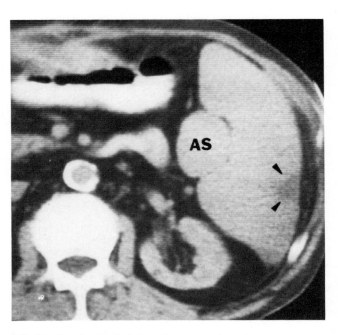

FIG. 25. Small splenic infarct (arrowheads) in patient with enlargement of spleen and accessory spleen (AS) due to myeloid metaplasia. The infarct is peripheral, wedge-shaped, and lower in density than surrounding splenic parenchyma. Note slight depression in splenic contour over the infarct.

Either CT or ultrasonography can be used to study the spleen in many situations. Both techniques can be used to document the presence and extent of splenomegaly. When the cause for splenic enlargement is not known, however, CT is the preferred technique because it is more likely to demonstrate conditions that may be responsible for the splenomegaly, such as lymphomatous enlargement of abdominal nodes.

Computed tomography and ultrasonography are also both useful in imaging focal masses within the spleen (52). In some patients, the cystic nature of a splenic mass suspected on CT can be confirmed by ultrasonography.

It would appear that at the present time, CT is the best radiologic method for screening patients with blunt abdominal trauma for the presence of splenic injury, and its use has decreased the need for abdominal arteriography and exploratory laparotomy. The sensitivity in detecting splenic injury by CT has been reported to be as high as 100% in the series reported to date (5,14,18,32,40,50). The noninvasive nature of the examination is a clear advantage over splenic angiography and the ability to examine the abdomen simultaneously for signs of hepatic, renal, retroperitoneal, or other trauma constitutes an advantage over radionuclide imaging (44). Although ultrasound can also be used to evaluate the possibility of splenic trauma, its sensitivity may not be as high (3) and it does not provide as clear a demonstration of some of the other areas of the abdomen and pelvis as can be obtained by CT.

REFERENCES

1. Alcorn FS, Mategrano VC, Petasnick JP, Clark JW: Contributions of computed tomography in the staging and management of malignant lymphoma. *Radiology* 125:717–723, 1977
2. Arcomano AP, Pizzolato NF, Singer R, Zucker SM: A unique type of calcification in chronic brucellosis. *AJR* 128:135–137, 1977
3. Asher WM, Parvin S, Virgilio RW, Haber K: Echographic evaluation of splenic injury after blunt trauma. *Radiology* 118:411–415, 1976
4. Beahrs JR, Stephens DH: Enlarged accessory spleens: CT appearance in postsplenectomy patients. *AJR* 135:483–486, 1980
5. Berger PE, Kuhn JP: CT of blunt abdominal trauma in childhood. *AJR* 136:105–110, 1981
6. Boldt DW, Reilly BJ: Computed tomography of abdominal mass lesions in children. *Radiology* 124:371–378, 1977
7. Breiman RS, Castellino RA, Harell GS, Marshall WH, Glatstein E, Kaplan HS: CT-pathologic correlation in Hodgkin's disease and non-Hodgkin's lymphoma. *Radiology* 126:159–166, 1978
8. Brinkley AB, Lee JKT: Cystic hamartoma of the spleen: CT and sonographic findings. *J Clin Ultrasound* 9:136–138, 1981
9. Burgener FA, Hamlin DJ: Histiocytic lymphoma of the abdomen: Radiologic spectrum. *AJR* 137:337–342, 1981
10. Clark RE, Korobkin M, Palubinskas AJ: Angiography of accessory spleens. *Radiology* 102:41–44, 1972
11. D'Altorio RA, Caro JY: Upside-down spleen as cause of suprarenal mass. *Urology* 11:422–424, 1978
12. Davidson ED, Campbell WG, Hersh T: Epidermoid splenic cyst occurring in an intrapancreatic accessory spleen. *Dig Dis Sci* 25:964–967, 1980
13. DeMaeyer P, Wilms G, Baert AL: Polysplenia. *J Comput Assist Tomogr* 5:104–105, 1981
14. Druy EM, Rubin BE: Computed tomography in the evaluation of abdominal trauma. *J Comput Assist Tomogr* 3:40–44, 1979
15. Eraklis AJ, Filler RM: Splenectomy in childhood: A review of 1413 cases. *J Pediatr Surg* 7:382–388, 1972
16. Favelukes HA: Calcific shadow in spleen of young man. *JAMA* 239:1177–1178, 1978
17. Federle MP: Abdominal trauma: The role and impact of computed tomography. *Invest Radiol* 16:260–268, 1981
18. Federle MP, Goldberg HI, Kaiser JA, Moss AA, Jeffrey RB, Mall JC: Evaluation of abdominal trauma by computed tomography. *Radiology* 138:637–644, 1981
19. Freeman MH, Tonkin AK: Focal splenic defects. *Radiology* 121:689–692, 1976
20. Frick MP, Feinberg SB, Loken MK: Noninvasive spleen scanning in Hodgkin's disease and non-Hodgkin's lymphoma. *Comput Tomogr* 5:73–80, 1980
21. Giuliano AE, Lim RC: Is splenic salvage safe in the traumatized patient? *Arch Surg* 116:651–656, 1981
22. Glazer GM, Axel L, Goldberg HI, Moss AA: Dynamic CT of the normal spleen. *AJR* 137:343–346, 1981
23. Gooding GAW: The ultrasonic and computed tomographic appearance of splenic lobulations: A consideration in the ultrasonic differential of masses adjacent to the left kidney. *Radiology* 126:719–720, 1978
24. Goodman PC, Federle MP: Splenorrhaphy: CT appearance. *J Comput Assist Tomogr* 4:251–252, 1980
25. Gordon DH, Burrell MI, Levin DC, Mueller CF, Becker JA: Wandering spleen—the radiological and clinical spectrum. *Radiology* 125:39–46, 1977
26. Grant E, Mertens MA, Mascatello VJ: Splenic abscess: Comparison of four imaging methods. *AJR* 132:465–466, 1979
27. Griscom NT, Harbreaves HK, Schwartz MZ, Reddish JM, Colodny AH: Huge splenic cyst in a newborn: Comparison with 10 cases in later childhood and adolescence. *AJR* 129:889–891, 1977
28. Harell GS: The current status of splenic computed tomography in patients with lymphoma. In: *Contrast Media in Computed Tomography,* ed. by R Felix, E Kazner, and OH Wegener, Amsterdam, Excerpta Medica, 1981, pp 237–242
29. Havron A, Seltzer SE, Davis MA, Shulkin P: Radiopaque liposomes: A promising new contrast material for computed tomography of the spleen. *Radiology* 140:507–511, 1981
30. Hunter TB, Haber K: Sonographic diagnosis of a wandering spleen. *AJR* 129:925–926, 1977
31. Isikoff MB, White DW, Diaconis JN: Torsion of the wandering spleen, seen as a migratory abdominal mass. *Radiology* 123:36, 1977
32. Jeffrey RB, Laing FC, Federle MP, Goodman PC: Computed tomography of splenic trauma. *Radiology* 141:729–732, 1981
33. Joshi SN, Wolverson MK, Cusworth RB, Nair SG, Perrillo RP: Complementary use of computerized tomography and technetium scanning in the diagnosis of accessory spleen. *Dig Dis Sci* 25:888–892, 1980
34. Koehler RE, Evens RG: The spleen. In: *Surgical Radiology,* ed. by JG Teplick and ME Haskin, Philadelphia, Saunders, 1981, pp 1064–1088
35. Koga T, Morikawa Y: Ultrasonographic determination of the splenic size and its clinical usefulness in various liver diseases. *Radiology* 115:157–161, 1975
36. Korobkin M, Moss AA, Callen PW, DeMartini WJ, Kaiser JA: Computed tomography of subcapsular splenic hematoma. *Radiology* 129:441–445, 1978
37. Krudy AG, Dunnick NR, Magrath IT, Shawker TH, Doppman JL, Spiegel R: CT of American Burkitt Lymphoma. *AJR* 136:747–754, 1981
38. Levy JM, Wasserman PI, Weiland DE: Nonsuppurative gas formation in the spleen after transcatheter splenic infarction. *Radiology* 139:375–376, 1981
39. Long JA, Doppman JL, Nienhaus AW, Mills SR: Computed tomographic analysis of beta-thalassemia syndromes with hemochromatosis: Pathologic findings with clinical and laboratory correlations. *J Comput Assist Tomogr* 4:159–165, 1980

40. Mall JC, Kaiser JA: CT diagnosis of splenic laceration. *AJR* 134:265−269, 1980

41. Mategrano VC, Petasnick J, Clark J, Bin JC, Weinstein R: Attenuation values in computed tomography of the abdomen. *Radiology* 125:135−140, 1977

42. Moss AA, Freidman MA, Brito AC: Determination of liver, kidney and spleen volumes by computed tomography: An experimental study in dogs. *J Comput Assist Tomogr* 5:12−14, 1981

43. Moss ML, Kirschner LP, Peereboom G, Ferris RA: CT demonstration of a splenic abscess not evident at surgery. *AJR* 135: 159−160, 1980

44. Nebesar RA, Rabinov KR, Potsaid MA: Radionuclide imaging of the spleen in suspected splenic injury. *Radiology* 110: 609−614, 1974

45. Okuda K, Taguchi T, Ishihara K, Konno A: Intrasplenic pseudocyst of the pancreas. *J Clin Gastroenterol* 3:37−41, 1981

46. Pearson HA, Johnston D, Smith KA, Touloukian RJ: The born again spleen. Return of splenic function after splenectomy for trauma. *N Engl J Med* 298:1389−1392, 1978

47. Perlmutter S, Jacobstein JG, Kazam E: Splenic uptake of ⁹⁹ᵐTc-Diphosphonate in sickle cell disease associated with increased splenic density on computerized transaxial tomography. *Gastrointest Radiol* 2:77−79, 1977

48. Piekarski J, Federle MP, Moss AA, London SS: CT of the spleen. *Radiology* 135:683−689, 1980

49. Redman HC, Glatstein E, Castellino RA, Federal WA: Computed tomography as an adjunct in the staging of Hodgkin's disease and non-Hodgkin's lymphoma. *Radiology* 124: 381−385, 1977

50. Reich NE, Haaga JR: Current cases and concepts. *Comput Axial Tomogr* 1:227−229, 1977

51. Scully RE, Galdabini JJ, McNeely BU: Case records of the Massachusetts General Hospital, Case 41-1976. *N Engl J Med* 295:828−834, 1976

52. Shirkhoda A, McCartney WH, Staab EV, Mittelstaedt CA: Imaging of the spleen: A proposed algorithm. *AJR* 135:195−198, 1980

53. Smidt KP: Splenic scintigraphy: A large congenital tissue mimicking splenic hematoma. *Radiology* 122:169, 1977

54. Smulewicz JJ, Clement AR: Torsion of the wandering spleen. *Dig Dis* 20:274−279, 1975

55. Stephens DH, Sheedy PF, Hattery RR, MacCarty RL: Computed tomography of the liver. *AJR* 128:579−590, 1977

56. Stiris MG: Accessory spleen versus left adrenal tumor: Computed tomographic and abdominal angiographic evaluation. *J Comput Assist Tomogr* 4:543−544, 1980

57. Vermess M: Computed tomography of the liver and spleen with iodinated fat emulsion. In: *Contrast Media in Computed Tomography,* ed. by R Felix, E Kazner and OH Wegener, Amsterdam, Excerpta Medica, 1981, pp 63−68

58. Vermess M, Chatterji DC, Doppman JL, Grimes G, Adamson RH: Development and experimental evaluation of a contrast medium for computed tomographic examination of the liver and spleen. *J Comput Assist Tomogr* 3:25−31, 1979

59. Vermess M, Doppman JL, Sugarbaker P, Fisher RI, Chatterji DC, Luetzeler J, Grimes G, Girton M, Adamson RH: Clinical trials with a new intravenous liposoluble contrast material for CT of the liver and spleen. *Radiology* 137:217−222, 1980

60. Vermess M, Inscoe S, Sugarbaker P: Use of liposoluble contrast material to separate left renal and splenic parenchyma on computed tomography. *J Comput Assist Tomogr* 4:540−542, 1980

61. Vermess M, Javadpour N, Blayney DW: Post splenectomy demonstration of splenic tissue by computed tomography with liposoluble contrast material. *J Comput Assist Tomogr* 5:106−108, 1981

62. Vick CW, Simeone JF, Ferrucci JT, Wittenberg J, Mueller PR: Pancreatitis-associated fluid collections involving the spleen: Sonographic and computed tomographic appearance. *Gastrointest Radiol* 6:247−250, 1981

63. Westcoll JL, Krufky EL: The upside-down spleen. *Radiology* 105:517−521, 1972

64. Wick MR, Rife CC: Paratesticular accessory spleen. *Mayo Clin Proc* 56:455−456, 1981

Chapter 10

Retroperitoneum

Joseph K. T. Lee

The retroperitoneum, bounded anteriorly by the parietal peritoneum and posteriorly by the transversalis fascia, extends from the diaphragm superiorly to the level of the pelvic viscera inferiorly. At the level of the kidneys, the retroperitoneal space is divided into three compartments—the perirenal surrounded by the anterior and posterior pararenal spaces. Two types of viscera exist in the retroperitoneal space: the true embryonic retroperitoneal organs (i.e., the adrenal glands, kidneys, ureters, and gonads), and those structures closely attached to the posterior abdominal wall and only partly covered by the peritoneum (i.e., aorta, inferior vena cava, pancreas, portions of the duodenum, colon, lymph nodes, and nerves).

In the past, the evaluation of most retroperitoneal structures by conventional radiography has been difficult. Since the advent of CT, direct noninvasive demonstration of normal and pathologic retroperitoneal anatomy has become possible with a level of clarity unsurpassed by any other available imaging method (42,48,81) (Fig. 1). Diagnostic scans can be obtained in almost all but the leanest patients because there is normally abundant fat in the retroperitoneum profiling the normal structures. In this chapter, discussion will be limited to diseases involving the great vessels, lymph nodes, psoas muscles, as well as primary retroperitoneal tumors. Diseases related to other solid retroperitoneal organs, such as the kidneys, the adrenals, and the pancreas, are covered in separate chapters. Inflammatory diseases (i.e., abscesses) will be dealt with separately in Chapter 11.

AORTA

Normal Anatomy

The abdominal aorta begins at the aortic hiatus of the diaphragm and usually extends along the ventral aspect of the lumbar spine to the level of the fourth lumbar vertebra, where it divides into the two common iliac arteries. On CT scans, the aorta appears as a circular soft tissue density in a paravertebral location. The caliber of the abdominal aorta decreases as it progresses distally toward the bifurcation. The major branches arising from the abdominal aorta that can be seen on a CT scan include the celiac trunk, the superior mesenteric artery, and renal arteries (43). Although the origin of the inferior mesenteric artery can be identified on CT scans in over 90% of cases, it rarely can be traced more than 1 cm beyond its origin.

The noncalcified aortic wall cannot be distinguished from its intraluminal blood on precontrast scans except in anemic patients. Whereas the attenuation value of the blood in the aortic lumen ranges from 50 to 70 Hounsfield units (HU) in normal subjects, it is considerably less in patients with a markedly reduced hematocrit. Thus, a visible, noncalcified aortic wall is a clue to the presence of anemia. Following intravenous administration of water-soluble iodinated contrast medium, the attenuation value of the aortic lumen can rise as high as +400 HU after a bolus injection.

Pathologic Conditions

Atherosclerosis

Atherosclerotic changes of the aorta can be detected on CT scans. These include calcification in the wall (Fig. 2), mild ectasia, and increased tortuosity. Although the aorta is usually located in a prevertebral position, it may either be parallel to the spine or even lie to the right of the vertebral column in patients with severe atherosclerosis. An atheromatous plaque or a thrombus may have a lower attenuation value than the flowing blood; it is best appreciated on postcontrast scans (Fig. 3).

Aortic Aneurysm

In the United States, abdominal aortic aneurysms are due mostly to atherosclerosis. Syphilitic or traumatic causes are uncommon. Aneurysms can be de-

1a,b

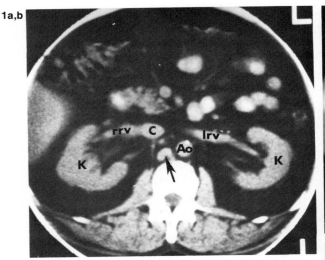

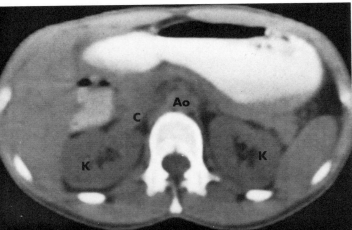

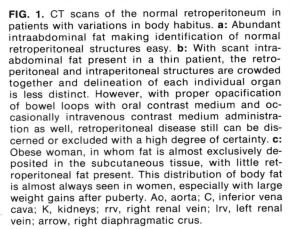

1c

FIG. 1. CT scans of the normal retroperitoneum in patients with variations in body habitus. **a:** Abundant intraabdominal fat making identification of normal retroperitoneal structures easy. **b:** With scant intraabdominal fat present in a thin patient, the retroperitoneal and intraperitoneal structures are crowded together and delineation of each individual organ is less distinct. However, with proper opacification of bowel loops with oral contrast medium and occasionally intravenous contrast medium administration as well, retroperitoneal disease still can be discerned or excluded with a high degree of certainty. **c:** Obese woman, in whom fat is almost exclusively deposited in the subcutaneous tissue, with little retroperitoneal fat present. This distribution of body fat is almost always seen in women, especially with large weight gains after puberty. Ao, aorta; C, inferior vena cava; K, kidneys; rrv, right renal vein; lrv, left renal vein; arrow, right diaphragmatic crus.

tected and differentiated from a tortuous aorta by CT regardless of the presence or absence of aortic wall calcification (Fig. 4). Measurements obtained on a CT scan correlate precisely with those found at surgery (3,38,68). The lumen size can be differentiated from the adjacent atheroma/thrombus following intravenous injection of contrast agent (60). The origin and the length of an aneurysm can be traced on serial cephalad and caudad scans.

The diagnosis of active leakage from an aneurysm is based on obscuration or displacement of the aorta by an irregular soft tissue density (the acute hematoma) with attenuation values between +40 and +70 HU; a portion of this mass may enhance after intravenous contrast material administration (Fig. 5). Similarly, a chronic aortic pseudoaneurysm can be imaged (Fig. 6).

Infected mycotic aneurysm can be diagnosed by CT if gas is seen within the wall of the aorta (69). Dissection of the aorta usually originates in the thoracic cavity, but sometimes extends into the abdomen. Its diagnosis is based on demonstration of displaced intimal calcifications, or the presence of an intimal flap with

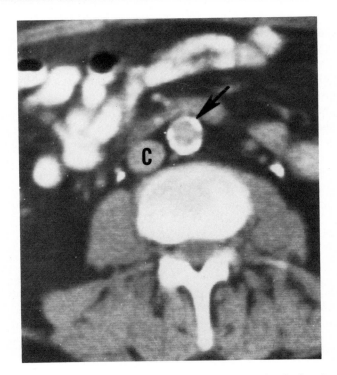

FIG. 2. Calcified wall (arrow) in a normal-sized abdominal aorta. C, inferior vena cava.

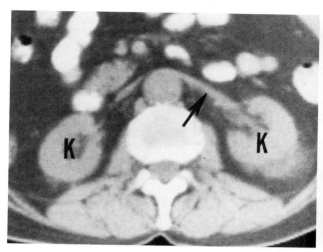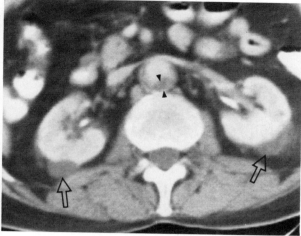

FIG. 3. Atheromatous plaque in a mildly ectatic aorta. **Left:** Precontrast scan. The atheromatous plaque cannot be distinctly separated from the aortic lumen. **Right:** Postcontrast scan. The irregular aortic lumen is clearly differentiated from the nonenhancing atheromatous plaque (arrowheads). The open arrows point to incidental renal cysts. Closed arrow, left renal vein; K, kidney.

enhancement of both the true and false lumina after intravenous administration of contrast media (27,39, 40,51). When the false lumen does not fill with contrast media, CT may be unable to differentiate a dissection from a fusiform aneurysm.

In patients with prior repair of abdominal aortic aneurysm, a collection of serous fluid can often be identified between the synthetic graft and the native aortic wall, which frequently is left in place (Fig. 7). When grafts become infected, small pockets of gas may be shown around the prosthesis on CT scans. These gas collections usually are multiple in number and posterior in location, and most often occur more than 10 days after the initial surgery (41). This is in contradistinction to "normal" gas collections seen in the postoperative period, which usually are single in number and anterior in location. Since the specificity

of this observation has not been documented, correlation with the patient's clinical status is required, and the performance of a needle aspiration for bacteriologic examination may be warranted.

Accuracy and Clinical Application

Although CT can detect the presence and the size of aortic aneurysms and their internal character with a high degree of accuracy (3,38,68), ultrasound still remains the procedure of choice in patients with suspected abdominal aortic aneurysms because of its ease of performance, non-ionizing radiation, lower cost, and the ability to obtain longitudinal scans as well as cross-sectional images. However, CT can be helpful in cases where ultrasound is unsuccessful either due to postsurgical scar tissue, obesity, or abundant bowel

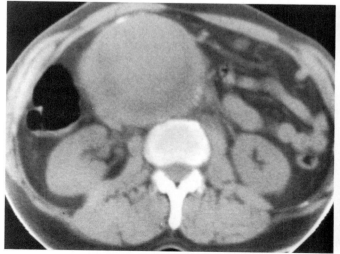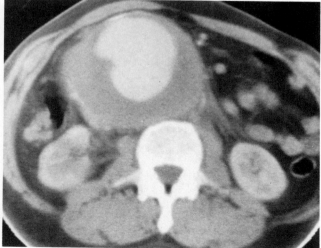

FIG. 4. Large abdominal aortic aneurysm. **Left:** Precontrast scan. The lumen of the aortic aneurysm has a higher attenuation value than its surrounding atheromatous plaque/thrombus. Note that only a minute portion of the wall of the abdominal aorta is calcified. **Right:** Postcontrast scan better defines the lumen of the aortic aneurysm.

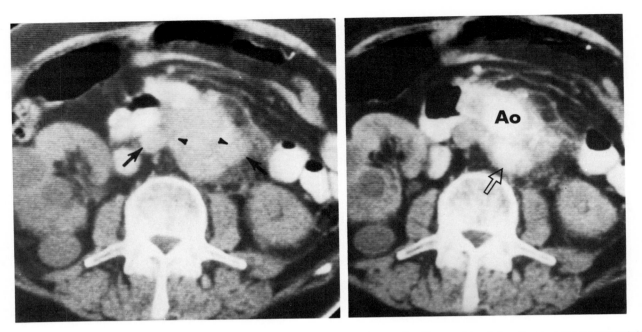

FIG. 5. Leaking aortic aneurysm. **Left:** Precontrast scan. Irregular masses (arrows) with near-blood density abut the faintly calcified aortic aneurysm (arrowheads) suggestive of recent hemorrhage. Incidentally, patient has multiple right renal cysts. **Right:** Scan obtained postbolus injection of intravenous contrast media shows an enhanced aortic lumen (Ao) with extravasation of contrast (open arrow) posteriorly. Fresh blood clot was found around the aneurysm at surgery.

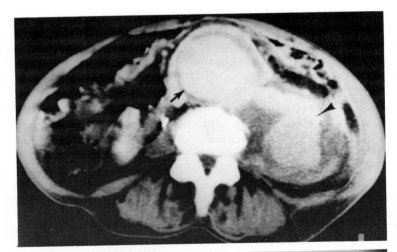

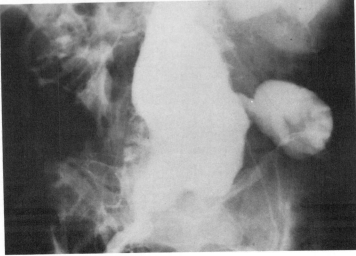

FIG. 6. Aortic aneurysm and associated pseudo-aneurysm. **Above:** Postcontrast CT scan demonstrates a large abdominal aortic aneurysm, extending posterolaterally into left paravertebral area. Note the centrally enhanced lumen in both the true (arrow) and false aneurysm (arrowhead). The lower density periphery represents either an atheroma or thrombus. The left psoas muscle is obscured secondary to the pseudoaneurysm. **Below:** The abdominal arteriogram shows findings similar to CT study.

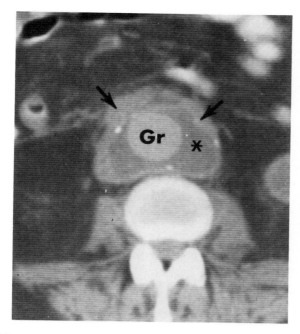

FIG. 7. A layer of fluid (∗) with near-water density is present between the native aortic wall (arrows) and the synthetic graft (Gr) in this patient who had an abdominal aortic aneurysm repaired several months ago.

gas. In our experience, CT is also superior to ultrasound in detecting infected aortic grafts and leaking abdominal aortic aneurysms. Associated anomalies, such as a horseshoe kidney and a retroaortic left renal vein, which may be important in the surgical management of abdominal aortic aneurysm, are more easily detected on CT.

INFERIOR VENA CAVA AND ITS TRIBUTARIES

Normal Anatomy

The inferior vena cava is formed by the two common iliac veins at the level of the fifth lumbar vertebra. From this point it ascends along the vertebral column to the right of the aorta to the level of the diaphragm and enters the chest terminating in the right atrium. Although it is in close proximity to the lumbar vertebral bodies in its most caudal position, it assumes a more ventral position at its cephalic end.

The shape, which may be round or flat, and the size of the inferior vena cava vary from patient to patient and even in the same patient at different levels. Performance of a Valsalva maneuver usually results in more distention of the inferior vena cava. The renal veins, which are located ventral to the renal arteries, often can be seen in their entirety entering the vena

cava. The left renal vein usually is longer than the right and passes across the midline between the abdominal aorta and the superior mesenteric artery. The main hepatic veins and their tributaries sometimes can be seen converging into the vena cava near the diaphragm. Normal caliber gonadal veins cannot be reliably identified on CT scans. Occasionally, they are enlarged in multiparous women and in men with varicoceles and thus will be apparent on CT scans (Fig. 8).

The attenuation value of the lumen of the inferior vena cava is similar to that of the abdominal aorta and thus varies with the hematocrit of the individual patient. However, in contrast to the aortic wall, the wall of the inferior vena cava is thin and rarely visible as a discrete structure even in severely anemic patients. The intrahepatic portion of the inferior vena cava usually can be identified on the noncontrast scans because it has a slightly lower density than the normal hepatic parenchyma.

Normal Variations

The precise knowledge of the various developmental anomalies of the venous system and the recognition of their CT appearances are of paramount importance lest they be misinterpreted as pathologic, possibly leading to unnecessary surgical evaluation.

The inferior vena cava is formed by the successive development and regression of three paired veins (19,20,73) (Fig. 9). Early in embryogenesis, the posterior supracardinal and more anterior subcardinal veins are formed. Later, the most caudal segment of the right supracardinal vein becomes the infrarenal vena cava. The middle segment joins with part of the right subcardinal vein to form the renal portion of the inferior vena cava. The cephalic portion of the inferior vena cava is formed from the efferent veins of the liver. The portion of the right supracardinal vein cephalad to the kidneys becomes the azygous vein; similarly, that portion on the left forms the hemiazygous system. The rest of the left cardinal system undergoes involution.

Interruption of normal regression of any of these venous structures results in different anomalies. Azygous vein continuation is an anomaly of the suprarenal segment. Circumaortic venous rings and retroaortic left renal vein involve the renal segment. Circumcaval ureter, transposition, and duplication of the inferior vena cava involve the infrarenal segment. The schematic representations of these various anomalies are shown in Fig. 10. Most of these venous anomalies can be confidently diagnosed by tracing their course on contiguous scans. If some confusion persists, the vascular nature of these structures can be proven by intravenous contrast material administration.

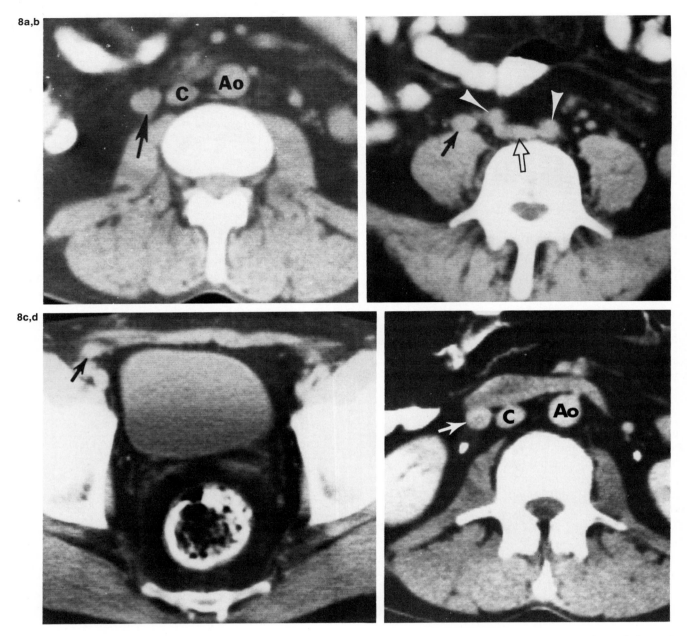

FIG. 8. An enlarged right gonadal vein in a man with an asymptomatic varicocele. **a:** Precontrast CT scan just below both kidneys shows an oval soft tissue density (arrow) lateral to the inferior vena cava (C). **b:** At the level of common iliac artery (arrowheads), an extra soft tissue density (arrow) lies anterior to the psoas muscle and lateral to the iliac artery. Open arrow points to the confluence of common iliac veins. **c:** At the level of acetabula, the soft tissue density (arrow) is seen near the inter-nal (deep) inguinal ring. The presence of such a soft tissue density over several scans indicates that this is a tubular structure. **d:** Postcontrast scan at a level slightly above (a) demonstrates the previously noted soft tissue structure (arrow) to enhance to a similar degree as the adjacent inferior vena cava (C), thus documenting its vascular nature. Serial scans and intravenous contrast material administration are often needed to clarify such complex venous anomalies. Ao, aorta; C, inferior vena cava.

Interrupted Inferior Vena Cava with Azygous/Hemiazygous Continuation

When the subcardinal vein fails to connect with the hepatic veins during the sixth fetal week, blood returns to the heart from the postrenal segment through the azygous/hemiazygous system and the hepatic veins drain directly into the right atrium (9,20,36). This anomaly usually occurs as an isolated lesion but occasionally can be associated with cardiac abnormalities or other visceral anomalies such as the asplenia and polysplenia syndromes.

On CT scans, a normal inferior vena cava is seen from the confluence of common iliac veins to the level of both kidneys. An intrahepatic segment of inferior vena cava, which lies anterior to the diaphragmatic

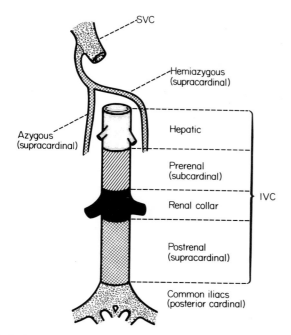

FIG. 9. A schematic diagram showing the precursors of different segments of the inferior vena cava.

crus and posterior to the caudate lobe of the liver, is absent. However, an enlarged azygous vein and often a hemiazygous vein as well can be seen in the retrocrural space on both sides of the aorta. The azygous vein can be further traced on more cephalic scans to the level where it arches anteriorly to join the superior vena cava or just below the level of the aortic arch (Fig. 11).

Circumaortic Left Renal Vein

There is a true vascular ring about the aorta in this anomaly. The preaortic left renal vein crosses from the left kidney to the inferior vena cava at the expected level of the renal veins. The additional retroaortic left renal vein(s) connects to the inferior vena cava by descending caudally and crossing the spine behind the aorta, usually one to two vertebrae below the level of the preaortic left renal vein (73). On CT scans, a normal left renal vein can be seen in its preaortic position. The anomalous retroaortic left renal vein is identified in a more caudal position.

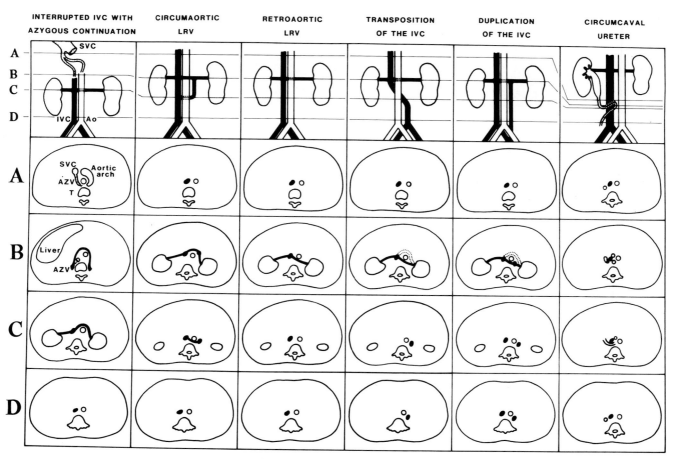

FIG. 10. A diagram showing the relationship of aorta, inferior vena cava, left renal vein in various congenital venous anomalies. (Modified from Royal and Callen, ref. 73.)

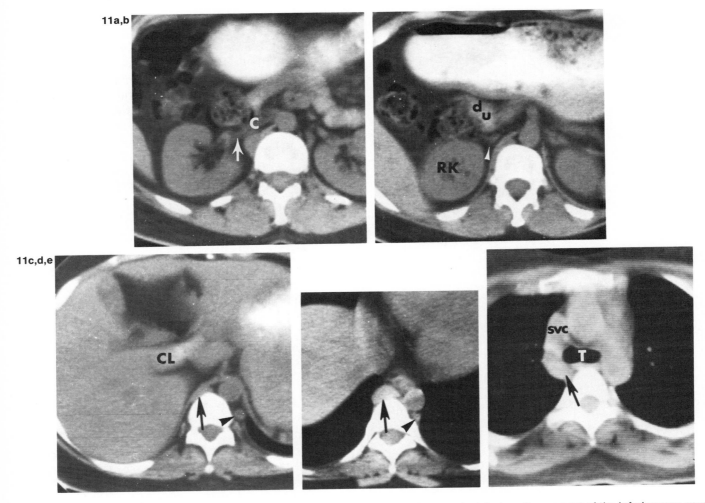

FIG. 11. Interrupted inferior vena cava with azygous/hemiazygous continuation. **a:** At the level of renal hilum, the right renal vein (white arrow) drains into the inferior vena cava (C). **b:** Scan through the upper pole of the right kidney (RK) shows absence of an inferior vena cava. Note that the right adrenal gland (white arrowhead) lies directly posterior to the descending duodenum (du). **c:** At the level of hepatic hilus, enlarged azygous (arrow) and hemiazygous (arrowhead) veins can be seen in the retro-crural space. An intrahepatic segment of the inferior vena cava, which is normally situated posterior to the caudate lobe of the liver (CL), is not present in this case. **d:** A more cephalic scan again demonstrating abnormally enlarged azygous (arrow) and hemiazygous veins (arrowhead). **e:** At the level of tracheal bifurcation (T), the enlarged azygous vein (arrow) drains into the superior vena cava (svc).

Retroaortic Left Renal Vein

In this anomaly, the anterior subcardinal veins regress completely and only the retroaortic supracardinal veins remain to connect the left kidney to the inferior vena cava (73,84). The retroaortic left renal vein (Fig. 12) can be seen either at the same level as a normal left renal vein or in a more caudal position, sometimes as low as the confluence of iliac veins.

Transposition of the Inferior Vena Cava

Anomalous regression of the right cardinal veins and persistence of the left cardinal system result in transposition of the inferior vena cava (19,73). In this entity, a single inferior vena cava ascends on the left side of the spine and crosses either anterior or posterior to the aorta at the level of the renal veins to ascend further to the right atrium on the right side of the spine (Fig. 13). The characteristic CT appearance is a single inferior vena cava to the right of the aorta at levels above the renal vein, a vascular structure either crossing anterior or posterior to the aorta at the level of the renal veins, and a large single inferior vena cava to the left of the spine at levels below the renal veins.

Duplication of the Inferior Vena Cava

In duplication of the inferior vena cava (Fig. 14) there is an inferior vena cava, albeit smaller than usual in size, along the right side of the spine (19,31,73). In addition, a left side inferior vena cava ascends to the level of the renal veins to join the right-sided inferior

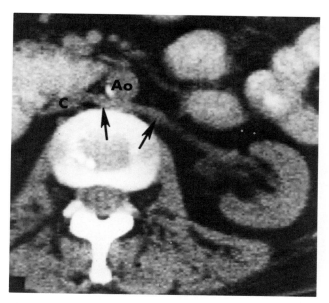

FIG. 12. Retroaortic left renal vein (arrows), which passes behind the aorta (Ao) to drain into the inferior vena cava (C).

vena cava through a vascular structure that may pass either anterior or posterior to the aorta at the level of the renal veins. Either vena cava can be the predominant vessel or they can be of equal size.

On CT scans, a single right-sided inferior vena cava is seen at levels above the renal veins. A vascular structure crossing either anterior or posterior to the aorta is seen at the level of the renal veins, and two vena cavae, one on each side of the aorta, are present below the level of the renal veins. A duplicated left inferior vena cava can be differentiated from a dilated left gonadal vein by following its course to the more caudal scans. While a duplicated left inferior vena cava ends at the level of common iliac veins, a dilated left gonadal vein can be traced further inferiorly to the level of the inguinal canal (73).

Circumcaval Ureter

Embryologically, circumcaval ureter results from anomalous regression of the most caudal segment of

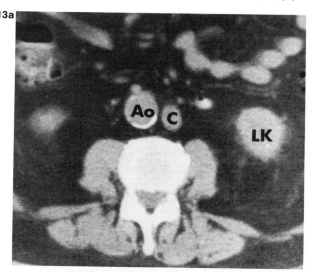

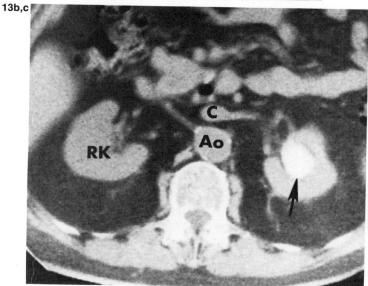

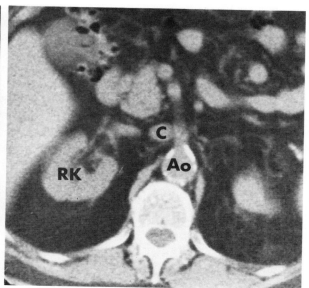

FIG. 13. Transposition of the inferior vena cava. **a:** CT scan below the level of renal veins showing the inferior vena cava (C) on the left side of the aorta (Ao). **b:** At the level of the renal veins, the inferior vena cava (C) crosses anterior to the aorta toward the right side. Left hydronephrosis (arrow) is secondary to a distal ureteral calculus. **c:** Cephalic to the level of renal veins, the inferior vena cava now lies on the right side of the aorta. RK, right kidney; LK, left kidney.

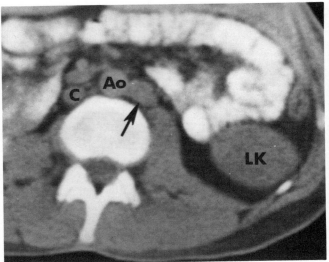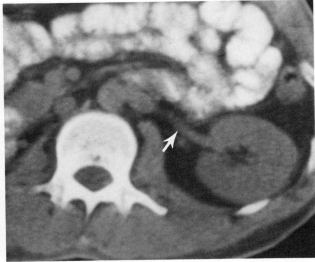

FIG. 14. Duplication of the inferior vena cava. **Left:** CT scan through the level of inferior pole of the left kidney (LK) shows an inferior vena cava (C) on the right side. In addition, a duplicated vena cava (arrow) is present on the left side of the aorta (Ao). **Right:** A more cephalic scan demonstrates the left renal vein (white arrow) draining into the left-sided inferior vena cava.

the supracardinal vein and persistence of the subcardinal vein. Consequently, the ureter passes behind and around the medial aspect of the inferior vena cava as it courses to the bladder.

As in other types of vena caval anomalies, circumcaval ureter may be discovered as an incidental radiographic finding. However, patients with this condition sometimes present with signs and symptoms related to right ureteral obstruction. Whereas asymptomatic patients or patients with minimal caliectasis require only occasional follow-up, patients with significant renal obstruction often require surgical correction.

Inasmuch as circumcaval ureter has a characteristic appearance on excretory urography (medial deviation of the upper one-third of the ureter with sharp turn toward the pedicle of the third or fourth lumbar vertebra producing a "reverse J" configuration), a definitive diagnosis by conventional imaging methods often requires concomitant opacification of the ureter and inferior vena cava, i.e., inferior cavography in conjunction with retrograde ureteral pyelography. Computed tomography can eliminate the need for venocavography in corroborating the diagnosis should this be considered necessary. With CT, the proximal right ureter can be seen coursing medially behind and then anteriorly around the inferior vena cava so as to encircle it partially. The distal ureter may be better distended and delineated with the aid of a lower abdominal compression device (35).

Pathologic Conditions

Venous Thrombosis

Tumoral and nontumoral thrombosis of the inferior vena cava can be identified but not differentiated from

each other on CT scans unless hypervascularity is shown in the tumoral thrombus by bolus CT angiography (62,79,85,88). Thrombosis of the renal and gonadal veins has been similarly documented (77). The involved segment of the vein can be either normal in caliber or substantially enlarged. Enlargement of the cava secondary to a thrombus can be strongly suggested on noncontrast-enhanced scans alone because dilatation is often more focal in cases of thrombosis in comparison to that due to increased blood flow or increased vascular resistance at the level of the diaphragm/right atrium. In cases of complete caval obstruction, paravertebral venous collaterals may also be identified by CT (67).

The definitive diagnosis of venous thrombosis by CT scans depends on demonstration of an intraluminal thrombus (Fig. 15). Whereas a fresh thrombus has a density similar to that of circulating blood, an old thrombus is of lower density than the surrounding blood on noncontrast scans. When the occlusion is complete, the involved segment remains unenhanced on postcontrast scans. In cases where the venous occlusion is partial, the thrombus appears as a low-density filling defect surrounded by iodine-containing blood. However, caution must be taken not to confuse true intraluminal defects from those caused by (a) influx of unopacified blood from large adjacent venous branches and (b) laminar flow phenomenon with the slower flowing enhanced blood staying closest to the wall and unopacified blood flowing centrally suggesting a luminal thrombus (4). The latter "defect" is commonly seen in the inferior vena cava at the end of a bolus injection when a foot vein is used (Fig. 16). With the current generation of scanners, there are probably few if any indications for administering contrast media via a foot vein injection.

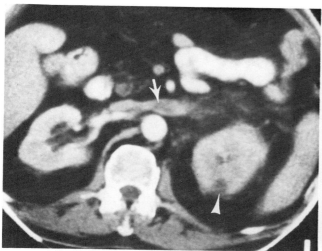
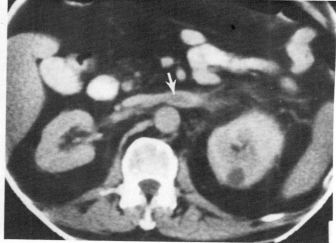

FIG. 15. Left renal vein thrombosis. Postcontrast CT scans (**left:** immediately following a bolus injection; **right:** after recirculation) show a thrombus (arrow) within a nondilated left renal vein. The patient also has a small left renal cyst (arrowhead).

Accuracy and Clinical Application

Although there are no data comparing the accuracy of CT and venography in detecting nontumoral thrombosis of the vena cava and its major branches, CT is reported to have similar overall accuracy in the detection of inferior vena cava and main renal vein invasion by renal cell carcinoma. In one study (88), the overall accuracy of CT was 93% in detecting inferior vena caval invasion and 82% in detecting main renal vein invasion. It is often harder to be certain of tumor thrombus in right renal vein, which is shorter than its counterpart on the left. Computed tomography is not able to detect tumor thrombus in intrarenal venous branches; however, this is of limited clinical significance since the presence of only intrarenal vein inva-

sion by tumor does not alter surgical management (88).

Because of its high degree of accuracy, CT usually can replace inferior vena cavography in detecting invasion of the main renal veins and inferior vena cava in patients with renal cell carcinoma. Although its role in the evaluation of patients with suspected nontumoral venous thrombosis is uncertain, recognition of its appearance on CT scan certainly will help in its diagnosis in cases where scans are obtained for other reasons.

LYMPH NODES

Normal Anatomy

Normal unopacified lymph nodes are routinely seen on CT scans. They appear as small soft tissue den-

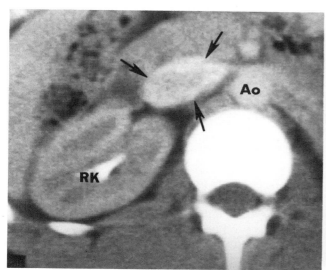
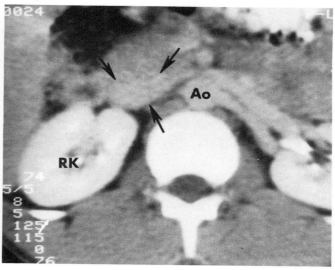

FIG. 16. Pseudothrombus secondary to laminar flow within the inferior vena cava. **Left:** Scan obtained 30 sec after a bolus injection of contrast medium into a foot vein shows residual opacified blood around the periphery of the inferior vena cava (arrows) with central lower density representing more rapidly flowing now unopacified blood. This appearance can be confused with an intraluminal thrombus. **Right:** Repeat scan the following day after rapid intravenous infusion of contrast media into an antecubital vein demonstrates the inferior vena cava (arrows) to be uniformly enhanced. Ao, aorta; RK, right kidney.

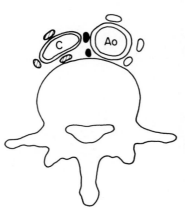

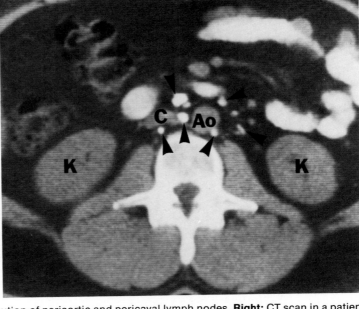

○ PERIAORTIC CHAIN
● INTERAORTO-CAVAL CHAIN
◑ PERICAVAL CHAIN

FIG. 17. **Left:** A schematic drawing denoting distribution of periaortic and pericaval lymph nodes. **Right:** CT scan in a patient following lymphangiography showing normal distribution of retroperitoneal lymph nodes (arrowheads). Ao, aorta; C, inferior vena cava; K, kidney.

sities, ranging from 3 to 10 mm in size. In the retroperitoneum, lymph nodes can be found adjacent to the anterior, posterior, medial, and lateral walls of the inferior vena cava and aorta (Fig. 17). Lymph nodes also can be found in the root of the mesentery and along the course of the major venous structures draining to the inferior vena cava and portal vein. In the pelvis, lymph nodes can be identified in close proximity with the iliac vessels. Although the internal architecture of a lymph node generally is not discernible on CT, fibrolipomatous changes have been shown on CT scans on rare occasion (Fig. 18).

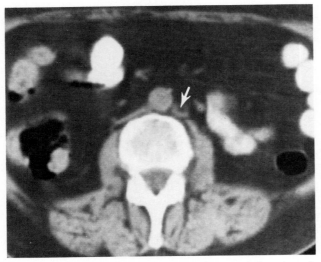

FIG. 18. Fibrolipomatous changes in a paraaortic lymph node. Note the central portion (arrow) of this lymph node has an attenuation value similar to retroperitoneal fat.

Pathologic Conditions

The diagnosis of retroperitoneal lymphadenopathy by CT is based on recognition of nodal enlargement, sometimes concomitant in far advanced disease with displacement or obscuration of normal structures (2,6,10,49,52,71,76). Except in unusually lean or cachectic patients, enlarged lymph nodes generally are well profiled by surrounding fat. In the abdomen and pelvis, lymph nodes are considered unequivocally abnormal if they exceed 2 cm in cross-section diameter (55). Lymph nodes in the retrocrural space are probably pathologic if they exceed 6 mm in size (13). An isolated abdominal or pelvic lymph node between 1 and 2 cm is regarded as a suspicious finding; clustering of nodes of this size should increase the index of suspicion (55). A lymphangiogram or a CT-guided percutaneous needle biopsy may be indicated in such problem cases.

The CT presentation of malignant lymphadenopathy may vary from (a) a small number of discrete enlarged lymph nodes to (b) a more conglomerate group of contiguous enlarged nodes similar in size to the aorta or inferior vena cava to (c) a large homogeneous mass, in which individual nodes are no longer recognizable, obscuring the contours of normal surrounding structures (Fig. 19). Massive enlargement of retroaortic and retrocaval nodes may cause anterior displacement of these vessels.

Because CT scanners are incapable of demonstrating intranodal architecture, lymph nodes that are normal in size but infiltrated with neoplastic cells cannot

19a,b

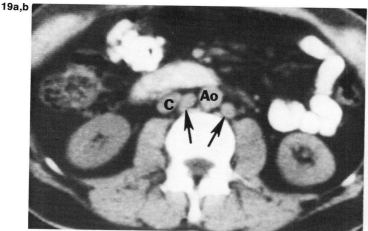
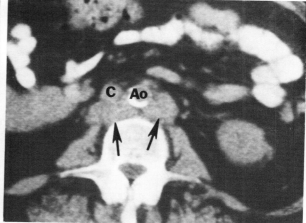

19c

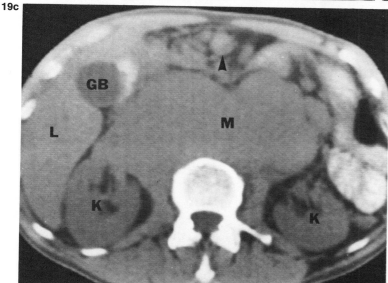

FIG. 19. Retroperitoneal lymphadenopathy in three different patients with lymphoma. **a:** Mild lymph node enlargement. Individual lymph nodes (arrows) are enlarged but their discrete outlines have been maintained. **b:** Moderate lymph node enlargement. Enlarged lymph nodes have coalesced to form a soft tissue mass (arrows), which is slightly larger than the adjacent aorta (Ao) and inferior vena cava (C). **c:** Massive lymph node enlargement is seen as a large, homogeneous soft tissue mass (M) resulting in total obscuration of the aorta and inferior vena cava. An enlarged mesenteric lymph node (arrowhead) is also present on this scan. GB, gallbladder; K, kidney; L, liver.

be distinguished as abnormal by CT. Furthermore, CT usually cannot differentiate between benign and malignant causes of lymph node enlargement. Diffuse lymph node enlargement secondary to viral or granulomatous disease cannot be differentiated from lymphoma based on CT findings alone (55), although the massive type of conglomeration described (Fig. 19c) almost never is seen with the benign conditions. Likewise, nodal enlargement secondary to metastatic disease can be virtually identical to that caused by lymphoma (Fig. 20). In one condition, Whipple's disease, a specific diagnosis may be possible. Although lymph node enlargement may occur, the attenuation value of the involved nodes often is quite low, ranging from +10 HU to +30 HU (59) (Fig. 21). This low density most likely is caused by the deposition of fat and fatty acids in the lymph nodes in this disease.

Other entities such as retroperitoneal fibrosis, perianeurysmal fibrosis, and false aortic aneurysm may also exhibit findings resembling malignant lymphadenopathy (1,11,82) (Figs. 22 and 23). Although

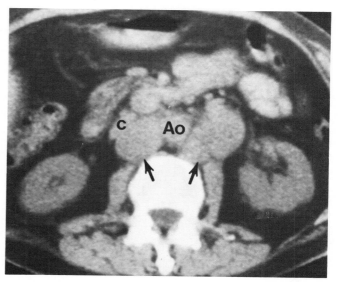

FIG. 20. Metastatic prostatic carcinoma. Enlarged paraaortic and paracaval lymph nodes (arrows) partially obscure the aorta (Ao) and inferior vena cava (c). This CT appearance is indistinguishable from lymphoma.

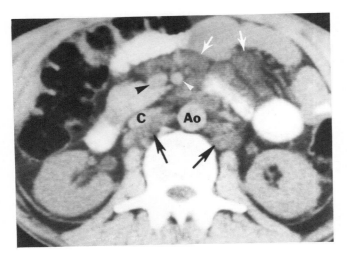

FIG. 21. Whipple's disease. Enlarged retroperitoneal (black arrows) and mesenteric lymph nodes (white arrows) are present. Note that the attenuation value of the lymph nodes is lower than that of adjacent vascular structures and psoas muscles. Ao, aorta; C, inferior vena cava; black arrowhead, superior mesenteric vein; white arrowhead, superior mesenteric artery.

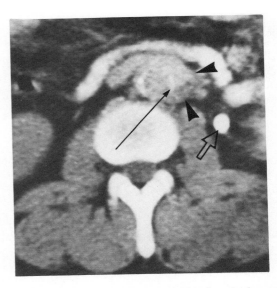

FIG. 22. Retroperitoneal fibrosis mimicking lymphadenopathy. Amorphous soft tissue densities (arrowheads) surround the aorta which can be identified by virtue of its calcified wall (long black arrow). This CT appearance is similar to those caused by malignant lymphadenopathy. The open arrow points to the dilated left ureter.

the inferior extent of the right crus of the diaphragm or vascular abnormalities (anomalies)—such as an enlarged gonadal vein (Fig. 8), a duplicated inferior vena cava, and a dilated azygous or hemiazygous vein—could conceivably be confused with an enlarged lymph node, scrutinizing of multiple contiguous scans and perhaps the concomitant use of intravenous iodinated contrast medium can separate these entities from lymphadenopathy.

Accuracy and Clinical Application

Lymphoma

The accuracy of CT in detecting intraabdominal and pelvic lymphadenopathy in patients with lymphoma has been studied by several groups of investigators since 1977. Results from these studies are generally influenced by the types of CT scanners used, expertise of the interpreters, and types of patients selected. The reported accuracy has ranged from 68 to 100%, with a false positive rate varying from 25 to 0% (2,6,7,10,26, 55,63,71,89). False positive cases are largely due to confusion with unopacified bowel loops or normal vascular structures, a problem that should be surmountable by rigorous attention to technique. False positive diagnosis also can be due to misinterpretation of lymphadenopathy secondary to benign inflammatory disease as malignant. False negative interpretations almost always are secondary to inability of recognizing replaced but normal-sized or minimally enlarged lymph nodes as abnormal. Although improvements in scanning techniques and equipment coupled with increasing experience in scan interpretation will undoubtedly result in higher diagnostic accuracy, lymph nodes that are involved with neoplastic disease but are of normal size will remain undetected by CT and account for most of the false negative interpretations.

Bipedal lymphangiography has been the technique employed in the past to investigate possible retroperitoneal lymph node abnormalities. However, the method is time-consuming, occasionally difficult to perform, and uncomfortable for the patient. In patients

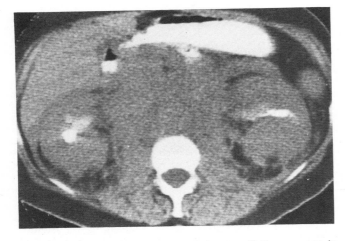

FIG. 23. Retroperitoneal fibrosis. A large soft tissue mass is present in the retroperitoneum resulting in total obscuration of the aorta and inferior vena cava. Also note the presence of mild hydronephrosis bilaterally. Streaky soft tissue densities posterior to both kidneys may be due to collateral vessels or previous renal inflammatory disease. This CT appearance is indistinguishable from that of malignant lymphadenopathy. Surgical biopsy yielded fibrosis.

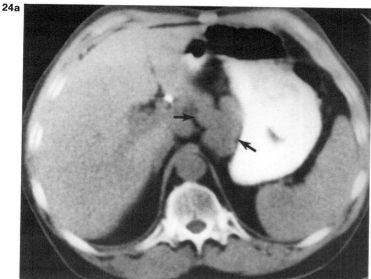

24a

24b,c

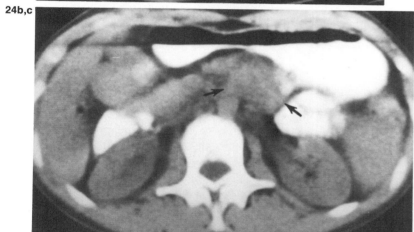
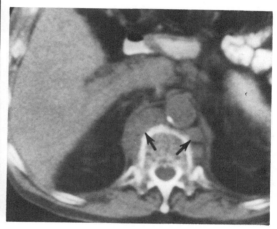

FIG. 24. Hodgkin's disease involving lymph nodes (arrows) in areas where lymphographic contrast medium does not reach. **a:** Left gastric. **b:** Celiac. **c:** Retrocrural. (Fig. 24c from Lee and Balfe, ref. 52, with permission.)

with chronic obstructive pulmonary disease, symptomatic radiation fibrosis, or congestive heart failure, lymphangiography may be medically contraindicated. The introduction of CT has provided a method for easy assessment of the retroperitoneal lymph nodes and for simultaneous evaluation of lymph nodes and organs elsehwhere in the abdomen. Efforts have been made by several investigators to compare the clinical efficacy of lymphangiography with that of CT. Although most investigators, including ourselves, found CT to have an accuracy comparable to lymphangiography in detecting retroperitoneal and pelvic lymph node involvement by lymphoma (6,7,26,30,89), others (15) showed lymphangiography to be a more accurate test. However, all groups found CT capable of detecting lymph nodes in areas where the lymphographic contrast medium does not reach, i.e., nodes around the celiac axis, retrocrural space, renal hilus, splenic and hepatic hila as well as in the mesentery (Figs. 24 and 25). Lymphomatous infiltration of various intraab-

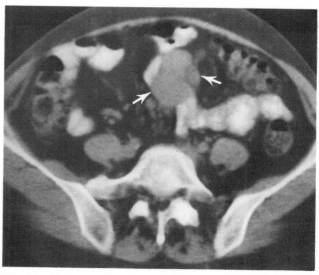

FIG. 25. Mesenteric lymphadenopathy (arrows) in non-Hodgkin's lymphoma. More cephalic scans revealed enlarged retrocrural and retroperitoneal lymph nodes. (From Lee and Balfe, ref. 52, with permission.)

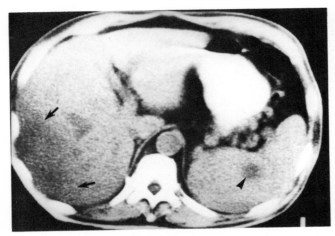

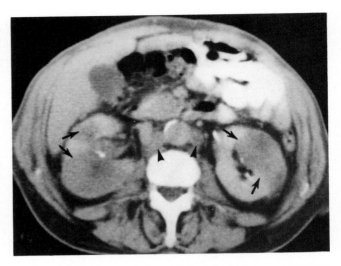

FIG. 26. Hepatic and splenic lymphoma. Low-density areas, due to Hodgkin's disease, are noted in the liver (arrows) and spleen (arrowhead). (From Lee and Balfe, ref. 52, with permission.)

FIG. 27. Renal involvement in histiocytic lymphoma. Postcontrast CT scan shows several low-density areas (arrows) in bilaterally enlarged kidneys. Mildly enlarged retroperitoneal lymph nodes (arrowheads) are also present.

dominal organs, such as the liver, the spleen, the kidneys, and the gastrointestinal tract, also have been seen on CT scans (Figs. 26–28). Such nodal and extranodal areas frequently are involved at presentation with the non-Hodgkin's lymphomas. Computed tomography clearly is superior to lymphangiography in delineating the exact extent of intraabdominal nodal involvement, usually because lymph nodes totally replaced by lymphoma are not opacified at all by lymphography.

There is nearly unanimous agreement (14,22,52) that CT should assume the primary radiologic role in staging patients with non-Hodgkin's lymphoma because of the tendency of these diseases to exhibit bulky lymphadenopathy in multiple sites and because of their high incidence of mesenteric lymph node involvement (greater than 50%). Lymphangiography need only be performed if the CT examination regarding the ret-

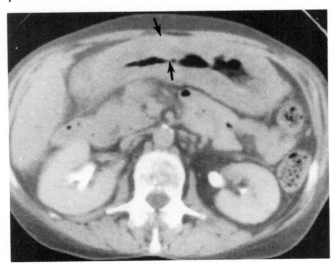

FIG. 28. Gastric lymphoma. Diffuse thickening of the gastric wall (arrows) is caused by histiocytic lymphoma. (From Lee and Balfe, ref. 52, with permission.)

roperitoneal lymph nodes is equivocal. In addition, other radiologic studies such as upper gastrointestinal series and barium enema are necessary only when specific symptoms of a patient suggest involvement of these organs.

However, controversy exists as to the proper role CT should play in the staging of Hodgkin's disease. Although some centers continue to use lymphangiography as a primary imaging method and use CT only as a complementary tool in abnormal cases, others including ourselves, have replaced lymphangiography with CT as the primary imaging method. A positive CT scan eliminates the need for a lymphangiogram. A negative CT scan can exclude nodal disease with a high degree of confidence. Lymphangiography certainly is valuable when the CT scans are equivocal and, following a negative CT scan, can be reassuring and on rare occasion may detect replaced but normal-sized lymph nodes. Staging laparotomy is still required for many patients at the time of initial presentation because of the inability of CT to detect microscopic disease in both lymph nodes and the spleen.

Our preference to use CT as a primary imaging method in the initial evaluation of patients with Hodgkin's disease is based on the following factors.

First, it has been suggested (44) that as many as 10% of involved lymph nodes in Hodgkin's disease are either of normal size or minimally enlarged and, therefore, will go undetected by CT scans. Because lymphangiography is capable of detecting alterations in intranodal architecture in a normal-sized lymph node, it is, therefore, assumed to be superior to CT in these areas. Review of the available data and our own experience indicates that such an occurrence is rare, certainly less than 1%. The ability to detect architec-

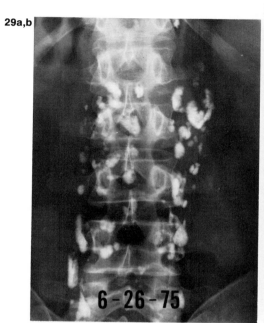

29a,b

6 - 26 - 75

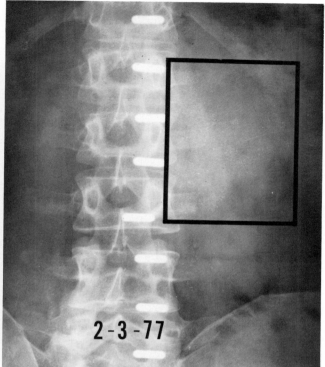

2 - 3 - 77

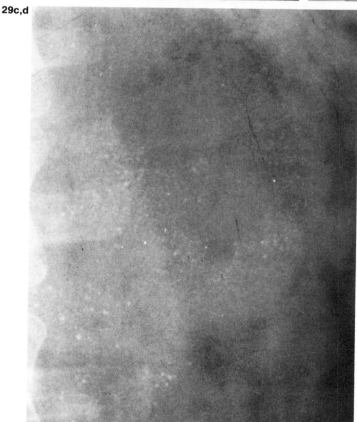

29c,d

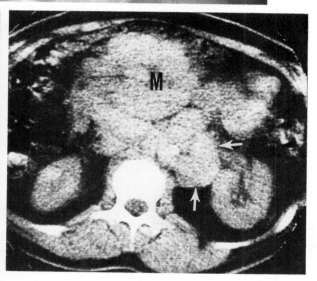

M

FIG. 29. Limitation of postlymphangiogram abdominal radiograph for long-term surveillence. **a:** The original lymphangiogram was normal in this patient with biopsy proven non-Hodgkin's lymphoma. **b:** A follow-up radiograph obtained 20 months later showed spreading of residual contrast material over a much larger area in the left upper quadrant. These changes are indicative of recurrent disease. The linear white lines overlying the spine were used as markers for obtaining CT scans in 1977, but are no longer necessary. **c:** A magnification view of the inset in (b) to better demonstrate the abnormality. **d:** A CT scan through the area of radiographic abnormality confirmed recurrent disease in the left paraaortic region (arrows). Massive mesenteric lymphadenopathy (M), unsuspected from the surveillance abdominal radiograph, is also demonstrated. The CT findings helped in planning of radiation ports in this patient.

tural alteration in normal-sized lymph nodes undoubt-edly increases the sensitivity of lymphangiography. However, this is achieved at the expense of the spec-ificity of the examination. Alterations in intranodal architecture by nonneoplastic processes cannot be re-liably differentiated from alterations caused by lymphomatous infiltration. The accuracy of a positive lymphangiogram in Hodgkin's disease is only 80%, even in the best hands (61). The theoretical advantage of lymphangiography, its ability to detect replaced but normal-sized lymph nodes, is further lessened by its inability to evelute lymph nodes in the higher abdomen at or above the level of the cisterna chyli. The un-opacified upper paraaortic and paracaval lymph nodes

are often affected first in patients who present with supradiaphragmatic disease (37).

Second, routine use of intraoperative abdominal radiographs to confirm removal of any suspicious lymph nodes shown on the preceding lymphangiogram has been proposed by some (44), but has not been a universally accepted practice. Planning of radiation ports based on information obtained from a lymphan-giogram should be replaced by CT since areas of ab-normality demonstrated on CT scans often exceed that on a lymphangiogram and the true three-dimensional cross-sectional format provided by CT is readily adapt-able for radiation therapy planning.

Third, the economical advantage of postlymphan-

30a,b

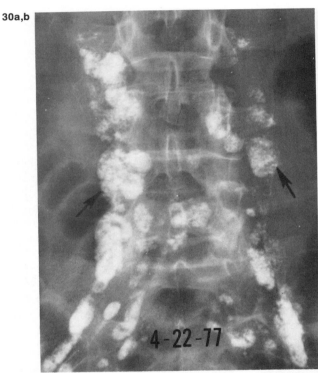
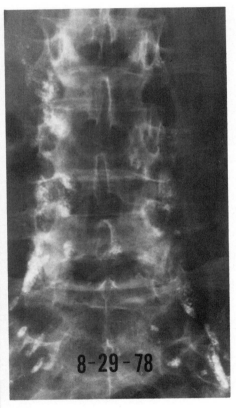

30c

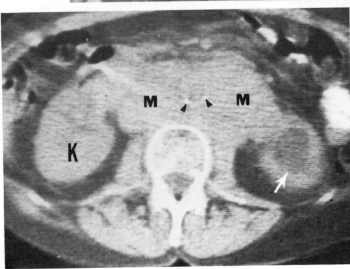

FIG. 30. Failure of a postlymphangiogram abdominal radiograph to detect recurrent disease. **a:** The initial lymphangiogram showed grossly abnormal paraaortic and paracaval lymph nodes (arrows) in this patient with biopsy proven non-Hodgkin's lymphoma. The patient was treated with chemotherapy and serial abdominal radio-graphs showed interval decrease in the size of opacified lymph nodes. **b:** A follow-up radiograph obtained 16 months later was interpreted as showing no evidence of recurrent disease. **c:** A CT examination obtained 2 days after the surveillance abdominal radiograph showed the unsuspected massive retroperitoneal lymphadenopathy (M) and left hydronephrosis (white arrow). The arrow-heads point to the calcified aortic wall, which is displaced anteriorly. K, kidney. (From Lee and Balfe, ref. 52, with permission.)

giogram abdominal radiographs as a means for following response to various forms of therapy is highly dependent on the frequency such radiographs are obtained. Although a surveillance abdominal radiograph is obtained every 2 to 4 weeks during the course of treatment in some centers, others (57) have found this practice of limited use. We have reported that a postlymphangiogram abdominal radiograph obtained 1 year after the initial study often contained inadequate residual contrast medium in the lymph nodes for accurate diagnosis. Since 50% of recurrence in Hodgkin's disease occurs more than 18 months after the initial treatment, postlymphangiogram abdominal radiographs are of limited use in long-term follow-up. Furthermore, even when there was apparently adequate residual contrast for diagnosis, the information on the surveillance radiograph was frequently misleading, resulting in underestimation of the amount of residual or recurrent disease or failure to detect any disease (Figs. 29 and 30).

Besides lymphangiography and CT, other noninvasive diagnostic tests (i.e., ultrasound and gallium scans) also have been reported to be of some value in the detection of abdominal lymphadenopathy. Ultrasound has been quite accurate in detecting retroperitoneal adenopathy (8); however, it is often difficult to obtain adequate scans of the lower abdomen because of bowel gas. In obese patients, examination of the retroperitoneal area by ultrasound also is difficult due to marked attenuation of the sound beam by the abundance of subcutaneous and mesenteric fat. The use of gallium-67 imaging in detecting intraabdominal nodal involvement by malignant lymphoma has been generally disappointing. In a large cooperative study (47), the true positive rate for detecting intraabdominal disease was 48%.

In addition to being used as an initial staging procedure, CT also has been used to follow response to various methods of treatment (Fig. 31). It should be emphasized that in patients with massive lymphadenopathy on the initial study, the follow-up scans may not always revert to normal even when patients are in complete clinical remission. Fibrotic changes secondary to prior radiation or chemotherapy may appear either as discrete, albeit smaller, soft tissue masses or as a thin sheath causing obscuration of the discrete outlines of the aorta and inferior vena cava (Fig. 32). Unfortunately, CT is incapable of differentiating between viable residual neoplasm and such fibrotic changes caused by chemo- or radiotherapy (78). Additional follow-up studies or surgical/percutaneous biopsy are often necessary for such a differentiation. Despite this limitation, CT provides a more accurate delineation of progression or regression of the disease process than any other radiologic procedure (53).

Testicular Tumors

Testicular neoplasms are the most common solid cancers in male patients 15 to 34 years old, accounting for 12% of all cancer deaths in this group. Histologically, the germ cell testicular tumors are composed of different cell types. For therapeutic purposes, they are classified into seminomatous and nonseminomatous categories. Although most seminomas are treated by radiation therapy, most nonseminomatous tumors (and some seminomas now) are treated by retroperitoneal lymphadenectomy or chemotherapy (16). Accurate preoperative determination of tumor extent helps in the design of radiation ports for seminomas and in the choice of initial mode of treatment (surgery versus chemotherapy) in the nonseminomatous group.

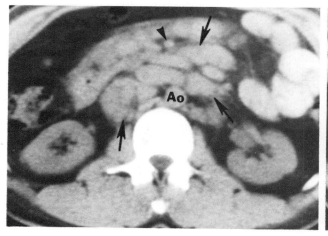 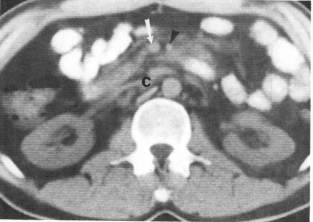

FIG. 31. Left: Initial CT scan in a patient with poorly differentiated lymphocytic lymphoma showed retroperitoneal and mesenteric lymphadenopathy (arrows). **Right:** A follow-up CT study after 6 courses of chemotherapy demonstrated near complete resolution of intraabdominal lymphadenopathy. Note that the inferior vena cava (C) and superior mesenteric vein (white arrow) can be much better appreciated on this examination. Ao, aorta; black arrowhead, superior mesenteric artery.

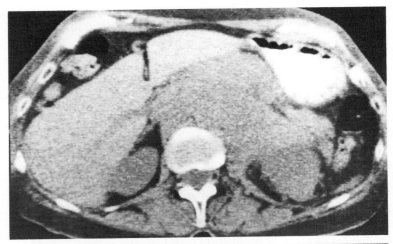

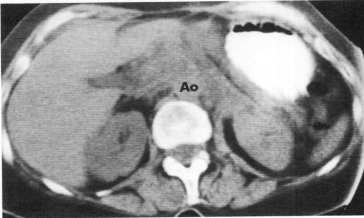

FIG. 32. Residual fibrosis following chemotherapy. **Above:** Initial scan in this patient with Hodgkin's disease shows massive retroperitoneal lymphadenopathy obscuring the aorta and inferior vena cava. Patient was started on chemotherapy and serial CT scans documented gradual improvement. **Below:** A follow-up study 2 years after the scan above demonstrates persistent residual soft tissue densities partially obscuring the aorta (Ao). Surgical biopsy of this area showed only residual fibrosis.

Testicular tumors tend to metastasize via the lymphatic system. A thorough understanding of the distribution and pattern of lymphatic spread by testicular cancer will be helpful in interpretation of CT findings. In general, the testicular lymphatics, which follow the course of the testicular arteries/veins, drain directly into the lymph nodes in or near the renal hilus (Fig. 33). These lymph nodes (sentinel nodes) lie lateral to the lumbar nodes and are usually not opacified by bipedal lymphangiography (17). After involvement of these sentinel nodes, the lumbar paraaortic nodes will become involved (unilaterally or bilaterally) followed by spread to the mediastinal and supraclavicular nodes or hematogenous dissemination to the lungs, liver, and brain.

Data from a large surgical series showed nodal metastases from the right testis tend to be midline, with primary zones of involvement being the interaortocaval, precaval, and preaortic lymph node groups (23) (Fig. 34). Although previous studies showed that the lymphatic drainage from the right testis not infrequently "crosses over" to the left side without involving the ipsilateral side, involvement of contralateral left paraaortic node(s) without concomitant involvement of

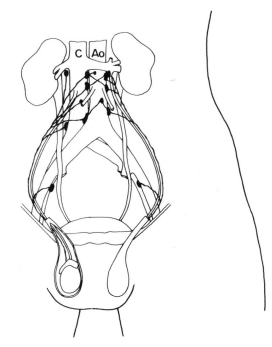

FIG. 33. A schematic diagram showing lymphatic drainage from the testis and epididymis. The testis primarily drains into lymph nodes at or below the level of renal hilum whereas the epididymis drains into the distal aortic or proximal iliac nodal group.

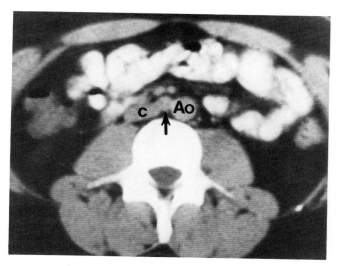

FIG. 34. Nodal metastases from embryonal cell carcinoma of right testis. CT scan below both kidneys shows a single 2 cm interaorto-caval lymph node (arrow). Metastases from the right testis have a predilection for this nodal chain. Ao, aorta; c, inferior vena cava.

interaortocaval nodes in patients with a right-sided testicular tumor was not found. If lymph nodes in the right renal hilar region are normal in size, then lymph nodes in the right suprahilar area are always uninvolved.

Nodal metastases from the left testis show a predilection for left paraaortic followed by preaortic and interaorto-caval nodal groups (Fig. 35). In contrast to right-sided testicular drainage, left suprahilar nodes have been found to be involved even when renal hilar nodal groups are grossly normal. However, the contralateral hilar nodes are always free of disease if the ipsilateral lymph nodes are not involved.

Although both testes have lymphatic channels to the ipsilateral external iliac nodes, isolated involvement of the external iliac, inguinal, and femoral nodes is most common when the primary drainage routes have been altered by previous inguinal surgery. Also, if the tumor locally involves the epididymis, spread may occur via lymphatic routes that normally drain the epididymis to the distal aortic or proximal common iliac group.

35a

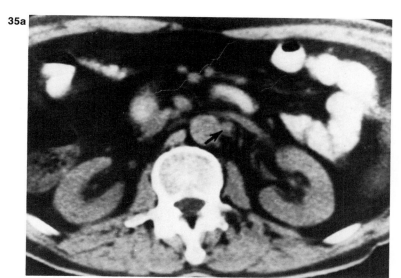

FIG. 35. Nodal metastases from embryonal cell carcinoma of left testis. Enlarged lymph nodes (arrows) are noted in the left paraaortic and interaorto-caval chain at several levels. **a:** CT scan through renal hilus. **b:** CT scan through lower pole of both kidneys. **c:** CT scan below both kidneys.

35b,c

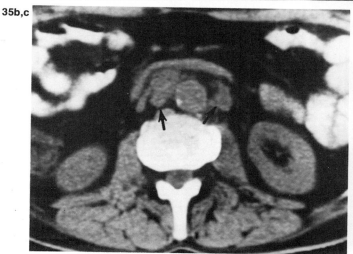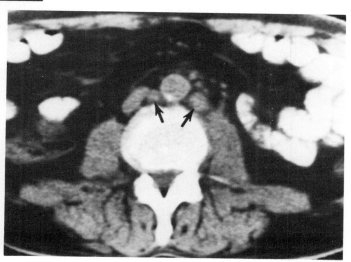

The overall accuracy achieved by CT examinations performed on early model scanners (scanning time 10–18 sec) compares very favorably with that of lymphangiography (12,25,28,54,58,74,83). The reported accuracy of CT is in the range of 70 to 90%. With recent improvements in CT equipment resulting in better spatial resolution and increased contrast sensitivity coupled with increasing experience in scan interpretation, the results from CT should be even better. Furthermore, because testicular tumors first metastasize to lymph nodes at the renal hilar level, a nodal group not normally opacified with bipedal lymphangiography, CT has a definite advantage in detecting early metastases to these lymph nodes. Similarly, CT is superior to lymphangiography in delineating the exact extent of the tumor mass, knowledge important in the planning of radiation therapy (Fig.

36). Computed tomography also can be used to detect metastases to extralymphatic organs such as the liver and the lung. Lymphangiography has a theoretical advantage over CT in detecting neoplastic replacement in normal-sized lymph nodes.

Although ultrasound has been found to be as accurate in detecting retroperitoneal testicular nodal metastases in some series (12), it is often difficult to obtain adequate scans of the lower abdomen because of bowel gas. In obese patients, examination of the retroperitoneal area by ultrasonography also is difficult due to marked attentuation of the sound beam by the abundance of subcutaneous and mesenteric fat.

Computed tomography is the preferred method in staging patients with known testicular neoplasms. Lymphangiography should be reserved for cases where the CT scans are equivocal or negative. Since

36a,b

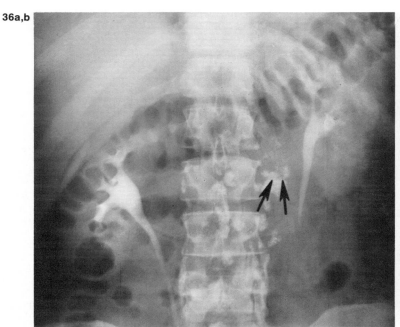

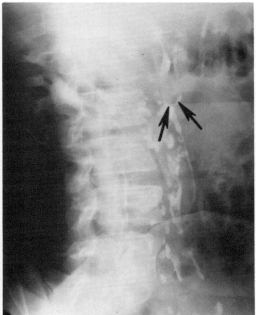

36c

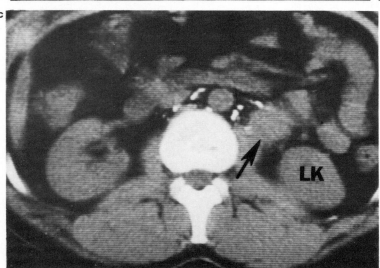

FIG. 36. Metastatic retroperitoneal lymphadenopathy in a patient with left testicular seminoma. Anteroposterior **(a)** and left posterior oblique **(b)** views of the abdomen from a bipedal lymphangiogram show a well-defined peripheral filling defect involving at least one left paraaortic lymph node (arrows) at the level of the second lumbar vertebra, compatible with nodal metastasis. **c:** CT scan demonstrates a large metastatic mass (arrow) not opacified by the preceding lymphangiogram. LK, left kidney.

over 90% of the nonseminomatous testicular tumors produce alpha-feto protein (AFP) or the beta subunit of human chorionic gonadotropin (β-HCG), serial determination of serum levels of these tumor markers is an extremely accurate method to follow therapeutic response and to detect possible recurrence (45,50). Computed tomography can be used to confirm the lesion anatomically when such markers become positive. Since the great majority of pure seminoma do not produce either HCG or AFP, CT has become the procedure of choice in following response to chemotherapy and radiation therapy in this group of patients (45, 54). As described previously, fibrotic changes secondary to prior radiation or chemotherapy cannot be differentiated from viable residual neoplasm (78) (Fig. 37). Additional follow-up studies or biopsy are often necessary for such a differentiation.

Other Metastatic Diseases

Nodal metastases from other primary tumors likewise can be detected on CT scans when the involved lymph nodes are enlarged. Because of its ability to evaluate the liver, adrenals, and abdominal lymph nodes simultaneously, CT has been used as part of an abdominal oncologic survey in patients with known malignancy, such as melanoma and colon carcinoma. Computed tomography is also used to document suspected recurrence or follow response to various treatments in these patients.

In contrast to lymphoma, nodal metastases from primary epithelial cancer of the genitourinary tract frequently cause replacement without enlarging the lymph node, a condition not discernible on CT scans (56). Furthermore, metastases to the pelvic lymph nodes

37a

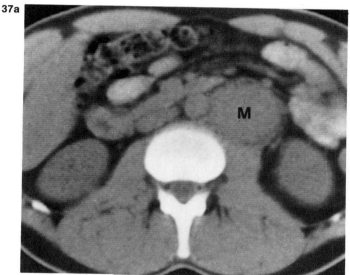

37b,c

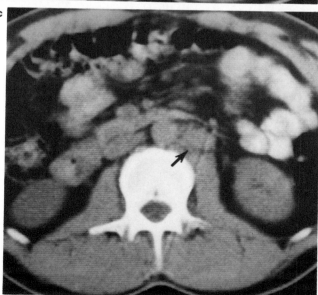

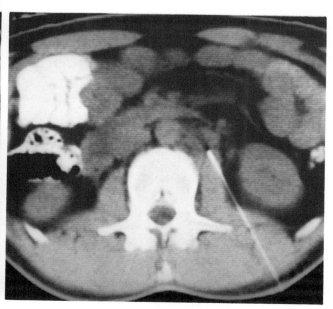

FIG. 37. Fibrotic changes following radiation therapy for metastatic seminoma. **a:** Initial CT scan shows markedly enlarged left paraaortic nodes (M). Following radiation therapy, serial scans (not shown) documented gradual regression of the disease. **b:** A follow-up study 14 months after (a) demonstrates residual soft tissue densities (arrow) at the site of original metastases. Differentiation between residual viable neoplasm and radiation fibrosis was considered impossible based on CT findings alone. **c:** Percutaneous needle biopsy of the mass under CT guidance (scan done prone) revealed fibrosis.

usually antedate involvement of retroperitoneal lymph nodes in these cases. The role of CT in primary epithelial carcinoma of the genitourinary tract will be covered in the chapter on the pelvis.

RETROPERITONEAL HEMORRHAGE

Retroperitoneal hemorrhage occurs most commonly in patients on anticoagulant therapy following trauma or as a complication of an aortic aneurysm or a retroperitoneal tumor. Bleeding into the retroperitoneal space has been reported to occur in a high percentage of patients following translumbar aortography (5,18) and percutaneous renal biopsy (72). It can also occur in patients with a bleeding diathesis or vasculitis (75).

Although acute onset of abdominal pain and development of an abdominal mass in association with a falling hematocrit are suggestive of retroperitoneal hemorrhage, clinical signs and symptoms may be ambiguous, delayed, or misleading. The diagnosis of retroperitoneal hemorrhage by plain abdominal radiographs lacks both sensitivity and specificity.

Computed tomography is an accurate noninvasive imaging method for detecting retroperitoneal hemorrhage (24,33,75). On CT scans, it appears as an abnormal soft tissue density, either well localized or diffusely enlarging the retroperitoneal space (75). Its location and attenuation characteristics depend on the source and duration of the hemorrhage.

Hemorrhage following renal biopsy is centered around the traumatized kidney, whereas those associated with a leaking abdominal aortic aneurysm (Fig. 5) or translumbar aortography will surround the aorta before extending into the surrounding retroperitoneum. An acute hematoma (approximately +70 HU) has a higher attenuation value than circulating blood because clot formation and retraction cause greater concentration of red blood cells. Progressive breakdown of red blood cells and removal of proteinaceous elements by the phagocytes result in lower attenuation levels within a chronic hematoma (+20 to +40 HU) (66).

The appearance of retroperitoneal hemorrhage on CT is by no means pathognomonic. An acute or a subacute hematoma can be confused with a retroperitoneal tumor; a chronic hematoma may have a similar appearance to an abscess, lymphocele, cyst, or urinoma. Differentiation among these entities often requires correlation with the patient's clinical history. The use of serial scanning, with decreasing size and attenuation value of the retroperitoneal mass, are reassuring signs that a diagnosis of hematoma is correct in cases where the clinical support is equivocal (21).

RETROPERITONEAL FIBROSIS

Retroperitoneal fibrosis, a disease process often insidious in its clinical presentation, is characterized pathologically by fibrous tissue proliferation along the posterior aspect of the retroperitoneal cavity causing displacement or encasement of blood vessels and ureters. Although most of the reported cases are idiopathic, certain drugs such as methysergide, primary or metastatic tumors, aneurysms, and aneurysm surgery have all been associated with similar pathologic alterations in the retroperitoneum (1,64,86). In cases where retroperitoneal fibrosis is associated with an aortic aneurysm, a heterogeneous population of leukocytes, i.e., polymorphonuclear leukocytes, lymphocytes, and plasma cells, can be found within the perianeurysmal tissues. Therefore, it has been suggested that perianeurysmal fibrosis may be the end result of an exaggerated inflammatory response to luminal thrombi or their breakdown products permeating the aortic wall (1). The lack of any hemosiderin-laden macrophages in the periaortic tissues negates the possibility of prior dissection or rupture (64).

The CT appearance of retroperitoneal fibrosis is quite variable. Although some have no detectable abnormality, others present as single or multiple soft tissue masses or as a sheath of soft tissue density with obscuration and displacement of the aorta and inferior vena cava (11,32) (Figs. 22 and 23). The latter two CT appearances are quite similar to those of primary retroperitoneal tumor or malignant lymphadenopathy (11,80). That enhancement of this fibrotic reaction may occur after intravenous contrast material administration has been emphasized (1,86).

PRIMARY RETROPERITONEAL TUMORS

Retroperitoneal tumors tend to be quite large when first suspected clinically because only when they reach such size are adjacent structures affected that produce symptoms (Fig. 38). The diagnosis of tumors arising from retroperitoneal tissues is readily accomplished with CT even when they are relatively small (80,81). Such neoplasms, usually sarcomas, appear on CT generally as soft tissue density masses that displace, compress, or obscure the normal retroperitoneal structures. Provided that some perivisceral fat is present, CT can accurately define the size, extent, and composition of the tumors as well as their effect on neighboring structures (Fig. 39). Adjacent organs may be invaded, but clear planes of separation cannot always be seen. Predictions as to definite invasion of normal structures, with implications toward surgical resectability, should be offered with caution.

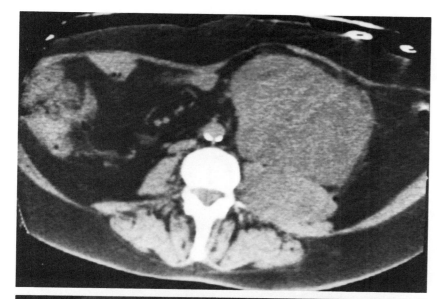

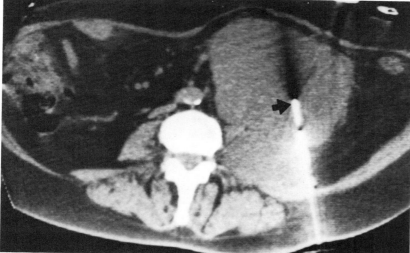

FIG. 38. Primary retroperitoneal sarcoma. **Above:** CT scan (done in the prone position) shows a large soft tissue mass extending from anterior abdominal wall to paraspinal area. Despite the tumor size, the patient had few symptoms. **Below:** Specimen from a percutaneous needle biopsy of the mass under CT guidance revealed undifferentiated sarcoma. Arrow points to the needle tip.

Although most solid retroperitoneal tumors have attenuation values similar to muscle tissue, a specific histologic diagnosis occasionally can be suggested based on unique CT findings. Lipomas appear as sharply marginated, homogeneous masses with CT densities equal to normal fat. A lymphangioma with high fat content can simulate a lipoma on CT scans (34).

With the exception of an exceedingly rare very well-differentiated liposarcoma, which is difficult to distinguish from a lipoma even at surgery and on pathologic examination, malignant liposarcomas can be distinguished from a benign lipoma by CT (34,87). Liposarcomas usually are inhomogeneous, poorly marginated, or infiltrative and have CT numbers greater than the patient's normal fat. They also may exhibit contrast enhancement. Three distinct CT patterns have been described in the literature (34). The solid pattern has CT numbers greater than +20 HU;

the mixed pattern has discrete fatty areas less than −20 HU and other areas greater than +20 HU; and a pseudocystic pattern has a homogeneous density between +20 HU and −20 HU. These CT patterns reflect the amount and distribution of fat within the liposarcomas. The well-differentiated liposarcoma with abundant mature fat generally still has a mixed pattern; poorly differentiated tumors with little fat are seen as the solid pattern and are indistinguishable on CT scans from other soft tissue density neoplasms. The pseudocystic pattern, near that of water, results from averaging of a homogeneous mixture of fat and solid connective tissue.

Tissue necrosis and cystic degeneration with areas of tumor approaching water in attenuation value are particularly common in leiomyosarcoma.

Computed tomography should be the procedure of choice in screening patients with suspected primary

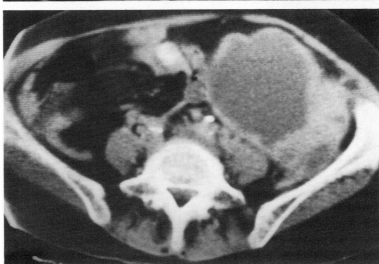

FIG. 39. Poorly differentiated retroperitoneal sarcoma. Postcontrast CT scans show a large irregular mass occupying almost the entire left side of the abdomen. The mass contains several areas of lower density compatible with necrosis. Note that the mass is closely associated with the aorta (Ao) and also has extended across midline to produce right hydronephrosis. The left kidney (LK) is displaced posteriorly. White arrowhead, dilated left ureter.

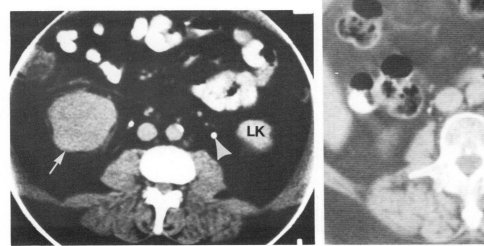

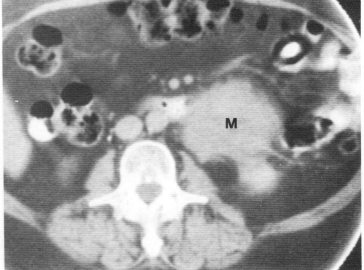

FIG. 40. Clarification of abnormal findings on conventional radiographs. Two patients were referred for CT because of lateral deviation of the lower pole of the left kidney and left ureter on excretory urography. **Left:** Abundant retroperitoneal fat accounts for abnormal urographic findings in this patient who has a carcinoma of the right kidney (arrow). LK, left kidney; white arrowhead, left ureter. **Right:** A large retroperitoneal soft tissue mass (M), subsequently shown to be due to a primary retroperitoneal leiomyosarcoma, is the explanation for renal and ureteral deviation.

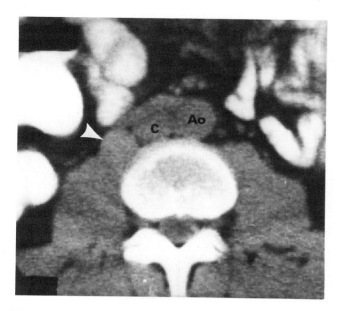

FIG. 41. The psoas minor muscle (arrowhead), prominent in some muscular individuals on CT, should not be confused with an enlarged lymph node. Ao, aorta; C, inferior vena cava.

retroperitoneal tumors either because of abnormal findings on physical examination or other radiologic studies (Fig. 40); its accuracy is exceedingly high, quite comparable to that in patients with retroperitoneal lymphoma or metastatic testicular cancer. In patients with known primary retroperitoneal tumors, CT can be used to assess response to treatment and to document possible recurrence.

PSOAS

Normal Anatomy

The psoas major, psoas minor, and iliacus muscles are a group of muscles that function as flexors of the thigh and trunk. The psoas major muscle originates from fibers arising from the transverse processes of the twelfth thoracic vertebra as well as all lumbar vertebrae. The muscle fibers fuse and pass inferiorly in a paraspinal location. As it exits from the pelvis, the psoas major assumes a more anterior location, merging with the iliacus to become the iliopsoas muscle. The iliopsoas passes beneath the inguinal ligament to insert on the lesser trochanter of the femur. At its superior attachment, the psoas muscle passes beneath the arcuate ligament of the diaphragm. The psoas muscle is in a fascial plane that directly extends from the mediastinum to the thigh.

The psoas minor is a long slender muscle, located immediately anterior to the psoas major. It arises from the sides of the bodies of the twelfth thoracic and first lumbar vertebrae and from the fibrocartilage between them. It ends in a long flat tendon, which inserts on the iliopectineal eminence of the innominate bone.

On CT scans, the normal psoas major muscles are delineated clearly in almost every patient as paired paraspinal structures. The proximal portion of the psoas muscle is triangular in shape, whereas the distal end has a more rounded appearance. The size of the psoas major muscle increases in a cephalo-caudad direction. When visible, especially in young muscular individuals, the psoas minor appears as a small, rounded, soft tissue mass anterior to the psoas major (Fig. 41). Caution must be taken not to confuse this muscle with an enlarged lymph node. The sympathetic trunk as well as the lumbar veins and arteries are sometimes seen as small soft tissue densities located just medial to the psoas muscles and lateral to the lumbar spine. However, differentiation between an artery, a vein, and a nerve in this location is not possible on noncontrast scans.

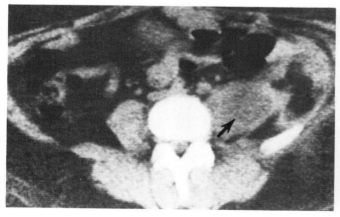

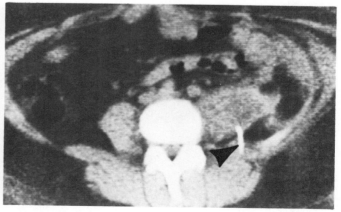

FIG. 42. Psoas abscess. Fifty-two-year-old woman with prior left nephrectomy presented with generalized malaise, low-grade fever, and leukocytosis. **Left:** The left psoas muscle was enlarged and contained several areas of lower density (arrow). Although no gas bubbles were seen within the muscle, a CT diagnosis of psoas abscess was made in view of clinical history. **Right:** After needle aspiration yielded pus, an 8.3 french pigtail catheter (arrowhead) with multiple side holes was inserted into the abscess cavity for drainage under CT guidance.

Pathologic Conditions

Inflammatory Lesions

Infection within the psoas muscle is commonly due to direct extension from contiguous structures such as the spine, kidney, bowel loops, and the pancreas. With the decreasing incidence of tuberculous involvement of the spine, the majority of psoas abscesses now encountered are of pyogenic origin. On CT scans, the involved psoas muscle is often diffusely enlarged, usually with central areas of lower density (0 to 30 HU) (46,65,70) (Fig. 42). The size and the extent of the abscess usually can easily be delineated; visualization of the abscess frequently can be improved on the scans by intravenous administration of urographic contrast material. Although uniform enlargement of a psoas muscle with areas of lower density is not specific for an inflammatory process, demonstration of gas bubbles within the psoas muscle is virtually pathognomonic of an abscess.

Other Conditions

The psoas muscle can be secondarily affected by other disease processes, including those originating in adjacent retroperitoneal structures. Although the psoas may be involved in spontaneous hemorrhage (Fig. 43), a hematoma in this muscle can also result from a leaking aortic aneurysm. As mentioned previously, the CT attenuation value of a hematoma varies from about +20 to +70 HU, depending on its age. A hematoma, abscess, or neoplasm, with or without central necrosis, all can have an identical CT appearance.

Lymphomas and other malignant retroperitoneal neoplasms can result in enlargement or obscuration of

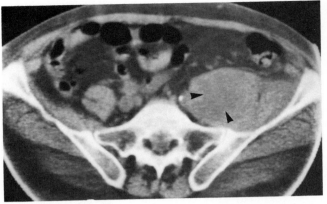

FIG. 44. Non-Hodgkin's lymphoma involving the left psoas muscle. CT scan from a patient with left back pain and fever demonstrates markedly enlarged left psoas muscle with areas of lower attenuation value (arrowheads). The CT findings are nonspecific and can be confused with hemorrhage or infection involving the psoas muscle. A definitive diagnosis was made by surgical biopsy.

the psoas muscle (Fig. 44). On occasion, it may be impossible to separate masses that invade the psoas from masses contiguous but without actual invasion of the psoas.

Besides infiltrative diseases, atrophy of the psoas muscle secondary to neuromuscular disorders can be similarly shown. A uniform decrease in the size of the muscle bulk on the involved side is seen (Fig. 45). On occasion, it also has a lower density due to partial fatty replacement of the muscle.

Accuracy and Clinical Application

The plain radiograph is neither sensitive nor specific in the assessment of disease processes involving the

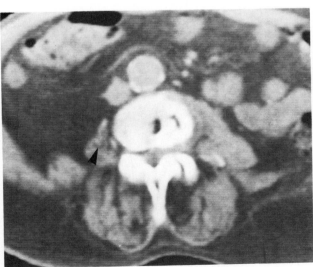

FIG. 45. Atrophy of the right psoas muscle in a patient with long-standing right hemiparesis. The right psoas muscle is not only smaller in size but also contains areas of lower attenuation value (arrowhead) consistent with partial fatty replacement. Air in the adjacent intervertebral disc space is also present.

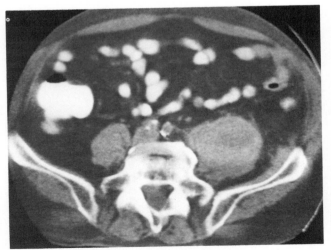

FIG. 43. Acute psoas hematoma secondary to anticoagulant therapy. The left psoas muscle is not only larger but also has a higher attenuation value than its counterpart on the right. Acute hematoma has higher attenuation value than normal muscles.

psoas muscle. Both psoas margins may be poorly visualized or not visualized in a substantial number of normal subjects (29). Furthermore, pathologic conditions involving the medial aspect of the psoas muscle cannot be initially identified on plain radiographs. Although ultrasound is also capable of demonstrating the normal and abnormal psoas muscle, this examination is often difficult or incomplete due to overlying bowel gas. In addition, sonography may be difficult to perform successfully in obese patients. It is the general consensus that CT should be the imaging method of choice in patients with real or suspected pathology involving the psoas muscles (65,70).

REFERENCES

1. Aiello MR, Cohen WM: Inflammatory aneurysm of the abdominal aorta. *J Comput Assist Tomogr* 4:265–267, 1980
2. Alcorn FS, Mategrano VC, Petasnick JP, Clark JW: Contributions of computed tomography in the staging and management of malignant lymphoma. *Radiology* 125:717–723, 1977
3. Axelbaum SP, Schellinger D, Gomes NM, Ferris RA, Hakkal HG: Computed tomographic evaluation of aortic aneurysms. *AJR* 127:75–78, 1976
4. Barnes PA, Bernardino ME, Thomas JL: Flow phenomenon mimicking thrombus: A possible pitfall of the pedal infusion technique. *J Comput Assist Tomogr* 6:304–306, 1982
5. Bergman AB, Neiman HL: Computed tomography in the detection of retroperitoneal hemorrhage after translumbar aortography. *AJR* 131:831–833, 1978
6. Best JJK, Blackledge G, Forbes WStC, Todd IDH, Eddleston B, Crowther D, Isherwood I: Computed tomography of abdomen in staging and clinical management of lymphoma. *Br Med J* 2:1675–1677, 1978
7. Blackledge G, Best JJK, Crowther D, Isherwood I: Computed tomography in the staging of patients with Hodgkin's disease: A report on 136 patients. *Clin Radiol* 31:143–148, 1980
8. Brascho DJ, Durant JR, Green LE: The accuracy of retroperitoneal ultrasonography in Hodgkin's disease and non-Hodgkin's lymphoma. *Radiology* 125:485–487, 1977
9. Breckenridge JW, Kinlaw WB: Azygos continuation of inferior vena cava: CT appearance. *J Comput Assist Tomogr* 4:392–397, 1980
10. Breiman RS, Castellino RA, Harell GS, Marshall WH, Glatstein E, Kaplan HS: CT-pathologic correlations in Hodgkin's disease and non-Hodgkin's lymphoma. *Radiology* 126:159–166, 1978
11. Brun B, Laursen K, Sorensen IN, Lorentzen JE, Kristensen JK: CT in retroperitoneal fibrosis. *AJR* 137:535–538, 1981
12. Burney BT, Klatte EC: Ultrasound and computed tomography of the abdomen in the staging and management of testicular carcinoma. *Radiology* 132:415–419, 1979
13. Callen PW, Korobkin M, Isherwood I: Computed tomographic evaluation of the retrocrural prevertebral space. *AJR* 129:907–910, 1977
14. Castellino RA, Marglin S, Blank N: Hodgkin disease, the non-Hodgkin lymphomas, and the leukemias in the retroperitoneum. *Semin Roentgenol* 15:288–301, 1980
15. Castellino RA, Noon M, Carroll BA, Hoppe RT, Young SW, Blank N, Marglin SI, Harell GS: Lymphography, computed tomography and ultrasound in staging Hodgkin's disease and non-Hodgkin's lymphoma. *Prog Lymphol* (in press)
16. Catalona WJ: Current management of testicular tumors. *Surg Clin North Am* (in press)
17. Chiappa S, Uslenghi C, Bonadonna G, et al: Combined testicular and foot lymphangiography in testicular carcinomas. *Surg Gynecol Obstet* 123:10–14, 1966
18. Chuang VP, Fried AM, Chen CQ: Computed tomographic evaluation of para-aortic hematoma following translumbar aortography. *Radiology* 130:711–712, 1979
19. Chuang VP, Mera CE, Hoskins PA: Congenital anomalies of the inferior vena cava. Review of embryogenesis and presentation of a simplified classification. *Br J Radiol* 47:206–213, 1974
20. Churchill RJ, Wesby G III, Marsan RE, Moncada R, Reynes CJ, Love L: Computed tomographic demonstration of anomalous inferior vena cava with azygous continuation. *J Comput Assist Tomogr* 4:398–402, 1980
21. Cisternino SJ, Neiman HL, Malave SR Jr: Diagnosis of retroperitoneal hemorrhage by serial computed tomography. *J Comput Assist Tomogr* 3:686–688, 1979
22. Crowther D, Blackledge G, Best JJK: The role of computed tomography of the abdomen in the diagnosis and staging of patients with lymphoma. *Clin Hematol* 83:567–591, 1979
23. Donohue JP, Zachary JM, Maynard B: Distribution of nodal metastases in non-seminomatous testis cancer. *J Urol* (in press)
24. Druy EM, Rubin BE: Computed tomography in the evaluation of abdominal trauma. *J Comput Assist Tomogr* 3:40–44, 1979
25. Dunnick NR, Javadpour N: Value of CT and lymphography: Distinguishing retroperitoneal metastases from non-seminomatous testicular tumors. *AJR* 136:1093–1099, 1981
26. Earl HM, Sutcliffe SBJ, Fry IK, Tucker AK, Young J, Husband J, Wrigley PFM, Malpas JS: Computerised tomography (CT) abdominal scanning in Hodgkin's disease. *Clin Radiol* 31:149–153, 1980
27. Egan TJ, Neiman HL, Herman RJ, Malave SR, Sanders JH: Computed tomography in the diagnosis of aortic aneurysm dissection or traumatic injury. *Radiology* 136:141–146, 1980
28. Ehrlichman RJ, Kaufman SL, Siegelman SS, Trump DL, Walsh PC: Computerized tomography and lymphangiography in staging testis tumors. *J Urol* 126:179–181, 1980
29. Elkin M, Cohen G: Diagnostic value of the psoas shadow. *Clin Radiol* 13:210–217, 1962
30. Ellert J, Kreel L: The role of computed tomography in the initial staging and subsequent management of the lymphomas. *J Comput Assist Tomogr* 4:368–391, 1980
31. Faer MJ, Lynch RD, Evans HO, Chin FK: Inferior vena cava duplication: Demonstration by computed tomography. *Radiology* 130:707–709, 1979
32. Fagan CJ, Larrieu AJ, Amparo EG: Retroperitoneal fibrosis: Ultrasound and CT features. *AJR* 133:239–243, 1979
33. Federle MP, Goldberg HI, Kaiser JA, Moss AA, Jeffrey RB, Mall JC: Evaluation of abdominal trauma by computed tomography. *Radiology* 138:637–644, 1981
34. Friedman AC, Hartman DS, Sherman J, Lautin EM, Goldman M: Computed tomography of abdominal fatty masses. *Radiology* 139:415–429, 1981
35. Gefter WB, Arger PH, Mulhern CB, Pollack HM, Wein AJ: Computed tomography of circumcaval ureter. *AJR* 131:1086–1087, 1978
36. Ginaldi S, Chuang VP, Wallace S: Absence of hepatic segment of the inferior vena cava with azygous continuation. *J Comput Assist Tomogr* 4:112–114, 1980
37. Glatstein E, Guernsey JM, Rosenberg SA, Kaplan HS: The value of laparotomy and splenectomy in the staging of Hodgkin's disease. *Cancer* 24:709–718, 1969
38. Gomes NM, Hufnagel CA: CT scanning: A new method for the diagnosis of abdominal aortic aneurysms. *J Cardiovasc Surg* 20:511–515, 1979
39. Goodwin JD, Herfkens RL, Skioldebrand CG, Federle MP, Lipton MJ: Evaluation of dissections and aneurysms of the thoracic aorta by conventional and dynamic CT scanning. *Radiology* 136:125–133, 1980
40. Gross SC, Barr I, Eyler WR, Khaja F, Goldstein S: Computed tomography in dissection of the thoracic aorta. *Radiology* 136:135–139, 1980
41. Haaga JR, Baldwin N, Reich NE, Beven E, Kramer A, Weinstein A, Havrilla TR, Seidelmann FE, Namba AH, Parrish CM: CT detection of infected synthetic grafts: Preliminary report of a new sign. *AJR* 131:317–320, 1978
42. Haaga J, Reich NE: Retroperitoneum. In: *Computed Tomography of Abdominal Abnormalities*, ed. by J Haaga and NE Reich, St. Louis, Mosby, 1978, pp 128–152
43. Haaga J, Reich NE: Aorta and vena cava. In: *Computed To-*

mography of Abdominal Abnormalities, ed. by J Haaga and NE Reich, St. Louis, Mosby, 1978, pp 153–176

44. Harell GS, Breiman RS, Glatstein EJ, Marshall WH, Castellino RA: Computed tomography of the abdomen in the malignant lymphomas. *Radiol Clin North Am* 15:391–400, 1977

45. Javadpour N, Doppman JL, Bergman SM, Anderson T: Correlation of computed tomography and serum tumor markers in metastatic retroperitoneal testicular tumor. *J Comput Assist Tomogr* 2:176–180, 1978

46. Jeffrey RB, Callen PW, Federle MP: Computed tomography of psoas abscesses. *J Comput Assist Tomogr* 4:639–641, 1980

47. Johnston GS, Go MF, Benna RS, Larson SM, Andrews GA, Hubner KF: Gallium-67 citrate imaging in Hodgkin's disease: Final report of cooperative group. *J Nucl Med* 18:692–698, 1977

48. Korobkin M, Callen PW, Fisch AE: Computed tomography of the pelvis and retroperitoneum. *Radiol Clin North Am* 17:301–318, 1979

49. Kreel L: The EMI whole body scanner in the demonstration of lymph node enlargement. *Clin Radiol* 27:421–429, 1976

50. Lange PH, Fraley EE: Serum alpha-fetoprotein and human chorionic gonadotropin in the treatment of patients with testicular tumors. *Urol Clin North Am* 4:383–406, 1977

51. Larde D, Belloir C, Vasile N, Frija J, Ferrane J: Computed tomography of aortic dissection. *Radiology* 136:147–151, 1980

52. Lee JKT, Balfe DM: Computed tomographic evaluation of lymphoma patients. *CRC Crit Rev Diagn Imaging* (*in press*)

53. Lee JKT, Levitt RG, Stanley RJ, Sagel SS: Utility of body computed tomography in the clinical follow-up of abdominal masses. *J Comput Assist Tomogr* 2:607–611, 1978

54. Lee JKT, McClennan BL, Stanley RJ, Sagel SS: Computed tomography in the staging of testicular neoplasms. *Radiology* 130:387–390, 1978

55. Lee JKT, Stanley RJ, Sagel SS, Levitt RG: Accuracy of computed tomography in detecting intraabdominal and pelvic adenopathy in lymphoma. *AJR* 131:311–315, 1978

56. Lee JKT, Stanley RJ, Sagel SS, McClennan BL: Accuracy of CT in detecting intraabdominal and pelvic lymph node metastases from pelvic cancers. *AJR* 131:675–679, 1978

57. Lee JKT, Stanley RJ, Sagel SS, Melson GL, Koehler RE: Limitations of the post-lymphangiogram plain abdominal radiograph as an indicator of recurrent lymphoma: Comparison to computed tomography. *Radiology* 134:155–158, 1980

58. Lein HH, Kolbenstvedt A, Kolmannskog F, Liverud K, Aakhus T: Computer tomography, lymphography, and phlebography in metastases from testicular tumors. *Acta Radiol [Diagn] (Stockh)* 21:505–512, 1980

59. Li DKB, Rennie CS; Abdominal computed tomography in Whipple's disease. *J Comput Assist Tomogr* 5:249–252, 1981

60. Machida K, Tasaka A: CT patterns of mural thrombus in aortic aneurysms. *J Comput Assist Tomogr* 4:840–842, 1980

61. Marglin S, Castellino R: Lymphographic accuracy in 632 consecutive, previously untreated cases of Hodgkin disease and non-Hodgkin lymphoma. *Radiology* 140:351–353, 1981

62. Marks WM, Korobkin M, Callen PW, Kaiser JA: CT diagnosis of tumor thrombosis of the renal vein and inferior vena cava. *AJR* 131:843–846, 1978

63. Marshall WH, Breiman RS, Harell GS, Glatstein E, Kaplan HS: Computed tomography of abdominal paraaortic lymph node disease: Preliminary observations with a 6 second scanner. *AJR* 128:759–764, 1977

64. Megibow AJ, Ambos MA, Bosniak MA: Computed tomographic diagnosis of ureteral obstruction secondary to aneurysmal disease. *Urol Radiol* 1:211–215, 1980

65. Mendez G, Isikoff MB, Hill MC: Retroperitoneal processes involving the psoas demonstrated by computed tomography. *J Comput Assist Tomogr* 4:78–82, 1980

66. New PFJ, Aronow S: Attenuation measurements of whole blood and blood fractions in computed tomography. *Radiology* 121:635–640, 1976

67. Pagani JJ, Thomas JL, Bernardino ME: Computed tomographic manifestations of abdominal and pelvic venous collaterals. *Radiology* 142:415–419, 1982

68. Perrett LV, Sage MR: Computed tomography of abdominal aortic aneurysms. *J Surg* 48:275–277, 1978

69. Pripstein S, Cavoto FV, Gerritsen RW: Spontaneous mycotic aneurysm of the abdominal aorta. *J Comput Assist Tomogr* 3:681–683, 1979

70. Ralls PW, Boswell W, Henderson R, Rogers W, Boger D, Halls J: CT of inflammatory disease of the psoas muscle. *AJR* 134:767–770, 1980

71. Redman HC, Glatstein E, Castellino RA, Federal WA: Computed tomography as an adjunct in the staging of Hodgkin's disease and non-Hodgkin's lymphomas. *Radiology* 124:381–385, 1977

72. Rosenbaum R, Hoffsten PE, Stanley RJ, Klahr S: Use of computerized tomography to diagnose complications of percutaneous renal biopsy. *Kidney Int* 14:87–92, 1978

73. Royal SA, Callen PW: CT evaluation of anomalies of the inferior vena cava and left renal vein. *AJR* 132:759–763, 1979

74. Safer ML, Green JP, Crews QE Jr, Hill DR: Lymphangiographic accuracy in the staging of testicular tumors. *Cancer* 35:1603–1605, 1975

75. Sagel SS, Siegel MJ, Stanley RJ, Jost RG: Detection of retroperitoneal hemorrhage by computed tomography. *AJR* 129:403–407, 1977

76. Schaner EG, Head GL, Doppman JL, Young RC: Computed tomography in the diagnosis, staging, and management of abdominal lymphoma. *J Comput Assist Tomogr* 1:176–180, 1977

77. Shaffer PB, Johnson JC, Bryan D, Fabri PJ: Diagnosis of ovarian vein thrombophlebitis by computed tomography. *J Comput Assist Tomogr* 5:436–439, 1981

78. Soo CS, Bernardino ME, Chuang VP, Ordonez N: Pitfalls of CT findings in post-therapy testicular carcinoma. *J Comput Assist Tomogr* 5:39–41, 1981

79. Steele JR, Sones PJ, Heffner LT Jr: The detection of inferior vena cava thrombosis with computed tomography. *Radiology* 128:385–386, 1978

80. Stephens DH, Sheedy PF, Hattery RR, Williams B: Diagnosis and evaluation of retroperitoneal tumors by computed tomography. *AJR* 129:395–402, 1977

81. Stephens DH, Williamson B Jr, Sheedy PF II, Hattery RR, Miller WE: Computed tomography of the retroperitoneal space. *Radiol Clin North Am* 15:377–390, 1977

82. Sterzer SK, Herr HW, Mintz I: Idiopathic retroperitoneal fibrosis misinterpreted as lymphoma by computed tomography. *J Urol* 122:405–406, 1979

83. Thomas JL, Bernardino ME, Bracken RB: Staging of testicular carcinoma: Comparison of CT and lymphangiography. *AJR* 137:991–996, 1981

84. Turner RJ, Young SW, Castellino RA: Dynamic continuous computed tomography: Study of retroaortic left renal vein. *J Comput Assist Tomogr* 4:109–111, 1980

85. VanBreda A, Rubin BE, Druy EM: Detection of inferior vena cava abnormalities by computed tomography. *J Comput Assist Tomogr* 3:164–169, 1979

86. Vint VC, Usselman JA, Warmath MA, Dilley RB: Aortic perianeurysmal fibrosis: CT density enhancement and ureteral obstruction. *AJR* 134:577–580, 1980

87. Waligore MP, Stephens DH, Soule EH, McLeod RA: Lipomatous tumors of the abdominal cavity: CT appearance and pathologic conditions. *AJR* 137:539–545, 1981.

88. Weyman PJ, McClennan BL, Stanley RJ, Levitt RG, Sagel SS: Comparison of computed tomography and angiography in the evaluation of renal cell carcinoma. *Radiology* 137:417–424, 1980

89. Zelch MG, Haaga JR: Clinical comparison of computed tomography and lymphangiography for detection of retroperitoneal lymphadenopathy. *Radiol Clin North Am* 17:157–168, 1979

Chapter 11

Abdominal Wall and Peritoneal Cavity

Robert G. Levitt

ABDOMINAL WALL

Normal Anatomy

The anterior abdominal wall is composed of several layers: skin, superficial fascia, subcutaneous fat, anterolateral and midline (rectus) muscle groups, transversalis fascia, extraperitoneal fat, and peritoneum. In the average adult with sufficient body fat, the subcutaneous fat layer and individual muscles can be identified on CT scans (Fig. 1) (11). The aponeuroses of the three anterolateral muscles (external oblique, internal oblique, and transversus) unite at the lateral border of the rectus muscle to form the Spigelian fascia, which splits to become the anterior and posterior rectus sheaths. The paired rectus muscles are joined in the midline by the junction of these fascial sheaths to form the linea alba, which is 4 to 6 mm in width. At the level of the anterior superior iliac spine, an inguinal

canal is formed, which extends to the pubic tubercle. The anterior wall of the canal is the aponeurosis of the external oblique muscle and the posterior wall is the transversalis fascia (Fig. 2) (10).

Pathologic Conditions

Hernias

Although the diagnosis of hernia almost always can be established clinically, CT may be useful in specific instances in differentiating a hernia from a mass within the abdominal cavity. Herniation of intraperitoneal fat and bowel through fascial defects in the abdominal wall is easily identifiable on CT scans. A ventral hernia is produced when the linea alba is disrupted and fat and bowel herniate anteriorly through the defect and sometimes laterally over the rectus sheath (Fig. 3). Weaknesses in the internal oblique and transversus aponeuroses of the Spigelian fascia allow peritoneal contents to herniate beneath an intact external oblique muscle, producing a Spigelian hernia.

When peritoneal contents herniate through the entrance (deep inguinal ring) to the inguinal canal, an in-

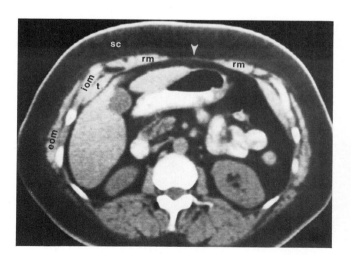

FIG. 1. Normal anatomy of the anterior abdominal wall. The subcutaneous fat layer and individual muscles of the anterolateral muscle group are identified. The paired rectus muscles are joined in the midline by the linea alba (arrowhead), which is attenuated in this obese patient. sc, subcutaneous fat layer; eom, external oblique muscle; iom, internal oblique muscle; t, transversus muscle; rm, rectus muscle.

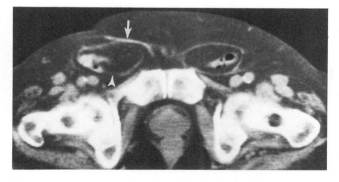

FIG. 2. Inguinal hernia. Bowel opacified with oral contrast material has herniated into both inguinal canals. The aponeurosis of external oblique muscle (arrow) and the aponeurosis of the transversus muscle (arrowhead) form the anterior and posterior walls of the canal, respectively.

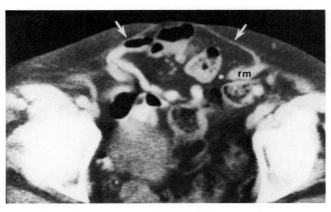

FIG. 3. Ventral hernia. Intraperitoneal fat and bowel herniate anteriorly through a fascial defect in the linea alba (arrows) to produce a ventral hernia. rm, rectus muscle.

guinal hernia results (Fig. 2). A femoral hernia develops when contents protrude lateral to the inguinal canal between the external oblique muscle insertion on the superior pubic ramus and the superior ramus itself adjacent to the femoral artery and vein (10).

Hematoma

An anterior abdominal wall hematoma most often occurs secondary to anticoagulant therapy. The diagnosis is clinically suspected because of abdominal wall pain, a palpable mass, discoloration of the anterior abdominal wall, or a falling hematocrit. Computed tomography may be performed for corroboration of the diagnosis, to assess the extent of hematoma, and to determine if a concomitant intra-abdominal or retroperitoneal hematoma also is present.

The CT appearance of such a hematoma is that of an abnormal mass, often elliptical in shape, within one or more layers of the anterior abdominal wall, enlarging, obliterating, or displacing normal structures. The hematoma may remain localized or may dissect along fascial planes laterally and inferiorly. An acute abdominal wall hematoma has a density equal to or

greater than the soft-tissue density of the abdominal muscles (Fig. 4), due to the high protein content of hemoglobin. As the hematoma matures, the progressive breakdown and removal of protein within red blood cells reduces the hematoma's attenuation value (29). By about 4 weeks after the initial bleeding episode, the density of the hematoma may approach that of serum. A fibroblastic and vascular membrane grows around the hematoma and, on occasion, part of a chronic hematoma, especially its periphery, may calcify (Fig. 5).

Inflammation/Infection

Inflammation within the anterior abdominal wall, usually secondary to surgery, trauma, or altered host defense (e.g., diabetes), produces several nonspecific findings on CT scans. Streaky soft-tissue densities, localized masses of varying density, and masses that dissect along fascial planes may all be seen.

An anterior abdominal wall abscess usually presents as an abnormal mass, most frequently with a lower density central zone. The peripheral zone or wall of the abscess may enhance after intravenous iodinated contrast material administration. Gas within the mass may be formed by gas-producing organisms (Figs. 6 and 7). Although gas production allows a specific CT diagnosis of abscess, it is seen in a minority of patients with abdominal wall abscess. Needle aspiration may be necessary to confirm the diagnosis of abscess when only an abnormal mass is identified in the clinical setting of possible infection or inflammation. In addition, gas in a partially open abdominal wall wound or gas in a fistula connecting bowel to the skin surface may simulate the appearance of a gas-containing abscess.

Neoplasm

Primary neoplasms, both benign and malignant, as well as secondary metastases, can occur within the abdominal wall. These tumors are generally discov-

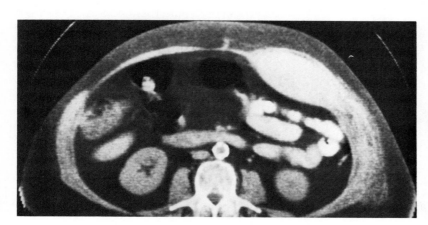

FIG. 4. Acute abdominal wall hematoma. Relatively high attenuation value elliptical mass enlarges left rectus muscle and dissects laterally along fascial planes.

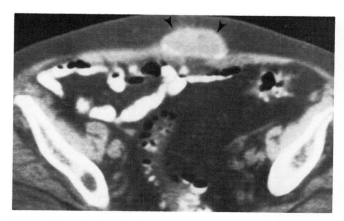

FIG. 5. Organized abdominal wall hematoma (arrowheads) with peripheral calcification.

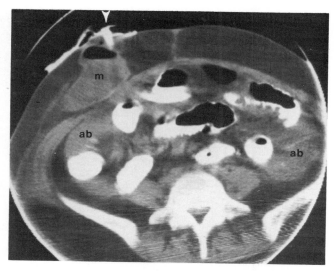

FIG. 7. Abdominal wall abscess. Mass (m) containing air-fluid level in anterior abdominal wall at ileostomy site (arrowhead) in patient with ulcerative colitis and postoperative fever. Lack of surrounding inflammatory changes may be due to concomitant steroid therapy. Prior to CT, the mass was thought clinically to represent a hernia at the ileostomy site. Several interloop abscesses (ab) are also noted within peritoneal cavity.

ered by inspection and palpation. However, small tumors or tumors in obese patients may be overlooked and discovered incidentally by CT. Computed tomography may also be valuable in defining the extent of palpable lesions for the purpose of placing radiotherapy ports and assessing the effectiveness of chemotherapy. Recurrence after surgical excision may be identified (9).

Abdominal wall tumors typically appear as soft-tissue density nodules or masses (Fig. 8). Desmoids are benign neoplasms consisting of accumulations of fibrous tissue, which commonly originate within the rectus sheath in parous women. These tumors can also involve the mesentery and may be very difficult to excise completely surgically (4). Sarcomas are the most common of the primary malignancies involving the abdominal wall, followed by lymphomas (Fig. 9).

Hematogenously borne metastases may seed the abdominal wall; sometimes the abdominal wall becomes involved with secondary neoplasm by direct spread from other metastatic sites. An "omental cake" produced by metastatic carcinoma, most typically of ovarian origin, may grow directly into the abdominal wall and can involve the umbilicus (Figs. 10–12). Differentiation of abdominal wall neoplasm from abscess or hematoma may not be possible using CT criteria alone and clinical correlation is mandatory.

PERITONEAL CAVITY

Normal Anatomy

The walls of the peritoneal cavity, as well as abdominal and pelvic organs contained within, are lined with peritoneum, an areolar membrane covered by a single row of mesothelial cells. Folds of peritoneum connect structures within this cavity (Fig. 13). A fold connecting the stomach to another structure is called an omentum; the lesser omentum joins the stomach to the liver, whereas the greater omentum joins the stomach to the transverse colon (gastrocolic segment) and then passes downward in front of the small bowel. A mesentery is a layer of peritoneum that connects the small bowel (small bowel mesentery) or transverse colon (transverse mesocolon) to the posterior abdominal wall (14). Normally, these peritoneal folds are not directly imaged by CT, but fat, lymph nodes, and vessels contained within them can be identified. However, when

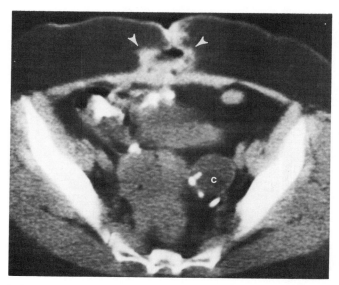

FIG. 6. Anterior abdominal wall abscess. Mass containing air-fluid level (arrowheads) present within previous incisional site. Cystic left ovarian mass (c) incidentally noted.

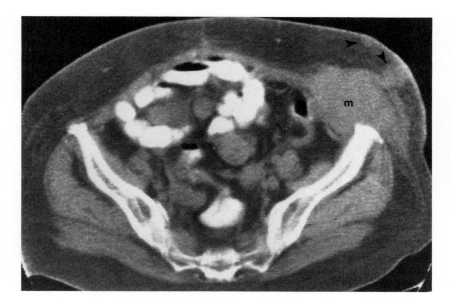

FIG. 8. Abdominal wall metastases from ovarian carcinoma. A palpable left lower quadrant mass (m) is identified to be within the abdominal wall rather than intraperitoneal in location. Additional unsuspected small subcutaneous metastases (arrowheads) are seen.

peritoneal folds become thickened by transudative ascites, inflammatory exudate, or neoplasm, they do become outlined (Fig. 14).

The transverse mesocolon divides the abdominal cavity into supra- and infra-mesocolic compartments (Fig. 15). The infra-mesocolic compartment is further subdivided into spaces of unequal size by the obliquely oriented root of the small bowel mesentery. A smaller right infracolic space is bounded inferiorly by the junction of the small bowel mesentery and ascending colon, whereas a larger left infracolic space is open toward the pelvis except where bounded by the sigmoid mesocolon. The pelvis, which is the most dependent part of the peritoneal cavity in both the erect and supine positions, also has compartments: the midline

cul-de-sac or pouch of Douglas (rectovaginal pouch in a woman and rectovesical pouch in a man) and the lateral paravesical recesses. These compartments are continuous with both paracolic gutters, the peritoneal recesses lateral to the ascending and descending colon (26).

The natural flow of intraperitoneal fluid is directed by gravity and variations in intra-abdominal pressure due to respiration along pathways determined by this compartmentalization. Understanding the course of flow facilitates CT identification and localization of intraperitoneal abscesses and metastases. An abscess usually forms and a mesenteric metastasis usually

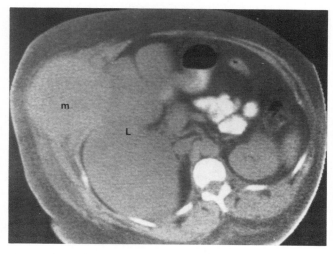

FIG. 9. Abdominal wall lymphoma. Mass (m) within anterior abdominal wall distorts anterolateral muscle group and extends along fascial planes. The liver (L) is extrinsically compressed.

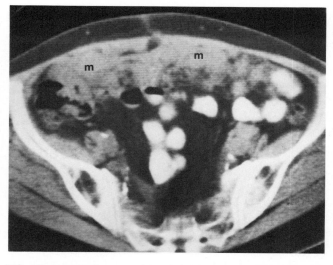

FIG. 10. Neoplastic spread to abdominal wall from omentum. Soft tissue density omental mass (m) due to metastatic ovarian carcinoma grows directly into anterior abdominal wall, obliterating the normal fat plane in this area and displacing bowel posteriorly.

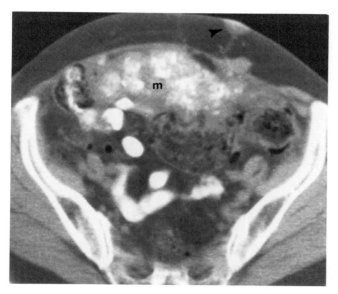

FIG. 11. Involvement of abdominal wall by neoplasm. Calcified "omental cake" (m) due to metastatic ovarian carcinoma separates bowel from the abdominal wall and grows into an incisional scar (arrowhead).

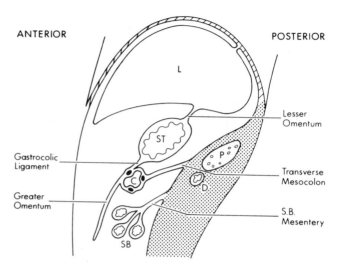

FIG. 13. Folds of peritoneum connect structures within the peritoneal cavity. L, liver; ST, stomach; SB, small bowel; P, pancreas.

grows in those sites where natural flow permits infected fluid or malignant ascites to pool.

Intraperitoneal fluid in the infra-mesocolic compartment migrates into the pelvis (Fig. 15). Fluid in the left infracolic space flows down alongside the rectum, but is frequently arrested by the sigmoid mesocolon before it descends into the pelvis. In the right infracolic space, flow is directed from recesses in the small bowel mesentery to the region of the ileocecal junction, where the root of the small bowel mesentery joins the ileum (Fig. 14). A pool of fluid forms at the mesenteric root with subsequent overflowing into the

pouch of Douglas and lateral paravesical recesses (Fig. 16). Once fluid has reached the pelvis, it can move upward in the paracolic gutters with changes in abdominal pressure during respiration. The major flow is along the right paracolic gutter into the right subhepatic and/or subphrenic space. Spread of fluid across the midline to the left subphrenic space is prevented by the coronary and falciform ligaments of the liver. Flow up the left paracolic gutter is slow and weak and its cephalad extension is usually limited by the left phrenicocolic ligament (26). Because an abscess develops where infected intraperitoneal fluid pools—the pelvis, right subhepatic space, and right subphrenic

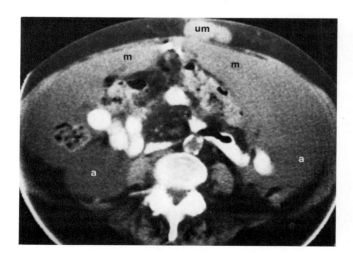

FIG. 12. Spread of metastatic neoplasm to abdominal wall. Metastatic appendiceal carcinoma (m) involving the omentum and periumbilical region (um). Ascites (a) also present.

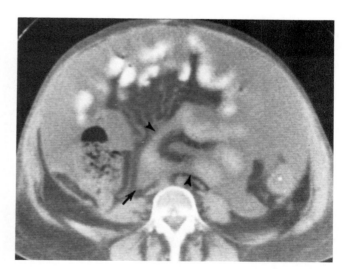

FIG. 14. Small bowel mesentery outlined by ascites. Ascites thickens the mesenteric leaves (arrowheads) and helps to identify the insertion of mesenteric root (arrow) near the ileocecal junction.

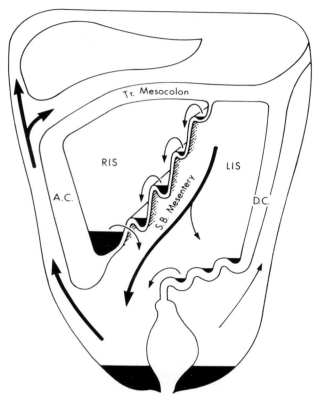

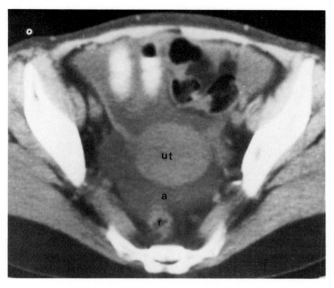

FIG. 16. Ascites in pouch of Douglas. The uterus (ut) is surrounded by ascites (a), filling the cul-de-sac. r, rectum.

FIG. 15. Compartmentalization of the peritoneal cavity. Peritoneal reflections divide the peritoneal cavity into several spaces. RIS, right infracolic space; LIS, left infracolic space; A.C., ascending colon; D.C., descending colon.

Pathologic Conditions

Intraperitoneal Abscess

space—are the most common sites (24). Similarly, the most common sites for pooling of malignant ascites and subsequent fixation and growth of mesenteric metastases are the pouch of Douglas, the lower small bowel mesentery near the ileocecal junction, the sigmoid mesocolon, and the right paracolic gutter (26).

A few decades ago, an abdominal abscess was usually the result of intraperitoneal spread from a perforated appendix, peptic ulcer, diverticulitis, or cholecystitis. Today such a complication most often results from surgery in the upper abdomen. Biliary, gastric, or duodenal surgery and resection of the right colon for carcinoma are common causes for right subphrenic and right subhepatic abscesses (24). Left subphrenic abscesses usually develop after breakdown of surgical anastomoses, or following gastric operations and splenectomies (15). Pelvic abscesses may occur

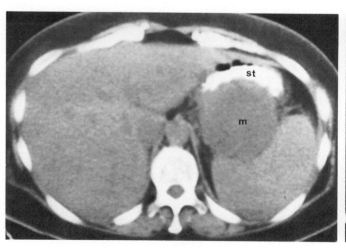

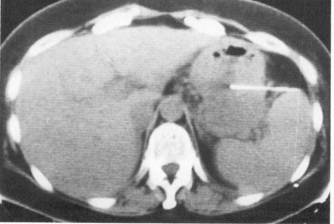

FIG. 17. Left subphrenic abscess. **Left:** Mass (m), slightly lower in attenuation value than the spleen, displaces the contrast material-filled stomach (st) anteriorly. **Right:** Diagnosis of abscess established by percutaneous needle aspiration.

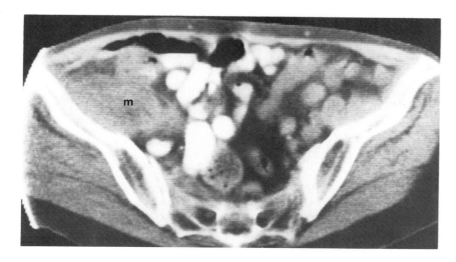

FIG. 18. Appendiceal abscess. Soft-tissue density mass (m) in right side of pelvis displaces contrast material-filled bowel loops medially and obscures the right iliopsoas muscle.

following pelvic surgery, or as a sequela of generalized peritonitis, appendicitis, or pelvic inflammatory disease (e.g., tubo-ovarian abscess). Secondary infection of a necrotic neoplasm or benign cyst can also lead to abscess formation.

In the past, the clinical course of intraperitoneal abscess was often complicated and rapidly fatal. Now abscesses most often present insidiously with nonspecific symptoms—such as fever, malaise, and abdominal discomfort—most likely due to the partially mitigating effects of concurrently administered antibiotics (24). Nevertheless, abdominal and pelvic abscesses continue to produce high morbidity and mortality (2). Thus early diagnosis and prompt drainage of abscesses remains essential.

CT findings.

In its earliest stage, when an abscess consists of a focal accumulation of neutrophils in a tissue or organ seeded by bacteria, a mass with an attenuation value near soft tissue is generally seen (Figs. 17–19). Use of

intravenous contrast media may aid identification of a small intraperitoneal abscess by increasing the density difference between normal surrounding tissues that enhance and the non-enhancing abscess itself. As the abscess matures, some normal cells and neutrophils undergo liquefactive necrosis and highly vascularized connective tissue proliferates around this central necrotic region. At this stage, the abscess usually has a low CT density central region surrounded by a higher density rim that may enhance after intravenous contrast material administration (Figs. 20 and 21) (3). The necrotic central zone may contain gas if the bacteria involved are gas producers. This gas, which occurs in about 25% of cases (7,35), usually appears as small bubbles, but occasionally an air-fluid level may be identified within the abscess (Figs. 22 and 23).

Most of these CT findings are not specific for an abscess. A similar central low attenuation value can be found with other masses—such as simple or complicated cysts, necrotic neoplasms (Fig. 24), urinomas, seromas (Fig. 25), hematomas, or other postoperative fluid collections (Fig. 26). Necrotic neoplasms, as well, may have a wall that contrast material enhances (7). Although fascial plane thickening, which often extends well beyond the lesion, may be seen in an abscess, this sign, too, is nonspecific, and may occur with intra-abdominal hemorrhage or neoplastic infiltration (35). Even the CT demonstration of gas within a mass is not specific for an abscess. An infected necrotic neoplasm (Fig. 27) or a pancreatic pseudocyst, which spontaneously communicates with bowel, also may contain gas. Since a specific diagnosis of abscess based solely on the CT findings often is not possible, correlation with the clinical history is imperative (Figs. 24 and 25). Sometimes only a differential diagnosis will be possible. Tissue sampling, such as by percutaneous needle aspiration, may be required for definitive diagnosis. By obtaining a specimen of fluid for Gram stain

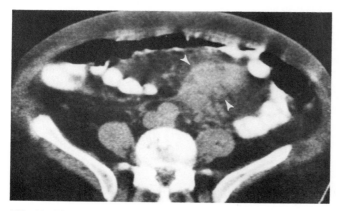

FIG. 19. Mesenteric abscess from diverticulitis. Soft-tissue density mass (arrowheads) is present within the mesentery.

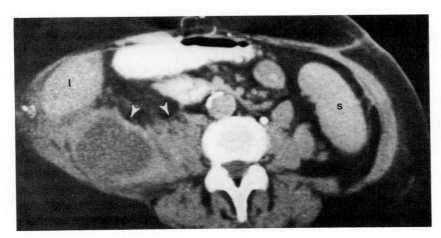

FIG. 20. Psoas abscess. The right psoas muscle and posterior pararenal space are enlarged by a mass (arrowheads) that has a low density central region surrounded by a higher density rim. l, liver; s, tip of an enlarged spleen.

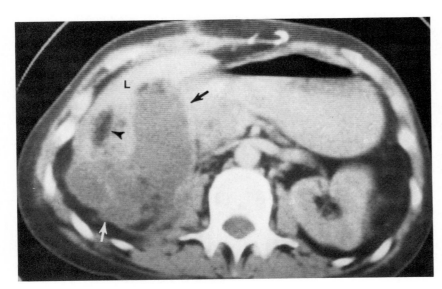

FIG. 21. Subhepatic abscess post right nephrectomy. Large inhomogenous mass (arrows) with low density central region and higher density rim posteroinferior to the liver (L). Intraperitoneal fat (arrowhead) adjacent to the liver is displaced by the abscess.

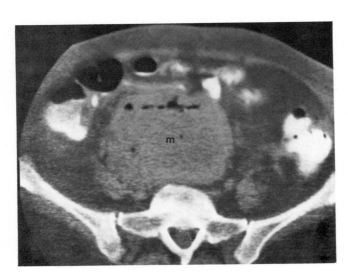

FIG. 22. Pelvic abscess secondary to perforated sigmoid carcinoma. Large soft-tissue density mass (m) contains multiple gas bubbles, some of which form small air-fluid levels.

23a,b

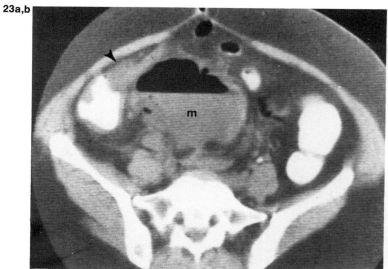

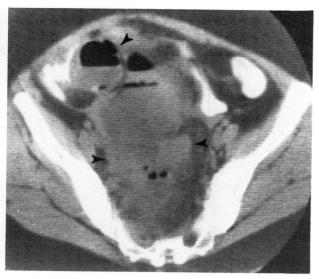

23c

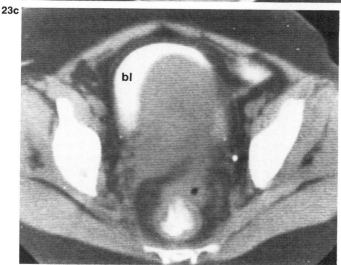

FIG. 23. Appendiceal abscess. **a:** Scan at level of pelvic inlet reveals a large soft-tissue density mass (m) containing an air-fluid level. Wall of adjacent bowel is thickened (arrowhead). **b:** Scan 6 cm inferiorly shows that mass (arrowheads) extends deep into the pelvis. **c:** Caudad, the mass extends into the pouch of Douglas and extrinsically compresses the urinary bladder (bl).

and culture from such a lesion under CT or ultrasound guidance, the presence or absence of an abscess usually can be quickly established. In many instances, a catheter can be inserted to provide definitive percutaneous drainage (Fig. 28) if an abscess is present (12,15,33). The technical details of CT-guided abscess drainage are described in Chapter 2.

CT accuracy in intraperitoneal abscess.

Accuracy in the detection of abdominal abscess is about 95% using current state-of-the-art CT scanners (16,35). False positive diagnoses can occur when either normal structures (fluid filled stomach or intestinal loop) are mistaken for abscess (Figs. 29 and 30). The proper use of abundant oral contrast to opacify the alimentary tract aids identification of the bowel and should eliminate this type of error. As previously em-

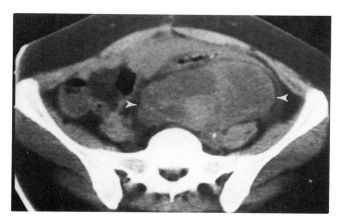

FIG. 24. Metastatic leiomyosarcoma. Large pelvic mass (arrowheads) has several areas of near-water attenuation value due to necrosis.

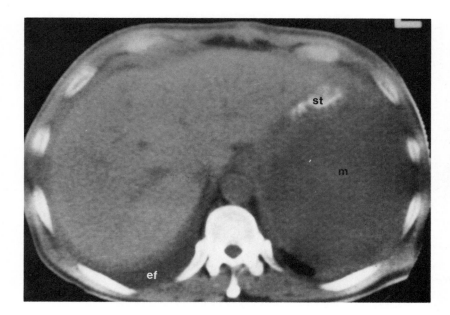

FIG. 25. Post-splenectomy seroma. Large near-water density left upper quadrant mass (m) compresses contrast material-filled stomach (st) anteriorly. Percutaneous needle aspiration demonstrated that this mass represented seroma rather than abscess. A right pleural effusion is present (ef).

phasized, other abnormal masses (hematoma, cyst, necrotic neoplasm) may mimic abscess, and vice versa.

Clinical application of CT in suspected intraperitoneal abscess.

Radiologic evaluation of the patient with suspected abdominal abscess should generally begin with a conventional radiographic examination of the abdomen. Subsequently, [67]gallium citrate radionuclide imaging, ultrasound, or CT may be potentially beneficial. Each of these techniques has its own advantages and disadvantages; combining them in certain circumstances may increase sensitivity and specificity (18,20,23).

Radionuclide imaging with [67]gallium citrate produces a unique view of the entire body in a single image, but often requires 24 to 72 hr to complete the study. Difficulty can be encountered in differentiating an abdominal abscess(es) from normal colonic activity (18). In addition, increased focal activity is not specific for an abscess, and can occur with neoplasms, vasculitis, or simple inflammation (3,20).

An ultrasound examination usually can be performed faster than CT, and on patients who are uncooperative. The ability to scan easily in multiple planes makes ultrasound the procedure of choice in a clinically suspected abscess involving the liver or right subphrenic space or subhepatic space. Real time scanning has reduced the level of skill required to perform and interpret a sonographic examination. Nevertheless, a major limitation of sonography remains the effect of gas and fat on the ultrasonic beam. Bowel gas can interfere with the demonstration of an abscess, particularly one deep within the abdomen (6).

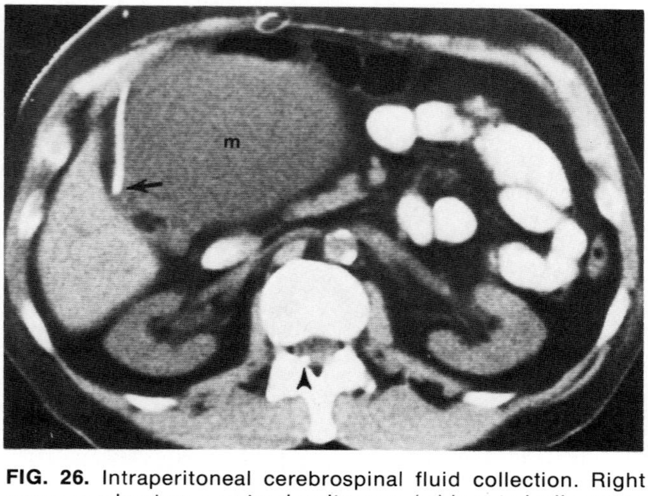

FIG. 26. Intraperitoneal cerebrospinal fluid collection. Right upper quadrant near-water density mass (m) is noted adjacent to the tip (arrow) of a lumbo-peritoneal shunt tube. The other end of the shunt is seen within spinal canal (arrowhead).

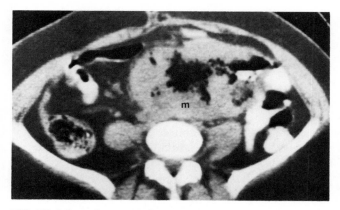

FIG. 27. Infected mesenteric metastasis. A large necrotic leiomyosarcoma (m) containing gas and oral contrast material is seen adjacent to an invaded loop of small bowel.

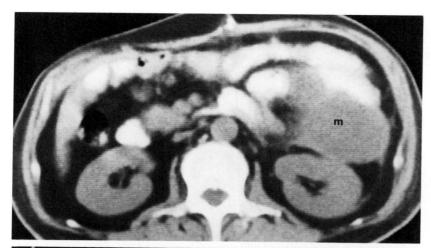

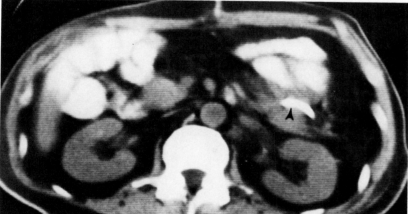

FIG. 28. Percutaneous catheter drainage of abscess. **Above:** A soft-tissue density mass (m) is present in the mesentery adjacent to small bowel loops in a patient postcolectomy for ulcerative colitis. **Below:** Scan at same level following percutaneous catheter (arrowhead) drainage shows marked decrease in the size of the abscess.

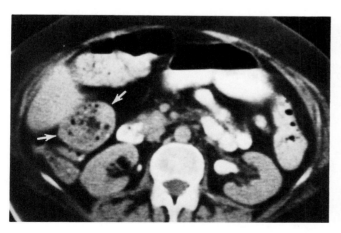

FIG. 29. Normal variant: ascending colon in Morrison's pouch. Ascending colon (arrows) is present within the posterosuperior extent of the right subhepatic space. Avoidance of mistaking this normal variant for an abscess within Morrison's pouch should be possible by carefully examining serial scans to trace the colon, or by opacifying the ascending colon with orally or rectally administered contrast medium.

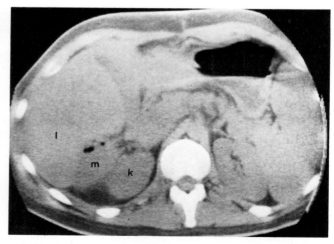

FIG. 30. Subhepatic abscess. Mass (m) containing gas in right subhepatic space. l, liver; k, kidney.

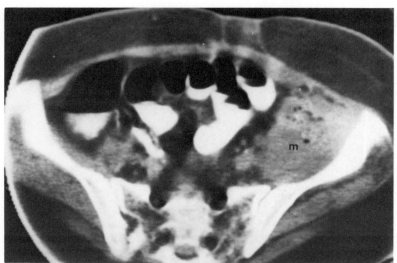

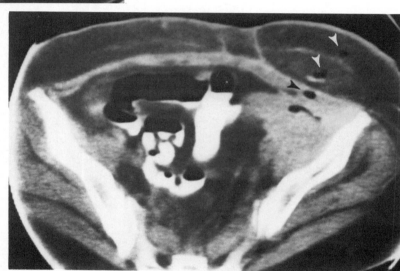

FIG. 31. Iliopsoas abscess. **Top:** Scan through upper sacrum shows a mottled mass (m) containing air within left iliopsoas muscle. **Center:** Scan 2 cm inferiorly shows the iliopsoas abscess, but also shows gas (arrowheads) within the anterior abdominal wall. **Bottom:** Scan at level of urinary bladder reveals that abscess (m) has dissected along the iliopsoas muscle to involve the hip.

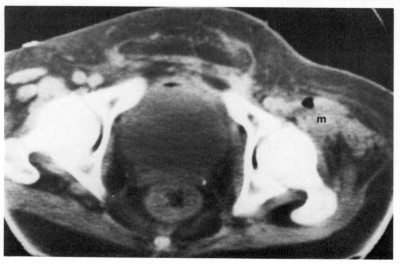

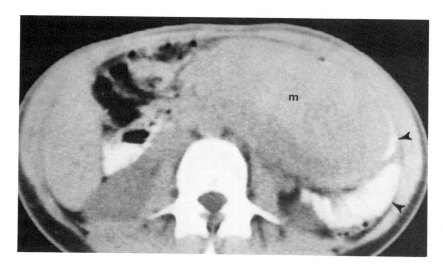

FIG. 32. Mesenteric desmoid. Well-circumscribed soft-tissue density mass (m) occupies left mid-abdomen and displaces adjacent bowel loops (arrowheads).

Gas-containing abscesses may be confused with a loop of bowel containing gas. In postoperative patients, wounds and drains may preclude the required freedom in optimal placement of the transducer.

Using fast CT scanners, a satisfactory examination of the abdomen and pelvis can be obtained in almost all patients (20), even seriously ill postoperative patients, many of whom have wounds, dressings, ostomy sites, and large amounts of bowel gas. Computed tomographic evaluation can be completed within minutes rather than the several hours to days required by radionuclide imaging. In addition, anatomic information about the extent and relationship to surrounding organs of a detected abscess(es), so vital to any therapeutic decision, is much more accurately depicted by CT (Figs. 23 and 31).

The following approach generally is recommended in evaluating the patient with suspected abdominal abscess. Computed tomography is preferred as the initial imaging procedure in patients who are acutely ill and/or have localizing abdominal signs. Exceptions include the suspicion of a right upper quadrant abscess (subphrenic, subhepatic, or hepatic) or a left subphrenic abscess when the spleen is present; in these instances, ultrasound is the preferred technique. If the CT examination of the entire abdomen and pelvis is unequivocally normal, abscess can be confidently excluded. If the CT examination is equivocal, ultrasonography may provide valuable information. Similarly, if an ultrasound study of the right upper quadrant is not entirely normal, CT may be performed.

In those patients with a suspected abdominal abscess who are not acutely ill and have no localizing signs, radionuclide imaging is suggested as the screening technique. If the examination is normal, no further radiologic evaluation is usually indicated. If focal increased gallium activity is present, a CT or ultrasound examination is performed, depending on the location of increased gallium activity (20), for documentation and assessment of the extent of a possible abscess.

Primary Neoplasm

Benign and malignant primary neoplasms of the peritoneum are rare. A mesenteric desmoid tumor arising from fibrous tissue in the mesentery usually appears on CT as a fairly well-circumscribed soft-tissue mass (Fig. 32), which displaces adjacent visceral structures (4). The CT appearance of a carcinoid tumor and its local metastases only somewhat resembles a mesenteric desmoid (see Fig. 47, Chapter 12). This mass, typically located in the right lower quadrant, often has linear soft-tissue densities, representing a desmoplastic response, radiating from the mass (31). A primary peritoneal mesothelioma usually grows by infiltration along the peritoneal surfaces; focal plaque-like masses and thickening of the mesenteric leaves may occur (37,38). Ascites is a frequent accompaniment, and is often loculated (Fig. 33).

Metastatic Neoplasm

Metastatic carcinoma and non-Hodgkin's lymphoma are the most common malignant neoplasms involving the peritoneum. Metastases usually arise from the stomach, colon, or ovary, and less often from the pancreas, biliary tract, or uterus (1,8). Mesenteric and omental deposits may not cause symptoms until they grow large enough to displace organs or cause intestinal obstruction. Prior to CT such metastases usually were not recognizable radiographically until they were quite large, with partial small bowel obstruction usually prompting barium studies of the gastrointestinal

33a

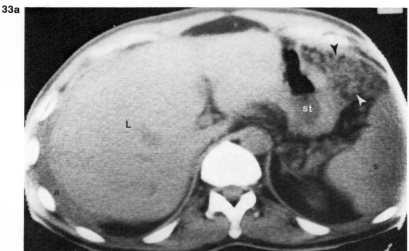

FIG. 33. Peritoneal mesothelioma. **a:** Scan through upper abdomen shows thickening of mesentery within lesser sac (arrowheads) and loculated ascites (a) around the liver (L). st, stomach; s, spleen. **b:** Scan through lower abdomen shows thickening of mesenteric leaves (arrowheads) including the mesenteric root (arrow). **c:** Scan through upper pelvis shows loculated ascites (a) surrounded by the mesothelioma (arrowheads) infiltrating the mesentery.

33b,c

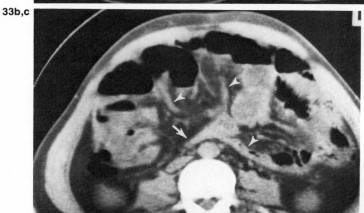 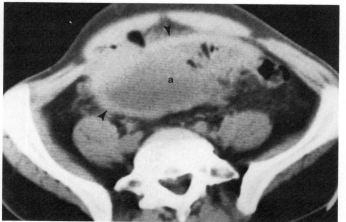

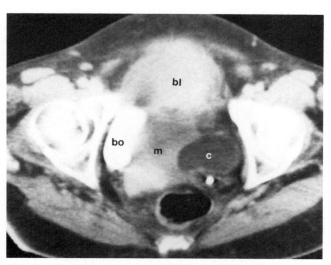

FIG. 34. Direct spread of metastatic neoplasm. Scan at acetabular level shows a cystic left ovarian carcinoma (c) infiltrating the contiguous pelvic fat with soft-tissue density neoplasm (m). The urinary bladder (bl) and an opacified loop of small bowel (bo) are displaced by the infiltrating neoplasm.

tract. Now mesenteric and omental masses, often as small as 1 cm in diameter, can be detected with CT before bowel obstruction occurs.

Detection of such small masses requires rigorous attention to CT technique. It is particularly important to opacify all small bowel loops with oral contrast material so that unopacified bowel is not mistaken for mesenteric tumor. Five hundred milliliters of an oral contrast agent, such as 2% barium suspension of E-Z CAT®, should be given at least 1 hr prior to the examination in order to opacify the distal small bowel. Another 500 ml of contrast material should be given approximately 15 min prior to the examination to opacify the stomach and proximal small bowel. If bowel cannot confidently be distinguished from a mesenteric mass, additional scans through the suspicious region can be obtained at closely collimated intervals. Generally, these scans are obtained after more oral contrast has been given. On occasion, a redundant sigmoid colon in the pelvis can cause confusion. If this occurs, a dilute solution of barium can be administered per rectum to exclude a pelvic mass.

Metastatic neoplasm can disseminate through the peritoneal cavity via four different pathways: direct spread through mesenteric and ligamentous attachments, intraperitoneal seeding, lymphatic extension, and embolic hematogenous dissemination (27). Many neoplasms metastasize predominantly by one particular route producing characteristic CT findings.

Direct spread along peritoneal surfaces.

Malignant neoplasms arising in the genital organs and gastrointestinal tract often break through the primary organ's capsule and spread along the contiguous visceral peritoneum to invade the wall of adjacent bowel. Infiltration of surrounding fat by soft-tissue density may be identified (Fig. 34) and bowel loops may be encased within the metastatic deposit. Neoplasms can also involve segments of the bowel at some distance from the primary tumor by spreading along the peritoneal pathways. Soft-tissue thickening of the mesenteric pathway leading from the primary tumor to bowel may be identified on CT scans. Carcinoma of

the stomach can spread down the gastrocolic ligament to the superior border of the transverse colon, whereas carcinoma of the transverse colon can spread up this ligament to involve the stomach (see Fig. 67, Chapter 12). Similarly, carcinoma of the pancreas may extend directly along the transverse mesocolon to involve the posteroinferior border of the transverse colon. The transverse mesocolon can also serve as the conduit for the spread of carcinoma of the hepatic flexure to the paraduodenal area (see Fig. 66, Chapter 12) (27).

Diffuse neoplastic infiltration of the greater omentum can produce a distinctive CT appearance. A soft-tissue mass is seen separating the colon or small intestine from the anterior abdominal wall, with obliteration of the normal fat plane in the area. Such "omental cakes" are most frequently produced by metastatic ovarian adenocarcinoma (Figs. 10–12) but may also occur with other neoplasms, e.g., colon carcinoma.

Another unusual CT appearance results when a mucinous cyst-adenocarcinoma of the ovary or appendix ruptures into the peritoneal cavity, resulting in pseudomyxoma peritonei (Fig. 35). The peritoneum and omentum may become diffusely involved with large amounts of mucinous material, which produce

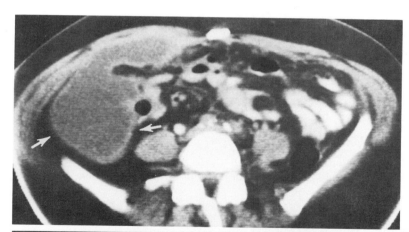

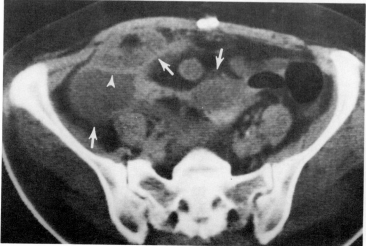
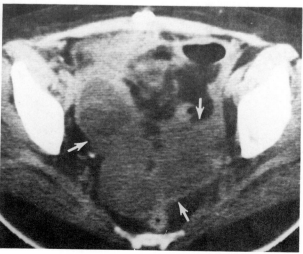

FIG. 35. Pseudomyxoma peritonei secondary to mucinous cystadenocarcinoma of the appendix. CT scans at 4-cm intervals through the pelvis reveal contiguous cystic masses of near-water attenuation value (arrows). The walls (arrowhead) of these masses are thin, and the CT appearance is similar to loculated ascites.

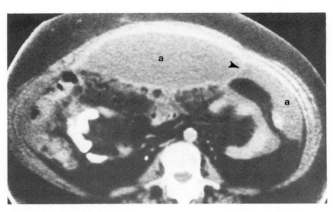

FIG. 36. Loculated malignant ascites. Low density ascites (a) with septation (arrowhead) due to metastatic endometrial carcinoma located anteriorly within the abdomen.

masses of relatively low attentuation value in the pelvis or abdomen on CT scans (22). If the walls of these cystic masses are thin, the CT picture may be similar to that produced by loculated ascites (Figs. 36 and 37), most frequently induced by non-mucin-producing ovarian cystadenocarcinoma. Scalloping of the liver margin by extrinsic pressure of the gelatinous masses and failure of bowel loops to float up toward the anterior abdominal wall may be useful in differentiating pseudomyxoma peritonei from ascites (32).

Intraperitoneal seeding.

Intraperitoneal seeding of neoplasm depends on the natural flow of fluid within the peritoneal cavity. The primary neoplasm usually arises in stomach, colon, or pancreas in men, whereas the genital system, most commonly the ovaries, is the usual source of the primary neoplasm in women. On CT scans, seeded me-

tastases appear as soft-tissue masses (Figs. 38–40), frequently associated with ascites, at one or more of the specific sites of normal pooling—the pouch of Douglas, the lower small bowel mesentery near the ileocecal junction, the sigmoid mesocolon, and the right paracolic gutter. If the metastases are very small, loculated ascites may be the only CT sign of intraperitoneal seeding (Figs. 36 and 37). Conversely, large peritoneal and mesenteric metastases may be identified in the absence of ascites (Fig. 40). Such large foci of metastatic carcinoma may have areas of decreased density within them, presumably due to necrosis (5).

Lymphatic dissemination.

Lymphatic extension plays a minor role in dissemination of metastatic carcinoma within the mesentery (25), but is the major mode of spread of lymphoma to mesenteric lymph nodes (17). Mesenteric lymph node involvement at the time of presentation occurs in approximately 50% of patients with non-Hodgkin's lymphoma but only 5% of patients with Hodgkin's disease (13). Identification of mesenteric lymph node disease is vitally important, because it almost always implies the need for chemotherapy, sometimes in conjunction with radiation therapy.

When mesenteric nodes are involved by carcinoma or lymphoma, they may appear as a single mass or as multiple soft-tissue mass(es) (Fig. 41) (21). Masses as small as 1 cm are detectable; masses over 2 cm in diameter should be routinely recognizable, except possibly in a very lean patient. A large confluent mass of lymphomatous mesenteric nodes may surround the superior mesenteric artery, producing a "sandwich-like" appearance (28). A multiplicity of soft-tissue masses or retroperitoneal lymph node enlargement is

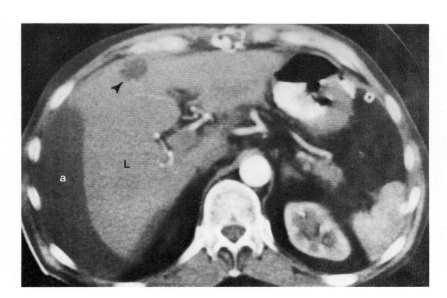

FIG. 37. Loculated ascites. Post-contrast scan shows low density ascites secondary to gastric carcinoma (a) located between the abdominal wall and the posterolateral margin of the liver (L). A liver metastasis is also noted (arrowhead).

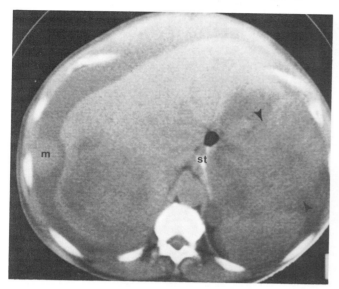

FIG. 38. Intraperitoneal seeding of metastatic neoplasm. Metastatic ovarian carcinoma is responsible for the round soft-tissue density mass (m) adjacent to parietal peritoneum and ascites over lateral aspect of right lobe liver. Additional soft-tissue density masses (arrowheads) fill the lesser sac; the partially contrast material-filled stomach (st) is displaced medially. Metastases within the liver and spleen are also noted.

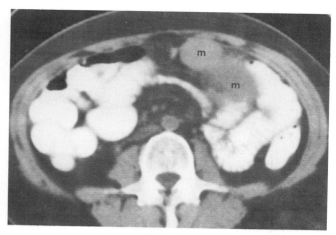

FIG. 40. Intraperitoneal seeding of mesentery. Soft-tissue mesenteric masses (m) due to metastatic uterine leiomyosarcoma adjacent to the lower jejunum. At surgery invasion of the bowel and the parietal peritoneum of the abdominal wall was found.

helpful in differentiating metastatic disease and lymphoma from a primary peritoneal tumor, such as a desmoid. When lymphoma disseminates to peritoneal surfaces other than the mesentery, the CT appearance may be indistinguishable from metastatic carcinoma (Fig. 42).

Embolic metastases.

Tumor emboli may be carried within the mesentery via the mesenteric arteries to the antimesenteric border of bowel where the cells implant and subsequently grow into intramural tumor nodules (27). Such lesions can extend to the bowel lumen and may eventually develop central ulceration. Melanoma and carcinoma of the breast or lung are the most common neoplasms to spread in this manner. These embolic metastases may produce thickening of mesenteric leaves (Fig. 43) or focal bowel wall thickening on CT; sometimes recognizable ulceration is present. Ulcerating small bowel lymphomas may have a somewhat similar CT appearance but usually a much larger exophytic soft-tissue mass is present (30).

Clinical Application of Imaging Procedures in Metastatic Disease of the Peritoneal Cavity

Conventional barium studies of the gastrointestinal tract provide only indirect signs of mesenteric disease, such as fixation, separation, angulation, and tethering of adjacent small bowel loops. These radiographic signs are not specific for mesenteric metastases and similar findings have been described in patients with prior radiation, retractile mesenteritis, tuberculosis, intramural hemorrhage, and inflammatory bowel disease. In contrast to barium gastrointestinal studies, which depend on inferential signs, gray scale ultrasound directly images metastatic mesenteric and peritoneal deposits. On sonography, they appear as nodular, sheetlike, or irregular solid masses with variable echogenicity (36). Using ultrasound, superficial peritoneal or omental masses are readily detected. Peritoneal nodules as small as 2 to 3 mm have been imaged in patients with a large amount of ascites because the peritoneal lining can be clearly seen within the echo-free ascitic fluid (36). However, it is more

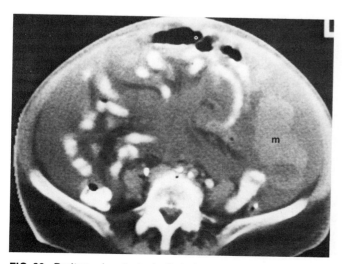

FIG. 39. Peritoneal metastasis. Soft-tissue density mass (m) with ascitic fluid near the sigmoid mesocolon due to metastatic endometrial carcinoma.

41a,b

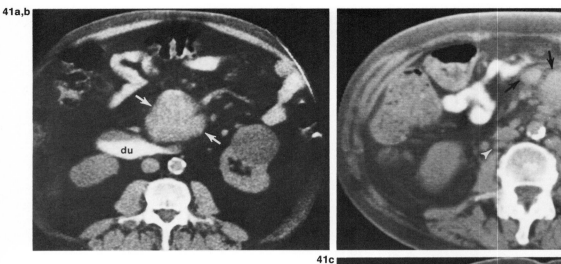

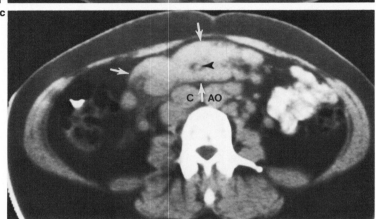

41c

FIG. 41. Involvement of the mesentery in patients with lymphoma. **a:** Solitary soft-tissue density mesenteric mass (arrows) near duodenum (du). Incidental left renal cyst is noted. **b:** Multiple enlarged lymph nodes (arrows) in mesentery near the ligament of Treitz are seen. Associated retroperitoneal lymph node enlargement (arrowheads) also is present. **c:** A large confluent mass of lymphomatous mesenteric nodes (arrows) "sandwiches" the superior mesenteric artery (arrowhead). Associated retroperitoneal lymphadenopathy is also present. AO, aorta; C, inferior vena cava.

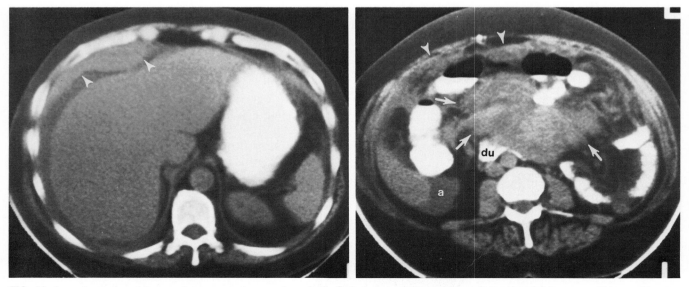

FIG. 42. Lymphoma involving peritoneum and mesentery. **Left:** Soft-tissue peritoneal mass (arrowheads) is seen within ascites surrounding the liver. **Right:** Scan 8 cm caudad shows lymphoma infiltrating the mesentery (arrows), compressing the third duodenum (du). Ascites (a) within the hepatorenal space and infiltration of the omentum by lymphoma (arrowheads) also present.

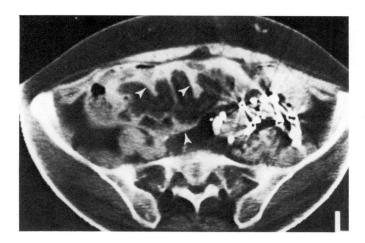

FIG. 43. Embolic metastases from breast carcinoma. Thickening of mesenteric leaves (arrowheads) is seen. Residual barium is present within several colonic diverticula.

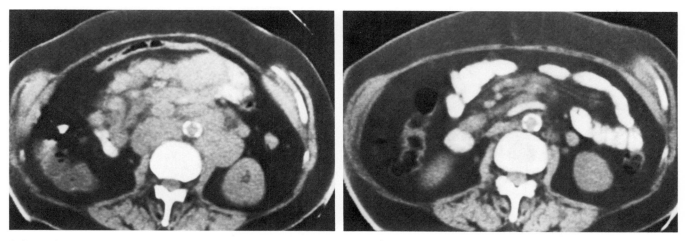

FIG. 44. Regression of enlarged mesenteric lymph nodes. **Left:** Marked mesenteric and retroperitoneal lymph node enlargement due to non-Hodgkin's lymphoma is present. **Right:** Following chemotherapy, nearly complete regression of enlarged nodes. Scans over the next year showed no change and the slight lymph node enlargement is felt to represent residual fibrosis.

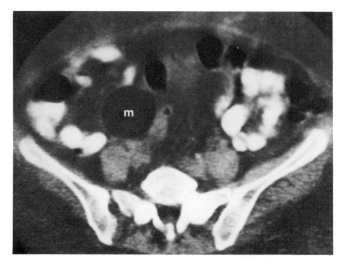

FIG. 45. Mesenteric lipoma. Homogenous fat density mass (m) with thin wall noted.

difficult to detect centrally placed mesenteric masses by ultrasound because the sonic beam cannot adequately penetrate bowel gas and excessive mesenteric fat (6).

A CT examination of the abdomen and pelvis is the preferred initial radiologic examination in the patient with known or suspected mesenteric or peritoneal metastases. Unlike ultrasound, the quality of CT scans is not degraded by excessive bowel gas or mesenteric fat. Furthermore, CT provides a better display of the peritoneal/mesenteric masses and their neighboring organs. An abnormal CT examination usually eliminates the need for barium studies. In addition, CT scans are an excellent method to follow the progression or regression of mesenteric involvement during therapy (Fig. 44) (19). In patients in whom bowel obstruction is suggested by CT or clinical findings, preoperative barium studies may be useful to determine the level of obstruction. If the CT examination is normal and metastases to bowel loops are still suspected (e.g., hematemesis or melena is present), barium studies may be indicated.

Miscellaneous Lesions

Mesenteric cysts and lipomas are uncommon lesions. Cysts are usually found in the mesentery of the ileum or the mesocolon of the cecum, transverse colon, or sigmoid colon (34). The CT findings in a simple mesenteric cyst are that of a nonenhancing near-water density mass with an imperceptible wall. The cyst is pliable and may conform to adjacent structures. Complicated cysts (e.g., chylous, infected, or hemorrhagic cysts) may have higher density contents and a contrast-enhancing wall. Lipomas (Fig. 45) have a similar configuration as simple cysts but their attenuation value is near that of fat rather than water.

Hematomas in the mesentery are similar on CT to those occurring elsewhere. A fresh mesenteric hematoma presents as a high-density mass on CT. As the hematoma matures, its density decreases.

Retractile mesenteritis, a rare abnormality of unknown etiology, is characterized by fibro-fatty thickening of the small bowel mesentery. On CT it may appear as a localized fat density mass containing areas of increased density (31).

REFERENCES

1. Ackerman LV: *Atlas of Tumor Pathology. Fasciles 23 and 24: Tumors of the Retroperitoneum, Mesentery and Omentum.* Washington, D.C., Armed Forces Institute of Pathology, 1954
2. Altemeier WA, Culbertson WR, Fullen WD, Shook, CD: Intra-abdominal abscesses. *Am J Surg* 125:70–79, 1973
3. Aronberg DJ, Stanley RJ, Levitt RG, Sagel SS: Evaluation of abdominal abscess with computed tomography. *J Comput Assist Tomogr* 2:184–187, 1978
4. Baron RL, Lee JKT: Mesenteric desmoid tumors: Computed tomographic and sonographic appearance. *Radiology* 140: 777–779, 1981
5. Bernardino ME, Jing BS, Wallace S: Computed tomography diagnosis of mesenteric masses. *AJR* 132:33–36, 1979
6. Bree RL, Schwab RE: Contribution of mesenteric fat to unsatisfactory abdominal and pelvic ultrasonography. *Radiology* 140:773–776, 1981
7. Callen PW: Computed tomographic evaluation of abdominal and pelvic abscesses. *Radiology* 131:171–175, 1979
8. Daniel O: The differential diagnosis of malignant disease of the peritoneum. *Br J Surg* 39:147–156, 1951
9. Dunnick NR, Schaner EF, Doppman JL: Detection of subcutaneous metastases by computed tomography. *J Comput Assist Tomogr* 2:275–279, 1978
10. Engel JM, Deitch EE: Sonography of the anterior abdominal wall. *AJR* 137:73–77, 1981
11. Fisch AE, Brodey PA: Computed tomography of the anterior abdominal wall: Normal anatomy and pathology. *J Comput Assist Tomogr* 5:728–733, 1981
12. Gerzof SG, Robbins AH, Johnson WC, Burkitt DH, Nabseth DC: Percutaneous catheter drainage of abdominal abscesses: A five year experience. *N Engl J Med* 305:653–657, 1981
13. Goffinet DR, Castellino RA, Kim H, Dorfman RF, Fuks Z,

Rosenberg SA, Nelsen T, Kaplan HS: Staging laparotomies in unselected previously untreated patients with non-Hodgkin's lymphomas. *Cancer* 32:672–681, 1973
14. Grant JCB, Basmajian JV: *Grant's Method of Anatomy.* Baltimore, William and Wilkins, 1972, pp 209–225
15. Haaga JA, Craig G, Weinstein AJ, Cooperman AM: New interventional techniques in the diagnosis and management of inflammatory disease within the abdomen. *Radiol Clin North Am* 17:485–513, 1979
16. Halber MD, Daffner RH, Morgan CL, Trought WS, Thompson WM, Rice RP, Korobkin M: Intra-abdominal abscess: Current concepts in radiology evaluation. *AJR* 133:9–13, 1979
17. Kaplan HS: Hodgkin's disease: Biology, treatment, prognosis. *Blood* 57:813–822, 1981
18. Korobkin M, Callen PW, Filly RA, Hoffer PB, Shimsak RR, Keesel HY: Comparison of computed tomography, ultrasonography, and gallium-67 scanning in the evaluation of suspected abdominal abscess. *Radiology* 128:89–93, 1978
19. Lee JKT, Levitt RG, Stanley RJ, Sagel SS: Utility of body computed tomography in the clinical follow-up of abdominal masses. *J Comput Assist Tomogr* 2:607–611, 1978
20. Levitt RG, Biello DR, Sagel SS, Stanley RJ, Aronberg DJ, Robinson ML, Siegel BA: Computed tomography and ^{67}Ga citrate radionuclide imaging for evaluating suspected abdominal abscess. *AJR* 132:529–534, 1979
21. Levitt RG, Sagel SS, Stanley RJ: Detection of neoplastic involvement of the mesentery and omentum by computed tomography. *AJR* 131:835–838, 1978
22. Mayers GB, Chuang VP, Fisker RG: CT of pseudomyxoma peritonei. *AJR* 136:807–808, 1981
23. McNeil BJ, Sanders R, Alderson PO, Hessel SJ, Finberg J, Siegelman SS, Adams DF, Abrams HL: A prospective study of computed tomography, ultrasound, and gallium imaging in patients with fever. *Radiology* 139:647–653, 1981
24. Meyers MA: *Dynamic Radiology of the Abdomen: Normal and Pathologic Anatomy.* New York, Springer-Verlag, 1976, p 1
25. Meyers MA: *Dynamic Radiology of the Abdomen: Normal and Pathologic Anatomy.* New York, Springer-Verlag, 1976, p 47
26. Meyers MA: Distribution of intra-abdominal malignancy seeding: Dependency on dynamics of flow and ascitic fluid. *Am J Roentgenol Radium Ther Nucl Med* 119:198–206, 1973
27. Meyers MA, McSweeney J: Secondary neoplasms of bowel. *Radiology* 105:1–11, 1972
28. Mueller PR, Ferrucci JT, Harben WP, Kirkpatrick RH, Simeone JF, Wittenberg J: Appearance of lymphomatous involvement of the mesentery by ultrasonography and body computed tomography: The "sandwich" sign. *Radiology* 134:467–473, 1980
29. New PF, Aronow S: Attenuation measurements of whole blood and blood fractions in computed tomography. *Radiology* 121:635–640, 1976
30. Pagani JJ, Bernardino ME: CT-radiographic correlation of ulcerating small bowel lymphomas. *AJR* 136:998–1000, 1981
31. Seigel RS, Kuhns LR, Borlaza GS, McCormick TL, Simmons JL: Computed tomography and angiography in ileal carcinoid tumor and retractile mesenteritis. *Radiology* 134:437–440, 1980
32. Seshill MB, Coulam CM: Pseudomyxoma peritonei: Computed tomography and sonography. *AJR* 136:803–806, 1981
33. van Sonnenberg E, Ferrucci JT, Mueller PR, Wittenberg J, Simeone JF: Percutaneous drainage of abscesses and fluid collections: Technique, results, and applications. *Radiology* 142:1–10, 1982
34. Warfield JO: A study of mesenteric cysts with a report of two recent cases. *Ann Surg* 96:329, 1932
35. Wolverson MK, Jaganna IB, Sundaram M, Joyce PF, Riaz MA, Shields JB: CT as a primary diagnostic method in evaluating abdominal abscess. *AJR* 133:1089–1095, 1979
36. Yeh HC: Ultrasonography of peritoneal tumors. *Radiology* 133:419–424, 1979
37. Yeh HC, Chahinian AP: Ultrasonography and computed tomography of peritoneal mesothelioma. *Radiology* 135:705–712, 1980
38. Whitley NO, Brenner DE, Antman KH, Grant D, Aisner J: CT of peritoneal mesothelioma: Analysis of eight cases. *AJR* 138:531–535, 1982

Chapter 12

Alimentary Tract

Matthew A. Mauro and Robert E. Koehler

Barium examinations and endoscopy are proven, time-honored primary methods of evaluating gastrointestinal diseases; however, CT can make several contributions to the radiologic study of the gastrointestinal tract, some quite unique. Barium studies and endoscopy both are essentially limited to examination of the surface, caliber, and contour of the bowel lumen and can provide only indirect information regarding intramural or extrinsic abnormalities. They remain the methods of choice for the initial detection of alimentary tract disease. Although CT can also be used to evaluate the lumen, albeit in less detail, its major contribution consists of directly visualizing the bowel wall and the adjacent tissues and organs. Being distinctly better than barium ''luminography'' in the evaluation of extraluminal abnormalities, CT is particularly useful in (a) staging gastrointestinal malignancies for treatment planning, (b) detecting and staging postoperative gastrointestinal tumor recurrence, (c) assessing tumor response to therapy, (d) evaluating the cause for gastrointestinal organ displacement, (e) clarifying intramural and extrinsic impressions detected by barium studies or endoscopy, and (f) evaluating palpable abdominal masses previously assessed by barium examinations. Occasionally large masses are seen on CT in patients with unimpressive findings on barium examinations.

A uniform CT staging system has been proposed for primary alimentary tract tumors and their recurrences (29) and will be followed in the ensuing discussion.

Stage 1. Intraluminal mass without wall thickening
Stage 2. Wall thickening (focal or diffuse) with no extramural tumor extension
Stage 3. Wall thickening with contiguous spread to adjacent tissue with or without regional lymph node involvement; rectal lesions are further subdivided into Stages 3A, without pelvic sidewall involvement, and 3B with pelvic sidewall involvement
Stage 4. Distant metastatic spread.

In general, Stage 1 and 2 lesions are resectable for cure, and CT outlines the precise location and size of the tumor. Stage 3 and 4 lesions are unresectable for cure, and CT is used by radiation therapists for treatment planning.

Additionally, knowledge of the CT appearance of the normal alimentary tract allows discovery of previously unsuspected gastrointestinal abnormalities on scans performed for other reasons. The images of the bowel loops on the CT scans should be carefully evaluated as well as the specific organs in question. Familiarity with the position, shape, and density of the normal gastrointestinal tract and its many anatomic variations on CT is important so as not to mistake them for masses or other abnormalities. Attention to the technique of opacifying the bowel lumen with oral contrast material is essential in dealing with the variable and ever-changing morphology of the alimentary tract. A great many interpretive errors stem from lack of care in distinguishing normal bowel from presumed intraabdominal abnormalities. A discussion of useful methods for opacifying each segment of the gastrointestinal tract is given in Chapter 2.

ESOPHAGUS

Normal Anatomy

The esophagus is usually well seen throughout its course. In all but very thin or emaciated individuals, the paraesophageal fat is visible as an interface between the esophagus and adjacent connective tissue, vascular, and cardiac structures. The cervical portion of the esophagus lies near the midline, directly posterior to the trachea (Fig. 1). Unlike the thoracic esophagus, the cervical esophagus usually does not contain swallowed air on the CT scans performed in the supine position. At the thoracic inlet, the esophagus lies posterior and slightly to the left of the trachea, and the fat between these two structures is

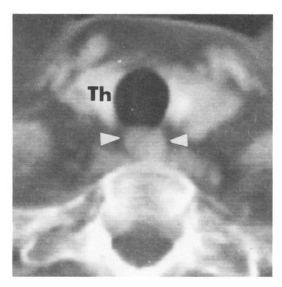

FIG. 1. Normal cervical esophagus (arrowheads) at the level of the thyroid gland (Th). There is usually no visible air in the lumen at this level.

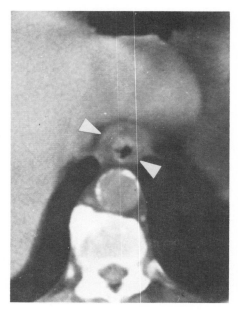

FIG. 3. Herniation of fat (arrowheads) surrounding distal esophagus.

often thin and not visible. Occasionally the esophagus is more lateral than usual and lies directly to the left of the trachea (3). Lower down, the esophagus is intimately related to the posterior surface of the left mainstem bronchus, but is separated from it by a fat plane. The esophagus pierces the diaphragm anterior to the aorta and to the left of the midline.

Small amounts of gas are present in the thoracic esophagus in about 65% of normal patients (9,12). The presence of a fluid level, fluid-filled lumen, or a luminal diameter greater than 10 mm is unusual and gener-

ally indicates the presence of an obstruction or severe esophageal dysmotility. The wall of the esophagus can easily be measured when there is either air or orally administered contrast in the lumen. Although the thickness of the normal esophageal wall varies with the degree of distention (Fig. 2), a thickness greater than 5 mm is usually abnormal when the lumen is well seen (5,31).

It is not uncommon to see either a fat or soft tissue density structure in the chest just above the esophageal hiatus representing herniated abdominal fat or gastric cardia, respectively (Fig. 3). If such a mass causes confusion but is thought likely to repre-

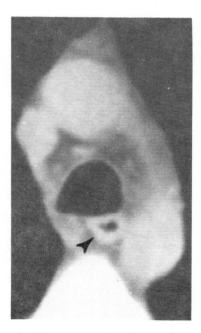

FIG. 2. The wall of the normal thoracic esophagus (arrowhead) appears thick due to incomplete distention.

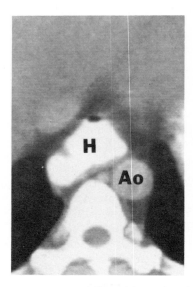

FIG. 4. A contrast material-filled hiatus hernia (H) is seen antero-medial to the aorta (Ao).

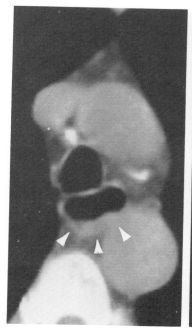
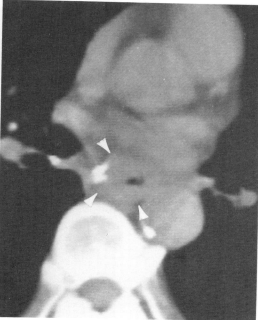

FIG. 5. Carcinoma of the midthoracic esophagus. **Left:** Just above the esophageal narrowing there is dilatation of the air-filled esophageal lumen and slight thickening of the posterior wall of the esophagus (arrowheads). **Right:** Scan through the bulk of the tumor shows a narrow eccentric lumen with a diffusely thickened esophageal wall (arrowheads). Calcification to the right of the esophagus lies within a granulomatous mediastinal lymph node.

sent a hiatus hernia, several swallows of oral contrast material can be given while scanning to opacify the herniated stomach (Fig. 4). When there is a need to see the esophageal lumen, such as when evaluating an obstruction, a tumor, or the esophageal wall thickness, a swallow of contrast material given just before each scan may be helpful.

Pathology

Neoplasia

The major use of CT in studying the esophagus is for the evaluation of known esophageal malignancy.

Computed tomography yields information on tumor size, extension, and resectability heretofore only obtained at thoracotomy. The CT findings of carcinoma of the esophagus include (a) intraluminal mass, (b) esophageal wall thickening, often sufficient to cause a soft tissue mass, (c) dilatation of the lumen with or without a fluid level proximal to an obstructing tumor, (d) obliteration of the fat between the esophagus and an adjacent structure such as the left atrium or aorta, (e) sinus tract or fistula to the tracheobronchial tree, (f) irregular or eccentric lumen, and (g) metastatic disease, especially enlargement of mediastinal, retrocrural, left gastric, or celiac lymph nodes, or low density masses in the liver (Figs. 5–14) (5,31).

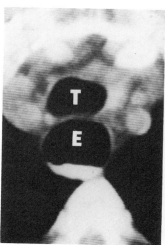
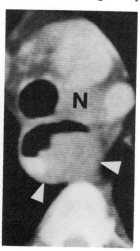

FIG. 6. Esophageal carcinoma with proximal dilatation. **Left:** Abnormally dilated esophagus (E) with an air/contrast material level proximal to the carcinoma. T, trachea. **Right:** A scan several centimeters lower reveals the carcinoma as an asymmetrically thickened esophageal wall (arrowheads). A metastatic node (N) is present adjacent to the trachea.

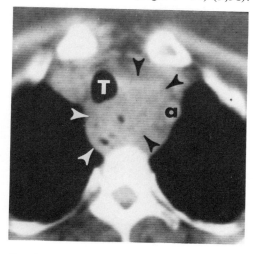

FIG. 7. Esophageal carcinoma. The esophageal tumor (arrowheads) has directly extended between the trachea (T) and left subclavian artery (a). Note the anterolateral deviation of the trachea. Tumor extension into adjacent tissues obviates a surgical cure.

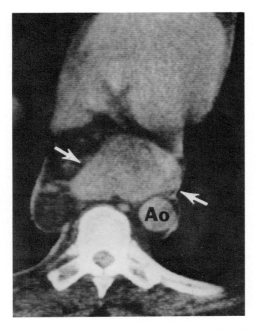

FIG. 8. Diffuse thickening of the esophageal wall due to esophageal carcinoma. The wall is so thick that the esophagus appears as a soft tissue mass (arrows). Note that the fat surrounding the esophagus is intact and that the tumor is not in direct contact with the adjacent aorta (Ao).

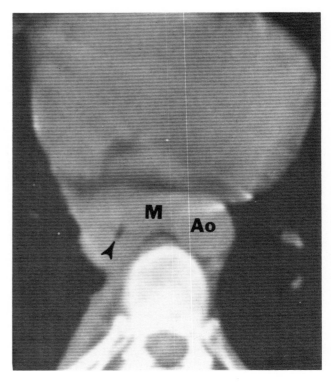

FIG. 10. Direct extension of esophageal carcinoma (M) to invade the adjacent aorta (Ao). Note the trace of air within the narrow esophageal lumen (arrowhead).

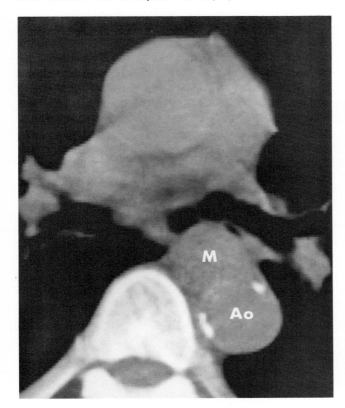

FIG. 9. Esophageal carcinoma. Obliteration of the fat plane between the mass (M) and the adjacent descending aorta (Ao) correlated with the finding of aortic wall invasion by tumor at thoracotomy.

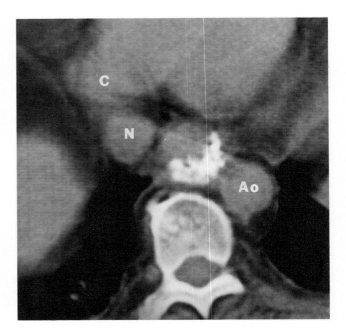

FIG. 11. Contrast material within the irregular eccentric lumen of an esophageal carcinoma. Enlargement of the adjacent mediastinal lymph node (N) indicates lymphatic spread of tumor. Ao, aorta; C, vena cava.

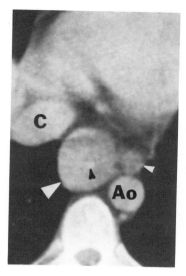

FIG. 12. Carcinoma of the esophagogastric junction. A circumferentially thick-walled distal esophagus (large arrowhead) is present. The contrast-material-filled narrowed lumen (black arrowhead) is only faintly visible. A para-esophageal lymph node (small white arrowhead) is enlarged. Ao, aorta; C, vena cava.

Although esophagography and endoscopy remain the primary methods for the initial discovery of esophageal malignancy, a few Stage 2 carcinomas have been reported to have been first detected by CT in patients being scanned for other reasons. Approximately 85% of patients with esophageal carcinoma have Stage 3 or 4 disease at presentation (31). Since esophageal carcinoma is usually advanced at the time of detection, CT findings are abnormal in virtually all

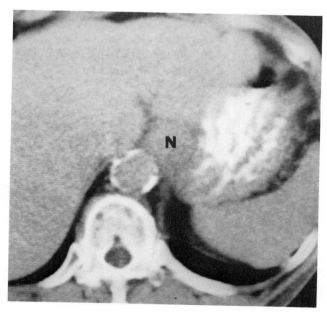

FIG. 13. Esophageal carcinoma. Scans through the upper abdomen show an enlarged left gastric lymph node (N) in the gastrohepatic ligament, indicating metastatic spread.

patients, most showing a soft tissue mass or focal wall thickening with an eccentric lumen. Most errors in interpretation occur in cachectic patients and in those with previous mediastinal surgery or radiation (5,31). Severely cachectic individuals often lack the normal fat planes around the esophagus, and surgery and radiation can alter the density of these fat planes. In all of these situations it can be difficult or impossible to stage esophageal carcinoma accurately by its CT appearance. In our experience, many of the patients with esophageal carcinoma are cachectic and may have scans where tumor invasion into adjacent structures cannot be confidently predicted.

Computed tomography is useful in detecting intra-abdominal nodal metastases from esophageal carcinoma. False positive errors can result from confusing diaphragmatic crura or fluid-filled bowel loops with enlarged nodes or by misinterpreting an enlarged hyperplastic (benign) node as a malignant nodal deposit (5). False negative errors are due to the inability of CT to show microscopic nodal metastases.

Benign tumors of the esophagus may appear as intraluminal masses, focal areas of wall thickening, or discrete mediastinal masses. Most are leiomyomas and are spherical or ovoid in shape. They are of soft tissue density and tend to be well marginated, showing no disruption of surrounding fat (Fig. 15). Differentiation from early malignancy is not always possible. An esophageal duplication cyst appears as a well-marginated, usually near-water density, spherical mass contiguous with the esophagus with preserved surrounding fat planes.

Inflammation

Computed tomography has not yet been shown useful in the evaluation of inflammatory diseases of the esophagus. Early experience suggests that when dealing with extensive lesions of the esophagus, CT demonstration of diffuse wall thickening with preserved fat planes implies benign inflammatory disease (5).

Miscellaneous

Varices appear as lobulated or rounded, tubular densities in the distal paraesophageal and perigastric locations, especially just anterior to the esophagus as it passes through the diaphragm (Fig. 16). Serial scans immediately after an intravenous bolus of contrast material are helpful in distinguishing varices, which enhance, from enlarged lymph node or neoplasia (4). When varices are suspected, careful attention should be directed toward the CT appearance of the coronary

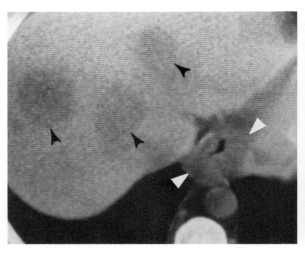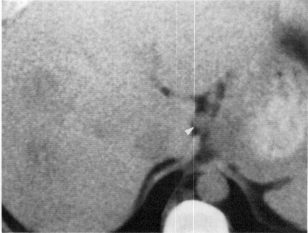

FIG. 14. Stage 4 distal esophageal carcinoma. **Left:** Thickened esophageal wall (white arrowheads) with eccentric lumen and numerous liver metastases (black arrowheads). **Right:** An enlarged lymph node (arrowhead) in the gastrohepatic ligament.

vein, splenic hilar veins, umbilical vein, and other potential portosystemic collaterals. The size and shape of the liver and spleen may also give clues to the presence of cirrhosis and portal hypertension (see Chapter 7).

STOMACH

Normal Anatomy

Opacification of the stomach with oral contrast material is mandatory for careful CT evaluation. Ideally, 500 ml of a 1.5% barium sulfate suspension is administered 30 min prior to the examination. An additional 200 to 400 ml is given just prior to scanning. Orally administered effervescent agents can also be used to help distend the stomach. If evaluation of the stomach is the prime concern, 1.0 mg of glucagon may be given intravenously just prior to the exam. Glucagon-induced hypotonia allows for more complete and longer lasting gastric distention.

With adequate distention, the normal gastric wall is almost always less than 1 cm in thickness (Fig. 17) (2,21). It is important that the thickness of the wall is measured from the depths of the crevices between the fugal folds to the serosal border as outlined by adjacent fat (Fig. 18). A lack of perigastric fat can hinder accurate measurements of thickness. The stomach should be empty at the time of the examination because undigested food can simulate gastric wall thickening or an intraluminal mass.

On CT the gastric wall sometimes appears thickened in the region of the esophagogastric junction and, to a

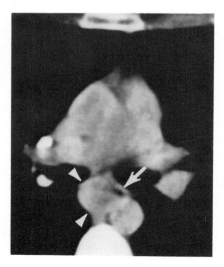

FIG. 15. Esophageal leiomyoma. Well-circumscribed round mass (arrowheads) displaces lumen (arrow) to the left.

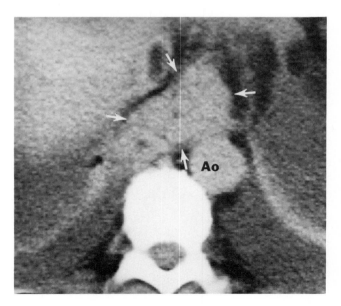

FIG. 16. Esophageal varices in a patient with cirrhosis. Multiple spherical densities (arrows) similar in attenuation to the adjacent aorta (Ao), surround the distal esophagus in a postintravenous-enhanced scan.

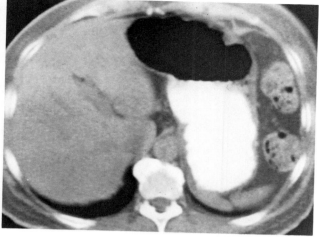
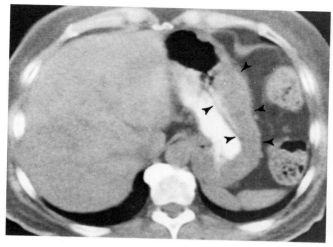

FIG. 17. Normal stomach. Contrast material fills the gastric lumen. **Left:** With incomplete distention the gastric wall (between arrowheads) appears thickened. **Right:** With additional contrast material, the stomach is more distended and the wall no longer appears thickened. Measurements of wall thickness should be made with adequate distention. (From Balfe et al., ref. 2, with permission.)

lesser extent, the antrum. The stomach wall is, in fact, usually thickest near the esophagogastric junction and nearly 40% of normal patients show either focal thickening or a focal mass-like structure in that region on CT (Fig. 18) (2,23). In addition, due to the transverse orientation of the stomach in the region of the cardia, the CT scanning plane can intersect the gastric wall tangentially producing the appearance of a pseudotumor. The transverse cleft of the liver, the fissure of the ligamentum venosum, often points to the esoph-

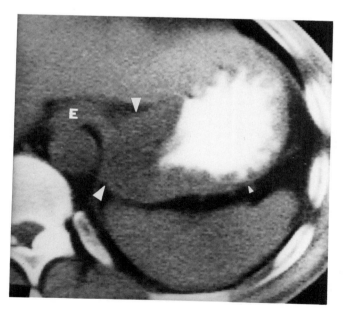

FIG. 18. Normal gastroesophageal junction. Note apparent abnormal thickness of gastric wall (large arrowheads) in this region due to tangential orientation of CT slice with respect to stomach. Thickened appearance extends from esophagus (E) to cardia. Small arrowhead indicates crevice between adjacent rugae illustrating a point where wall thickness can be measured. (From Balfe et al., ref. 2, with permission.)

agogastric junction on CT scans (23). If focal gastric wall thickening and the transverse cleft are seen on the same or adjacent slices, a pseudotumor should be suspected. If the patient drinks additional contrast material, the lumen in this area will distend, indicating normal anatomy. Similarly, due to the transverse orientation of the antrum, a false thickening may also be seen in that area (Fig. 19) (2).

Occasionally, the fundus will remain unopacified after oral contrast material administration when the patient is studied in the standard supine position. This is particularly true in patients with a cascade stomach because oral contrast material given in the erect or sitting position either bypasses a portion of the fundus or rapidly empties out of the fundus before the patient lies down. This can lead to the appearance of a soft tissue density (unopacified fundus) just to the left of the spine that may be mistaken for a mass (16). A gastric diverticulum near the esophagogastric junction may produce a similar finding and mimics the appearance of a paraspinal mass such as an adrenal tumor. If one suspects such a density to be unfilled gastric fundus or diverticulum, additional oral contrast material administered while the patient lies supine in the scanner will opacify this portion of the stomach and alleviate the problem (Fig. 20).

Pathology

Neoplasia

The contribution of CT to the evaluation of gastric tumors is primarily in staging and treatment planning, measurement of response to therapy, and the detection of recurrence. In selected cases, CT will also be helpful in the differential diagnosis of a gastric lesion.

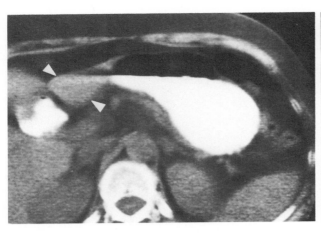
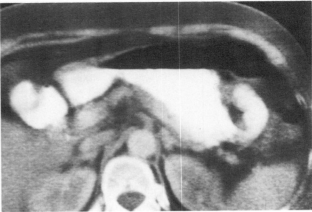

FIG. 19. Normal stomach. Tangential passage of the plane of the CT slice can cause pseudothickening of the gastric wall in the antrum. **Left:** Apparent thickening (arrowheads) of antral wall. **Right:** Normal appearance after more contrast is given. (From Balfe et al., ref. 2, with permission.)

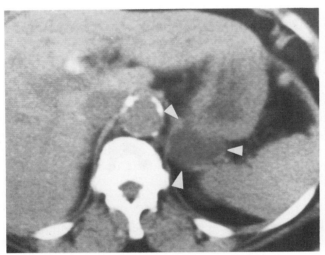
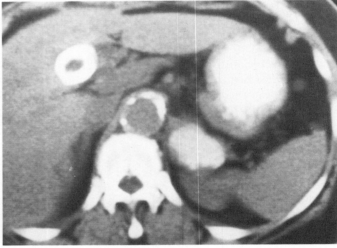

FIG. 20. Confusing appearance in a patient studied to evaluate the possibility of an adrenal mass. **Left:** Apparent mass (arrowheads) with low density center. **Right:** Administration of oral contrast material while the patient was supine showed that the mass represents a portion of the stomach, a subsequently proven diverticulum of the gastric cardia. A calcified gallstone is also seen.

Adenocarcinoma of the stomach may show concentric thickening of the wall, focal wall thickening, or intraluminal masses (Figs. 21–24). Obliteration of the perigastric fat planes is a reliable CT indicator of extragastric spread of tumor. Common sites of direct tumor extension include the esophagus, pancreas, gastrocolic ligament to the colon, gastrohepatic ligament to the liver, and gastrosplenic ligament to the spleen. The left gastric, gastroepiploic, celiac, retrocrural, peripancreatic, and splenic hilar regional nodal groups are commonly involved (Figs. 25 and 26). Distant metastases to the liver, ovary, adrenal, kidney, and peritoneum also occur (2,21,30).

Although difficult to distinguish from carcinoma solely on the basis of gastric involvement, lymphomatous masses tend to be bulky and cause a lobular inner contour to the gastric wall representing the thickened gastric rugae (Fig. 27). However, gastric lymphoma may also produce smooth, concentric wall thickening

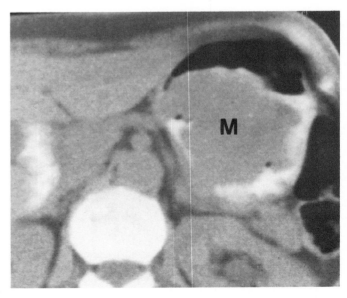

FIG. 21. Gastric adenocarcinoma. A large intraluminal mass (M) is evident.

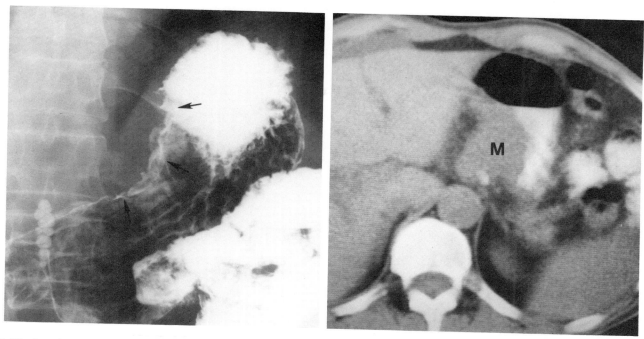

FIG. 22. Gastric carcinoma missed on upper gastrointestinal series. **Left:** Irregularity and mass effect (arrows) along lesser curvature appreciated only in retrospect. **Right:** Obvious mass (M) evident by CT.

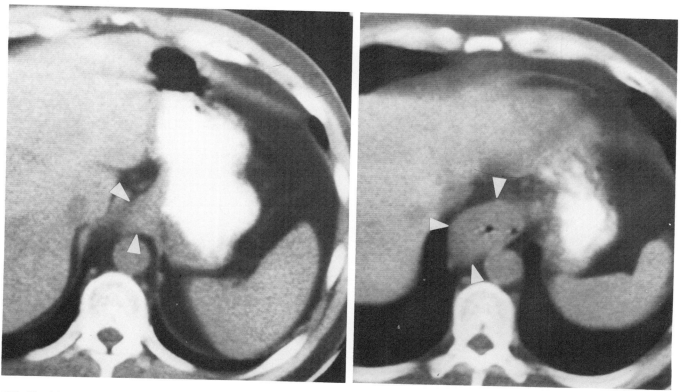

FIG. 23. Adenocarcinoma of the cardioesophageal junction. **Left:** The thickened gastric wall (arrowheads) looks much like a normal variant but proved to be neoplastic. **Right:** Scan 2 cm cephalad shows esophageal extension of tumor (arrowheads).

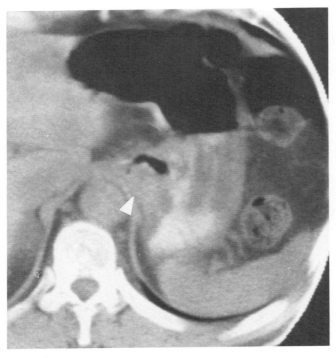

FIG. 24. Gastric adenocarcinoma. The tumor causes thickening and irregularity of the posterior wall of the cardia (arrowhead).

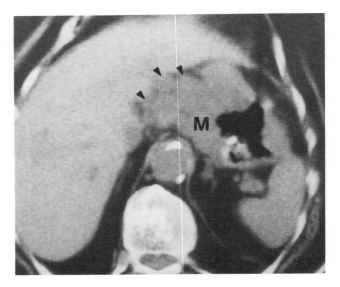

FIG. 25. Spread of gastric carcinoma (M) to left gastric lymph nodes (arrowheads).

or a focal mass (Figs. 28 and 29). More importantly, other signs of lymphoma (splenomegaly and diffuse retroperitoneal and mesenteric lymphadenopathy), when present, suggest the correct histologic diagnosis (Fig. 30).

Leiomyosarcomas are largely extraluminal tumors usually ranging 4 to 14 cm in diameter, which can often be distinguished from carcinoma or lymphoma on CT. When small, the primary gastric lesion generally is well circumscribed and intramural in location and may be indistinguishable from a leiomyoma (Fig. 31). Leiomyosarcomas may contain small foci of calcification and often have well-defined, spherical, low-density areas within the tumor representing either

areas of necrosis and liquefaction or a cystic component to the tumor (Figs. 32 and 33) (2). Unlike adenocarcinoma of lymphoma, regional lymph node involvement is rare whereas metastases to the liver and lung are common. The hepatic deposits may also show discrete, focal, low-density areas, as seen in the primary tumor (33).

Although greater than 90% of gastric adenocarcinomas, lymphomas, and leiomyosarcomas cause wall thickening greater than 1 cm, a similar appearance can also be seen with metastases to the gastric wall (Fig. 34) and even with benign inflammatory conditions involving the stomach. Therefore, with disease limited to the stomach, CT cannot reliably distinguish adenocarcinoma, lymphoma, gastric wall metastasis, and inflammatory disease. Only when the secondary signs of neoplasia are present can benign disease be excluded.

After the tumor has been detected, staged, and

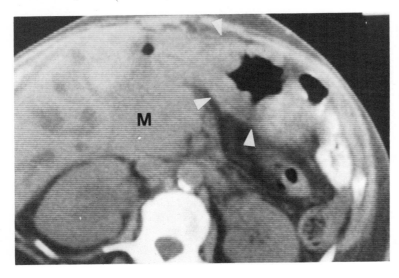

FIG. 26. Gastric adenocarcinoma (arrowheads) causing concentric thickening of the gastric wall. A large metastatic mass (M) involving the porta hepatis and peripancreatic nodes is causing biliary obstruction.

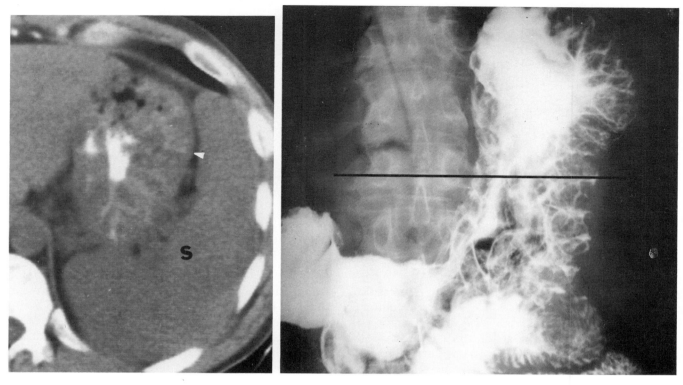

FIG. 27. Gastric lymphoma. **Left:** CT shows diffuse rugal thickening with normal wall thickness measured from the depths of the contrast material-filled crevices between rugal folds (arrowheads). Splenomegaly (S) is also present. **Right:** Barium examination showing the diffuse rugal thickening (line indicates level of CT).

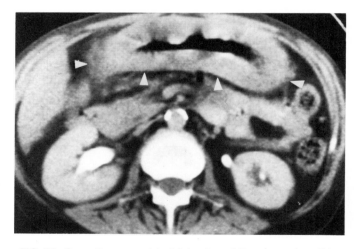

FIG. 28. Smooth, concentric thickening of the stomach wall by histiocytic lymphoma (arrowheads).

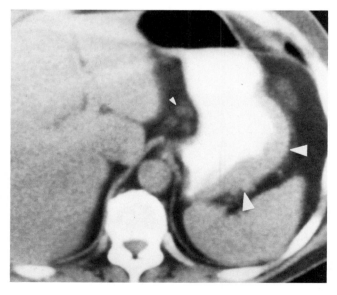

FIG. 29. Gastric lymphoma appearing as focal thickening of the greater curvature (large arrowheads). Pseudothickening does not occur in this area when the stomach is well distended. Note slight enlargement of left gastric lymph nodes (small arrowhead).

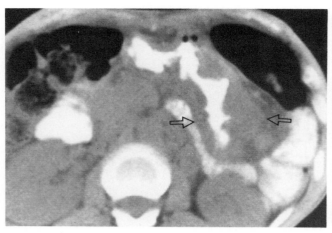
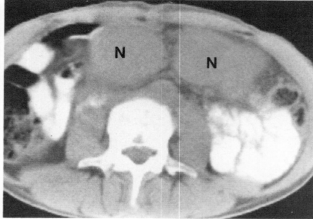

FIG. 30. **Left:** Gastric lymphoma (arrows). There is gross distortion of the gastric lumen with a fairly smooth outer wall. **Right:** The presence of mesenteric and periaortic nodal enlargement is a clue to the correct histologic diagnosis. N, enlarged mesenteric nodes.

treated, CT is useful in evaluating the response to radiation therapy and the detection of recurrent tumor (Fig. 35). A base-line postoperative CT examination is frequently needed for comparison to detect early recurrences and distinguish them from normal postoperative changes. The base-line examination should be obtained at least 1 month after surgery, allowing the immediate postoperative tissue changes to subside. A CT-directed needle biopsy of suspicious soft tissue masses can provide histologic confirmation of recurrent tumor.

Cases of suspected carcinoma on barium studies with indeterminate or negative findings at endoscopy can also benefit from CT evaluation (16). Computed tomography may show the abnormality on the barium

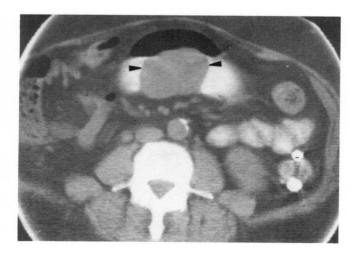

FIG. 31. Gastric leiomyosarcoma. CT scan shows an intramural tumor (arrowheads) with intact perigastric fat planes. A metastasis was seen in the liver on higher level scans.

examination to be caused by an intramural or extrinsic tumor in cases in which superficial endoscopic biopsies would be negative. Therefore, CT can help differentiate extrinsic disease invading the stomach from a primary gastric lesion. A typical example would be adenocarcinoma or an inflammatory mass of the pancreas with involvement of the stomach (Fig. 36). Computed tomography can also demonstrate that extrinsic gastric compression is due to normal variations of adjacent organs (particularly spleen and liver) or simply abundant intraabdominal fat (Fig. 37).

Benign gastric neoplasms, if evident, appear as well-marginated intraluminal masses or discrete mural nodules with intact fat planes (30). Occasionally, in the case of a lipoma, a negative CT attenuation value [−50 to −100 Hounsfield units (HU)] in a well-circumscribed homogeneous lesion will allow a specific histologic diagnosis (27).

Inflammatory

The CT appearance of the stomach is normal in most patients with inflammatory peptic disease but focal or diffuse wall thickening may be seen (2,30). Inflammatory wall thickening is generally less than 2 cm whereas neoplastic thickening is often greater than 2 cm. The finding of extragastric extension of a mass or distant metastases indicates the presence of a neoplastic process. Pneumoperitoneum and extravasation of orally administered contrast material into the greater or lesser peritoneal cavity can be seen with perforated gastric ulcers.

The Zollinger-Ellison syndrome can be suggested by the CT findings of thickened gastric rugae, increased secretions in the lumen, and thickening of

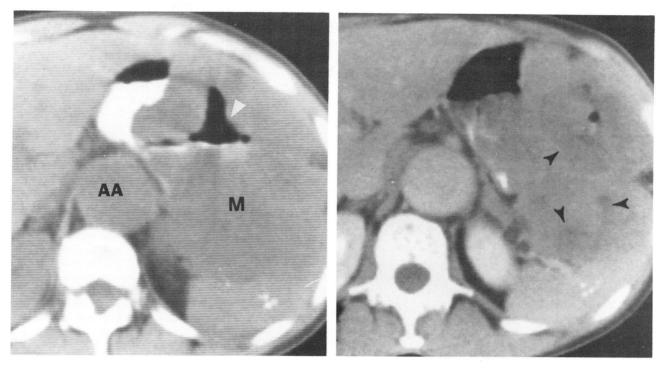

FIG. 32. Gastric leiomyosarcoma. **Left:** Large mass (M) is primarily extragastric. There is contrast material in the distorted gastric lumen and a trace of contrast material in an excavation (arrowhead) within the tumor. An abdominal aortic aneurysm (AA) is also present. **Right:** After intravenous contrast material, low density areas (arrowheads) characteristic of leiomyosarcoma are evident within the mass.

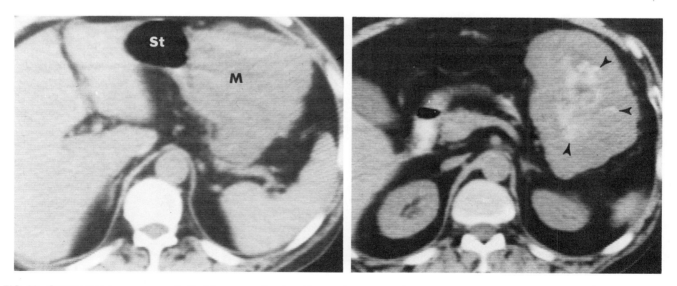

FIG. 33. Gastric leiomyosarcoma. **Left:** A large, predominantly extraluminal mass (M) arises from the greater curvature of the stomach (St). **Right:** At a more caudal level, areas of fresh hemorrhage (arrowheads) are present in the mass. (Case courtesy of Dr. Gene Davis.)

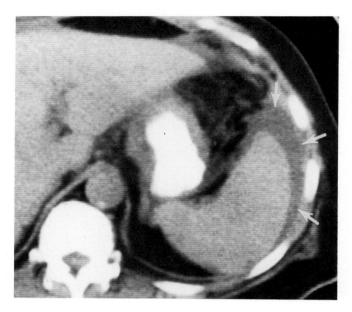

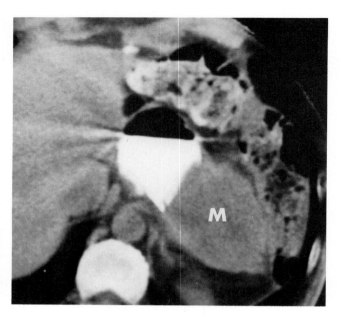

FIG. 34. Diffuse thickening of the gastric wall in a patient with metastatic spread of breast cancer to the stomach. Ascitic fluid (arrows) is also present around the spleen.

FIG. 35. Recurrent gastric carcinoma (M) after partial gastrectomy.

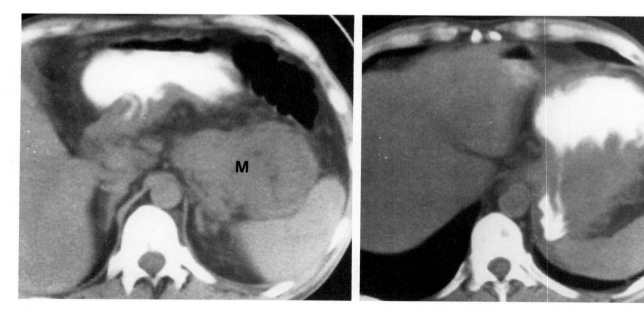

FIG. 36. Pancreatitis affecting the stomach. **Left:** A large inflammatory mass (M) lies behind the stomach. **Right:** Four centimeters cephalad, the gastric wall is involved with thickening of the rugal folds.

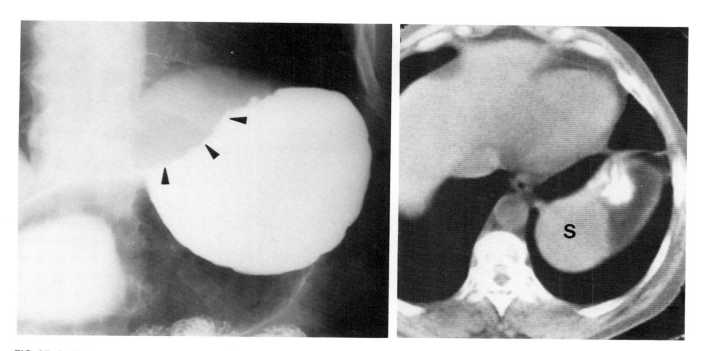

FIG. 37. Left: Impression on gastric fundus (arrowheads) of uncertain significance on upper gastrointestinal series. **Right:** CT showed the finding to be due to the spleen (S), which lay higher and more medial than usual.

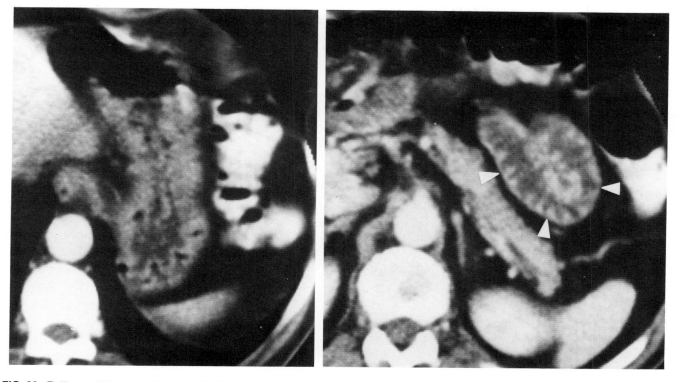

FIG. 38. Zollinger-Ellison syndrome. **Left:** The gastric rugae are prominent and there is fluid in the stomach. **Right:** Fold thickening is also obvious in the jejunum (arrowheads). A gastrinoma was never found. (Case courtesy of Dr. Thomas Lawson.)

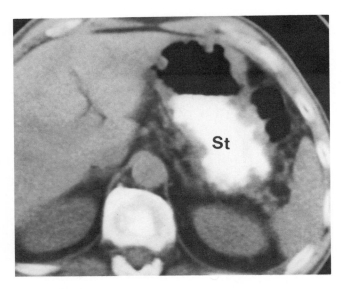

FIG. 39. Nonuniform, lobular thickening of rugal folds in the stomach (St) in a patient with hypertrophic gastritis.

the valvulae conniventes of the proximal small bowel (Fig. 38). The finding of thickened rugal folds alone is less specific, but can suggest some form of hypertrophic gastritis (Fig. 39).

DUODENUM AND SMALL INTESTINE

Normal Anatomy

The duodenum is intimately related to the pancreas with the second, or descending, portion cradling the pancreatic head and the third and fourth portions coursing along the inferior edge of the body and tail of the pancreas. The second portion of the duodenum lies just medial to the gallbladder and liver, anterior to the right kidney and adrenal, and posterior to the proximal transverse colon and mesocolon. The common bile duct crosses the posterior surface of the duodenal bulb and descends along the medial aspect of the second portion to the ampulla of Vater. The horizontal portion of the duodenum crosses the midline posterior to the superior mesenteric artery and inferior to the left renal vein (Fig. 40).

There are several anatomic variants and normal postoperative appearances that should not be mistaken for significant abnormalities. Small intestine may be interposed between the liver or stomach and the anterior abdominal wall simulating an omental mass or intraperitoneal air. Single, round collections of air or orally administered contrast material are occasionally seen medial to the duodenum within the "C" loop and usually represent duodenal diverticula (Fig. 41). Malrotation of the small intestine shows an incomplete horizontal portion of the duodenum with abnormal location of the duodenal-jejunal junction and proximal small bowel located in the right upper abdomen rather than in the left (Fig. 42).

Nonopacified small intestinal loops may mimic the appearance of an abdominal mass, a problem avoided by the use of sufficient oral contrast material (see Chapter 2). Scanning of the patient in different positions, such as prone or lateral decubitus, or at different times may also be used to induce movement of contrast material or air into questionable regions or to demonstrate change in position of bowel loops, thereby distinguishing them from enlarged lymph nodes or other masses (24).

Nonopacified loops are particularly prone to be mistaken for disease in several postoperative situations. After left nephrectomy, small bowel may occupy the renal fossa, mimicking recurrent tumor. Similarly, colon or jejunum may lie in the left upper

FIG. 40. Normal horizontal portion of duodenum (arrowhead) passing anterior to the aorta and posterior to the mesenteric vessels.

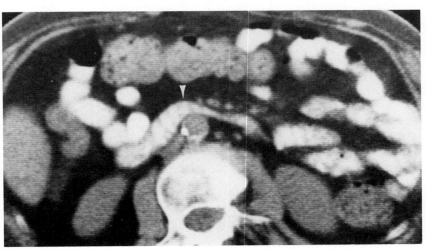

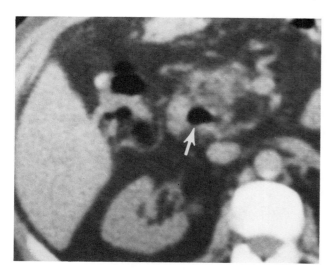

FIG. 41. Gas collection (arrow) just medial to second portion of duodenum lies in a duodenal diverticulum. Gas or ingested contrast material in this area should not be mistaken for signs of perforation or distal common bile duct calculus, respectively.

quadrant and lesser sac after splenectomy. Bowel can be seen in the porta hepatis after biliary-enteric anastomosis, mimicking tumor or adenopathy in that area. After abdominal hysterectomy, ileal loops usually lie deep in the pelvis. In such patients, contrast opacification of these loops and the placement of a vaginal tampon should permit correct interpretation of the CT findings (24).

There have been no published studies quantifying normal small bowel wall thickness, fold thickness, or luminal diameter as seen on CT. In general, the normal luminal diameter does not exceed 3 cm. Small bowel fold and wall thickness vary considerably with the degree of distention, appearing thicker when the bowel is not distended. Bowel wall thickness should only be assessed when the lumen is well defined (Fig. 43). If the bowel is collapsed or filled only with physiologic juices, the lumen often cannot be defined, and the bowel wall cannot be measured. With a moderately distended lumen, neither the bowel

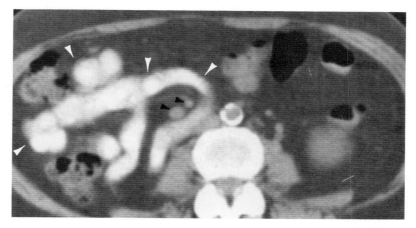

FIG. 42. Congenital nonrotation of small intestine. Jejunum and distal duodenum (white arrowheads) lie in right upper abdomen. Note rightward displacement of superior mesenteric vessels (black arrowheads) and normal colon position.

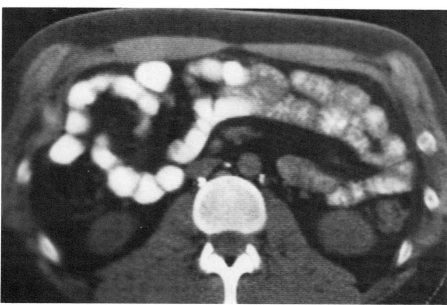

FIG. 43. Normal small intestine. Note delicate feathery folds in proximal jejunum in left abdomen and less prominent fold pattern in mid small bowel lying on the right. Lymphangiographic contrast in retroperitoneal nodes.

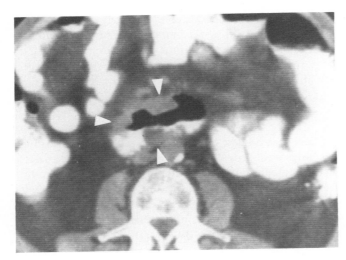

FIG. 44. Primary adenocarcinoma of the duodenum. A lobulated annular mass (arrowheads) encircles the horizontal portion of the duodenum.

wall nor the mucosal folds should appear thicker than 3 mm (13). The finding of thickened mucosal folds in patients in whom the bowel wall thickness is equivocal supports the suspicion that the bowel is truly abnormal.

Pathology

Neoplasia

Adenocarcinoma, lymphoma, leiomyosarcoma, and carcinoid tumors are the most common primary small bowel malignancies in decreasing order of frequency. Computed tomography can demonstrate the obstruction caused by an adenocarcinoma by showing dilated bowel proximal and nondilated loops distal to the tumor. The tumor mass itself can be seen if it is large enough (Fig. 44). Mesenteric extension and other intraabdominal spread of tumor can usually be shown better by CT than by other radiologic methods. Tumor recurrence and response to therapy can also be evaluated by CT (Fig. 45).

Lymphoma may affect the small bowel primarily or as part of systemic involvement. Five patterns of small bowel involvement have been described: (a) multiple nodules, (b) mural infiltration (Fig. 46), (c) polypoid mass, (d) an endo-exoenteric form with excavation and fistula, and (e) mesenteric invasion with extraluminal mass (25). The endo-exoenteric form appears on CT as an irregular soft tissue mass with low density areas that may fill with contrast material. Mesenteric masses usually appear as round, oval, or lobulated shadows (33). The infiltrative form causes thickening of the valvulae conniventes and bowel wall. Localized bowel wall thickening is, of course, not specific for tumor and can be seen in a number of benign entities such as radiation enteritis, granulomatous enteritis, and bowel wall hemorrhage. Again, an advantage of CT is its ability to detect disease in other areas of the abdomen, especially the liver, spleen, kidneys, adrenals, and mesenteric and retroperitoneal lymph nodes. Multiple sites of intestinal involvement, occurring in 10 to 20% of patients with intestinal lymphoma, or associated nodal enlargement strongly suggest that bowel wall thickening seen on CT is due to lymphoma (17).

Leiomyosarcomas show largely extraluminal growth with stretching of associated bowel loops. Low-density areas of necrosis, ulceration, or fistula formation can also be seen within the mass (17). Differentiation from leiomyoma is difficult unless metastases

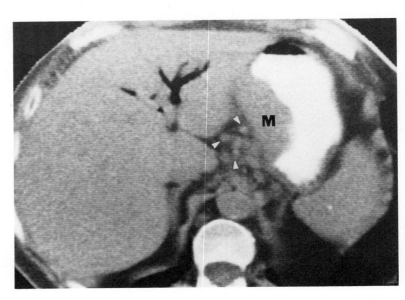

FIG. 45. Recurrent duodenal carcinoma after Whipple procedure. There is a mass (M) in the gastric wall and enlargement of lymph nodes (arrowheads) in the left gastric chain. Air in biliary tree is due to prior choledochoenterostomy.

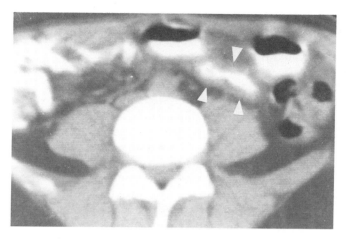

FIG. 46. Localized histiocytic lymphoma of small intestine. The ileal wall is uniformly thickened (arrowheads) in the affected segment.

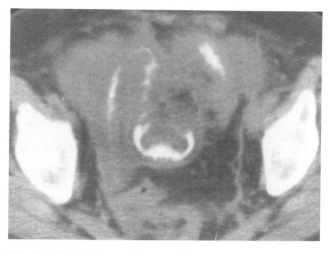

FIG. 48. Metastatic ovarian carcinoma encasing the small bowel. Note the narrowed lumen and thickened valvulae conniventes and bowel wall as well as the large irregular masses projecting from the serosal surface of the bowel. The appearance is typical of metastatic ovarian cancer.

are evident, but necrosis and fistula formation favor malignancy. Leiomyosarcoma may also be indistinguishable from lymphoma.

Carcinoid tumors are usually small and are rarely seen on CT. However, their mesenteric metastases and the resulting desmoplastic response in the surrounding mesentery can be seen and appear as a well-defined right lower abdominal mass with neurovascular bundles radiating toward it (Fig. 47) (36). Small bowel obstruction can also be seen but is, of course, not specific. Similar findings can be encountered in patients with retractile mesenteritis, a disease of unknown etiology characterized by fibrofatty thickening of the mesentery, and in patients with peritoneal mesothelioma (11).

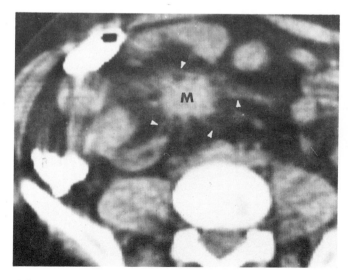

FIG. 47. Carcinoid tumor. A soft tissue mass (M) with radiating linear densities (arrowheads) represents a mesenteric metastatic deposit from an intestinal carcinoid tumor. The radiating linear densities are the distorted neurovacular bundles within the mesentery. (Case courtesy of Dr. Craig Coulam.)

Metastatic disease often affects the small bowel and duodenum via hematogenous or intraperitoneal routes or by direct spread. The CT appearances of small bowel metastases include mural nodules with or without obstruction, diffuse bowel wall thickening, encasement of loops within a large mesenteric mass (Fig. 48), and an excavating mass with small bowel loops running through it (34). Due to its proximity to multiple neighboring organs, the duodenum is often involved by direct extension of tumor. Computed tomography may be the best radiological method for distinguishing primary duodenal tumor from invasion by an adjacent malignancy. The most common pattern of spread is from the pancreas, but carcinoma of the stomach, gallbladder, bile duct, right kidney, right adrenal, and colon can all involve the duodenum by contiguous spread (28).

A leiomyoma, especially the subserosal type, can occasionally be identified as a soft tissue mass adjacent to bowel loops. A well-defined tumor of homogeneous fatty density, −50 to −100 HU, can be confidently diagnosed as a lipoma (27).

Inflammation

Computed tomography plays little role in patients with clinically obvious peptic disease of the duodenum. However, some complications of peptic ulcer disease, particularly extraperitoneal duodenal perforation, have been detected by this method (8). Extraluminal gas is commonly confined to the right anterior pararenal space, but the associated inflammatory process may break through the renal fascia and spread into the adjacent perirenal space.

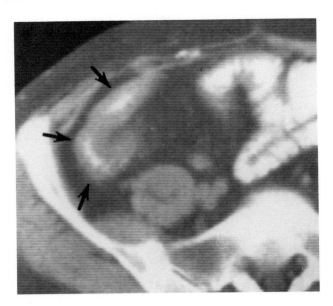

FIG. 49. Recurrent ileal Crohn's disease after right colectomy. The wall of the involved segment (arrows) is diffusely thickened and the lumen is narrowed.

Computed tomography occasionally plays a role in the evaluation of patients with Crohn's disease in whom the discovery and delineation of abdominal abscesses or inflammatory masses can otherwise be difficult. Bowel wall and mesenteric thickening in regional enteritis can also be demonstrated (Fig. 49). Radiation enteritis, intestinal hemorrhage, and lymphatic obstruction cause similar wall thickening (Fig. 50) (34). Computed tomography can be useful in the evaluation of abdominal fistulae when conventional radiographic techniques fail to clarify either the route or the compartmental location of the process. Injection of the fistulous tract with water soluble contrast media followed by scans covering the suspected areas of involvement demonstrate the course of the fistula and associated cavities (1).

The findings of thickened jejunal folds, increased intestinal fluid content, and thickened gastric rugae should suggest the Zollinger-Ellison syndrome in the appropriate clinical setting (Fig. 38). In such cases, particular attention to the pancreas and duodenal wall should be made in search of an underlying gastrinoma. However, most lesions in the duodenal wall are characteristically small and are not likely to be seen on CT. Whipple's disease can also produce thick, nodular folds in the small intestine. Of particular note in this condition is the peculiar appearance of the enlarged retroperitoneal and mesenteric lymph nodes, which are of unusually low density, presumably due to the lipid-laden histiocytes within them (Fig. 51) (22).

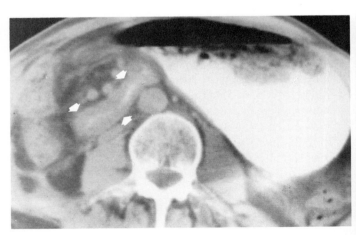

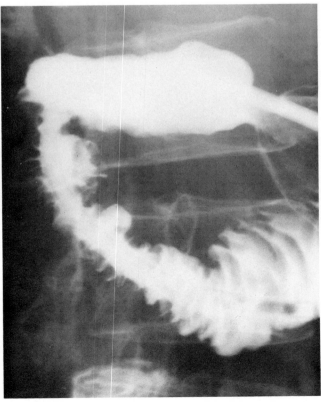

FIG. 50. Radiation duodenitis after treatment of Ewing's sarcoma of a lower right rib. **Above:** There is a thickened bowel wall (arrows) and resulting partial gastric outlet obstruction. **Right:** Thickened folds are seen on the barium examination.

51a,b

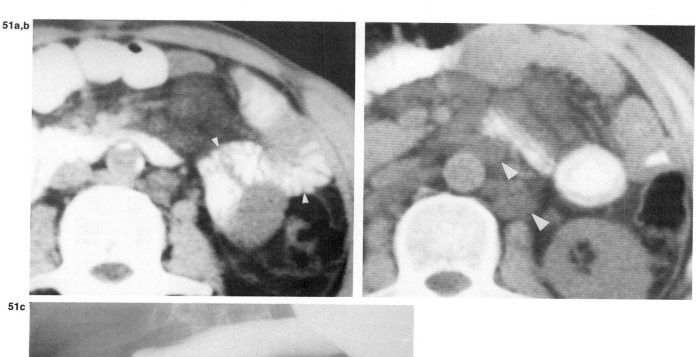

51c

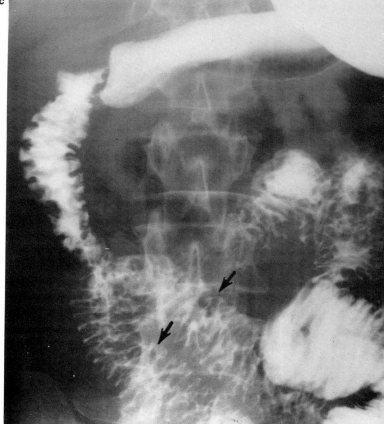

FIG. 51. Whipple's disease. **a:** There are thickened proximal jejunal folds (arrowheads). **b:** Characteristic low density lymph nodes are present in the para-aortic region (arrowheads) as well as in the mesentery. **c:** Barium study demonstrates the thickened jejunal folds (arrows).

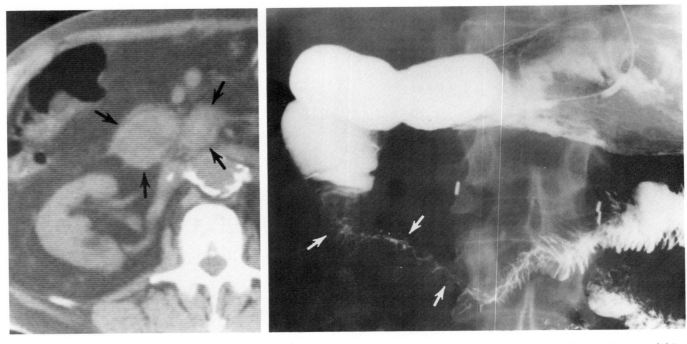

FIG. 52. Postoperative hematoma of third portion of duodenum 2 weeks after aortic aneurysmectomy. **Left:** CT scan just caudal to uncinate process of pancreas shows thickened duodenum (arrows) with central low density area. **Right:** Barium study shows high grade mechanical obstruction (arrows). A gastrojejunostomy was required.

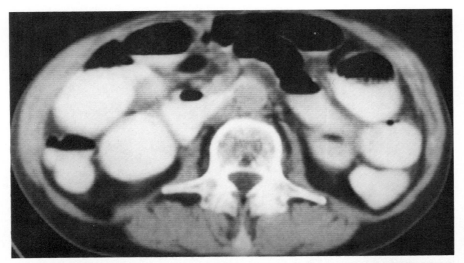

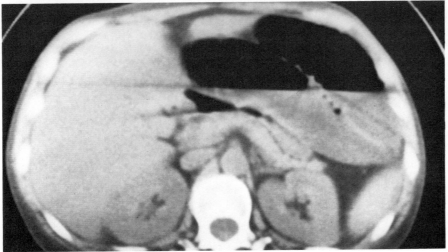

FIG. 53. Mechanical small bowel obstruction due to adhesions in two patients. **Top:** There are numerous dilated segments filled with gas and contrast material. **Bottom:** Contrast material was not given but the dilated, fluid-filled bowel is still evident.

Trauma

Computed tomography is a very sensitive method for detecting extraperitoneal gas due to traumatic duodenal perforation (8,15). Due to the fixed retroperitoneal position of the second, third, and fourth portions, most duodenal perforations are extraperitoneal with gas escaping into the right or left anterior pararenal space. An associated inflammatory process may also be seen, and one should search for evidence of trauma to other abdominal organs. Traumatic intramural hematoma, most commonly seen after blunt trauma to the duodenum, appears as a focal mass with attenuation value equal to or greater than adjacent soft tissue or as diffuse wall and fold thickening (Fig. 52). As in other organs, the hematoma gradually approaches the density of serum—20 to 30 HU—over the next several weeks.

Miscellaneous

Obstruction

The small bowel does not normally contain large amounts of fluid or air. Their presence suggests adynamic ileus or mechanical obstruction (Fig. 53). Although CT is certainly not the primary radiologic means of diagnosing small bowel obstruction, it can at times be useful in elucidating the etiology. Occasionally CT has been requested for confusing abdominal symptoms, and obstruction may be noted. Mesenteric masses may be encountered, appearing as soft tissue densities either effacing or encasing bowel loops.

Intussusception has a typical CT appearance. The individual layers of bowel wall, contrast material, and mesenteric fat can often be identified (Figs. 54 and 55). As seen in cross-section, the intussusception is composed of an outer layer of bowel wall (the intussuscipiens) with a thin layer of orally administered contrast material just inside. Within the outer layer of contrast material resides the intussusceptum. Because the mesentery is attached to only a portion of the bowel, the mesenteric fat accompanying the intussusceptum is seen on only a portion of its circumference. Where mesenteric fat is present, the two bowel walls (2 and 3 in Fig. 54a and b) that comprise the intussusceptum are individually seen, being separated by the invaginated mesenteric fat. On the side of the intussusception, which does not have invaginated mesenteric fat, the two adjacent bowel walls (2 and 3 in Fig. 54a and b) cannot be distinguished on CT. Therefore, where mesenteric fat is seen, three individual layers of bowel wall can be identified, whereas in portions of the intussusception, where mesenteric fat is not present, only

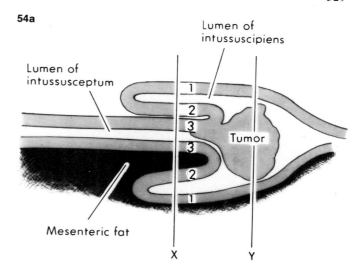

54a

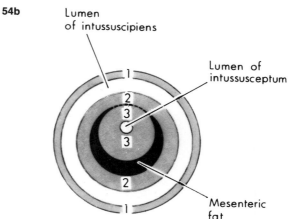

54b

FIG. 54. Intussusception. **a:** Diagram of a longitudinal section through an intussusception. 1, wall of intussuscipiens; 2 and 3, folded layers of bowel wall that comprise the intussusceptum. Note how invaginated mesenteric fat is attached to one side of the intussusceptum and separates the wall of the intussusceptum into two individual layers. **b:** Diagram of cross-section of an intussusception at level X in (a). Note eccentric lumen of intussusceptum. Where mesenteric fat is present, three distinct layers (1, 2, and 3) can be seen. Only two layers are visible where there is no mesenteric fat because layers 2 and 3 cannot be distinguished.

two layers are visible. Due to the asymmetrical location of the invaginated mesenteric fat, the lumen of the intussusceptum is often eccentrically positioned (Fig. 56) (35,37).

The afferent loop syndrome in which there is retention of bile and pancreatic juices in an obstructed afferent loop after gastrojejunostomy can also be demonstrated on CT (Fig. 57). Findings include an upper abdominal, cystic mass, often U-shaped, in which the distal portion passes behind the superior mesenteric artery (19). Mild dilatation of the biliary tree may also be present. The obstructed loop can simulate a pseudocyst, but the identification of a portion of the cystic mass passing posterior to the superior mesenteric artery in a

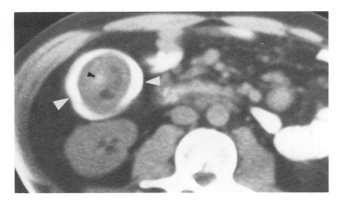

FIG. 55. Ileocolic intussusception. As diagrammed in Fig. 54b, this cross-sectional view shows contrast material in the ascending colon (white arrowheads) surrounding the intussuscepted ileum and associated mesenteric fat. A tiny amount of contrast material is seen in the ileal lumen (black arrowhead). Lymphoma of the ileum formed the leading mass.

post-gastrectomy patient should suggest the proper diagnosis. Afferent loop obstruction usually occurs at the anastomosis or as the loop traverses the transverse mesocolon.

Hernias

The role of CT in the evaluation of patients known or suspected of having an abdominal hernia, particularly of the ventral or incisional type, includes: (a) detection of the hernia in obese patients who are difficult to examine clinically, (b) differentiation of hernia from tumor or other mass, and (c) preoperative evaluation of unusually large hernias. The contents of the hernia can be seen, whether they are small bowel, colon, omental fat, solid organs such as the liver or spleen, or a cyst or tumor. The abdominal wall defect and hernia contents can be seen clearly even though no hernia may be palpable. Occasionally a palpable hernia will be mistaken clinically for a tumor, in which case CT may clarify the situation. With exceptionally large hernias, the CT appearance can give the surgeon a better appreciation of the size and extent of the abdominal defect as well as the hernia's contents to help surgical planning (see Chapter 6).

COLON

Normal Anatomy

The ascending and descending portions of the colon are usually well seen, being surrounded by extraperitoneal fat in the anterior pararenal space. The transverse colon lies anteriorly in the midabdomen and is distinguishable from the small intestine by

its haustrations and by the bubbly appearance of its fecal contents. The transverse colon is suspended from the retroperitoneum in front of the pancreas by the transverse mesocolon, which extends along the anterior surface of the pancreas from just inferior to the ampulla of Vater to a point superior to the ligament of Treitz (28). Normally, the transverse mesocolon is not visible by CT, but it may serve as a pathway along which pancreatic tumor or inflammatory disease can spread to the colon, in which case it appears as a band-like horizontal structure superior to the transverse colon. The superior surface of the transverse colon is connected to the greater curvature of the stomach by the gastrocolic ligament, which may also act as a pathway for spread of disease. The hepatic flexure and proximal transverse colon are closely related to the inferior surface of the liver and gallbladder and to the anterior aspect of the duodenum and upper pole of the right kidney, and can be affected by direct spread of disease from these organs (28).

Gas and fluid are normally present in the colon; however, colonic distention and air/fluid levels seen on CT hold the same significance as on plain abdominal radiographs. With sufficient fluid, air, or contrast material in the lumen, the colonic wall thickness can be evaluated and is usually less than 5 mm (38). It is occasionally helpful to opacify the colonic lumen with contrast material to avoid mistaking nonopacified large bowel, particularly the sigmoid colon, for a mass lesion. This is accomplished either by administering oral contrast material well in advance of the study or by giving an enema of dilute contrast material just prior to scanning.

Anatomic variations of colonic position should be kept in mind. The transverse colon, for example, can descend well into the pelvis or extend anterior and superior to the liver. The ascending and descending portions of the colon may be suspended by a mesentery, lack extraperitoneal fixation, and lie more medially within the abdomen than usual. Failure of complete colonic rotation will lead to a superiorly situated cecum. Portions of the left colon fill the left renal fossa in patients with left renal agenesis or after left nephrectomy. A vacant right renal fossa may be filled with portions of the right colon as well as duodenum or liver. The presence of contrast material in the colon will help identify these variations.

Pathology

Neoplasia

Adenocarcinoma of the colon generally appears as a spherical or circumferential soft tissue mass (Fig. 58) (26). Large tumors may show a central low den-

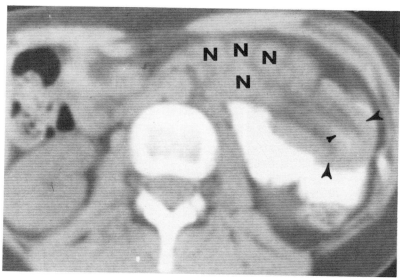

FIG. 56. Entero-enteric intussusception due to
metastatic melanoma. **Top:** Longitudinal view of
intussusception. A small amount of contrast
material (small arrowhead) outlines the lumen of
the intussusceptum. Large arrows indicate the
intussuscipiens. Mesenteric fat adjacent to the
intussusceptum is also seen. Note the mesenteric lymphadenopathy (N). **Center:** At a more
caudal level, the intussusception is seen in
cross-section. Note the eccentric lumen of the
intussusceptum (small arrowhead) and mesenteric fat (large arrowhead) on one side. **Bottom:**
Two centimeters caudal to the center scan. The
leading tumor mass (Tu) is seen within the intussuscipiens as diagrammed by level Y in Fig. 54a.

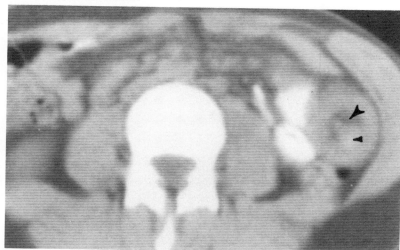

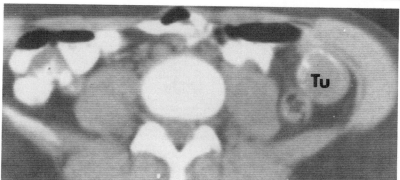

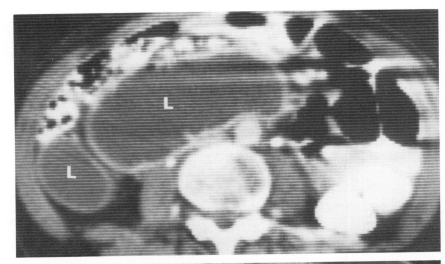

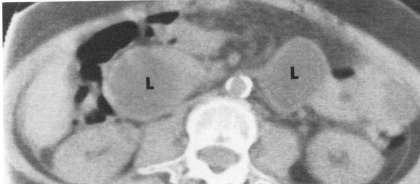

FIG. 57. Characteristic CT appearance of afferent loop obstruction in two patients due to recurrent gastric carcinoma in each. **Top:** Obstructed fluid-filled duodenal loop (L) mimics cystic masses. (Case courtesy of Drs. Frank Mainser and Barbara Rolfing.) **Bottom:** Second and fourth portions of dilated duodenal loop (L) seen in cross-section. Note absence of air in obstructed segment in both patients.

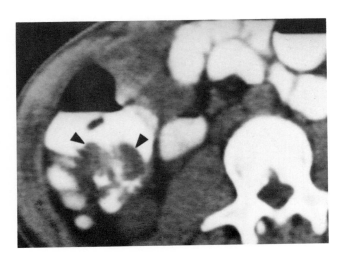

FIG. 58. Polypoid cecal carcinoma (arrowheads) adjacent to ileocecal valve.

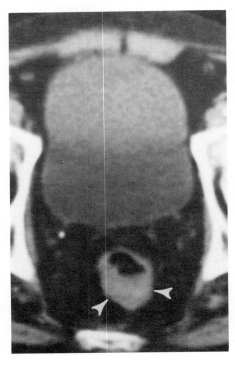

FIG. 59. Rectal carcinoma—Stage 2. Asymmetric posterior rectal wall thickening (arrowheads) is present. No evidence of tumor extension into adjacent pelvic structures.

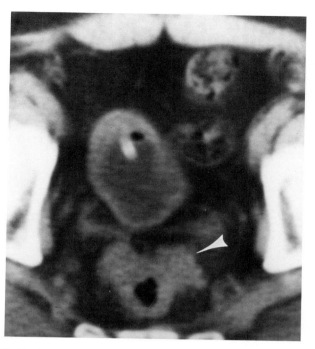

FIG. 60. Bilobed thickening of rectal wall (arrowhead) in patient with rectal adenocarcinoma. There is a catheter in the bladder.

sity area representing necrosis. Occasionally, the primary lesion may contain gas and be indistinguishable from diverticulitis with pericolonic abscess. Lesions of the rectum and rectosigmoid are seen as asymmetrical or circumferential thickening of the bowel wall with deformation and narrowing of the lumen (Figs. 59 and 60) (38). Other findings include extension of tumor into pericolonic fat, invasion of adjacent structures, lymphadenopathy, adrenal or liver metastases, hydronephrosis, ascites, and masses in the abdominal wall or mes-

entery. Obliteration of the margin between the colon and an adjacent structure may indicate local extension of tumor. Common sites of local extension from rectosigmoid carcinoma include the pelvic musculature, bladder, prostate, seminal vesicles, and ovaries (38). Obliteration of the fat plane between the muscle group and the mass and enlargement of the muscle adjacent to the mass indicate muscular involvement by tumor.

Spread into neighboring viscera may be difficult to predict confidently because the tumor mass may be visually inseparable from a structure and yet not actually invade it (14). Enlarged lymph nodes usually indicate the presence of nodal metastases. CT-directed aspiration biopsy of suspicious nodes can help when distinction from benign hyperplasia is important. Direct bony invasion can be diagnosed especially when there is frank cortical disruption (Fig. 61).

Computed tomography is both accurate and sensitive in the detection and staging of recurrent rectosigmoid carcinoma. Recurrent tumor following rectosigmoid anastomosis most commonly appears as focal rectal wall thickening with or without extension of mass into adjacent muscles, organs, bone, or pelvic sidewalls (32). Barium enema and endoscopy are of little use in the detection of pelvic recurrence in patients who have undergone abdominoperineal resection for rectal carcinoma. It is particularly in this clinical setting that CT has become the preferred method for detecting local recurrence (7,14,20,32,39). Recurrent tumor following abdominoperineal resection usually appears as a homogeneous globular soft tissue mass, which may undergo central necrosis and show a low density center simulating an abscess (Figs. 62–64). The recurrences are generally detectable when they are at least 1.5 cm in diameter. Uncomplicated

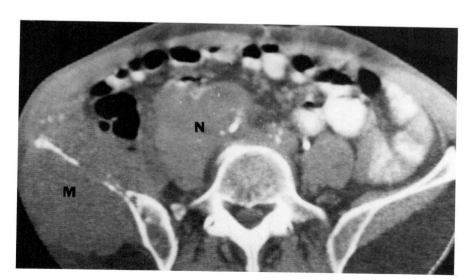

FIG. 61. Recurrent colonic carcinoma after right colectomy. A large mass (M) is destroying the right ilium and there is marked retroperitoneal lymph node enlargement (N).

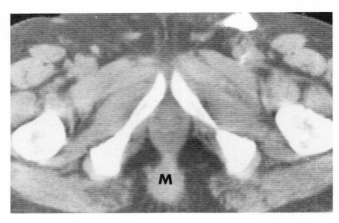

FIG. 62. Small nodule of recurrent tumor (M) after abdomino-perineal resection for carcinoma of the rectum.

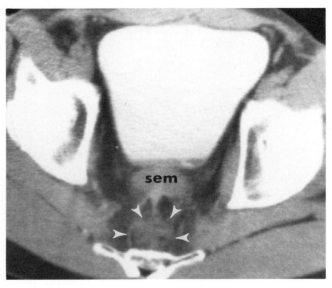

FIG. 63. Recurrent adenocarcinoma after abdominoperineal resection. Small recurrence (arrowheads) lies just anterior to sacrum. Tissue just behind the bladder is the seminal vesicles (sem).

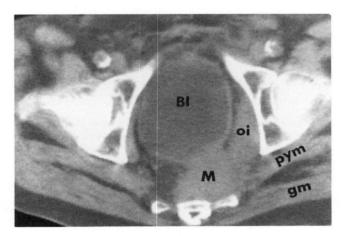

FIG. 64. Recurrent tumor—Stage 3b. The soft tissue mass (M) anterior to the sacrum represents a recurrence following abdominoperineal resection for carcinoma of the rectosigmoid. The mass is invading the posterior wall of the bladder (Bl), obturator internus (oi), and pyriformis (pym) muscles and extends to the left pelvic sidewall. gm, gluteus maximus.

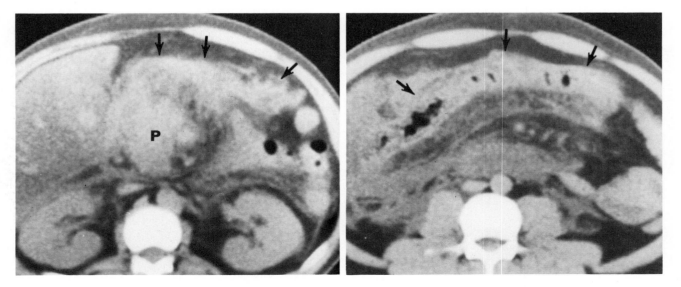

FIG. 65. Acute pancreatitis with spread of inflammatory reaction through transverse mesocolon to colon. **Left:** The head of the pancreas (P) is ill defined and enlarged. The transverse mesocolon (arrows), normally not seen on CT, is inflamed and appears as a thick soft tissue density anterior to the pancreas. **Right:** Scan 4 cm lower shows transverse colon (arrows) enveloped in inflammatory reaction.

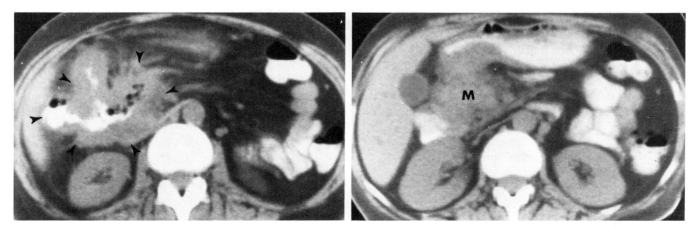

FIG. 66. Carcinoma of the hepatic flexure. **Left:** A large soft tissue mass (arrowheads) surrounds and distorts the hepatic flexure. **Right:** Four centimeters cephalad, the mass (M) is seen to extend into the head of the pancreas and the posterior surface of the gastric antrum. Initially, this case was thought to represent pancreatitis with involvement of the colon.

postoperative fibrosis usually does not produce a discrete mass as does recurrent neoplasm (20). However, patients with draining fistulae or abscesses may have soft tissue or low density masses. CT-directed needle aspiration biopsy can prove useful in problem cases. Routine postoperative scans may be helpful in detecting even smaller recurrences amid the normal postoperative changes. Base-line postoperative scans should probably not be performed until at least 2 to 4 months after operation to allow signs of postoperative bleeding and edema to subside (32). Further discussion of the postoperative changes is found in Chapter 15.

Adjacent muscles are invaded in approximately 70% of patients with recurrent tumor after abdomino-

perineal resection (14). It is important to remember that distant metastases may occur without evidence of local recurrence. The overall accuracy of CT for detecting recurrent tumor in patients after abdominoperineal resection is greater than 90% (7,14,20,39). False positive interpretations usually arise from mistaking relocated pelvic organs, small bowel loops, or postoperative fibrosis for recurrent tumor.

Computed tomography can often be used to differentiate a primary colonic process from a process secondarily involving the colon, such as pancreatic cancer or inflammatory disease, which has extended down the transverse mesocolon (Figs. 65 and 66) or gastric carcinoma extending through the gastrocolic ligament

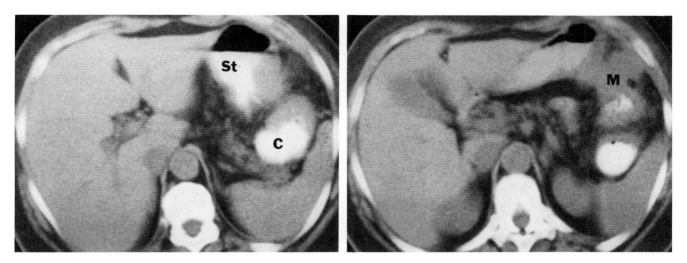

FIG. 67. Stage 3 carcinoma of splenic flexure with spread through gastrocolic ligament to stomach. **Left:** There is thickening of the wall of the colon (C) and adjacent stomach (St). **Right:** The mass (M) bridges the space between the colon and stomach. At operation the tumor involved the muscular but not the mucosal layers of the stomach.

(Fig. 67). The sigmoid colon and ileocecal region are common sites for metastatic intraperitoneal deposits, but other areas of the colon can be affected as well. Mural and mesenteric masses (Fig. 68) and stretched colonic loops can be seen.

Bulky masses, either single or multiple, or diffuse bowel nodularity and wall thickening can be seen with colonic lymphoma (Figs. 69 and 70). When present, splenomegaly and marked retroperitoneal or mesenteric adenopathy help make the diagnosis.

Colonic lipomas, lipomas of the ileocecal valve, or lipomatous infiltration of the valve can be identified and classified on CT by their characteristic low CT attenuation number (Fig. 71) (27). Other benign colonic tumors, if visible, appear as soft tissue density masses.

Inflammation

Computed tomography can be of use in the evaluation of several of the complications of diverticulosis and inflammatory bowel disease, such as abscess and fistula. Pericolonic abscesses due to tumor, diverticulitis, or appendicitis can be imaged (Fig. 72). A pericolonic diverticular abscess will appear as a mass with a thick wall of soft tissue density and a low density center that may contain gas (Fig. 73) or, if in communication with the lumen, contrast material. Uncomplicated diverticulosis of the colon may show a thickened colonic wall on CT due to the circular muscular hypertrophy (Fig. 74). Air- or contrast-material-filled diverticula can also be seen and should not be mistaken for air in the bowel wall or a perforation. An appendiceal abscess is, of course, most frequently located in the right lower quadrant but may occur in the cul-de-sac or right upper abdomen. Computed tomography will demonstrate an oval-to-round mass

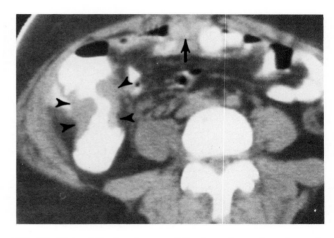

FIG. 68. Metastatic carcinoma of the breast causing circumferential thickening (arrowheads) of the colonic wall. A portion of an omental cake (arrow) is also present.

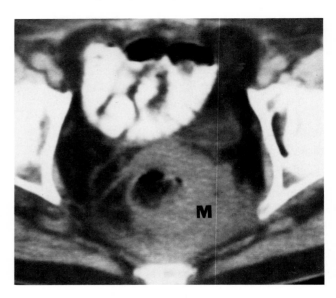

FIG. 69. Bulky mass (M) of lymphoma involving rectum and adjacent pelvic musculature.

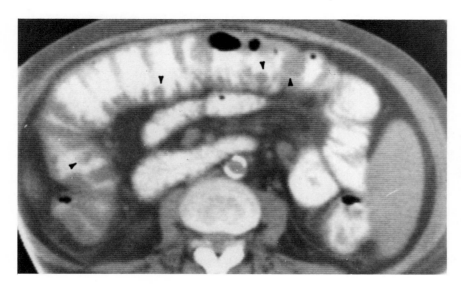

FIG. 70. Diffuse histiocytic lymphoma of the colon. There are nodules (arrowheads) of various sizes and thickening of the colon wall and interhaustral folds.

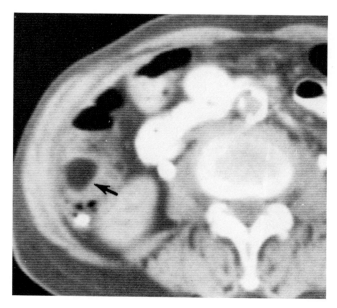

FIG. 71. Lipomatous infiltration of ileocecal valve (arrow) appears as a circumscribed cecal mass with density similar to subcutaneous fat.

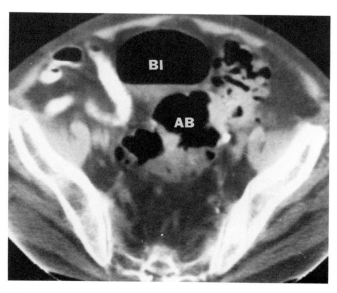

FIG. 73. Diverticulitis. There is a large gas-containing pericolonic mass representing a diverticular abscess (AB). Gas in the bladder (BI) indicates a colo-vesical fistula.

with a low density center that may contain gas and occasionally a densely calcified appendicolith.

A thick-walled colon can be seen in patients with Crohn's colitis (Fig. 75), pseudomembranous colitis, and colitis cystica profunda (Fig. 76) (11). Proctitis may appear on CT as a uniformly thickened rectal wall with a narrow lumen.

Miscellaneous

Obstruction

Mechanical obstruction of the colon can be identified on CT by the differential colonic distention proximal and distal to the site of obstruction. Occasionally the etiology of the obstruction can be ascertained. A primary obstructing malignancy can be seen as a soft tissue mass with or without a narrow, irregular lumen that has been opacified with contrast material (26). Tumors secondarily invading the colon can be seen, and their sites of origin may be determined. Ileocolic intussusception can be easily identified because of its characteristic CT appearance (35,37) described in the section on the small intestine (Figs. 54 and 55). In adults, 50% of colonic

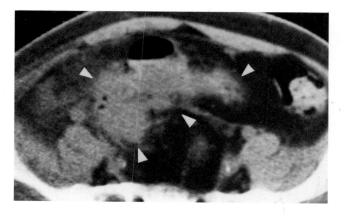

FIG. 72. Perforated sigmoid carcinoma. The inflammatory process (arrowheads) infiltrates the adjacent mesenteric fat.

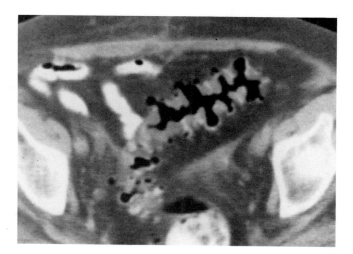

FIG. 74. Diverticulosis of sigmoid colon with associated thickening of circular colonic muscle. Air in diverticula should not be confused with air in the colonic wall.

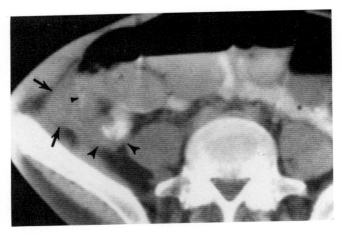

FIG. 75. Recurrent Crohn's disease in a patient who has undergone partial ileal resection with ileal-ascending colon anastomosis. A thickened and narrowed distal ileal segment (large arrowheads) is present along with an inflammatory mass (arrows) with a small sinus tract (small arrowhead) faintly opacified with contrast material.

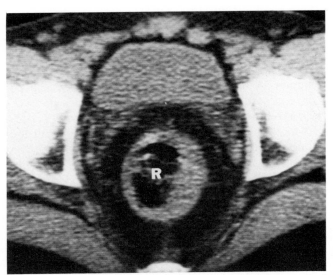

FIG. 76. Concentric but asymmetrical thickening of the wall of the rectum (R) in a young man with colitis cystica profunda.

intussusceptions are caused by malignant tumors, which are themselves occasionally imaged as a soft tissue mass within the intussuscipiens (35). A lipoma of the ileocecal valve is the most common benign tumor responsible for intussusception and may occasionally be seen as a well-defined mass within the intussuscipiens with characteristic fatty CT attenuation values.

Radiation

The CT findings in radiation effects on the distal colon include: (a) mural thickening of the irradiated segment, (b) widening of the presacral space, (c) increased perirectal fat, (d) thickening of perirectal fibrous tissue, and (e) fibrotic connections between the rectum and sacrum (Fig. 77) (7). The increased presacral space (greater than 1 cm) alone is a nonspecific finding and may be seen in normal patients. If there is significant increase in perirectal fat without fibrosis or bowel wall thickening, pelvic lipomatosis should be considered. Perirectal fibrous tissue is not seen or is barely visible in normal individuals. The asymmetrical increase in perirectal fibrous tissue found after radiation helps distinguish radiation proctitis from the asymmetrical appearance of recurrent tumor or postoperative fibrosis. Rarely, a similar symmetric appearance can be seen in extension of prostatic cancer or following extensive perirectal inflammatory disease. After radiation, the combination of increased perirectal fat and thickened perirectal fascia can produce a "halo effect" about the rectum, with the rectum itself being thick walled and narrow (7).

Ischemia

Ischemic bowel can be identified on CT by linear or punctate collections of gas in the bowel wall (Fig.

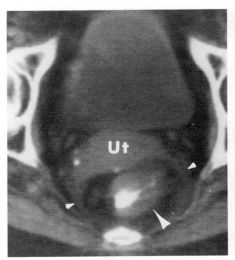
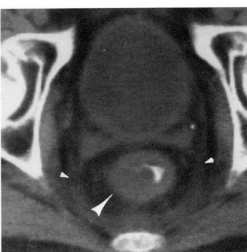

FIG. 77. Radiation proctitis. **Left:** Radiation for carcinoma of colon has resulted in irregular thickening of the rectal wall (large arrowhead) and prominence of the perirectal fascia (small arrowheads). Ut, uterus. **Right:** Similar findings in another patient after radiotherapy of prostatic carcinoma. Large arrowhead indicates rectal wall; small arrowheads indicate perirectal fascia.

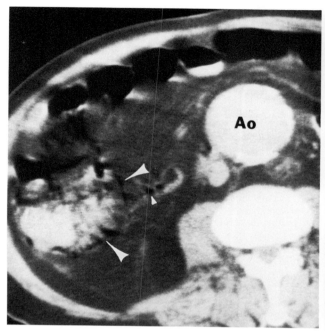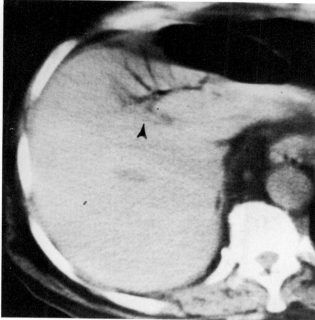

FIG. 78. CT performed for evaluation of acute abdominal pain in patient with known abdominal aortic aneurysm. **Left:** The aorta (Ao) is dilated but there is no sign of rupture. Intramural gas in the cecal wall (large arrowheads) and gas in mesenteric veins (small arrowhead) indicate colonic ischemia which was proved at operation. **Right:** Gas is also present in portal venous branches (arrowhead). (Case courtesy of Dr. Avery B. Brinkley, Jr.)

78). Gas can also extend into mesenteric and portal veins.

REFERENCES

1. Aspestrand F: Demonstration of thoracic and abdominal fistulas by computed tomography. *J Comput Assist Tomogr* 4:536–537, 1980
2. Balfe DM, Koehler RE, Karstaedt N, Stanley RJ, Sagel SS: Computed tomography of gastric neoplasms. *Radiology* 140:431–436, 1981
3. Cimmino CV: The esophageal-pleural stripe: An update. *Radiology* 140:609–613, 1981
4. Clark KE, Foley WD, Lawson TL, Berland LL, Maddison FE: CT evaluation of esophageal and upper abdominal varices. *J Comput Assist Tomogr* 4:510–515, 1980
5. Daffner RH, Halber MD, Postlethwait RW, Korobkin M, Thompson WM: CT of the esophagus. II. Carcinoma. *AJR* 133:1051–1055, 1979
6. Doubleday LC, Bernardino ME: CT findings in the perirectal area following radiation therapy. *J Comput Assist Tomogr* 4:634–638, 1980
7. Frommhold W, Hubener KH: The role of computerized tomography in the after care of patients suffering from a carcinoma of the rectum. *Comput Tomogr* 5:161–168, 1981
8. Glazer GM, Buy JN, Moss AA, Goldberg HI, Federle MP: CT detection of duodenal perforation. *AJR* 137:333–336, 1981
9. Goldwin RL, Heitzman ER, Proto AV: Computed tomography of the mediastinum. *Radiology* 124:235–241, 1977
10. Goodman PC, Federle MP: Pseudomembranous colitis. *J Comput Assist Tomogr* 4:403–404, 1980
11. Grant D, Aisner J: CT of peritoneal mesothelioma: Analysis of eight cases. *AJR* 138:531–535, 1982
12. Halber MD, Daffner RH, Thompson WM: CT of the esophagus: I. Normal appearance. *AJR* 133:1047–1050, 1979
13. Herlinger H: Small bowel. In: *Double Contrast Gastrointestinal Radiology with Endoscopic Correlation,* ed. by I Laufer, Philadelphia, Saunders, 1979, pp 448–454
14. Husband JE, Hodson NJ, Parsons CA: The use of computed tomography in recurrent rectal tumors. *Radiology* 134:677–682, 1980
15. Karnaze GC, Sheedy PF, Stephens DH, McLeod RA: Computed tomography in duodenal rupture due to blunt abdominal trauma. *J Comput Assist Tomogr* 5:267–269, 1981
16. Kaye MD, Young SW, Hayward R, Catellino RA: Gastric pseudotumor on CT scanning. *AJR* 135:190–193, 1980
17. Koehler RE: Neoplasms of the small bowel. In: *Alimentary Tract Radiology,* ed. by AR Margulis and HJ Burhenne, St. Louis, Mosby, 1982
18. Kressel HY, Callen PW, Montagne JP, Korobkin M, Goldberg HI, Moss AA, Arger PH, Margulis AR: Computed tomographic evaluation of disorders affecting the alimentary tract. *Radiology* 129:451–455, 1978
19. Kuwabara Y, Nishitani H, Numaguchi Y, Kamoi I, Matsuura K, Saito S: Afferent loop syndrome. *J Comput Assist Tomogr* 4:687–689, 1980
20. Lee JKT, Stanley RJ, Sagel SS, Levitt RG, McClennan BL: CT appearance of the pelvis after abdomino-perineal resection for rectal carcinoma. *Radiology* 141:737–741, 1981
21. Lee KR, Levine E, Moffat RE, Bigongiari LR, Hermreck AS: Computed tomographic staging of malignant gastric neoplasms. *Radiology* 133:151–155, 1979
22. Li DKB, Rennie CS: Abdominal computed tomography in Whipple's disease. *J Comput Assist Tomogr* 5:249–252, 1981
23. Marks WM, Callen PW, Moss AA: Gastroesophageal region: Source of confusion on CT. *AJR* 136:359–362, 1981
24. Marks WM, Goldberg HI, Moss AA, Koehler PR, Federle MP: Intestinal pseudotumors: A problem in abdominal computed tomography solved by directed techniques. *Gastrointest Radiol* 5:155–160, 1980
25. Marshak RH, Lindner AR, Maklansky D: Lymphoreticular disorders of the gastrointestinal tract: Roentgenographic features. *Gastrointest Radiol* 4:103–120, 1979

26. Mayes GB, Zornoza J: Computed tomography of colon carcinoma. *AJR* 135:43–46, 1980

27. Megibow AJ, Redmond PE, Bosniak MA, Horowitz L: Diagnosis of gastrointestinal lipomas by CT. *AJR* 133:743–745, 1979

28. Meyers MA: *Dynamic Radiology of the Abdomen.* New York, Springer-Verlag, 1976

29. Moss AA, Margulis AR, Schnyder P, Thoeni RF: A uniform, CT-based staging system for malignant neoplasms of the alimentary tube. *AJR* 136:1251–1252, 1981

30. Moss AA, Schnyder P, Candardjis G, Margulis AR: Computed tomography of benign and malignant gastric abnormalities. *J Clin Gastroenterol* 2:401–409, 1980

31. Moss AA, Schnyder P, Thoeni RF: Margulis AR: Esophageal carcinoma: Pretherapy staging by computed tomography. *AJR* 136:1051–1056, 1981

32. Moss AA, Thoeni RF, Schnyder P, Margulis AR: Value of computed tomography in the detection and staging of recurrent rectal carcinomas. *J Comput Assist Tomogr* 5:870–874, 1981

33. Noon MA, Young SW, Castellino RA: Leiomyosarcoma metastatic to the liver: CT appearance. *J Comput Assist Tomogr* 4:527–530, 1980

34. Pagani JJ, Bernardino ME: CT-radiographic correlation of ulcerating small bowel lymphomas. *AJR* 136:998–1000, 1981

35. Parienty RA, Lepreux JF, Gruson B: Sonographic and CT features of ileocolic intussusception. *AJR* 136:608–610, 1981

36. Seigel RS, Kuhns LR, Borlaza GS, McCormick TL, Simmons JL: Computed tomography and angiography in ileal carcinoid tumor and retractile mesenteritis. *Radiology* 134:437–440, 1980

37. Siegelman SS: *CT Diagnosis of Intussusception.* Presented at the Fifth Annual Course of the Society of Computed Body Tomography, Tarpon Springs, Florida, 1982

38. Thoeni RF, Moss AA, Schnyder P, Margulis AR: Detection and staging of primary rectal and rectosigmoid cancer by computed tomography. *Radiology* 141:135–138, 1981

39. Zaunbauer W, Haertel M, Fuchs WA: Computed tomography in carcinoma of the rectum. *Gastrointest Radiol* 6:79–84, 1981

Chapter 13

Kidney

Bruce L. McClennan and Joseph K. T. Lee

Computed tomography (CT) has been used to image a spectrum of renal diseases. The impact of CT on diagnostic uroradiology has been substantial and a clear view of the utility of CT scanning in the diagnosis of urologic disease is emerging (26,46,48,77,101,115,117, 127). Because of the cross-sectional anatomic display possible with CT, areas previously considered "blind" to most imaging techniques can now be demonstrated. The anterior and posterior surfaces of the kidney and the medial (hilar) and lateral aspects of the kidney as they relate to the renal vascular pedicle can be clearly imaged. In addition, the paranephric fascial compartments are vividly displayed. The nonvisualized kidney at urography is no longer as enigmatic a problem since CT is able to demonstrate the site and cause of most cases of obstructive hydronephrosis. Azotemia is no longer the stumbling block to adequate uroradiologic diagnosis, since CT can be performed in lieu of the urogram without the need for intravenous contrast material. Likewise, CT can serve to evaluate the kidneys in patients with contrast media sensitivity.

Computed tomography is superior to conventional radiography in resolving tissues with only minor differences in their attenuation values. Because of the increased contrast sensitivity, CT can differentiate a benign renal cyst from a solid renal mass. Computed tomography now has a specific acceptable role in the imaging decision tree for the renal mass (Fig. 1). Renal CT is quick and easy to perform, and free from operator dependence. It is noninvasive with little or no risk except that related to the use of intravenous, water soluble contrast material.

The indications for CT in the evaluation of patients with real or suspected renal diseases are continuously evolving (77). Table 1 lists the common and current indications for CT in modern uroradiologic practice. The effects on diagnostic processes and therapeutic management are seen daily. Computed tomography is frequently the only diagnostic imaging study required prior to definitive therapy. This chapter will focus on the problems outlined in Table 1, drawing largely on our experience at the Mallinckrodt Institute of Radiology as well as the published experience of others.

NORMAL ANATOMY

The cross-sectional anatomy of the normal kidney is clearly demonstrated by CT. The presence of perinephric and renal sinus fat provides the tissue contrast needed to define the renal contours and collecting system complex. Renal margins, especially along the anterior and posterior surfaces, are seen in their entirety, and visualization is more complete than is possible with urography and linear tomography. On noncontrast scans, the renal tissue density is uniform throughout with attenuation values measuring 30 to 60 Hounsfield units (HU) depending on patient hydration and hematocrit. Segments of the urine-filled renal pelvis and calyces with a near water density can be visualized on precontrast scans but are seen better after intravenous administration of contrast medium. The hilar vascular structures are frequently identified; when identified, the renal veins are anterior to the arteries and are usually of larger caliber (Fig. 2).

CONTRAST MEDIA UTILIZATION

In renal CT, intravenous contrast material is a fundamental requirement. It improves both lesion detection and definition, whether vascular or avascular (28,46). Contrast-medium-assisted CT provides a gross functional assessment of the kidney and relies on the physiologic phenomenon of contrast material excretion. Dynamic CT of the kidney takes advantage of the same urographic principles that relate to the appearance of the nephrogram and pyelogram (52). The functional information provided by contrast-medium-assisted renal CT may facilitate judgments concerning salvageability of an obstructed system by revealing the amount of residual functioning parenchyma. Some precontrast renal CT scans may be necessary for organ or lesion localization depending on availability of computed radiographic scouting capabilities. Precontrast scans are also required when the presence of calcification is suspected (28).

The methods of contrast material delivery for renal CT are either rapid intravenous bolus or intravenous

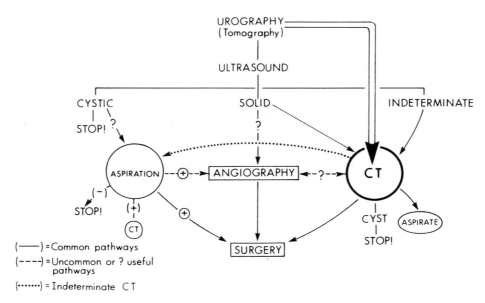

FIG. 1. Imaging evaluation of the renal mass. This flow chart describes the role of CT in the evaluation process for renal masses.

infusion techniques using a peripheral vein. Direct intraarterial injections are rarely, if ever, necessary. Rapid bolus injections (less than 15 sec) are by far the best method for contrast material delivery for most renal CT (70,133). Infusion techniques are usually reserved for opacification of major vascular structures such as the inferior vena cava, which may be opacified via a foot vein infusion when staging large, bulky renal cell carcinomas (124). Infusion techniques are also valuable when a large area must be studied. Small intravenous bolus injections of 10 to 40 cc of a 50 to 66% solution of contrast material are usually sufficient for assessment of mass enhancement or renal vascular integrity. Total doses of between 20 and 40 g of iodine given by the multiple, bolus technique are common in renal CT and in line with current urographic practice. Larger amounts of contrast material are rarely necessary under optimal scanning conditions (22,57).

The physiologic principles of contrast material excretion as they relate to urography can also be applied to CT. There is a linear relationship between iodine concentration and CT number (18,19). Therefore, an increase in plasma concentration of contrast material (iodine) will increase the CT number of the renal parenchyma taking into consideration method of delivery and time (18). A higher peak plasma concentration and therefore cortical CT number is achieved after a bolus injection of contrast material. The peak plasma concentration and renal cortical CT number achieved with infusion techniques are lower than with bolus injections but the peak is maintained longer (18,19). Scans performed with slower scanners or scans performed on trauma patients may require infusion methods of contrast material delivery for the above reasons.

The pharmacokinetics of intravenously administered contrast material seen with body CT is biphasic, that is, a rapid interstitial diffusion (total body effect) followed by slower, renal excretion (38). The renal handling of contrast material as observed by serial dynamic CT is really triphasic, namely, major vascular opacification (artery and vein) followed by a nephrogram and then, a pyelogram (Fig. 3). Some authors refer to these phases as bolus effect, nonequilibrium, and equilibrium, respectively (22). An intravenous bolus of contrast material delivered to the kidney first opac-

TABLE 1. *Indications for renal CT*

Renal masses
    Cyst, tumor, abscess, hematoma, cortical nodule (pseudotumor), calcification
Renal failure
    Hydronephrosis—degree and cause; parenchymal diseases
Juxtarenal processes (peri-, pararenal)
    Blood, pus, urine, lymph, effusion, tumor, fat, air
Oncologic management
    Tumor detection, staging, treatment planning, and follow-up
Miscellaneous
    Trauma, contrast media sensitivity, congenital anomalies, allografts

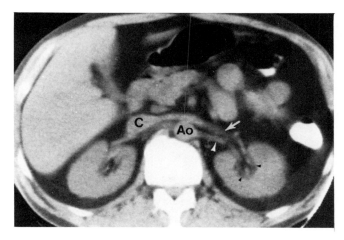

FIG. 2. Normal renal anatomy. Both kidneys are surrounded by abundant perinephric fat. The renal hilum (black arrowheads) generally contains fat and can, therefore, be differentiated from adjacent parenchyma. The renal vein (arrow) lies anterior to the renal artery (white arrowhead). Ao, aorta; C, inferior vena cava.

ifies the aorta and renal arteries. Interstitial diffusion is not as important a consideration as it may be in other organ systems because of the excretory nature of the kidney (57). The time density curve for each renal artery should parallel the aorta in the absence of significant renal artery stenosis or increased intrarenal vascular resistance (132). A CT renal angiogram will show the aorta, renal artery, and renal vein, followed immediately by an intense vascular nephrogram outlining the corticomedullary junction, which quickly becomes a tubular nephrogram identical to that seen during intravenous urography (Fig. 3). The attenuation value of the renal parenchyma may increase to 80 to 120 HU after contrast material administration. The degree of enhancement depends on the patient's renal function and the method of contrast material delivery.

The nephrogram as visualized by CT after a rapid bolus injection of contrast material is initially a vascular nephrogram with prompt (less than 1 min) demonstration of the cortical thickness (corticomedullary junction). In fact, the appearance time of the corticomedullary junction correlates well with renal functional impairment in that it has been shown to be delayed compared with the normal (normal = 67 ±1.3 sec) (52). The amount of normal cortex and its thickness as measured by CT are inversely proportional to the patient's age (52).

As contrast material reaches the tubules, medullary opacification occurs, usually between 1 and 3 min. Medullary opacification is greatest during this time period, that is, 1 to 3 min, and may be even denser (higher attenuation values) than cortex (18,19). The CT number of the cortical nephrogram is dose dependent in a linear fashion up to the maximum clearance values for the agent (18,19). The cation portion of the contrast medium molecule (sodium or meglumine salt)

does not seem to affect the CT number measured during the nephrogram. However, higher CT numbers were achieved in the medulla of a dog with sodium salts compared with meglumine salts (18,19). If this has diagnostic significance in humans is uncertain at this point.

A pyelogram develops at approximately the 2- to 3-min interval and progresses toward calyceal filling and distention similar to that observed urographically. Computed tomography allows the most optimal visual evidence of contrast material excretion by the kidney achieved to date. Intrarenal distribution can be documented and, in fact, quantified as to amount and percentage change in either the cortex or the medulla (18,19). This may have potential direct clinical use in evaluating medical renal diseases. Certainly poor excretion of contrast material due to renal failure or trauma to the kidneys or even excretion of lower doses of contrast material than would be required for optimal urography can be recorded using CT. Therefore, the amount of contrast material required for routine renal CT in patients with normal renal function may even be less than that required for conventional urography. Crude functional assessments can be made even in the face of severe renal failure, unilaterally or bilaterally, with or without intravenous contrast material since parenchymal thickness can be quickly estimated in both kidneys and potential salvageability determined.

Because of the improved spatial resolution of CT compared with radionuclide scanning, the assessment of real or suspected renal ischemia may be better using CT (49,90,132). Time density curves generated for the aorta and renal artery can detect renal artery stenosis in dogs; renal ischemia created by balloon occlusion of the renal artery can be easily detected especially when intravenous contrast material is used (49). The attenuation value (CT number) of the ischemic kidney actually increases, i.e. approximately 10 HU units, compared with control parenchymal values (49,125). Prolonged ischemia or actual frank renal infarction tends to lower CT numbers both before and after intravenous contrast material administration. The segmental nature of renal infarcts makes their CT detection straightforward in most cases (42,45) (Fig. 4). Renal vein thrombosis or aneurysm formation in the renal arteries can be shown effectively using contrast-material-assisted CT, often-times eliminating the need for more invasive vascular procedures. A "patchy" nephrogram that persists may actually be due to intrarenal vasoconstriction secondary to acute tubular necrosis (ATN) (54). Patchy nephrographic patterns have also been seen in trauma, bacterial nephritis, interstitial nephritis, lymphoma, and polyarteritis nodosa (93). Similarly, prolonged, diffusely dense nephrograms on CT have been seen in glomerulonephritis, leukemia, and urate nephropathy (76).

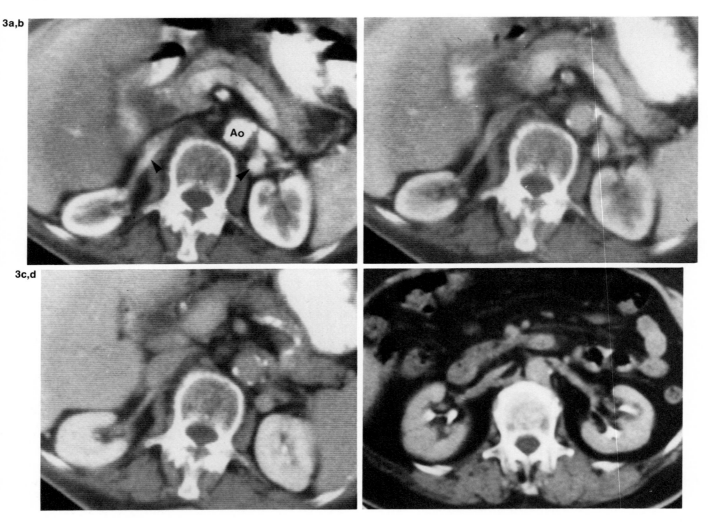

3a,b

3c,d

FIG. 3. a–c: Normal CT nephrogram following a bolus injection. **a:** Vascular phase. Note the aorta (Ao) and arterial branches (arrowheads) are densely opacified. The markedly enhanced renal cortex can be clearly differentiated from lower density medulla on this scan. **b:** Fifteen sec following scan (a) The density difference between renal cortex and medulla has decreased. **c:** Tubular nephrogram on scan obtained approximately 60 sec after the injection. The medulla now has enhanced to a similar degree as the renal cortex. **d:** Normal pyelogram in a different patient. The pyelocalyceal system is well opacified by contrast at this stage.

NORMAL VARIANTS AND CONGENITAL ANOMALIES

As with urography, knowledge of the varied CT presentations of congenital anomalies of the kidney and minor anatomical variants is essential to the understanding and diagnosis of renal pathology. Normal variations in renal anatomy, such as the dromedary (splenic) hump suggesting a renal mass or the extrarenal pelvis simulating hydronephrosis on ultrasound, should be easily recognizable by their CT patterns. Suspected mass lesions on urography are frequently just prominent, persistent fetal lobulations when imaged with CT (67). These parenchymal nodules will enhance with intravenous contrast material to the same degree as normal renal parenchyma (Fig. 5) and, when centrally placed, will stand out as the commonly

encountered column of Bertin. Such normal variations in renal morphology must be distinguished from pathologic processes and focal compensatory hypertrophy (6).

Common congenital anomalies of fusion such as horseshoe kidney (Fig. 6), cross-fused ectopy, and duplex kidneys as well as renal agenesis, hypoplasia, and simple ectopia all have characteristic CT appearances. Ptotic or frankly ectopic kidneys can be confusing when encountered on CT. Enlargement of the liver or the spleen will push the right or left kidney caudad and rotate it about its horizontal axis making it appear spuriously enlarged (Fig. 7). An excessive accumulation of retroperitoneal fat can also cause renal axis shift but this is commonly lateral with rotation about the vertical axis (101). Duplex kidneys with obstruction of one moiety (usually upper) may mimic renal mass lesions on precontrast CT scans (50) (Fig. 8). When a kidney is congenitally absent or ectopic or removed, the splenic flexure and pancreatic tail will fill the renal fossa on the left (Fig. 9) whereas the liver, duodenum, proximal small bowel, and hepatic flexure may fill the fossa on the right. Intravenous contrast material and oral contrast material opacifications are mandatory in these instances for accurate diagnosis.

The finding of a small or unilaterally hypoplastic kidney suggests some previously acquired insult. True congenital hypoplasia is rare and may be difficult to document.

A normal variant seen in the aging kidney is renal sinus lipomatosis (Fig. 10). Variably described to occur in between 0.6 and 1.25% of the adult population, this phenomenon can cause differential diagnostic difficulties (43). The quantity of renal sinus fat varies and the proportion between fibrous and fatty component also varies. Renal sinus lipomatosis can mimic

parapelvic cyst formation and even hydronephrosis on precontrast CT scans. Renal sinus lipomatosis may measure near-water density if only a small amount of sinus fat is present because of partial volume averaging or if fat and fibrous tissue are almost equally mixed. Occasionally, renal sinus lipomatosis and parapelvic cyst formation may even coexist. Since both renal sinus lipomatosis and parapelvic cysts are benign lesions, efforts to differentiate between these two entities may become just an academic exercise.

PATHOLOGIC CONDITIONS

Renal Masses

The impact of CT has been great in the diagnostic clarification of renal mass lesions (5,59,66,71,77). The

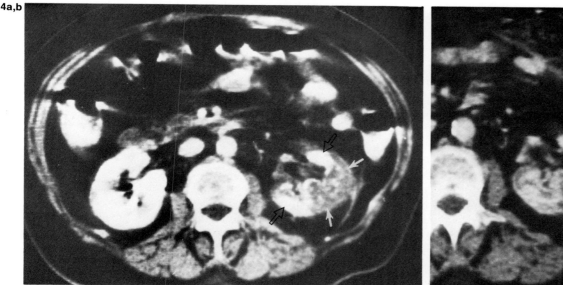

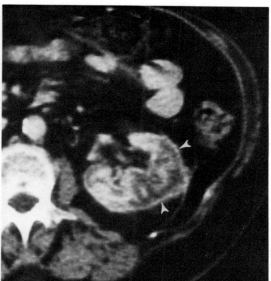

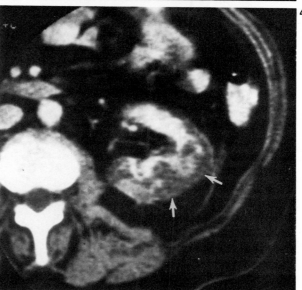

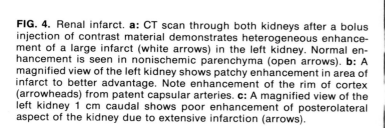

FIG. 4. Renal infarct. **a:** CT scan through both kidneys after a bolus injection of contrast material demonstrates heterogeneous enhancement of a large infarct (white arrows) in the left kidney. Normal enhancement is seen in nonischemic parenchyma (open arrows). **b:** A magnified view of the left kidney shows patchy enhancement in area of infarct to better advantage. Note enhancement of the rim of cortex (arrowheads) from patent capsular arteries. **c:** A magnified view of the left kidney 1 cm caudal shows poor enhancement of posterolateral aspect of the kidney due to extensive infarction (arrows).

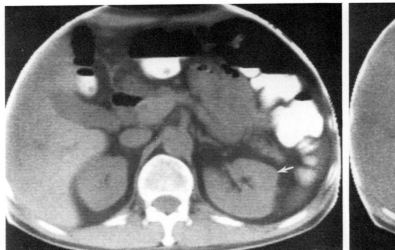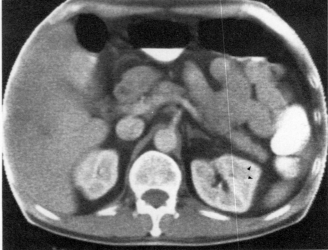

FIG. 5. Dromedary hump. **Left:** A prominent splenic (dromedary) hump (arrow) is seen in the left kidney. **Right:** After a bolus of contrast material, the dromedary hump is seen to enhance as normal renal parenchyma. A sharp corticomedullary junction exists in the area of the dromedary hump (arrowheads).

excretory urogram with routine tomography still remains the major screening test for *detection* of the renal mass, but, once detected, further *definition* and *diagnosis* are best performed using CT. Modern gray scale ultrasonography plays a significant role in the work-up of the renal mass, but the position of CT scanning in the evaluation of renal masses is much clearer (Fig. 1). The diagnostic accuracy of properly performed CT for separating cyst from neoplasm is extremely high, well over 90% in our experience (78, 101). The analysis of the CT image of a renal mass involves consideration of several features including mass size, shape (walls), location, number, internal density characteristics (attenuation value), contrast enhancement, and relationship to other organs. These features individually or collectively are considered when a CT

diagnosis of a renal mass is rendered. One must also relate these features to the individual scanner geometry, speed, resolution capability, and, of course, the patient's condition (78).

Renal Cystic Disease

Simple cysts.

The most common renal mass is the renal cyst (Fig. 11). Most cysts are cortical in location and are round in shape. They may be solitary or multiple and are often on the front or back surfaces of the kidneys (Fig. 12). Masses in these locations are extremely difficult to detect by excretory urography even with linear tomography. Cortical cysts increase in number with age and

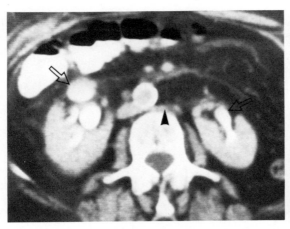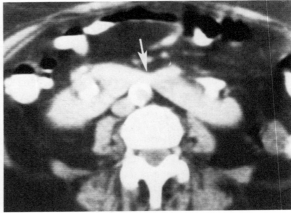

FIG. 6. Horseshoe kidney. **Left:** Postcontrast CT scan demonstrates malrotation of both upper poles at this level. The renal pelves (open arrows) are directed anteriorly. Minimal obstruction of the ureters, a common feature of horseshoe kidney, accounts for the caliectasis. Also of note is a retroaortic left renal vein (arrowhead). **Right:** The midline isthmus (arrow) enhances to the same degree as the rest of the kidney indicating that it is all functioning parenchyma.

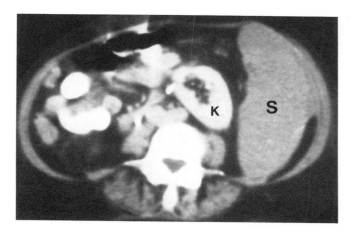

FIG. 7. Caudal displacement of left kidney (K) by a markedly enlarged spleen (S) in a patient with non-Hodgkin's lymphoma. The anteroposterior diameter of the kidney is increased due to rotation about its horizontal axis.

50% of patients over the age of 50 have one or more cortical cysts seen at autopsy. The requisite CT features for a benign renal cyst are as follows: (a) homogeneous near-water density, (b) no enhancement with contrast material, (c) no detectable wall (when cysts project be-

yond renal outline), (d) smooth interface with parenchyma.

When the above-listed criteria are strictly met, the CT diagnosis of a renal cyst is certain (78). It is our policy *not* to routinely aspirate all renal cysts since CT discovers a myriad of incidental renal cysts. In the asymptomatic patient, if the CT criteria are successfully met for a renal cyst, no further imaging studies are needed. Renal angiography, mass aspiration, and surgical exploration are reserved for those masses that cannot be confidently categorized as a simple cyst; this will be discussed further in the section on indeterminate renal masses (8,78).

Renal cysts are often small, less than 1 cm, but usually resolvable down to 5 mm in diameter using current generation CT scanners. Masses smaller than scan slice (collimator) thickness may be volume averaged leading to spurious attenuation measurements (21). Rarely, a renal cyst may have a higher than acceptable central attenuation value for the presumed fluid content even when studied with narrow collimation (2–5 mm). As experience has accumulated, it has become clear that CT numbers cannot be considered absolute values. A wide range of CT numbers has been ob-

8a,b

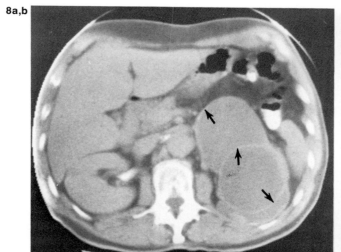 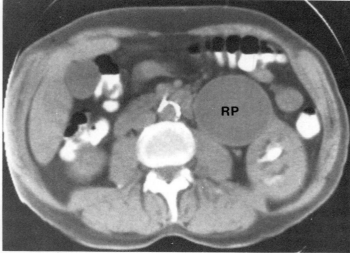

8c

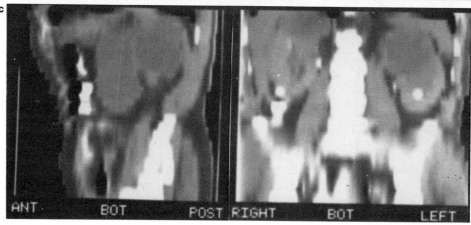

ANT.   BOT   POST RIGHT   BOT   LEFT

FIG. 8. Duplex left kidney with obstruction of upper pole moiety. a: A dilated, obstructed upper pole duplication is seen in the position of the left kidney. The lower pole of the left kidney is displaced inferiorly. Only rim enhancement (arrows) of the duplication is present. b: Two centimeters caudal the lower pole of the left kidney with dilated renal pelvis (RP) medial to it is shown. c: From left to right, sagittal and coronal reconstructions of left upper pole duplication.

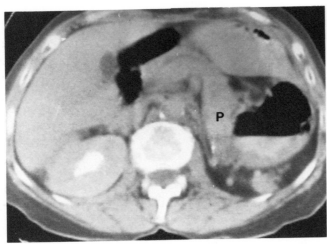
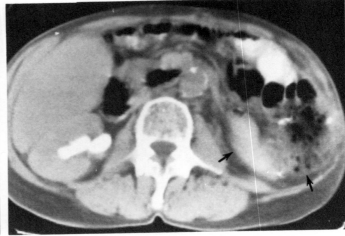

FIG. 9. Normal postnephrectomy changes. **Left:** The left kidney has been removed for renal cell carcinoma. Compensatory hypertrophy of the right kidney is seen. Note vertical orientation of body and tail of pancreas (P), a frequent finding after left nephrectomy. **Right:** Two centimeters caudal contrast-medium-filled small and large bowel loops (arrows) are seen in the left renal bed.

served for a given tissue type depending on various factors such as kVp and location within the scanning ring. Therefore, it is often valuable to compare the attenuation value of a renal mass with the density of a known standard, such as a paraspinal muscle in the same patient. Furthermore, the range of acceptable attenuation values for a benign renal cyst must be determined for each individual scanner. Our levels range from 0 to 20 HU using an EMI 7070 body scanner. Overreliance on exact measurements, however, can lead to diagnostic errors, but every effort should be made to assure correct measurements in a confusing lesion. Recalibration and phantom water measurements may occasionally be necessary.

Although rare, a simple renal cyst may have a higher attenuation value than normal renal parenchyma on noncontrast enhanced CT scans (Fig. 13) (25). High attenuation cysts are often solitary but also can be

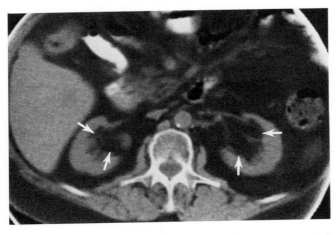

FIG. 10. Renal sinus lipomatosis. There is increased amount of renal sinus fat (arrows) bilaterally causing compression of the renal hilar vessels and pylocalyceal system.

seen in polycystic kidneys (61). The cysts are noncalcified and contain fluid of varying character. Some contain thick, dark, crankcase oil-like fluid whereas others have clear yellow-orange fluid. Because renal cyst fluid is in limited equilibrium with urine, the theory that intravenous contrast material may account for some high central attenuation measurements has been suggested. Shanser and co-workers analyzed aspirated renal cyst fluid 24 to 96 hr after performance of excretory urography (109). They compared the iodine concentration with serum samples obtained simultaneously. Iodine was found to enter a renal cyst after excretory urography, remaining there for at least 96 hr. The iodine levels in the cyst fluid, however, were insufficient to cause measurable differences in the attenuation value of the cyst fluid pre- and postcontrast and would not account for a cyst appearing solid on CT.

If a renal cyst is cortical in location and of sufficient size to project beyond the renal margin, the wall of the cyst should be imperceptible. A parenchymal spur or beak may be seen on CT similar to the beak of compressed renal parenchyma seen on nephrotomography. If the renal cyst is polar, transverse CT scans may be obtained through the spur or beak of renal parenchyma (108) and result in a pseudo-thick wall appearance. Care must be taken to obtain scans through that portion of the renal cyst outside the true confines of the kidney. Direct coronal scans or coronal/sagittal reconstruction may resolve this problem of the pseudo-thick wall sign. If the wall is definitely thick, then the diagnosis may still be a renal cyst, but it would have to be a "complicated" renal cyst, i.e., infected cyst, hemorrhagic cyst, or cystic neoplasm, but not the true "blue-domed" cyst familiar to the urologic surgeon (8). Tumor in the wall of a cyst or a "cystic" neoplasm has been seen but the walls have been focally or uni-

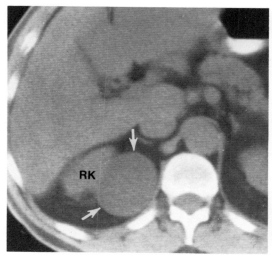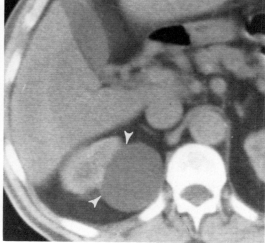

FIG. 11. Simple renal cyst. **Left:** Precontrast CT scan demonstrates a well-marginated mass (arrows) arising from the medial aspect of the upper pole of the right kidney (RK). The attention value of this mass was +4 HU. **Right:** Postcontrast scan demonstrates no enhancement within the mass. The interface between the kidney and the mass is sharp and smooth (arrowheads). These CT features are characteristic of a benign renal cyst.

formly thick. An intrarenal cyst has been reported with a tiny benign hemangioma at its base not visible using early generation CT scanners (118). Even with state of the art CT scanners, a small tumor in the wall or at the base of a cyst could go undetected, if the slice level did not pass directly through the lesion or volume averaging obscured it (84,86). If microscopic hematuria was the initial reason for the examination, selective magnification renal arteriography might be an appropriate next imaging method in the search for an occult lesion.

Peripelvic/parapelvic cysts.

Parapelvic cysts or parapelvic uriniferous pseudocysts are thought to be either lymphatic in origin or acquired lesions secondary to prior obstruction with subsequent urine extravasation. Parapelvic renal cysts display the same CT features as cortical renal cysts. They have a near-water attenuation value and can be multiple or multilocular (Fig. 14). Parapelvic cysts will displace or replace renal hilar fat. Areas of compressed renal tissue, hilar vessels, or contiguous calyces may simulate a thick wall. Parapelvic cysts may be bilateral and, on rare occasion, may communicate with the renal sinus or collecting system. On noncontrast CT scans, parapelvic cysts may often mimic hydronephrosis or a large extrarenal pelvis; scans after administration of intravenous contrast medium easily solve this problem.

Adult polycystic kidney disease.

Adult polycystic kidney disease is almost invariably bilateral although unilateral involvement has been described (61,62) (Figs. 15–17). Patients with this dis-

ease often present without evidence of renal failure. Abdominal mass or hypertension may be the clinical finding. In patients with a known diagnosis, the search for focal neoplastic change or abscess often prompts CT evaluation.

The cysts vary in size and are usually seen throughout the entire substance of the kidney. Although most cysts in polycystic kidney disease are near-water density, some of them have higher attenuation values, presumably due to inspissated mucoid content (Fig. 15). Asymmetrical renal involvement is common (Fig. 17). Other organ involvement, such as the liver, the spleen, and the pancreas, can be evaluated similarly. Because ionizing radiation should be avoided when possible, US is the procedure of choice in the routine follow-up of patients with polycystic kidney disease and in initial screening of their family members. Computed tomog-

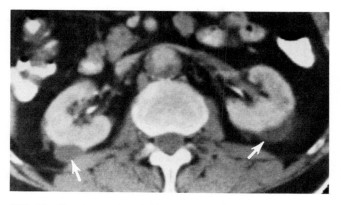

FIG. 12. Simple renal cyst. Postcontrast CT scan shows small cortical cysts (arrows) arising from posterior surface of each kidney. Cysts in this location are extremely difficult to see on an excretory urogram.

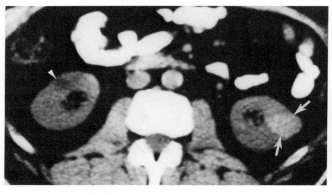
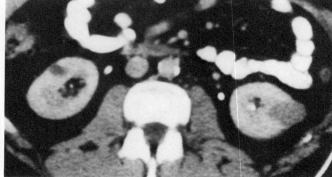

FIG. 13. Hyperdense renal cyst. **Left:** Precontrast CT scan shows a 2-cm mass (arrows) arising from the lateral aspect of the left kidney. The mass has a higher attenuation value than adjacent renal parenchyma. A smaller renal cyst (arrowhead) is present in the right kidney. **Right:** Postcontrast scan demonstrates a sharp interface between the nonenhanced mass and enhanced renal parenchyma. Because of the high attenuation value, which is atypical for a benign renal cyst, the left kidney was explored and the mass resected. Pathology: benign renal cyst.

raphy should be reserved for evaluation of possible hemorrhage or malignant transformation.

Von Hippel-Lindau disease.

Patients with Von Hippel-Lindau disease, with its frequent cystic renal involvement and, more importantly, frequent concurrent renal cell carcinoma, are optimally imaged with CT (65) (Fig. 18). Often, however, the renal cell carcinoma is diffuse throughout the kidney rather than a focal tumorous process. Compressed renal parenchyma may be difficult to differentiate from carcinomatous involvement, especially when cystic involvement is extensive.

Tuberous sclerosis.

Tuberous sclerosis, when it involves the kidney, is usually in the form of multiple hamartomas, commonly called angiomyolipomas (41,44,122,126). Cystic involvement is a part of the spectrum of this disease as well, but the cysts are usually small. CT differentiation of the cysts from small fatty tumors may be difficult if 1-cm collimation is used. Repeat scan using narrower

collimation, e.g., 2 or 5 mm, can often resolve this problem (Fig. 19). Furthermore, the need to separate cyst from small angiomyolipoma is in essence academic when renal involvement is diffuse. Renal failure is associated with tuberous sclerosis and can be severe. This is thought to be due to the cystic involvement of the kidney. In this case, confusion with adult polycystic kidney disease may exist, but the cysts in tuberous sclerosis rarely get larger than 3 cm.

Cystic disease of chronic dialysis.

A recently recognized cause of diffuse acquired cystic renal disease is chronic dialysis (53). The kidney not only decreases in overall mass and volume during the first 3 years of chronic dialysis, but also cystic degeneration occurs throughout the remaining native kidneys. In one study, the incidence of renal cysts was noted to increase considerably in patients who had been on dialysis more than 3 years in duration (53). In addition, there is also an increased incidence of renal and perirenal hemorrhage as well as an apparent increased incidence of adenoma or adenocarcinoma in these patients. Whether CT should be used for sur-

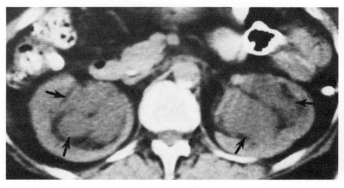
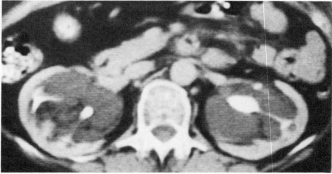

FIG. 14. Peripelvic/parapelvic cyst. **Left:** Multiple near-water density masses (arrows) are present in the renal sinus bilaterally. **Right:** Postcontrast scan accentuates the density difference between enhanced renal parenchyma and nonenhanced parapelvic cysts. Note compression of pyelocalyceal system and renal sinus fat by these cysts.

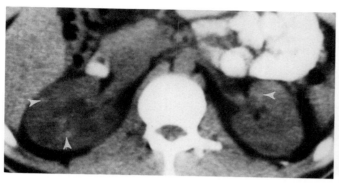
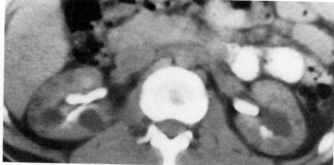

FIG. 15. Adult polycystic kidney disease—early stage. **Left:** Multiple small to medium sized cysts are present bilaterally in a young man with a family history of polycystic disease. Areas of high attenuation (arrowheads) believed to represent inspissated mucoid material or calcified walls can be seen in several cysts. **Right:** Postcontrast scan shows renal cysts more clearly.

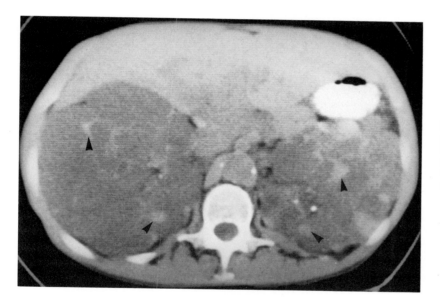

FIG. 16. Adult polycystic kidney disease—advanced stage. Both kidneys are markedly enlarged and contain numerous cysts of varying sizes. Only islands of functioning renal parenchyma (arrowheads) are left in a patient with renal failure.

FIG. 17. Adult polycystic kidney disease—asymmetric involvement. Postcontrast CT scan demonstrates extensive cystic involvement of the left kidney. Small cysts are present in the right kidney (arrowheads).

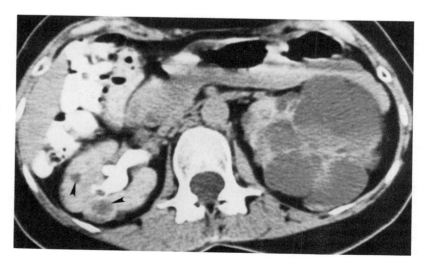

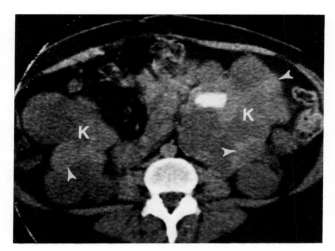

FIG. 18. Von Hippel-Lindau disease. Postcontrast CT scan shows both kidneys (K) to be enlarged with numerous cystic and solid masses. Enhancing areas (arrowheads) represent extensive renal cell carcinoma proven by angiography and surgery.

veillance purposes in these patients is yet to be determined.

Other renal cystic disease.

A multilocular cystic nephroma (MLCN) is a localized cystic disease of the kidney (88,98). On CT scans, it appears as a renal mass with thick walls and septations

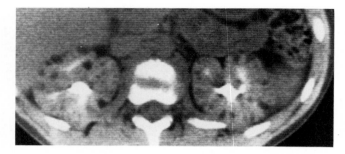

FIG. 19. Tuberous sclerosis. Postcontrast CT scan demonstrates numerous small fat density masses within both kidneys. Differentiation between a cyst and a small angiomyolipoma may be difficult if the mass is only a few millimeters in size. (From Totty et al., ref. 122, with permission.)

(88) (Fig. 20). Although not pathognomonic, CT demonstration of such a lesion in an asymptomatic adult female should suggest the diagnosis. Very rarely a cystic renal cell carcinoma may mimic the CT pattern of MLCN.

The CT appearance of multicystic dysplastic kidney has been limited to 2 isolated case reports (23,120); we also have encountered such a case (Fig. 21).

Renal Neoplasms

Adenocarcinoma.

Renal neoplasms, the most common of which are

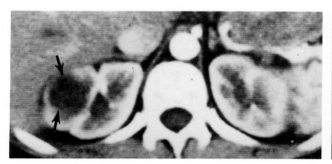
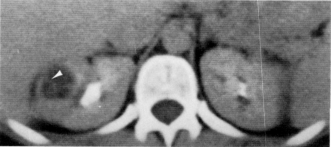

FIG. 20. Multilocular cystic nephroma. **Left:** CT scan obtained 15 sec after a bolus injection shows a bulging low-density mass (arrows) arising from the lateral aspect of the right kidney. Linear internal septations are faintly visible. **Right:** Delayed scan more clearly defines the margins of this moderately thick-walled cystic mass. Internal septations (arrowhead), commonly seen in this entity, are well delineated.

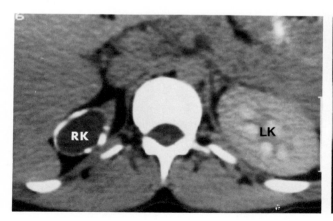
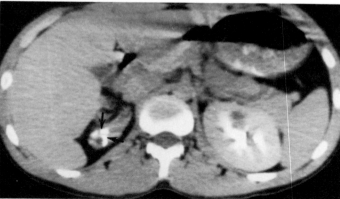

FIG. 21. Adult multicystic dysplastic kidney. **Left:** Postcontrast CT scan shows enlarged left kidney (LK) and the calcified cystic remnant of right kidney (RK). **Right:** One centimeter cephalad, clumps of calcification (arrows) are noted within the posterior aspect of the dysplastic right kidney.

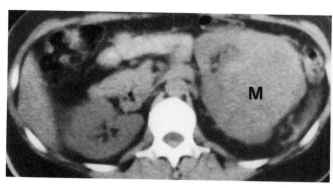
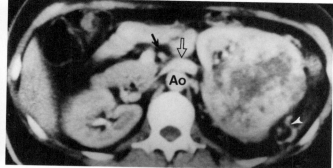

FIG. 22. Renal cell carcinoma. **Left:** Precontrast CT scan shows a large mass (M) arising from the posterolateral surface of the left kidney. The kidney is displaced anteromedially by it. The mass is essentially isodense compared to normal renal parenchyma. **Right:** Postcontrast scan following a bolus injection demonstrates nonuniform enhancement of the tumor. The central low-density area consists of necrotic, avascular tissue. In spite of its large size, the tumor remains confined within Gerota's fascia. The open arrow points to a normal appearing main left renal vein. Note the compression (nutcracker effect) of the left renal vein between the aorta (Ao) and superior mesenteric artery (black arrow). Arrowhead points to a large capsular vessel supplying the tumor.

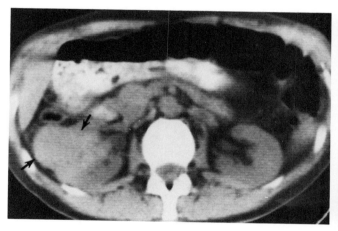
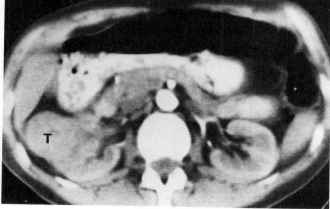

FIG. 23. Hyperdense renal cell carcinoma. **Left:** An irregular mass (arrows) with higher density than normal renal parenchyma is seen projecting from the lateral aspect of the right kidney. **Right:** Ten sec after a bolus injection of contrast material, a heterogeneous enhancement pattern is seen within the tumor (T). The interface between the tumor and surrounding normal renal parenchyma is rather indistinct.

adenocarcinomas, are diagnosed on CT scan by the distortion created in the renal outline, collecting system, or renal sinus fat (Fig. 22). The criteria for the diagnosis of a renal tumor by CT include: (a) Often heterogeneous attenuation value close to but normally less than that of renal parenchyma ($N = 20-30$ HU). Less commonly, the tumor may appear denser than normal renal parenchyma on precontrast images (Fig. 23). (b) Definite contrast enhancement, but always less than the surrounding normal parenchyma in both the nonequilibrium (nephrogram) and equilibrium (pyelogram) phases. Transient, marked enhancement can be seen during the arterial phase of ''CT angiography,'' when a bolus technique is used. (c) Unsharp interface with the surrounding renal parenchyma but encapsulation is occasionally seen. When encapsulated the wall is thick and irregular. (d) Secondary characteristics, such as renal vein or renal artery enlargement, nodular areas of soft tissue attenuation within the perinephric space, enlarged

regional lymph nodes, gross invasion of the inferior vena cava or main renal vein, and hepatic metastases (Figs. 24–28).

Based on these criteria, CT is highly accurate in the diagnosis of renal cell carcinoma (64,68). In one study, CT interpretation was correct in 59 of 62 cases of renal cell carcinoma with 3 indeterminate cases (124). Because bilateral renal cell carcinomas do occur on occasion, careful analysis of the contralateral kidney in patients with renal cell carcinoma cannot be overemphasized. Since a tissue specific diagnosis is not possible with CT, differentiation between a primary renal cell carcinoma and an extensive retroperitoneal tumor invading the kidney may be difficult. Other entities, such as lymphoma, adrenal carcinoma, metastatic disease, or xanthogranulomatous pyelonephritis, may on occasion exhibit CT features similar to a renal cell carcinoma.

Besides being used for initial diagnosis, CT also can

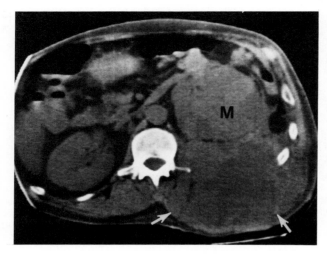

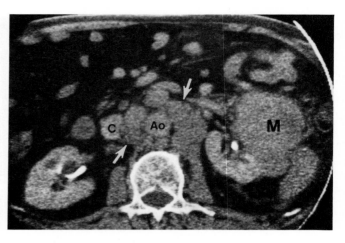

FIG. 24. Renal cell carcinoma invading contiguous tissue spaces. A large tumor mass (M) is present in the left kidney. In addition, there is direct infiltration of the musculature of the back (arrows). The extent of this malignancy could not be appreciated by either physical examination or arteriography. (From Weyman et al., ref. 124, with permission.)

FIG. 25. Renal cell carcinoma with lymph node metastases. Multiple enlarged retroperitoneal lymph nodes (arrows) are present in this patient with a primary left renal cell carcinoma (M). The aorta (Ao) and inferior vena cava (C) are displaced by the large lymph nodes. (From Weyman et al., ref. 124, with permission.)

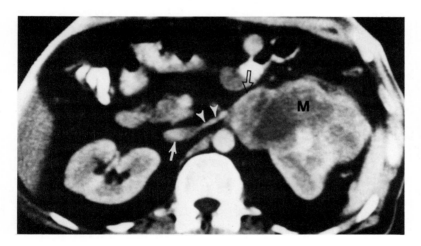

FIG. 26. Renal cell carcinoma with renal vein invasion. A large necrotic tumor mass (M) arising from the anterior surface of the left kidney extends medially to involve the proximal portion of the left renal vein (open arrow). Note that the distal portion of the left renal vein (arrowheads) is normal in size. The inferior vena cava (arrow) is also normal.

be used to delineate the extent of renal cell carcinoma (124). Although Robson's classification[1] of renal cell carcinoma is used by many investigators (94), it has the problem of including perirenal extension with lymph node and renal vein involvement in the same clinical stage (Stage III). Lymph node metastasis confers a very bad prognosis but renal vein involvement alone is no worse than perirenal extension confined to Gerota's fascia (112). A more precise preoperative staging is made possible by CT.

On CT scans, tumor extension beyond the renal confines is recognized as an indistinct tumor margin with strands (webs) of soft tissue density extending into the perirenal fat (Fig. 24). Irregular or streaky densities into the perirenal space may be seen in the absence of true tumor spread because of collateral vascular supply, edema, or thickening of connective tissue septa. Minute amounts of perirenal extension or microscopic invasion are often not visible on CT scans. Since radical nephrectomy includes en bloc removal of the kidney, perirenal fat, and Gerota's fascia, such minor degrees of perirenal involvement do not alter surgical treatment. Since Gerota's fascia can be visualized in most individuals using current generation CT scanners, caution must be used when interpreting thickening of Gerota's fascia as indicative of tumor involvement in the absence of frank tumor invasion of adjacent organs. Local or diffuse thickening of Gerota's fascia is a *nonspecific* sign. In fact, a lack of correlation between tu-

---

[1] Robson's classification of renal cell carcinoma: I, tumor confined within the renal capsule; II, Perirenal extension but not beyond Gerota's fascia; III, perirenal extension, lymph node involvement and venous invasion, and; IV, adjacent or distant organ involvement.

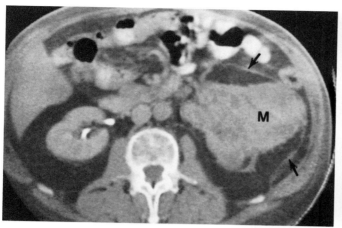

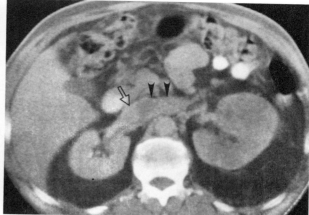

FIG. 27. Renal cell carcinoma with left renal vein invasion. **Left:** A large carcinoma (M) of the left kidney is present. Thickening of Gerota's fascia is also seen (arrows). **Right:** Postcontrast scan 2 cm cephalad shows a dilated left renal vein filled with tumor thrombus (arrowheads). The thrombus extends to the inferior vena cava (open arrow).

28a

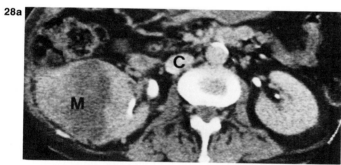

FIG. 28. Renal cell carcinoma with inferior vena cava and hepatic metastases. **a:** A large necrotic tumor (M) is seen arising from the lateral surface of the right kidney. Note that the inferior vena cava (C) is normal size. **b:** Scan 3 cm cephalad shows an irregular, low density metastasis (black arrowheads) in the left lobe of the liver. The right renal vein (white arrow) and inferior vena cava (black arrow) are markedly enlarged due to tumor invasion. **c:** Scan 6 cm more cephalad better demonstrates the venous tumor thrombus (open arrow). (From Weyman et al., ref. 124, with permission.)

28b,c

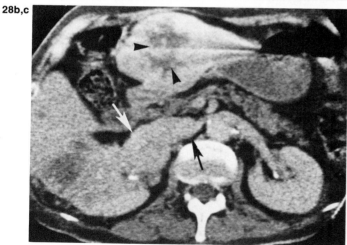

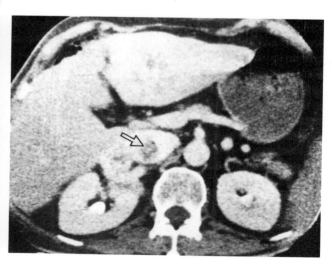

mor size and extracapsular extension previously noted in angiographic series also exists using CT today (17, 58,91,124).

The presence of lymph node metastases confers a poor prognosis in renal cancer, and routine lymphadenectomy is part of the surgical treatment in many cases (122) (Fig. 25). Lymph nodes less than 1 cm in diameter can be identified with CT and are considered normal. Nodes in the 1- to 2-cm range, especially if numerous in the renal hilar area, would be regarded with suspicion but are considered indeterminate by size criteria alone, and nodes greater than 2 cm are almost always enlarged by tumor. Enlarged nodes due to reactive hyperplasia and normal size nodes containing microscopic foci of tumor are the common causes of false positive and false negative CT interpretations, respectively. Care must be taken not to confuse lymph nodes with enlarged venous collaterals.

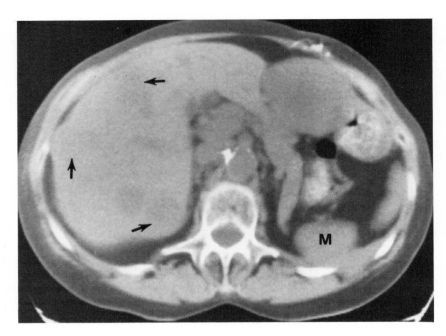

FIG. 29. Recurrent renal cell cancer. A globular mass (M) in the left renal fossa is present after nephrectomy for renal cell carcinoma. Low density areas (arrows) in liver represent metastases.

Bolus injections of contrast material and serial contiguous scans can usually make this distinction.

Renal venous involvement by renal cell carcinomas also has been considered a poor prognostic sign (Figs. 26 and 27). Computed tomography can detect major renal vein involvement in most cases, unless the vein is compressed or displaced by extensive local tumor, especially on the right side, where the renal vein is short. False positive studies may occur with bland thrombosis of the renal vein. Venography would be more accurate for assessing *intrarenal* venous involvement than CT alone, but such involvement does not affect the surgical approach. Careful scanning at the level of the renal veins with the judicious use of bolus injections of contrast material is necessary to assess venous integrity when staging patients with renal cell carcinoma. A tendency for the left renal vein to be compressed between the aorta and the superior mesenteric artery, the so-called "nutcracker" phenomenon, must be recognized because mild proximal dilatation of the left renal vein may occur in these instances and should not be confused with tumor involvement. When any doubt as to renal venous patency exists, venography should be performed (74).

Tumor thrombus in the inferior vena cava is almost always easy to detect (Figs. 27 and 28) by CT (33, 74, 116). Bolus or foot vein infusions of contrast material will often be necessary with large tumors. Large bulky tumors on the right side may be hard to evaluate due to caval displacement and compression. The foot vein infusion method will help identify intraluminal tumor thrombus, often showing cephalic extent and may allow distinction of intraluminal tumor thrombus from extrinsic compression by lymph nodes. Although multi-

planar reconstruction has been reported to be useful in assessing the inferior vana cava in renal cancer (113), it is rarely, if ever, needed in our experience. Caution should be used when evaluating equivocal inferior vena caval involvement in cases of renal cell carcinoma, since a laminar flow phenomenon in the inferior vana cava, often encountered with a foot vein infusion, may cause an apparent filling defect (10,40,113). As the contrast material layers against the periphery of the inferior vana cava, the faster flowing central column of blood can cause a "doughnut" like appearance to be seen with noncontrast enhanced flowing blood representing the hole in the doughnut (see Fig. 16 in Chapter 10).

When compared with renal arteriography, CT has proven more accurate and sensitive than angiography in detecting perirenal extension, more sensitive in assessing lymph node involvement, and equally accurate in detecting main renal vein and vena cava involvement (124). Although some still contend that angiographic evaluation is required for all renal cell carcinomas, it is rarely necessary for the initial diagnosis, and the surgical approach is rarely altered by angiography. In many institutions today urologic surgeons are routinely operating on renal cell carcinomas based on the information from CT scans alone. Renal angiography should be reserved for the equivocal CT case or where vascular anatomy is essential for angiographic embolization or surgical planning, such as local resection in a solitary kidney, a horseshoe kidney, or in patients with Von Hippel-Lindau disease or adult polycystic kidney disease.

In addition to the initial diagnosis and staging of renal cell carcinoma, CT also plays an important role in the follow-up of these patients who are treated with surgi-

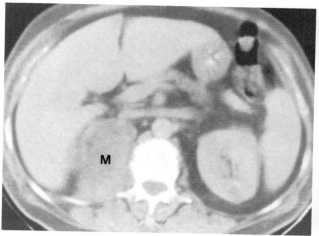 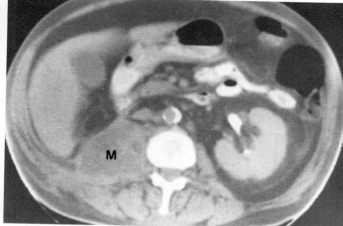

FIG. 30. Recurrent renal cell cancer. **Left:** A large mass (M) fills the renal fossa on the right in this patient with a prior radical right nephrectomy for carcinoma. Compensatory hypertrophy of the left kidney is present. **Right:** Two centimeters caudal, the tumor mass (M) is noted to invade the right psoas. Percutaneous biopsy confirmed recurrence.

cal resection (1,14). Those patients who are at increased risk of postoperative recurrence benefit most from follow-up CT. Extensive bulky renal tumors and lymph node or ipsilateral adrenal metastases all place the patient at risk for recurrence. Early detection of local recurrence would allow prompt surgical resection. The features that suggest tumor recurrence are a large soft tissue mass in the renal fossa clearly separate from contrast-medium-filled loops of bowel, enlargement or irregularity of the psoas muscle on the side of resection, and other local organ involvement (Figs. 29 and 30). Bowel loops and the tail of the pancreas can fill the vacant left renal fossa postoperatively (Fig. 9). A displaced spleen (or accessory spleens), scar tissue, and abscess all have been seen to mimic postoperative recurrence of tumor in patients with renal cell cancer.

Renal cell carcinoma treated with angiographic embolization will have a characteristic CT appearance depending on the time interval after infarction. Early, within the first 48 hr, persistence of trapped contrast material (staining) will be seen along with frequently branching peripheral air collections. Later, 5 to 7 days after embolization, the air collection becomes more central depending on the extent of infarction and necrosis. The overall kidney size tends not to change significantly from the preembolization state (13,128).

Transitional cell carcinomas.

Transitional cell carcinomas are the next most common renal neoplasm after adenocarcinoma. The role of CT in the uroradiologic evaluation of patients with real or suspected transitional cell carcinomas of the pelvis and ureter is twofold. First, CT is used to solve the diagnostic problem of a radiolucent filling

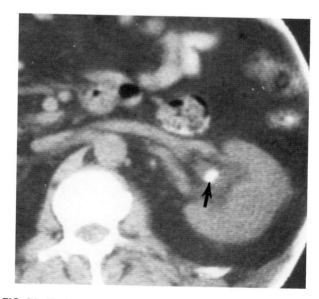

FIG. 31. Urate stone. A high-density calculus (arrow) (+110 HU) is present in the left renal pelvis. This corresponds to a radiolucent filling defect seen on a prior urogram.

defect in the renal pelvis or ureter seen by urography (92). Although CT cannot be histospecific, it can usually differentiate soft tissue masses from fresh blood clot or stone. Radiolucent stones, such as struvite or pure urate calculi, can be easily detected on CT scan because they have a density higher than soft tissue (Fig. 31) (20,31,107). Second, CT is often used to delineate the actual tumor extent after its initial diagnosis by excretory urography or retrograde pyelography. Since conservative surgery, i.e., local resection, is becoming a more popular therapy for transitional cell carcinoma, CT plays an important role in preoperative staging of

TABLE 2. *CT patterns of transitional cell carcinoma of the upper urinary tract*

Sessile mass		12 / 24
Ureteral wall thickening		5 / 24
Infiltrating renal mass		7 / 24

From Baron et al. (11), with permission.

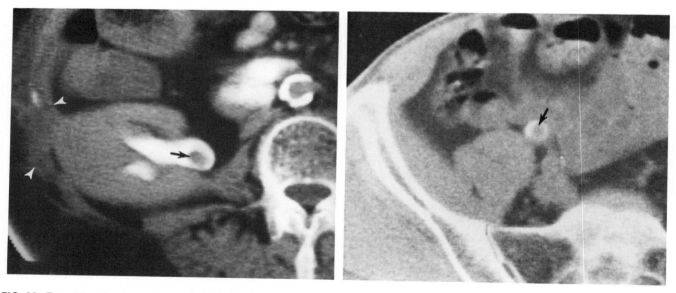

FIG. 32. Transitional cell carcinoma. **Left:** A fixed, sessile soft tissue mass (arrow) is seen in the right renal pelvis. This has been the most common CT pattern of transitional cell tumor in our experience. Soft tissue changes in right flank musculature (arrowheads) are secondary to previous ureterotomies for transitional cell carcinoma. **Right:** CT scan through distal right ureter in another patient demonstrates an intraluminal tumor with soft tissue attenuation value (arrow) surrounded by a rim of contrast medium. (From Baron et al., ref. 11, with permission.)

transitional cell tumors similar to that described for renal cell cancers (11).

On CT scans, three patterns have been seen with transitional cell carcinoma involving the renal pelvis and ureter (Table 2) (11). They may appear as sessile, intraluminal masses (most common pattern) (Fig. 32), concentric or eccentric ureteral wall thickening (Fig. 33), or large infiltrating masses (Fig. 34). When it presents as a large infiltrating mass, it may locally invade the renal pelvis or obliterate the normal sinus fat planes around the pelvis and collecting system. In that case, CT alone will not be able to categorically distin-

guish transitional cell cancer from renal cell carcinoma or other infiltrating processes (7,11).

Transitional cell carcinomas may be solitary or multiple and the CT attenuation values approach soft tissue (muscle) having a range from 40 to 70 HU (11,97). Rarely, speckles of calcification may be seen associated with a transitional cell carcinoma (Fig. 35). The surface of the tumor may be smooth or irregular, depending on tumor architecture or presence of blood clots. Although characteristically avascular on angiography, CT may show slight contrast enhancement (Fig. 36). Pre- and postcontrast CT scans are both necessary

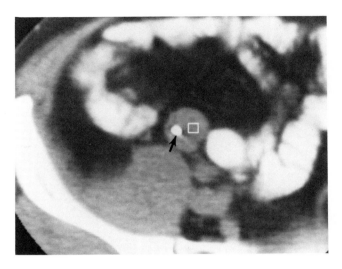

FIG. 33. Transitional cell carcinoma of the right ureter: semilunar pattern. The cursor is placed over eccentric portion of thickened ureteral wall. The arrow points to the eccentric ureteral stent. (From Baron et al., ref. 11, with permission.)

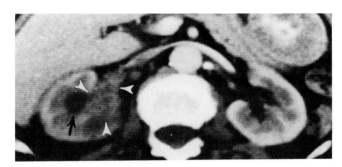

FIG. 34. Transitional cell carcinoma. CT scan obtained immediately following a bolus injection shows an irregular, right renal pelvic tumor (arrowheads) extending into upper pole collecting system posteriorly. Dilated anterior upper pole calyx is seen (arrow). Note that the tumor has an inhomogeneous appearance. (From Baron et al., ref. 11, with permission.)

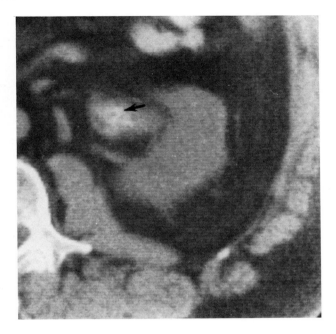

FIG. 35. Calcified transitional cell carcinoma. A soft tissue mass with amorphous calcification (arrow) is present in the left renal pelvis. Although most transitional cell carcinomas have attenuation values approaching soft tissue (40–70 HU), calcification may rarely be seen. (From Baron et al., ref. 11, with permission.)

for evaluation of transitional cell carcinomas, but only a small number of precontrast scans for localization and attenuation measurements are required. Serial bolus injection of small amounts of contrast material, 10 to 25 cc of a 60 to 66% solution, is routinely used in our practice since too dense opacification of the urine may obscure tumor involvement.

Computed tomography can be used to detect periureteric and intrarenal extension, and thus stage transitional cell carcinomas (Figs. 37 and 38). Computed tomography cannot differentiate tumors limited to the uroepithelial mucosa (Stage I[2]) from muscle wall invasion (Stage II), but the treatment is not significantly different for Stage I and II tumors of transitional cell origin. Computed tomography also will fail to detect tumor in normal size lymph nodes. Nonetheless, CT plays an important role in defining transitional cell car-

cinoma of the upper urinary tract and is an effective complementary imaging method to urography.

Lymphoma.

The kidneys are often displaced laterally by enlarged retroperitoneal lymph nodes in patients with known lymphoma (96). Primary renal infiltration without concomitant lymph node involvement is rare in both Hodgkin's disease and non-Hodgkin's lymphoma (96). However, renal involvement is not uncommon in patients with the far advanced stages of non-Hodgkin's lymphoma. On CT scans, renal lymphoma may appear as: (a) multinodular pattern (Fig. 39), (b) solitary mass with extrarenal extension (Fig. 40), (c) diffuse infiltrating pattern, and (d) extrarenal periureteric obstruction.

Although renal masses due to lymphoma have a CT appearance similar to masses of other etiologies, the correct diagnosis can be suggested in the newly presenting patient when there is associated widespread retroperitoneal or mesenteric lymphadenopathy (96).

Benign renal tumors.

Angiomyolipoma. Angiomyolipoma (AML) may occur as an isolated lesion, most commonly seen in

---

[2] Staging classification of transitional cell carcinoma: I, limited to uroepithelial mucosa and lamina propria; II, invasion to, but not beyond, the pelvic/ureteral muscularis layer; III, beyond the muscularis into adventitial fat or renal parenchyma; and IV, distant metastasis.

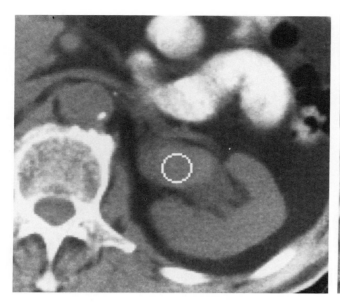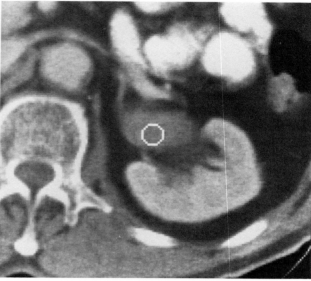

FIG. 36. Transitional cell carcinoma: contrast enhancement. **Left:** Precontrast CT scan shows a soft tissue mass (cursor) with attenuation value of +49 HU in the left renal pelvis. **Right:** Following a 25-cc bolus injection of iodinated contrast medium, the attenuation value of the tumor under cursor increased to +78 HU. (From Baron et al., ref. 11, with permission.)

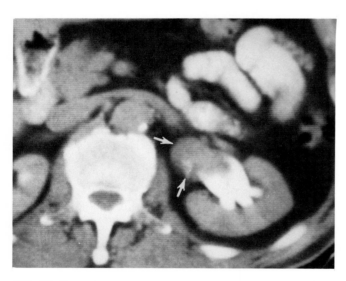

FIG. 37. Stage II transitional cell carcinoma. Postcontrast CT scan (same patient as Fig. 36) demonstrates a well-defined mass (arrows) in the left renal pelvis. No extrapelvic extension is seen.

middle-aged women, or as the renal manifestation of tuberous sclerosis (see Fig. 19), most frequently small, multiple, and bilateral. Histologically, it is composed of three main tissues: (a) large blood vessels, (b) smooth muscle, and (c) fat. The proportions of these components vary considerably from tumor to tumor.

On CT scans, AML appear as well-circumscribed, fat density masses either totally or partially within the renal parenchyma (44,122) (Fig. 41). In most cases enough fat is present within the tumor to allow a specific CT diagnosis. Intramural hemorrhage or a large muscular component to the AML may make it difficult to find the fat component on the CT scans (36). In cases in which the tumor is predominantly extrarenal

in location, differentiation between AML and a primary retroperitoneal liposarcoma invading the kidney may be difficult (Fig. 42). Very small lesions may be confused with cysts due to partial volume averaging (37,47). In children, Wilms' tumor may contain fatty tissue and thus simulate an AML on CT scans. Since the rare coexistence of renal cell carcinoma and AML in the same kidney or patient can occur, other more invasive studies, e.g., angiography, might be necessary for evaluating a solid, nonfatty renal tumor found at CT in patients with tuberous sclerosis.

Arteriovenous malformations. Large arteriovenous malformations (AVM), which may or may not be clinically suspected, will only be distinguished from a neoplasm on CT if the typically highly enhancing lesion is studied following a bolus injection of an intravenous contrast agent. The density of the flowing blood within the AVM will have the same concurrent density as that in the aorta. Curvilinear calcification within the wall of the mass associated with enlargement of the renal artery and renal vein to that side may be clues that an AVM or arteriovenous fistula is present (Fig. 43). If such a lesion is only studied after a drip infusion of contrast medium, the degree of enhancement of the lesion compared with the renal parenchyma may suggest a solid neoplasm and the true nature of the lesion will be apparent only if a subsequent arteriogram is performed.

Others. Renal fibromas (Fig. 44), adenomas, and hemangiomas appear as well-circumscribed, soft tissue density masses. They do not have unique CT features and thus a specific diagnosis is rarely made based on CT findings alone (60,83,129,130). Surgical exploration is often required for a definitive diagnosis in these cases.

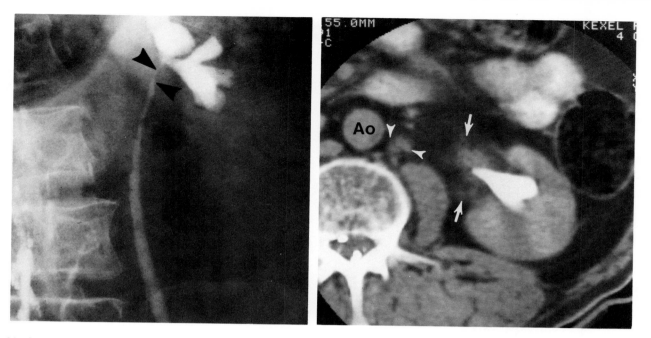

FIG. 38. Stage IV transitional cell carcinoma. **Left:** Retrograde pyelogram shows irregular constriction of the ureteral pelvic junction (arrowheads) causing dilatation of intrarenal collecting system. The exact tumor extent cannot be appreciated on this study. **Right:** Postcontrast CT scan through left renal pelvis demonstrates an extraureteral soft tissue mass with spiculations extending out into the perirenal fat (arrows). A cluster of minimally enlarged lymph nodes (arrowheads) is noted lateral to the aorta (Ao). (From Baron et al., ref. 11, with permission.)

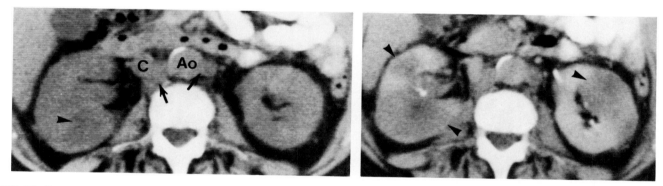

FIG. 39. Renal lymphoma. **Left:** Precontrast CT scan shows an ill-defined low-density area (arrowhead) in the slightly enlarged right kidney. The left kidney appears normal. Mildly enlarged paraaortic and paracaval lymph nodes are also seen (arrows). Ao, aorta; C, inferior vena cava. **Right:** After administration of intravenous contrast medium, the density difference between lymphomatous masses (arrowheads) and normal renal parenchyma is accentuated. Multiple areas of involvement not appreciated on precontrast scans are now evident.

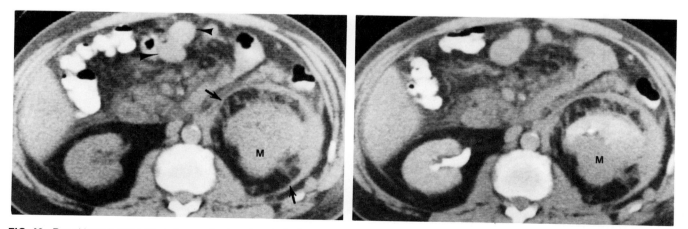

FIG. 40. Renal lymphoma with extrarenal extension. **Left:** A soft tissue mass (M) with an attenuation value similar to that of normal renal parenchyma is seen arising from the posterior surface of the left kidney. In addition, there is extrarenal involvement as evidenced by the thickened renal fascia (arrows) and streaky soft tissue densities in the perinephric space. Enlarged mesenteric lymph nodes (arrowheads) are also present. **Right:** Postcontrast scan accentuates the density difference between the lymphomatous mass (M) and the residual normal renal parenchyma.

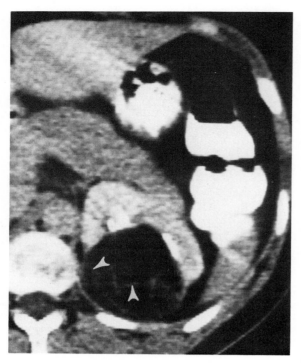

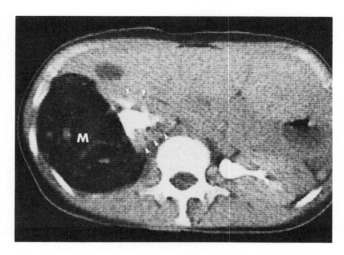

FIG. 42. Angiomyolipoma with a large extrarenal component. Postcontrast CT scan demonstrates a predominantly fatty mass (M) displacing the kidney (arrowheads) anteriorly and medially. When the tumor has a large extrarenal component as in this case, differentiation between AML and a primary retroperitoneal liposarcoma invading the kidney may be difficult. (From Totty et al., ref. 122, with permission.)

FIG. 41. Angiomyolipoma. A fat density mass with internal "septations" that represent blood vessels (arrowheads) occupies the posterior aspect of the left kidney.

43a,b,c

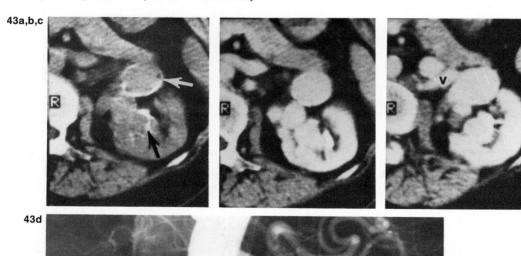

43d

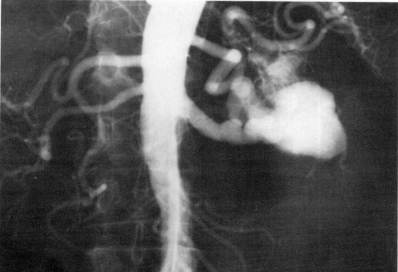

FIG. 43. Renal arteriovenous fistula. **a:** Precontrast scan shows an extensive, peripherally calcified lesion involving the hilar area of the left kidney (arrows). **b:** Immediately following a bolus injection of iodinated contrast medium, the calcified lesion enhances to the same extent as the aorta. **c:** One sec after scan (b) the dilated left renal vein (V) is opacified. The CT features are those of a large arteriovenous malformation. **d:** Abdominal aortogram confirms the CT findings. (Case courtesy of Larry Anderson, M.D., Everett, Washington.)

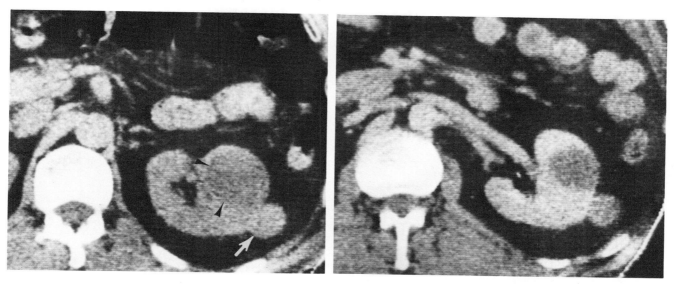

FIG. 44. Renal fibroma. **Left:** Precontrast CT scan shows a well-circumscribed 2-cm mass (arrow) arising from the posterolateral surface of the left kidney. The mass has the same attenuation value as the normal renal parenchyma. In addition, an intrarenal cyst (arrowheads) is present in the lateral aspect of the kidney, which is partial volume averaged. **Right:** Postcontrast scan demonstrates the cyst to a better degree. The cyst did not enhance; the fibroma enhanced to a lesser extent than normal renal parenchyma.

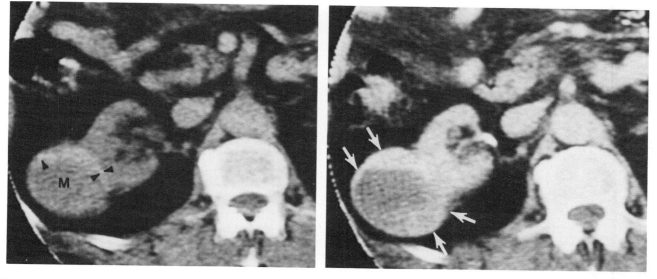

FIG. 45. Indeterminate renal mass. **Left:** Precontrast scan through right renal mass (M), which has high-density rim (arrowheads) and low attenuation center. **Right:** Postcontrast scan shows minimal rim enhancement (arrows). Diagnosis: papillary adenocarcinoma.

Indeterminate Masses

Some renal masses do not fit satisfactorily into the CT criteria of cyst, tumor, or abscess, even when correlated with pertinent history and physical examination, and are thus classified as indeterminate (8). Masses that display indeterminate CT features in a patient with an obvious urinary tract infection and sepsis most likely are abscesses and will be discussed in a later section. In one study in which 815 patients were referred for evaluation of one or more renal masses

nearly 8% of the renal masses detected by CT were considered indeterminate (8). The causes for indeterminate CT interpretations included: (a) technically indeterminate scans, (b) cyst-like masses without technical problems, and (c) solid masses with complex features.

Technically indeterminate renal masses were masses having many CT features of a simple cyst but one or more features not consistent with that diagnosis. Technical problems that resulted in an altered, con-

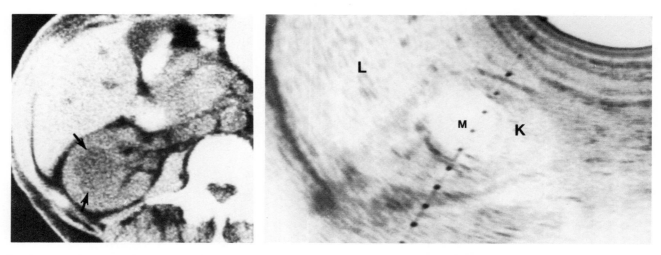

FIG. 46. Indeterminate renal mass—type II. **Left:** Noncontrast CT scan demonstrates a low density mass (+35 HU) (arrows) within the right kidney. **Right:** Longitudinal sonogram confirms the mass (M) to be cystic in nature. Percutaneous needle aspiration yielded pus. Mass resolved on antibiotic therapy. L, liver; K, kidney. (From Balfe et al., ref. 8, with permission.)

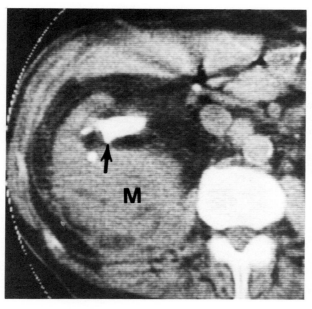

FIG. 47. Indeterminate renal mass—Type III. Noncontrast CT scan demonstrates a large right renal mass (M) extending into posterior pararenal space. A staghorn calculus (arrow) is seen in the right renal pelvis. The right kidney did not function on prior urogram. Diagnosis: XGPN with paranephric extension.

fusing CT image of the renal lesion were (a) a mass smaller than the scan collimator, (b) motion, causing gross artifacts and spuriously high attenuation values due to volume averaging, and (c) data poor, photopenic scans in large patients. Most of the cases in this category were studied using an 18-sec scanner. Current generation high-resolution, fast scanners should eliminate most of the problems that result in technically indeterminate renal masses, especially motion. However, suboptimal images may still occur in large

patients on current generation CT scanners if inappropriate ring size is used or if the mass is less than 1 cm. In resolving these technically indeterminate masses, ultrasound and needle aspiration have proven to be most helpful in our experience, as most of these masses were benign cysts. Angiography was usually of little help (8).

In the absence of scan artifacts or other technical problems, a cyst-like renal mass may still be considered indeterminate on CT scans because of the following features: (a) uniformly thick wall, (b) wall calcification, (c) central attenuation higher than a benign cyst (20–60 HU), and (d) irregular contour or poor delineation from surrounding tissues. High attenuation measurements and thickened walls were the most common features in our experience (Fig. 45). None of the masses in this second category displayed contrast enhancement but many were better defined after contrast material. Although several of these masses were found to be abscesses (Fig. 46) and benign or malignant cystic neoplasms, a large proportion proved to be complicated cysts. As in the last category, angiography was often not contributory whereas ultrasound and needle aspiration were most helpful in clarification of indeterminate masses in this category (8).

The last category of CT indeterminancy includes cases that closely resemble neoplasms but exhibit confusing CT features (8). Typically these are large, complex renal masses with ill-defined contours sometimes extending beyond the expected confines of the kidney into the perirenal spaces. Often, the extent of involvement of the perinephric space is out of proportion to the size of the primary lesion. Irregular contrast material enhancement and heterogeneous attenuation are common. Unlike typical renal cell carcinomas, the involvement of peripheral structures was ill-defined

48a,b

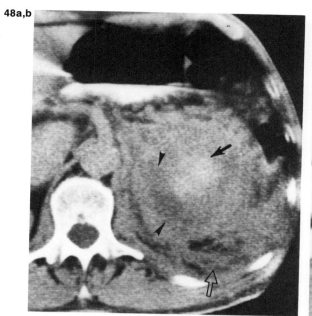
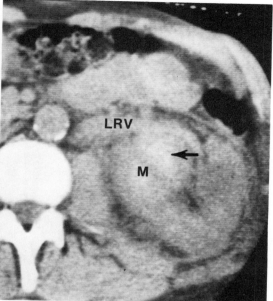

48c

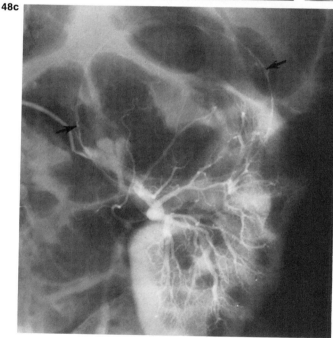

FIG. 48. Indeterminate renal mass—Type III. **a:** A large irregular mass with areas of high (arrow) and low (arrowheads) attenuation value is present in the upper pole of the left kidney in this patient with recent minor trauma to left flank. Amorphous soft tissue densities (open arrow) are also noted in the posterior pararenal space. **b:** Four centimeters caudal, a retroaortic left renal vein (LRV) is seen anterior to the mass (M) in the left kidney. High attenuation areas (arrow) within the mass represent hemorrhage. **c:** Selective left renal arteriogram reveals an avascular mass. Rim vascularity (arrows) is present. Diagnosis: necrotic renal cell carcinoma with intrarenal and perirenal hemorrhage. (From Balfe et al., ref. 8, with permission.)

rather than nodular in our experience. Secondary features, such as renal vein invasion or lymph node involvement, were absent. A majority of the lesions in this group were found to be xanthogranulomatous pyelonephritis (XGPN) or renal cell carcinomas complicated by extensive perirenal hemorrhage or urinoma (Figs. 47 and 48). Lesions in this category require surgical intervention for definitive diagnosis and treatment. Angiography and ultrasound, although frequently performed, rarely altered therapy in our experience (8).

The diagnostic strategy that has evolved from analyzing our indeterminate renal masses is designed to provide information sufficient for the decision of nonoperative versus operative management. The approach is as follows: (a) if an obvious technical difficulty is present and can be remedied, a repeat CT scan is performed. If not, ultrasound or aspiration is suggested. (b) If the mass or masses are cyst-like on CT but have any or all of the dissonant features previously described, e.g., thick wall, an ultrasound and needle aspiration of the mass is suggested (7). (b) If the mass has complex CT features and is apparently solid, even though not typical for neoplasm, surgical evaluation is indicated occasionally preceded by percutaneous bi-

KIDNEY

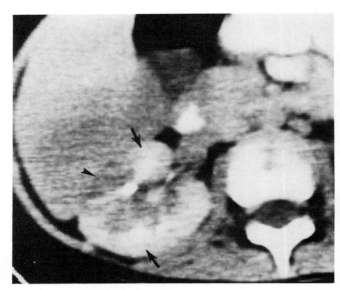 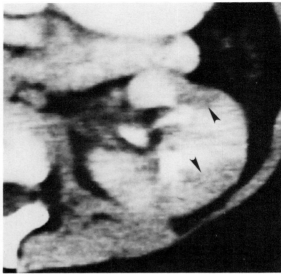

FIG. 49. Acute focal bacterial nephritis. **Left:** Postcontrast CT scan of right kidney shows "patchy" enhancement (arrows). Wedge-shaped areas of parenchyma that do not enhance (arrowhead) are involved by inflammation. Ultrasound examination was normal on two occasions. **Right:** The left kidney reveals similar changes in the nephrographic phase. The arrowheads point to the nonenhanced renal parenchyma.

opsy. Angiography is only recommended for cases in which renal sparing surgery is contemplated (7,8).

Inflammatory Masses

Acute.

When a patient presents with fever, chills, flank pain, and a focal mass or swollen kidney on excretory urography, inflammatory renal disease is strongly considered. A host of terms has been used to describe this clinical entity, including severe acute pyelonephritis, focal or suppurative pyelonephritis, acute bacterial nephritis, and acute lobar nephronia (51,63). Acute focal bacterial nephritis (AFBN) best describes the early, more edematous (solid) phase of a renal inflammatory process, usually caused by a gram negative organism. Although most patients with acute pyelonephritis will not come to CT, those patients with focal process(es) on excretory urography may be referred for CT examination to evaluate the possibility of frank renal or perirenal abscess.

On CT scans, AFBN appears as a focal mass, without definable walls, frequently wedge shaped, corresponding to the renal lobule (Fig. 49). The areas of involvement can be either isodense or slightly less dense than normal renal parenchyma on noncontrast scans. After intravenous contrast medium administration, there is patchy and inhomogeneous enhancement, similar to the striated nephrogram on excretory urography.

Whereas AFBN can be adequately treated with antibiotics alone resulting in complete resolution in most instances, it may, on rare occasion, progress into an abscess cavity, which then requires percutaneous or surgical drainage.

On CT scans, an abscess is often well defined, of lower density than normal renal parenchyma, and has a thick irregular wall (Fig. 50). Central contrast enhancement is absent, but the wall may exhibit variable degrees of contrast enhancement. In this regard, abscesses are very similar to centrally necrotic renal cell cancers, as seen with CT. Besides being capable of differentiating a renal abscess from AFBN, CT also provides detailed information as to the possible perinephric extension (Fig. 51) (69).

Chronic.

Xanthogranulomatous pyelonephritis is an interesting pathologic condition that results from chronic infection in an obstructed kidney (102) (Figs. 47 and 52). The usual CT appearance of XGPN includes these features: (a) a large calculus in the renal pelvis or collecting system; (b) absence of contrast material excretion in the kidney or area of focal involvement; (c) multiple nonenhancing, round areas within the medullary space having higher attenuation than urine, arranged in a hydronephrotic pattern; (d) discrete (solid) masses; and (e) frequent involvement of the perirenal space.

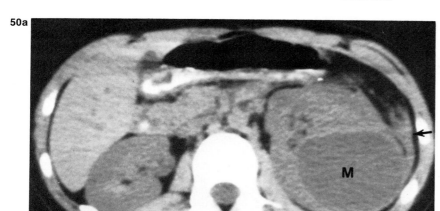

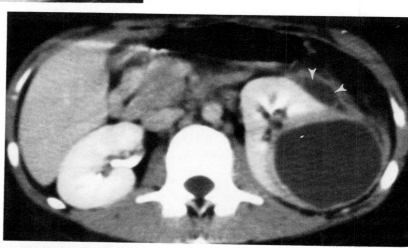

FIG. 50. Renal abscess with perirenal extension. **a:** Noncontrast enhanced CT scan shows a large, low-density mass (M) in the left kidney. Thickening of renal fascia (arrow) anterolaterally is present. **b:** After intravenous administration of contrast medium, a slightly enhanced thick wall is seen. The center of the mass remains unenhanced. Perinephric collection is seen anterior to kidney (arrowheads). **c:** Two centimeters caudal to **b**, a perirenal collection (arrowheads) and the thickening of renal fascia (arrow) are again noted.

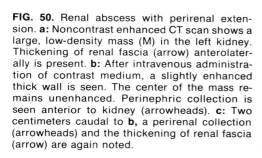

Large masses infiltrating the flank and air-containing intrarenal abscesses have also been seen with XGPN. This is not to be confused with emphysematous pyelonephritis, which presents a different CT picture, including gas within the collecting system, as well as in the surrounding perirenal spaces (102). A high attenuation, pyohydronephrosis may mimic XGPN, and only

pathologic evaluation will reveal the typical inflammatory changes and lipid-laden macrophages of XGPN. Although XGPN has not been shown to be a predisposing factor, concomitant XGPN and renal cell carcinoma has been reported (105).

Because XGPN may be focal, renal sparing surgery can be performed if the disease is suitably staged. A

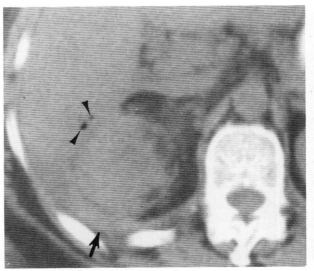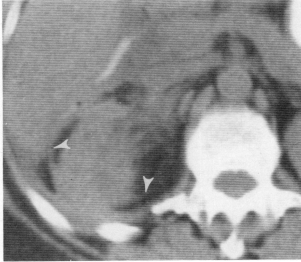

FIG. 51. Perirenal abscess. **Left:** Precontrast CT scan through upper pole of right kidney demonstrates two small air pockets (arrowheads) together with amorphous soft tissue densities (arrow) along the lateral surface of the right kidney. The renal outline is indistinct secondary to the inflammatory process in the perirenal space. **Right:** Scan 1 cm caudal, thickened renal fascia (arrowheads) and the renal outline are better delineated at this level.

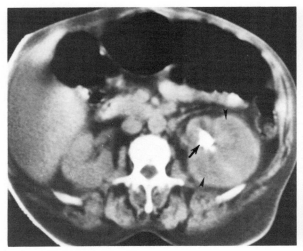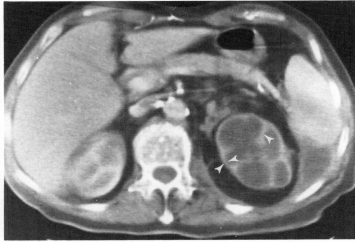

FIG. 52. XGPN. **Left:** Precontrast CT scan shows a staghorn calculus (arrow) in an enlarged left kidney. Central low-density areas (arrowheads) represent obstructed, dilated collecting system. **Right:** Immediate postcontrast scan shows hydronephrotic left kidney with only rims (arrowheads) of enhancing renal parenchyma surrounding low attenuation areas (dilated calyces).

staging system has been suggested similar to the staging criteria for renal cell carcinoma (72). Computed tomography can precisely define the full extent of XGPN and assist in the planning of surgical therapy.

Total fatty replacement of the kidney is a rare form of chronic renal inflammatory disease. Frequently this is seen in conjuction with the presence of a large staghorn calculus and XGPN. This condition can be well displayed on CT scan (Fig. 53). Extensive proliferation of renal sinus fat is thought to be the etiology, and pathologic examination reveals *no* remaining renal parenchyma.

Calcified Renal Masses

Calcification in a renal mass may appear in both benign or malignant conditions. It is important to stress that not all calcified renal masses fall into an indeterminate category (123). Because of the ability of CT to localize calcifications more accurately than conventional radiographic methods and to determine the cystic or solid composition of a mass, CT allows for the distinction of benign from malignant categories of calcified renal masses with more certainty.

Based on their CT appearances, calcified renal mass-

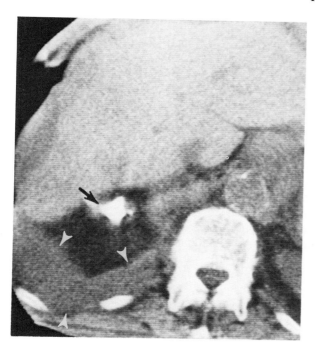

FIG. 53. Total fatty replacement of the kidney. A densely calcified staghorn calculus (arrow) is surrounded by fatty tissue totally replacing the renal parenchyma on the right. A crescent-shaped fluid collection (arrowheads) posterior to the kidney represents a perirenal abscess that was subsequently drained surgically.

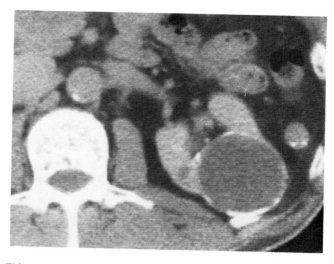

FIG. 55. Calcified renal cyst. A round, peripherally calcified mass with near water density center arises from the posterolateral surface of the left kidney. The mass exhibits no contrast enhancement. Calcified masses that fit these criteria are invariably benign.

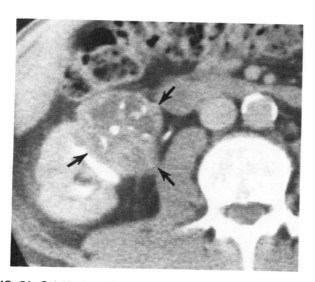

FIG. 54. Calcified renal cell carcinoma. Postcontrast CT scan shows an irregular soft tissue mass (arrows) with patchy enhancement and multiple central punctate calcifications arising from the anteromedial aspect of the right kidney. The presence of soft tissue mass surrounding calcifications on CT scans is highly suggestive of a malignant tumor.

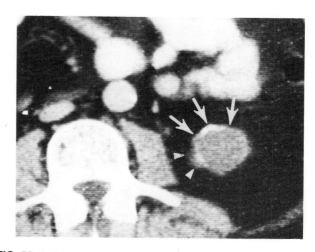

FIG. 56. Indeterminate calcified renal mass. Curvilinear calcification (arrows) is present along the anteromedial aspect of this left lower pole mass. Although the peripheral location of calcification suggests benignity, attenuation value (+30 HU) is higher than generally acceptable for a benign cyst. At surgery, this was proven to be a hemorrhagic cyst. Arrowheads, functioning renal tissue. (From Weyman et al., ref. 124, with permission.)

es can be categorized into the following three groups: (a) tumors of primarily soft tissue density, (b) cystic lesions with mural calcifications, and (c) indeterminate masses. The distinguishing feature of the cases in the soft tissue group is the presence of calcifications that are *not* truly peripheral in location (Fig. 54). Calcifications in this group are curvilinear, amorphous, punctate, or a combination thereof. There is always a soft tissue component to the mass outside the confines of the calcification. In other words, the calcification, even when appearing peripheral on radiographs, does not truly define the periphery of the renal mass. Although the correct diagnosis of renal cell carcinoma can be suspected by excretory urography in most cases on retrospective review, CT confirms the diagnosis and, further, provides valuable staging information (124). It should be noted that a calcified renal cell carcinoma has a better prognosis than a noncalcified renal cell carcinoma (106,123).

The major distinguishing features of the cystic lesions (group b) include the absence of any detectable soft tissue mass, other than the usually uniformly thick wall, and the homogeneous, near-water attenuation value of the fluid in the central area of the lesion (Fig. 55). The calcifications are largely curvilinear and occasionally punctate, but they all truly define the perimeter of the mass where present. The calcified cystic masses are mostly benign in our experience (123).

Renal hydatid cystic disease has strikingly similar CT features to the second group of calcified renal masses (39,55,75). Although extremely rare in this country, hydatid cystic disease is endemic in many parts of the world. Computed tomography can display the solitary or diffuse forms of renal involvement when present. The presence of daughter cysts within a larger cyst coupled with calcifications in the walls of the cysts is pathognomonic for this entity. The cysts have thin or thick walls that enhance with contrast material. The fluid content has a density higher than water (greater than 10 HU).

The indeterminate calcified renal masses are those with peripheral calcification and central attenuation values above those acceptable for uncomplicated fluid-filled cysts, with minimal or absent enhancement after administration of intravenous contrast material (Fig. 56). This group comprises a wide spectrum of pathological conditions ranging from papillary cystadenocarcinoma to hemorrhagic cyst. Other conditions such as adult Wilms' tumor, transitional cell carcinoma, and metastases all may have similar CT features (106,123). Although aneurysms, AVMs, and calcified angiomyolipomas also may have similar CT findings, these can be more precisely diagnosed by proper CT methodology.

Effect on the Diagnostic Process

The effect of CT on the diagnostic imaging evaluation of renal masses has been substantial. As the flow chart in Fig. 1 shows, invasive diagnostic procedures such as angiography and cyst aspiration have been markedly reduced. The character and extent of renal masses, whether malignant or inflammatory, have never been better illustrated than with CT. Computed tomography can actually replace ultrasound as the primary triage imaging method for masses detected by excretory urography and tomography. However, cost, radiation, availability, and time needed to perform the examination must be taken into account. There are circumstances in which CT should be the first diagnostic imaging study performed for evaluation of renal masses detected or suggested on a urogram. These include abnormalities on excretory urography that strongly suggest renal tumor, XGPN, or other inflammatory masses. When nephromegaly is associated with nonfunction, CT can often identify the specific cause or condition. Multiple renal masses, for example, adult polycystic kidney disease or multiple cortical cysts, may also be best imaged first with CT. Left upper pole renal masses or masses less than 1.5 cm in diameter, especially in obese patients, are difficult to examine by sonography and therefore should be studied first with CT. Additionally, most masses considered indeterminate or unresolvable by ultrasound can often be resolved using CT.

Figure 1 illustrates the common and alternative pathways for imaging the renal mass. Using such an imaging scheme in our practice, the actual number of angiograms and primary high-dose nephrotomograms performed has markedly declined.

Juxta Renal Processes

Many juxta renal processes began as primary renal processes. As diseases extend out from the kidney to involve contiguous areas, the CT appearance reflects the size, extent, and source of the process. Computed tomography can clearly delineate involvement of the extraperitoneal spaces around the kidney and often may provide a precise diagnosis (69). As illustrated in Chapter 6, CT can demonstrate the various fascial planes that divide the retroperitoneal area at the level of the kidneys into three separate compartments: an anterior pararenal, a perirenal, and a posterior pararenal space. The perirenal and posterior pararenal

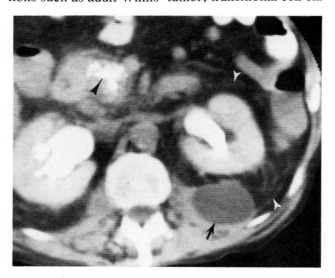

FIG. 57. Pancreatic pseudocyst involving posterior pararenal space. A low density mass (arrow) abuts the lateral surface of left psoas and quadratus lumborum muscles and displaces the left kidney anteriorly. This mass can be traced to be contiguous with the pancreas on more cephalic scans. Also note a cluster of calcifications (black arrowhead) within the pancreatic head and thickening of the renal fascia (white arrowheads). (Case courtesy of George Wilson, M.D., Columbia, Missouri.)

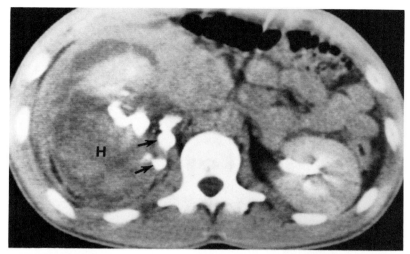

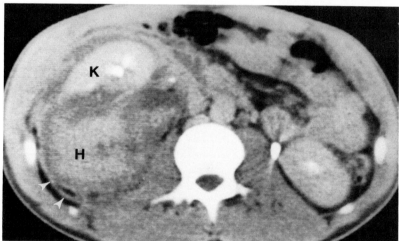

FIG. 58. Renal trauma. **Above:** Postcontrast CT scan demonstrates a large hematourinoma (H) from fracture through midpole of the right kidney. Extravasation of contrast material (arrows) is seen. The patient was in stable condition and treated conservatively. **Below:** Two centimeters caudal, a large hematoma (H) is noted with thickening of renal fascia (arrowheads). Remaining normal right kidney (K) is displaced anteriorly by hematoma.

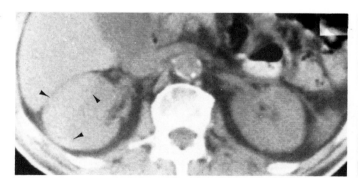

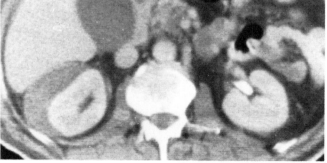

FIG. 59. Acute subcapsular hematoma. **Left:** A crescent-shaped collection (arrowheads) partially encircles and compresses the right kidney. The density of this collection is higher than nonenhanced renal parenchyma and is compatible with an acute bleed. **Right:** Postcontrast scan better demonstrates the outline of this extrarenal fluid collection due to marked enhancement of the normal renal parenchyma. Although the right kidney still remains in the nephrographic phase, contrast excretion into the pyelocalyceal system has occurred in the left kidney. The abnormally prolonged nephrogram is due to compression of right kidney by the subcapsular hematoma.

spaces are usually filled with fat, whereas the anterior pararenal space is most often only a potential space. The processes that frequently affect the extraperitoneal pararenal spaces are hemorrhage, infection (occasionally gaseous), urine or lymph extravasation, tumor spread, fat deposition, and pancreatic pseudocysts (extrapancreatic fluid collections) (59,89,100,104,111) (Fig. 57). Although the pattern of spread of the various types of effusions may be similar, CT is often able to detect the origin and nature of the extraperitoneal process.

Hemorrhage

Hemorrhage into the perirenal or posterior pararenal spaces may be extensive without causing any significant changes in conventional radiographs, including excretory urography. Trauma, either blunt or penetrating, is the most common cause of hemorrhage into perirenal space (Fig. 58) (85,95,100). In patients with penetrating injury, which includes renal biopsy, blood most commonly accumulates in the inferior perirenal space followed by posterior pararenal and subcapsular collections. Other causes of perirenal hemorrhage include arteritis, interstitial nephritis (lupus), cystic degeneration with chronic dialysis, anticoagulation, and small renal cell cancers. Although most aortic aneurysms rupture into the retroperitoneum, psoas muscles, or intraperitoneal compartment, blood may dissect into the perirenal compartment on rare occasions (2,3,12,103,119,131). On CT scans, a hematoma appears as a soft tissue mass either conforming to or enlarging the perirenal space (Fig. 59) (114). An acute hematoma measures 60 to 80 HU whereas chronic hematoma has an attenuation value in the 20 to 40 HU range (89).

Urinoma

Urinary extravasation into the perirenal spaces occurs spontaneously, secondary to urinary tract obstruction, after renal trauma including that resulting from interventional procedures (4,27,82). Computed tomography has been shown to be superior to excretory urography in defining the size and location of urinoma formation (27,82).

On CT scans, urinoma is a low-density mass with attenuation values ranging from −10 to +20 HU (see Fig. 15a in Chapter 15). The CT appearance of urinoma is similar to a chronic hematoma or an abscess. On rare occasions, the walls of urinomas may even calcify.

Abscesses

Most perirenal inflammatory disease is an extension of renal inflammatory disease and is generally confined within Gerota's fascia. However, aggressive infection may break through existing fascial planes and involve contiguous spaces or organs. A perirenal (perinephric) abscess has the same CT appearance as abscess elsewhere in the body. It is a low-density mass, usually with a thick irregular wall that may contrast enhance. Unless gas is present within the mass, an abscess can-

not be differentiated from a hematoma, a urinoma, or a necrotic neoplasm (9,24,80,81) (Figs. 50 and 51).

In addition to a dominant mass, thickening of Gerota's fascia and strands (webs) of soft tissue density are often present throughout the perirenal or pararenal fat. Similar CT features also can be seen in some cases of neoplastic disease (9,89).

Impaired Renal Function (Renal Failure)

Renal evaluation using CT to determine the size, location, and contour of the kidneys in the azotemic patient is feasible in almost all adult patients. However, due to its nonionizing radiation, ease of performance, and lower cost, gray scale ultrasonography is the procedure of choice in differentiating obstructive uropathy from renal parenchymal disease. Computed tomography is reserved for cases in which ultrasound is technically unsuccessful due to extreme obesity or cases in which ultrasound fails to define the level and etiology of renal obstruction (16,35).

A CT diagnosis of hydronephrosis can be made without the use of intravenous contrast medium (Fig. 60) although its identification is much easier on postcontrast scans. A small dose of contrast (10−20 cc of 50−60% solution) may be all that is required to separate parenchyma from dilated calyces.

On noncontrast enhanced CT scans, the dilated urine-filled calyces appear as areas of low attenuation value within a normal or enlarged renal silhouette. In pyonephrosis the attenuation value of the urine is usually higher. After intravenous contrast material, a faint nephrogram and pyelogram may be seen, often when not apparent at urography. The characteristic prolonged "obstructive nephrogram" is also occasionally seen on CT (Fig. 61). Persistent nephrograms may also be seen in patients with acute renal failure due to a variety of causes including acute glomerulonephritis,

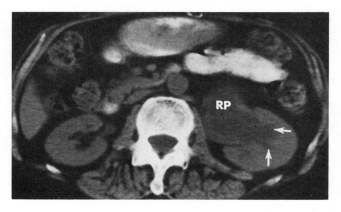

FIG. 60. Left hydronephrosis. A noncontrast enhanced CT scan shows a dilated, urine-filled left collecting system (arrows) communicating with a dilated renal pelvis (RP). A distal ureteral obstruction secondary to bladder carcinoma accounted for the hydronephrosis.

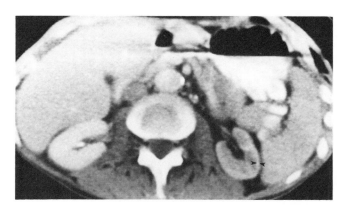

FIG. 61. Persistent nephrogram secondary to an obstructing ureteral calculus. Postcontrast CT scan demonstrates delayed and persistent nephrogram on the left. The renal cortex (arrowheads) is still denser than the renal medulla on the left whereas the entire renal parenchyma is of uniform density on the right.

leukemia, and ATN (77). Parenchymal thickness can easily be assessed, thus providing information regarding the potential salvageability of the obstructing process.

Besides hydronephrosis, a variety of renal parenchymal diseases that result in imparied renal function also have been evaluated with CT. Although chronic atrophic pyelonephritis often results in an irregular contour with deep cortical scars and calyceal distor-

tion (Fig. 62), renal ischemia leads to a small, smooth kidney (Fig. 63). Cystic diseases of the kidney and renal parenchymal calcifications, as in acute cortical necrosis, chronic glomerulonephritis (Fig. 64) end-stage renal tuberculosis (putty kidney) (Fig. 65), and end-stage renal oxylosis, similarly can be imaged by CT (110). The CT finding of small end-stage kidneys implies irreversibility and often terminates the imaging work-up of an azotemic patient (76) (Fig. 66).

Other Considerations

Renal Trauma

Trauma to the kidney as an isolated event or as a concomitant injury in the patient with multiple abdominal trauma is an everyday event. Motor vehicle accidents account for a large number of cases and patients in the younger age groups are frequently the victims. Most renal trauma today is of the blunt type. Penetrating abdominal injuries usually require rapid management with a minimum of radiologic evaluation; therefore experience with CT in penetrating injuries to the urinary tract is currently limited (29,30,73,121).

Conservative, nonoperative management of the renal trauma patient is becoming the rule in many institutions. Computed tomography is complementary to excretory urography in evaluating the extent of the

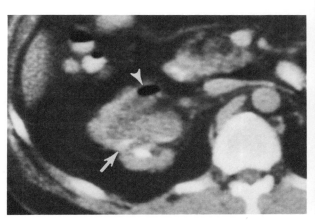 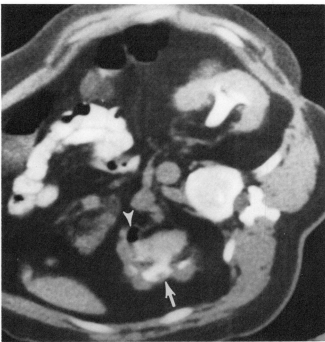

FIG. 62. Chronic atrophic pyelonephritis with acute exacerbation. **Left:** Precontrast supine CT scan shows a small and irregular right kidney with deep cortical scar (arrow) posterolaterally, findings compatible with chronic atrophic pyelonephritis. In addition, a gas bubble (arrowhead) is seen within the dilated pyelocalyceal system indicative of an acute infectious process caused by gas-forming organisms. **Right:** Scan obtained with patient in right lateral decubitus position confirms the gas bubble (arrowhead) to be within a dilated calyx. Arrow points to the deep cortical scar and blunted calyx.

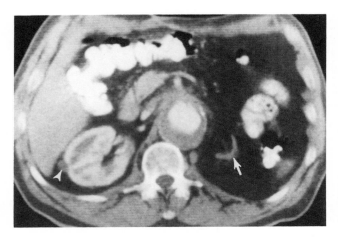

FIG. 63. Atrophic left kidney secondary to ischemia. A small but smooth left kidney (arrow) is present in this patient with a large abdominal aortic aneurysm. The presence of a large right kidney suggests that the ischemic insult to the left kidney is in the far distant and not recent past. Arrowhead points to a benign cortical cyst.

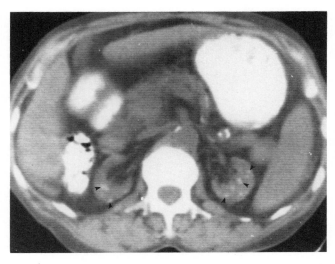

FIG. 64. End-stage renal disease due to chronic glomerulonephritis. Multiple calcific densities (arrowheads) are seen throughout both atrophic kidneys.

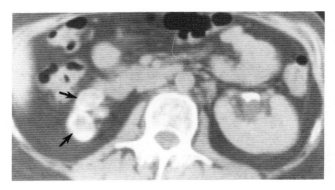

FIG. 65. End-stage renal tuberculosis. Postcontrast CT scan shows a small nonfunctioning right kidney with rim calcifications (arrows).

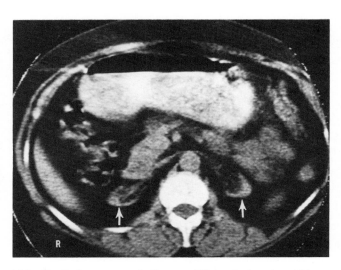

FIG. 66. End-stage renal disease. Bilateral shrunken kidneys (arrows) are noted in this adult male with severe renal failure of unknown etiology. The marked diminution of kidney size implies irreversibility and chronicity.

renal damage. If the intravenous urogram with tomography is technically satisfactory and normal, then there is little need for CT. However, in the patient with an unsatisfactory urogram or labile clinical conditions, i.e., persistent hematuria or declining hematocrit, a CT examination should be the next imaging study considered. Extravasation of urine may be detected by CT when not visible on a conventional urogram even with tomography (29). The presence and extent of subcapsular and perinephric hematoma or urinoma formation can be accurately depicted with CT (Fig. 58). Other associated abdominal injuries, particularly hepatic, splenic, and retroperitoneal, often are optimally displayed as well.

Renal Pelvis Filling Defects

The differential diagnosis of a filling defect in the renal pelvis includes a tumor, a blood clot, fungus ball,

and a radiolucent stone (34). Because of its improved contrast resolution compared with conventional radiography, CT is capable of differentiating among these entities based on differences in their attenuation values. Nonradioopaque calculi include urate, xanthine, cystine, matrix, or struvite stones. Due to the high effective atomic number (Z) of urate and cystine, the attenuation value of these calculi, often in the range of 300 to 600 HU, is sufficiently higher than soft tissue and therefore easily identifiable by CT scans (20,107) (Fig. 31).

An acute hematoma, often with an attenuation value of 70 HU, can be differentiated from uroepithelial tumors that have a density of soft tissue (40–50 HU).

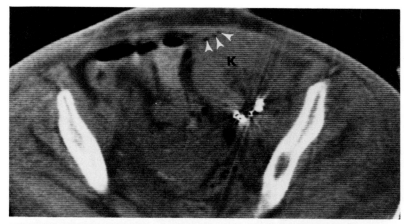

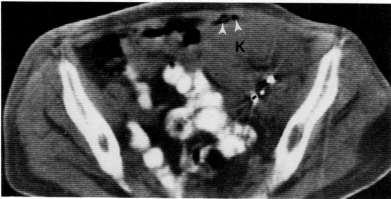

FIG. 67. Renal transplant. **Above:** CT scan of renal transplant 8 days after drain removal demonstrates small pockets of gas (arrowheads) anterior to the graft (K). **Below:** Scan 6 days after the scan above shows gas has increased (arrowheads). Wound dehiscence due to staphylococcus abscess occurred 4 days following this study.

However, if a mass has a soft tissue density, an exact histology of the tumor cannot be predicted based on CT findings.

Computed tomography significantly changes the work-up of the radiolucent filling defect in the renal pelvis or ureter seen at urography. More invasive procedures, such as retrograde pyelography, may frequently be obviated (11).

Renal Transplants

Radionuclide imaging and gray scale ultrasound are the procedures of choice in evaluating renal transplant patients with real or suspected complications. Computed tomography is reserved for cases in which ultrasound fails, because of either an open surgical wound or excessive overlying bowel gas (15,56,79,87, 99).

As previously mentioned, CT is capable of differentiating between acute hematoma, urinoma, or abscesses. Distinction between gas in an abscess from normal residual gas in the immediate postoperative bed can be difficult and a follow-up scan may be necessary in these situations (Fig. 67). While normal postoperative gas invariably decreases with time, gas in the abscess cavity has been shown to increase on serial scans.

REFERENCES

1. Alter AJ, Uehling DT, Zwiebel WJ: Computed tomography of the retroperitoneum following nephrectomy. *Radiology* 133:663–668, 1979
2. Alter AJ, Zimmerman S, Kirachaiwanich C: Computerized tomographic assessment of retroperitoneal hemorrhage after percutaneous renal biopsy. *Arch Intern Med* 140:1323–1326, 1980
3. Amendola MA, Tisnado J, Fields WR, Beachley MC, Vines FS, Cho SR, Turner MA, Konerding KF: Evaluation of retroperitoneal hemorrhage by computed tomography before and after translumbar aortography. *Radiology* 133:401–404, 1979
4. Anderson KA, Tanagho EA: Unusual presentation of chronic ureteral obstruction. *J Urol* 125:114–116, 1981
5. Baert AL, Marchal G, Staelens B, Coenen Y: CT evaluation of renal space occupying lesions. *Fortschr Roentgenstr* 126:285–291, 1977
6. Baert AL, Wackenheim A, Jeanmart L: Atlas of pathological computed tomography. In: *Abdominal Computed Tomography, Vol. 2.* New York, Springer-Verlag, pp 10–43, 1980
7. Balfe DM, McClennan BL, AufderHeide J: Multimodal imaging in evaluation of two cases of adenocarcinoma of the renal pelvis. *Urol Radiol* 3:19–23, 1981
8. Balfe DM, McClennan BL, Stanley RJ, Weyman PJ, Sagel SS: Evaluation of renal masses considered indeterminate by computed tomography. *Radiology* 142:421–428, 1982
9. Barlaza GS, Kuhns LR, Siegel RS, Rapp R: The posterior pararenal space: An escape route for retrocrural masses. *J Comput Assist Tomogr* 3:470–473, 1979
10. Barnes PA, Bernardino ME, Thomas JL: Flow phenomenon mimicking thrombus: A possible pitfall of the pedal infusion technique. *J Comput Assist Tomogr* 6:304–306, 1982
11. Baron RL, McClennan BL, Lee JKT, Lawson T: Transitional

cell carcinoma of the pelvis and ureter—CT evaluation. *Radiology* 144:125–130, 1982

12. Bergman AB, Neiman HL: Computed tomography in the detection of retroperitoneal hemorrhage after translumbar aortography. *AJR* 131:831–833, 1978

13. Bernardino ME, Chuang VP, Wallace S, Thomas JL, Soo CS: Therapeutically infarcted tumors: CT findings. *AJR* 136:527–530, 1981

14. Bernardino ME, deSantos LA, Johnson DE, Bracken RB: Computed tomography in the evaluation of post-nephrectomy patients. *Radiology* 130:183–187, 1979

15. Bia MJ, Baggish D, Katz L, Gonzalez R, Kliger AS, Rosenfield AT: Computed tomography in the diagnosis of pelvic abscesses in renal transplant patients. *JAMA* 246:1435–1437, 1981

16. Bosniak MA, Megibow AJ, Ambos MA, Mitnick JS, Lefleur RS, Gordon R: Computed tomography of ureteral obstruction. *AJR* 138:1107–1114, 1982

17. Bracken B, Jonsson K: How accurate is angiographic staging of renal carcinoma? *Urology* 14:96–99, 1979

18. Brennan RE, Curtis JA, Pollack HM, Weinberg I: Sequential changes in the CT numbers of the normal canine kidney following intravenous contrast administration. *Invest Radiol* 14:239–245, 1979

19. Brennan RE, Curtis JA, Pollack HM, Weinberg I: II. The renal medulla. *Invest Radiol* 14:239–245, 1979

20. Brown RC, Loening SA, Ehrhardt JC, Hawtrey CE: Cystine calculi are radioopaque. *AJR* 135:565–567, 1980

21. Buck DR, Dunnick NR, Doppman JL: Retrorenal cysts. *J Comput Assist Tomogr* 3:765–767, 1979

22. Burgener FA, Hamlin DJ: Contrast enhancement in abdominal CT: Bolus vs infusion. *AJR* 137:351–358, 1981

23. Christianson PJ, Clark MA, Meek J, Sharer W, Anclair PL, O'Connell KJ: Unusual case of dysgenetic renal cyst. *Urology* 19:447–449, 1982

24. Colley DP, Farrell JA, Clark RA: Perforated colon carcinoma presenting as a suprarenal mass. *Comput Tomogr* 5:55–58, 1981

25. Curry NS, Block G, Metcalf JS, Sens MA: Hyperdense renal mass: Unusual CT appearance of a benign renal cyst. *Urol Radiol* 4:33–36, 1982

26. Dailey ET, Rozanski RM, Kieffer SA, Dinn WM: Computed tomography in genitourinary pathology. *Urology* 12:95–105, 1978

27. Dunnick NR, Long JA, Javadpour N: Perirenal extravasation of urographic contrast medium demonstrated by computed tomography. *J Comput Assist Tomogr* 4:538–539, 1980

28. Englestad B, McClennan BL, Levitt RG: The role of precontrast images in CT of the kidney. *Radiology* 136:153–155, 1980

29. Federle MP, Cross RA, Jeffrey BB, Trunkey DD: Computed tomography in blunt abdominal trauma. *Arch Surg* 117:654–650, 1982

30. Federle MP, Goldberg HI, Kaiser JA, Moss AA, Jeffrey RB, Mall JC: Evaluation of abdominal trauma by computed tomography. *Radiology* 138:637–644, 1981

31. Federle MP, McAninch JW, Kaiser JA, Goodman PC, Roberts J, Mall JC: Computed tomography of urinary calculi. *AJR* 136:255–258, 1981

32. Feiner HD, Katz LA, Gallo GR: Acquired cystic disease of kidney in chronic dialysis patients. *Urology* 17:260–264, 1981

33. Ferris RA, Kirschner LP, Mero JH, McCabe DJ, Moss ML: Computed tomography in the evaluation of inferior vena caval obstruction. *Radiology* 130:7–10, 1979

34. Flechner SM, McAninch JW: Aspergillosis of the urinary tract: Ascending route of infection and evolving patterns of disease. *J Urol* 125:598–601, 1981

35. Forbes WSC, Isherwood I, Fawcitt RA: Computed tomography in the evaluation of the solitary or unilateral nonfunctioning kidney. *J Comput Assist Tomogr* 2:389–394, 1978

36. Friedman AC, Hartman DS, Sherman J, Lautin EM, Goldman M: Computed tomography of abdominal fatty masses. *Radiology* 139:415–429, 1981

37. Frija J, Larde D, Belloir C, Botto H, Martin N, Vasile N: Computed tomography diagnosis of renal angiomyolipoma. *J Comput Assist Tomogr* 4:843–846, 1980

38. Gardeur D, Lautrou J, Millard JC, Berger N, Metzger J: Pharmacokinetics of contrast media: Experimental results in dog and man with CT implications. *J Comput Assist Tomogr* 4:178–185, 1980

39. Gilsanz V, Lozano F, Jimenez J: Renal hydatid cysts: Communicating with collecting system. *AJR* 135:357–361, 1980

40. Goncharenko V, Gerlock AJ, Kadir S, Turner B: Incidence and distribution of venous extension in 70 hypernephromas. *AJR* 133:263–265, 1979

41. Gutierrez OH, Burgener FA, Schwartz S: Coincident renal cell carcinoma and renal angiomyolipoma in tuberous sclerosis. *AJR* 132:848–850, 1979

42. Haaga JR, Morrison SC: CT appearance of renal infarct. *J Comput Assist Tomogr* 4:246–247, 1980

43. Hadar H, Meiraz D: Renal sinus lipomatosis. Differentiation from space-occupying lesion with aid of computed tomography. *Urology* 15:86–90, 1980

44. Hansen GC, Hoffman RB, Sample WF, Becker R: Computed tomography diagnosis of renal angiomyolipoma. *Radiology* 128:789–791, 1978

45. Harris RD, Dorros S: Computed tomographic diagnosis of renal infarction. *Urology* 17:287–289, 1981

46. Harris RD, Seat SG: Value of computerized tomography in evaluation of kidney. *Urology* 12:729–732, 1978

47. Hartman DS, Goldman SM, Friedman AC, David CJ, Medewell JE, Sherman JL: Angiomyolipoma: Ultrasonic-pathologic correlation. *Radiology* 139:451–458, 1981

48. Havrilla TR, Reich NE, Seidelmann FE, Haaga JR: Computed tomography of the kidneys and retroperitoneum: Current status. *J Comput Assist Tomogr* 2:227–240, 1978

49. Heinz ER, Dubois PJ, Drayer BP, Hill R: A preliminary investigation of the role of dynamic computed tomography in renovascular hypertension. *J Comput Assist Tomogr* 4:63–66, 1980

50. Hinman CG, Older RA, Cleeve DM, Trought WS, Weinerth JL: Computerized tomographic diagnosis of massive hydronephrosis of duplicated system in an adult. *Urology* 12:92–94, 1978

51. Hoffman EP, Mindelzun RE, Anderson RU: Computed tomography in acute pyelonephritis associated with diabetes. *Radiology* 135:691–695, 1980

52. Ishikawa, I, Onouchi Z, Saito Y, Kitada H, Shinoda A, Ushitani K, Tabuchi M, Suzuki M: Renal cortex visualization and analysis of dynamic CT curves of the kidney. *J Comput Assist Tomogr* 5:695–701, 1981

53. Ishikawa I, Saito Y, Onouchi Z, Kitada H, Suzuke S, Kurihara S, Yuri T, Shinoda A: Development of acquired cystic disease and adenocarcinoma of the kidney in glomerulonephritic chronic hemodialysis patients. *Clin Nephrol* 14:1–6, 1980

54. Ishikawa I, Saito Y, Shinoda A, Onouchi Z: Evidence for patchy renal vasoconstriction in man: Observation by CT scan. *Nephron* 27:31–34, 1981

55. Ismail MA, Al-Dabagh MA, Al-Janabi A, Al-Moslih MI, Al-Ani MS, Rassam S, Fawzi AH, Shafik MA, Al-Rawas AY: The use of computerised axial tomography (CAT) in the diagnosis of hydatid cysts. *Clin Radiol* 31:287–290, 1980

56. Kittredge RD, Brensilver J, Pierce JC: Computed tomography in renal transplant problems. *Radiology* 127:165–169, 1978

57. Kormano M, Dean PB: Extravascular contrast material: The major component of contrast enhancement. *Radiology* 121:379–382, 1976

58. Lange EK: Arteriographic assessment and staging of renal cell carcinoma. *Radiology* 101:17–27, 1971

59. Lau SWL: Diagnosis of renal mass lesions. *Australas Radiol* 25:52–60, 1981

60. Lautin EM, Gordon PM, Friedman AC, McCormick JF, Fromowitz FB, Goldman MJ, Sugarman LA: Radionuclide imaging and computed tomography in renal oncocytoma. *Radiology* 138:185–190, 1981

61. Lawson TL, McClennan BL, Shirkhoda A: Adult polycystic kidney disease: Ultrasonographic and computed tomographic appearance. *JCU* 6:295–302, 1981

62. Lee JKT, McClennan BL, Kissane JM: Unilateral polycystic kidney disease. *AJR* 130:1165–1167, 1978

63. Lee JKT, McClennan BL, Melson GL, Stanley RJ: Acute focal bacterial nephritis: Emphasis on gray scale sonography and computed tomography. *AJR* 135:87–92, 1980

64. Levine E, Lee KR, Weigel J: Preoperative determination of abdominal extent of renal cell carcinoma by computed tomography. *Radiology* 132:395–398, 1979

65. Levine E, Lee KR, Weigel JW, Farber B: Computed tomography in the diagnosis of renal carcinoma complicating Hippel-Lindau syndrome. *Radiology* 130:703–706, 1979

66. Livingston WD, Collins TL, Novicki DE: Incidental renal mass. *Urology* 17:257–259, 1981

67. Love L, Churchill RJ, Reynes CJ, Moncada R, Demos T: CT of the kidney and perinephric space. *Semin Roentgenol* 16:277–289, 1981

68. Love L, Churchill RJ, Reynes CJ, Schuster GA, Moncada R, Berkow A: Computed tomography staging of renal carcinoma. *Urol Radiol* 1:3–10, 1979

69. Love L, Meyers MA, Churchill RJ, Reynes CJ, Moncada R, Gibson D: Computed tomography of extraperitoneal spaces. *AJR* 136:781–789, 1981

70. Love L, Reynes CJ, Churchill R, Moncada R. Third generation CT scanning in renal disease. *Radiol Clin North Am* 17:77–90, 1979

71. Magilner AD, Ostrum BJ: Computed tomography in the diagnosis of renal masses. *Radiology* 126:715–718, 1978

72. Malek RS, Elder JS: Xanthogranulomatous pyelonephritis: A critical analysis of 26 cases and of the literture. *J Urol* 119:589–593, 1978

73. Margulis A: Abdominal trauma: The role and impact of computed tomography. *Invest Radiol* 16:260–268, 1981

74. Marks WM, Korobkin M, Callen PW, Kaiser JA: CT diagnosis of tumor thrombosis of the renal vein and inferior vena cava. *AJR* 131:843–846, 1978

75. Martorana G, Giberti C, Pescatore D: Giant echinococcal cyst of the kidney associated with hypertension evaluated by computerized tomography. *J Urol* 126:99–100, 1981

76. McClennan BL: Current approaches to the azotemic patient. *Radiol Clin North Am* 17:197–211, 1979

77. McClennan BL, Fair WR: CT scanning in urology. *Urol Clin North Am* 6:343–373, 1979

78. McClennan BL, Stanley RJ, Melson GL, Levitt RG, Sagel SS: Computed tomography of the renal cyst—Is cyst aspiration necessary? *AJR* 133:671–675, 1979

79. McDonald JE, Lee JKT, McClennan BL, Melzer JS, Sicard GA, Etheredge EE, Anderson CB: Natural history of extraperitoneal gas after renal transplantation: CT demonstration. *J Comput Assist Tomogr* 6:507–510, 1982

80. McNeil BJ, Sanders R, Alderson PO, Hessel SJ, Finberg H, Siegelman SS, Adams DF, Abrams HL: A prospective study of computed tomography, ultrasound, and gallium imaging in patients with fever. *Radiology* 139:647–653, 1981

81. Medez G, Isikoff MB, Morillo G: The role of computed tomography in the diagnosis of renal and perirenal abscesses. *J Urol* 122:582–586, 1979

82. Mitty HA: CT for diagnosis and management of urinary extravasation. *AJR* 134:497–501, 1980

83. Morales A, Wasan S, Bryniak S: Renal oncocytomas: Clinical, radiological and histological features. *J Urol* 123:261–264, 1979

84. Navari RM, Ploth DW, Tatum RK: Renal adenocarcinoma associated with multiple simple cysts. *JAMA* 246:1808–1809, 1981

85. Noble MJ, Novick AC, Straffon A, Stewart BH: Renal subcapsular hematoma: A diagnostic and therapeutic dilemma. *J Urol* 125:157–160, 1981

86. Norfray JF, Chan PK, Failma R, Cross RR: Carcinoma in a renal cyst: Computed tomography diagnosis. *J Urol* 125:102–104, 1981

87. Novick AC, Irish C, Steinmuller D, Buonocore E, Cohen C: The role of computerized tomography in renal transplant patients. *J Urol* 125:15–18, 1981

88. Parienty RA, Pradel J, Imbert MC, Picard JD, Savant P: Computed tomography of multilocular cystic nephroma. *Radiology* 140:135–139, 1981

89. Parienty RA, Pradel J, Picard JD, Ducellier R, Lubrano JM, Smolarski N: Visibility and thickening of the renal fascia on computed tomograms. *Radiology* 139:119–124, 1981

90. Parker MD: Acute segmental renal infarction: Difficulty in diagnosis despite multimodality approach. *Urology* 18:523–526, 1981

91. Pillari G, Lee WJ, Kumari S, Chen M, Abrams HJ, Buchbinder, M, Sutton AP: CT and angiographic correlates: Surgical image of renal mass lesions. *Urology* 17:296–299, 1980/81

92. Pollack HM, Arger PH, Banner MP, Mulhern CB, Coleman BG: Computed tomography of renal pelvic filling defects. *Radiology* 138:645–651, 1981

93. Pope TL, Buschi AJ, Moore TS, Williamson BRJ, Brenbridge ANAG: CT features of renal polyarteritis nodosa. *AJR* 136:986–987, 1981

94. Robson CJ: The results of radical nephrectomy for renal cell carcinoma. *J Urol* 101:297–301, 1969

95. Rosenbaum R, Hoffsten PE, Stanley RJ, Klahr S: Use of computerized tomography to diagnose complications of percutaneous renal biopsy. *Kidney Int* 14:87–92, 1978

96. Rubin BE: Computed tomography in the evaluation of renal lymphoma. *J Comput Assist Tomogr* 3:759–764, 1979

97. Ryan KG, Hoch WH, Craven RM: Intraureteral tumor demonstrated by computed tomography. *J Comput Assist Tomogr* 3:474–477, 1979

98. Sadlowski RW, Smey P, Williams J, Taxy J: Adenocarcinoma in multilocular renal cyst. *Urology* 14:512–514, 1979

99. Sage MR, Pugsley DJ, Simmons KC: Computer tomography in the diagnosis of complication following renal transplantation. *Australas Radiol* 24:156–160, 1980

100. Sagel SS, Siegel MJ, Stanley RJ, Jost RG: Detection of retroperitoneal hemorrhage by computed tomography. *AJR* 129:403–407, 1977

101. Sagel SS, Stanley RJ, Levitt RG, Geisse G: Computed tomography of the kidney. *Radiology* 124:359–370, 1977

102. Sandler CM, Foucar E, Toombs BD: Xanthogranulomatous pyelonephritis with air-containing intrarenal abscesses. *Urol Radiol* 2:113–116, 1980

103. Sandler CM, Jackson H, Kaminsky RI: Right perirenal hematoma secondary to a leaking abdominal aortic aneurysm. *J Comput Assist Tomogr* 5:264–266, 1981

104. Schaner EG, Balow JE, Doppman JL: Computed tomography in the diagnosis of subcapsular and perirenal hematoma. *AJR* 129:83–89, 1977

105. Schoborg TW, Saffos RO, Urdaneta L, Lewis CW: Xanthogranulomatous pyelonephritis associated with renal cell carcinoma. *J Urol* 124:125–127, 1980

106. Scully RE, Mark EJ, McNeely BU: Case records of the Massachusetts General Hospital. Case 32-1981. *N Engl J Med* 305:331–336, 1981

107. Segal AJ, Spataro RF, Linke CA, et al: Diagnosis of nonopaque computed tomography. *Radiology* 129:447–450, 1978

108. Segal AJ, Spitzer RM: Pseudo thick-walled renal cyst by CT. *AJR* 132:827–828, 1979

109. Shanser JD, Hedgcock MW, Korobkin M: Transit of contrast material into renal cyst following urography or arteriography. Presented at the Society of Uroradiology meeting, New York, 1978

110. Shuman WP, Mack LA, Rogers RV: Diffuse nephrocalcinosis: Hyperechoic sonographic appearance. *AJR* 136:830–832, 1981

111. Siegelman SS, Copeland BE, Saba GP, Cameron JL, Sanders RC, Zerhouni EA: CT of fluid collections associated with pancreatitis. *AJR* 134:1121–1132, 1980

112. Skinner D, Vermillion CD, Colvin RB: The surgical management of renal cell carcinoma. *J Urol* 107:705–710, 1972

113. Smith WP, Levine E: Sagittal and coronal CT image reconstruction: Application in assessing the inferior vena cava in renal cancer. *J Comput Assist Tomogr* 4:531–535, 1980

114. Somogyi J, Cohen WN, Omar MM, Makhuli Z: Communica-

tion of right and left perirenal spaces demonstrated by computed tomography. *J Comput Assist Tomogr* 3:270–273, 1979

115. Stanley RJ, Sagel SS, Fair WR: Computed tomography of the genitourinary tract. *J Urol* 119:780–782, 1978

116. Steele JR, Sones PJ, Heffner LT: The detection of inferior vena caval thrombosis with computed tomography. *Radiology* 128:385–386, 1978

117. Stewart BH, James R, Haaga J, Alfidi RJ: Urological applications of computerized axial tomography: A preliminary report. *J Urol* 120:198–204, 1978

118. Summers JL: Hemangioma in the wall of a cyst. *J Urol* 118:529–530, 1977

119. Takahashi M, Tamakawa Y, Shibata A, Fukushima Y: Computed tomography of "page" kidney. *J Comput Assist Tomogr* 1:344–348, 1977

120. Takao R, Amamoto Y, Matsunaga N, Tasaki T, Kakimoto S, Ito M, Fujii H, Futagawa S, Sekine I: Computed tomography of multicystic kidney. *J Comput Assist Tomogr* 4:548–549, 1980

121. Toombs BD, Lester RG, Ben-Menachem Y, Sandler CM: Computed tomography in blunt trauma. *Radiol Clin North Am* 19:17–35, 1981

122. Totty WG, McClennan BL, Melson GL, Patel R: Relative value of computed tomography and ultrasonography in the assessment of renal angiomyolipoma. *J Comput Assist Tomogr* 5:173–177, 1981

123. Weyman PJ, McClennan BL, Lee JKT, Stanley RJ: CT of calcified renal masses. *AJR* 138:1095–1099, 1982

124. Weyman PJ, McClennan BL, Stanley RJ, Levitt RG, Sagel SS: Comparison of computed tomography and angiography in the evaluation of renal cell carcinoma. *Radiology* 137:417–424, 1980

125. White EA, Korobkin M, Brito AC: Computed tomography of experimental acute renal ischemia. *Invest Radiol* 14:421–427, 1978

126. Whittemore DM, Wendel RG: Bilateral involvement of renal hamartoma in two cases without tuberous sclerosis. *J Urol* 125:99–101, 1981

127. Williamson B, Hattery RR, Stephens DH, Sheedy PF: Computed tomography of the kidneys. *Semin Roentgenol* 13:249–255, 1978

128. Wilms G, Baert AL, Marchal G, Bruneel M: CT demonstration of gas formation after renal tumor embolization. *J Comput Assist Tomogr* 3:838–839, 1979

129. Wojtowicz J, Karwowski A, Konkiewicz J, Lukaszewski B: Renal oncocytoma. *J Comput Assist Tomogr* 3:124–125, 1979

130. Wolverson MK, Sundarum M, Heiberg E: Computed tomography of renal pseudotumor secondary to anticoagulant therapy. *Urol Radiol* 3:55–57, 1981

131. Yandow D, Wojtowycz M, Alter A, Crummy A: Detection of retroperitoneal hemorrhage after translumbar aortography by computerized tomography. *Angiology* 31:655–658, 1980

132. Young SW, Noon MA, Marincek B: Dynamic computed tomographic time-density study of normal human tissue after intravenous contrast administration. *Invest Radiol* 16:36–39, 1980

133. Young SW, Turner RJ, Castellino RA: A strategy for the contrast enhancement of malignant tumors using dynamic computed tomography and intravascular pharmacokinetics. *Radiology* 137:137–141, 1980.

Chapter 14

The Adrenals

Philip J. Weyman and Harvey S. Glazer

Computed tomography has become the primary imaging technique in suspected adrenal disease providing morphologic delineation of both normal and abnormal adrenal glands. In comparison to standard radiographic techniques, the greater contrast resolution and the ease with which the adrenals can be imaged render CT well suited for noninvasive examination of these small retroperitoneal organs with relatively low inherent radiographic contrast.

With the current generation of CT scanners and adherence to optimal scanning technique, both adrenal glands can be imaged in nearly every patient. Although both adrenals were seen in 55 to 90% of patients in earlier studies (5,22,27), both glands can be identified in up to 99% of examinations using currently available CT scanners (30,41). Failure to visualize the adrenal glands in earlier studies usually was due to a paucity of fat surrounding the gland in thin patients; this problem has been largely overcome by the improved spatial and contrast resolution of newer scanners. Initial screening, performed using 10-mm collimation and 10-mm scan intervals, will detect most adrenal masses. If this examination is equivocal or when small masses are suspected, such as in patients with hyperaldosteronism, narrower scan intervals and collimation should be used. Scanning with 5-mm collimation at 5-mm intervals reduces partial volume effects and improves spatial resolution. Orally administered contrast material is helpful to distinguish adjacent gastrointestinal structures and is given routinely. Iodinated intravenous contrast media may improve definition of the adrenal glands in thin patients by differential enhancement of adjacent organs. When given by bolus injection with rapid sequential scanning, intravenous contrast material also is useful to distinguish adjacent vascular structures (Fig. 1). Although not used routinely, intravenous contrast material should be given when the initial scans are equivocal.

NORMAL ANATOMY

The adrenal glands are thin retroperitoneal structures enclosed within Gerota's fascia and, except in very thin individuals, are surrounded by sufficient fat for CT identification. The right adrenal gland is commonly seen on scans beginning 1 to 2 cm above the upper pole of the right kidney and extends 3 to 4 cm caudally. The right adrenal lies immediately behind the inferior vena cava, between the right crus of the diaphragm medially, and the right lobe of the liver laterally. Because of the sparse amount of fat in this area, the right adrenal gland may be more difficult to visualize than the left. The left adrenal is seen at the same level or just caudal to the level of the right adrenal gland. It is usually more closely applied to the upper pole of the kidney than the right adrenal, and its cephalad extent is most often seen just anterior and medial to the upper pole of the left kidney. The pyramidal or triradiate shape of the adrenal glands results in a variety of cross-sectional appearances, depending on the orientation of the gland and the portion of the gland included in the cross-sectional image. The right adrenal most commonly displays an oblique linear configuration paralleling the crus of the diaphragm or an inverted V configuration (27,41) (Fig. 2). Triangular or K shapes are also encountered (Fig. 3). The left adrenal is most often seen as an inverted V or Y shape, but triangular or linear configurations also are seen (27,41) (Fig. 4). The shape of the adrenal glands on CT images is highly variable and different shapes are commonly seen in the same gland (30), depending on the level of the scan (Fig. 5).

The adrenal glands extend over 2 to 4 cm in craniocaudad direction and scans must be included through the entire gland since the gland may appear normal at one level but contain a small mass on a different section (Fig. 6). The length of the limbs of the adrenal glands on any cross-section is highly variable, and the limbs may measure up to 4 cm in length. Except at the apex of the gland where the limbs converge, the limbs of the adrenal glands have a uniform thickness with straight or concave margins. On any cross-section the normal thickness of the limbs perpendicular to their long axis is usually 5 to 7 mm (22) and measurements greater than 10 mm should be viewed with suspicion (22,27).

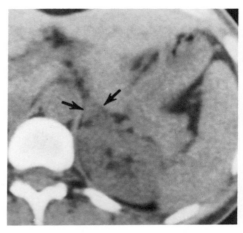

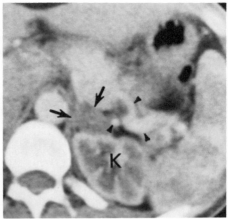

FIG. 1. A 33-year-old woman with primary aldosteronism. Left: Precontrast CT scan suggests enlargement of the left adrenal gland (arrows), but it is difficult to separate surrounding organs and vessels from the adrenal gland. Right: CT scan following 35-cc intravenous bolus injection of iodinated contrast medium more clearly separates the left adrenal (arrows) from the left kidney (K) and splenic vessels (arrowheads). Histologic examination of the surgical specimen disclosed an adenoma.

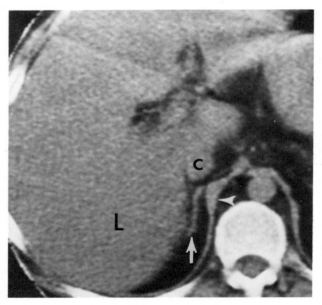

FIG. 2. Normal right adrenal gland. The long vertical limb of the right adrenal (arrow) is seen posterior to the inferior vena cava (C) between the crus of right hemidiaphragm (arrowhead) and right lobe of liver (L). (From Karstaedt et al., ref. 22, with permission from the publisher.)

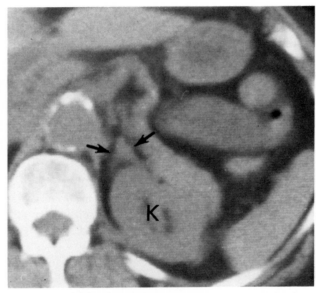

FIG. 4. Normal left adrenal gland. Triangular-shaped left adrenal gland (arrows) is seen anterior to left kidney (K).

PSEUDOTUMORS

When a suspected adrenal mass on CT is not clearly within the adrenal and separate from adjacent structures, administration of oral or intravenous contrast material may be useful to avoid misinterpretation of adjacent vascular or gastrointestinal structures as adrenal masses. Such "pseudotumors" occur predominantly in thin patients with little fat surrounding the adrenal glands. On the left, a prominent medial lobulation of the spleen or accessory spleen may produce a rounded density resembling an adrenal mass. In most cases, a splenic lobulation can be shown to be continuous with the spleen (Fig. 7) and the normal adrenal can be seen at a different level if narrow collimation is used. If confusion persists or if the normal gland cannot be identified, administration of intravenous contrast material will demonstrate equal enhancement of splenic pseudotumors and the remainder of the spleen. Liposoluble contrast agents, which are currently under investigation for selective enhancement of the liver and spleen, may aid in distinguishing these splenic "pseudotumors" (39). Adjacent duodenum, small

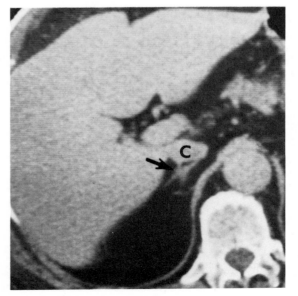

FIG. 3. Normal right adrenal gland. K shaped right adrenal gland (arrow) posterior to the inferior vena cava (C).

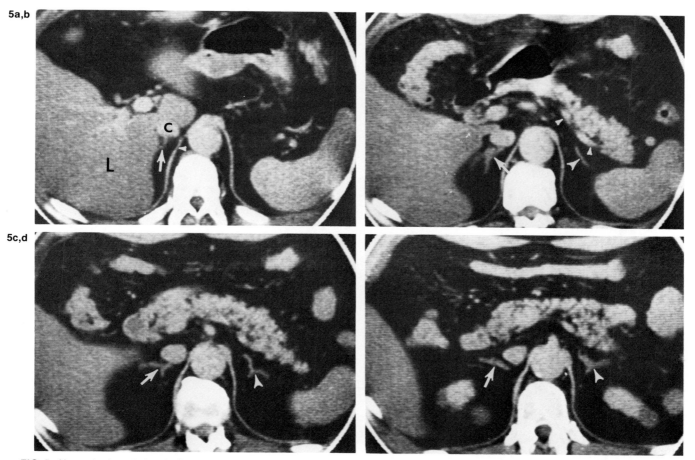

FIG. 5. Normal adrenal gland. (Serial consecutive slices at 1-cm intervals.) **a:** A portion of the lateral limb of the right adrenal (arrow) is seen posterior to the inferior vena cava (C) between the crus of right hemidiaphragm (arrowhead) and the right lobe of the liver (L). **b:** Normal inverted Y-shaped right adrenal (arrow) is seen, and one limb of the left adrenal (large arrowhead) is visible. Small arrowheads, splenic vein. **c:** A scan at a lower level shows the normal inverted Y-shaped right adrenal (arrow) and left adrenal (arrowhead). **d:** Only the lateral limb of the right adrenal (arrow) is demonstrated on this scan 1 cm inferior to (c). The left adrenal (arrowhead) is well visualized.

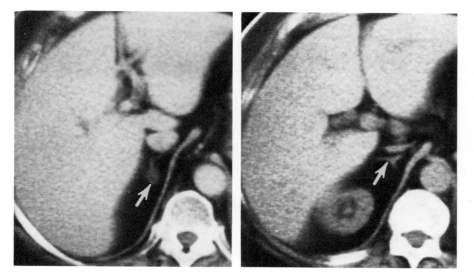

FIG. 6. Incidental nonfunctioning adenoma. CT scan was performed to evaluate abnormal liver function tests. There was no clinical or biochemical evidence of adrenal disease. **Left:** A 1-cm low density mass (arrow) is seen projecting from the medial limb of the right adrenal. Follow-up CT scan 5 months later showed no change in the size of the mass. **Right:** A normal right adrenal (arrow) is seen 2 cm inferiorly. (From Glazer et al., ref. 17, with permission from the publisher.)

bowel, a redundant posteriorly folded gastric fundus, or gastric diverticulum can simulate an adrenal mass, and administration of oral contrast agent (Fig. 8) is helpful in distinguishing these structures. In some in-

dividuals the close proximity of a tortuous splenic artery to the lateral limb of the left adrenal can produce the appearance of a small adrenal mass. Rapid sequential scans performed following bolus administra-

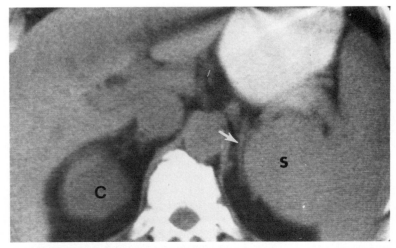

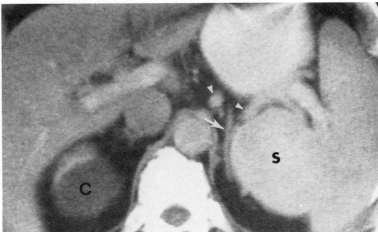

FIG. 7. Prominent splenic lobulation masquerading as an adrenal mass on excretory urogram. **Above:** CT scan demonstrates prominent medial splenic lobulation (S) accounting for suprarenal mass seen on prior intravenous urogram. The left adrenal (arrow) is seen just medial to the spleen (S). An incidental right renal cyst (C) is present. **Below:** After intravenous contrast material, CT scan demonstrates equal enhancement of the splenic lobulation and remainder of the spleen as well as enhancement of adjacent splenic vessels (arrowheads). Arrow, left adrenal; C, right renal cyst.

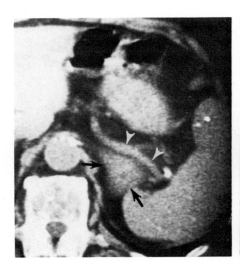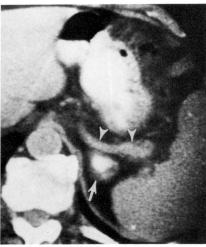

FIG. 8. Gastric pseudotumor. **Left:** CT scan shows a triangular-shaped soft tissue mass (arrows) posterior to the splenic artery (arrowheads) in the region of the left adrenal gland. **Right:** A repeat scan after administration of additional oral contrast material demonstrates the previously noted soft tissue mass to contain contrast material (arrow), thus representing a portion of gastric fundus. Arrowheads, splenic artery.

tion of intravenous contrast material can resolve this problem by demonstrating the dense blood pool enhancement of these adjacent vascular structures.

Pseudotumors are less common on the right but occasionally tortuous renal vessels can cause confusion.

Careful scanning, often using narrow collimation (5 mm) at contiguous intervals (5 mm) to delineate the normal adrenal gland or the use of intravenous contrast material to enhance vascular structures, can help avoid misinterpretation.

PATHOLOGIC CONDITIONS

A CT examination of patients with suspected adrenal disease has proved valuable not only due to the ability to detect adrenal masses, but also because of the ability to exclude such lesions by demonstration of normal adrenal glands. The diagnosis of adrenal hyperfunction is based on biochemical studies. Computed tomography is then used to localize a mass lesion or corroborate a clinical impression (absence of a mass or presence of hyperplasia). In most cases the CT findings are nonspecific but, when combined with appropriate biochemical tests, a specific histologic diagnosis often can be made. The accuracy of CT in diagnosing adrenal masses exceeds 90% (1,12,25). With recent refinements in scanning equipment resulting in greater spatial resolution and contrast sensitivity, combined with increased sophistication in conducting and interpreting the examination, the overall accuracy is expected to improve even further.

Adrenal masses as small as 5 mm in diameter can be detected by CT; focal enlargement within a portion of the adrenal gland produces a convexity to the normally concave or straight margins of one limb (Fig. 9). These masses may have attenuation values identical to the normal adrenal and detection of focal enlargement is then the only sign of adrenal neoplasm. Such focal convexity of the margins and focal enlargement is more significant than absolute measurements in detecting these small masses. Larger masses appear as rounded or oval densities in the location of the adrenal gland, often replacing or compressing the normal adrenal tissue, which is then not clearly identified (Fig. 10). With very large masses the primary site of origin

may be difficult to determine by CT. Large renal, hepatic, or primary retroperitoneal tumors may be indistinguishable from adrenal lesions because of obscuration of the usual organ boundaries on cross-sectional images. An adrenal origin may be established by biochemical testing if the lesion is a hormonally active adrenal tumor. In some cases, the vector of displacement of adjacent structures and location of the epicenter of the mass are helpful clues, such as anterior displacement of the inferior vena cava (Fig. 11), pancreas, and splenic vein by adrenal or renal lesions and posterior or medial displacement of the inferior vena cava by hepatic tumors.

In contradistinction to focal mass lesions, hyperplastic adrenal glands often demonstrate thickening of the limbs but usually maintain a normal adrenal configuration (Fig. 12). Hyperplasia also is bilateral, whereas adenomas and other primary adrenal mass lesions usually are unilateral with a normal ap-

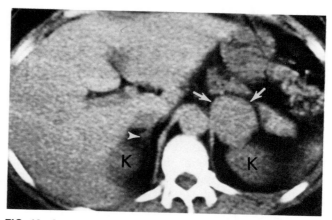

FIG. 10. Cushing's syndrome due to cortical adenoma. A 4-cm mass in the left adrenal (arrows) is seen posterior to the tail of the pancreas. The mass is similar in attenuation to the aorta and liver. K, kidney; arrowhead, normal right adrenal.

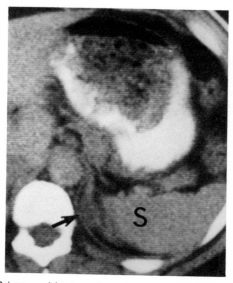

FIG. 9. Primary aldosteronism due to adrenal adenoma. A 1.5-cm low density mass (arrow) is present projecting from a limb of the left adrenal medial to the spleen (S).

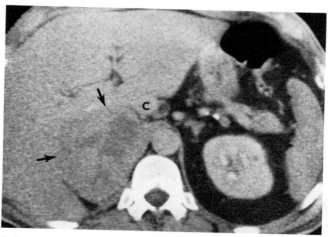

FIG. 11. Right adrenal metastasis (arrows) displacing the inferior vena cava (C) anteriorly in patient with prior simple nephrectomy for renal cell carcinoma.

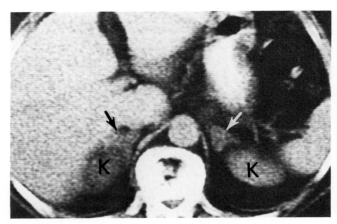 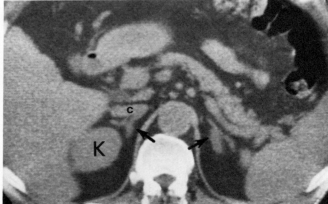

FIG. 12. Adrenal hyperplasia. **Left:** Cushing's syndrome with bilateral adrenal hyperplasia. Although the adrenal glands are enlarged (arrows), their normal configuration is maintained. K, kidneys. **Right:** In a different patient with Conn's syndrome, mild enlargement of both adrenals (arrows) is seen. Again note that the normal configuration is maintained. K, kidney; c, inferior vena cava.

pearing contralateral adrenal by CT. However, in as many as 50% of patients with clinical and biochemical evidence of adrenal hyperplasia, CT demonstrates normal adrenal glands (12,25). Since the normal thickness of the adrenal cortex is only 2 mm, a large increase in cortical thickness is necessary before hyperplasia can be detected by CT.

Hyperplasia may produce microscopic or macroscopic nodules on pathologic examination. Although these hyperplastic nodules are usually small (less than 5 mm in diameter), nodules may be as large as 2 cm (33) and can be detected by CT (25). Nodularity concomitant with bilateral adrenal enlargement should suggest adrenal hyperplasia rather than primary adrenal tumors since the contralateral adrenal cortical tissue is atrophic in the presence of a functioning tumor and will appear normal by CT. However, a single hyperplastic nodule with otherwise normal appearing adrenal glands cannot be distinguished from an adenoma by CT.

Occasionally mild to moderate enlargement of the adrenal glands is noted on CT in patients without clinical suspicion of adrenal pathology and without accompanying biochemical abnormalities. These findings almost never are of clinical significance. Nonspecific hyperplasia of the adrenal glands is known to occur pathologically and is associated with acromegaly (nearly 100%), hyperthyroidism (40%), hypertension with arteriosclerosis (16%), diabetes mellitus (3.4%), and a variety of malignant diseases (33). In addition to diffuse enlargement, nonfunctioning adenomas may also be detected incidentally, as will be discussed later.

In most patients with hypoadrenalism, the adrenal glands appear normal by CT. This is not unexpected as the adrenal medulla remains intact and atrophy of the cortex alone may not be detectable by CT. This is also the explanation for the normal appearing contralateral adrenal in patients with adenomas.

CUSHING'S SYNDROME

Endogenous Cushing's syndrome may be due to adrenal cortical hyperplasia (70%) secondary to pituitary (Cushing's disease) or less commonly ectopic ACTH stimulation. Adrenal cortical neoplasms, which may be either adenomas (20%) or carcinomas (10%), account for the remaining cases (33). In patients with Cushing's syndrome, 24-hr urinary cortisol excretion is elevated, and failure to suppress cortisol excretion by low dose dexamethasone administration (0.5 mg every 6 hr) confirms the diagnosis. If cortisol excretion then is not suppressed by high dose dexamethasone administration (2.0 mg every 6 hr), Cushing's syndrome usually is due to adrenal cortical neoplasm or ectopic ACTH production (7). Elevated plasma ACTH levels distinguish the latter etiology. Dexamethasone suppression testing prior to CT examination may be useful since CT is relatively insensitive in diagnosing hyperplasia but is an excellent method for localizing adrenal neoplasms.

Computed tomography has been highly accurate in localizing adrenal adenomas prior to surgery (11,12). Adenomas usually appear as well-defined homogeneous masses. These lesions may have a soft tissue density (Fig. 10) but, because of their high lipid content, approximately 40% exhibit attenuation values below that of soft tissue and often near that of water (32) (Fig. 13). In patients with appropriate biochemical abnormalities, these lesions, which are usually slightly inhomogeneous, should not be confused with adrenal cysts, which are rare. Calcification in adrenal adenomas may be encountered occasionally.

A normal CT examination in patients with biochemical evidence of Cushing's syndrome usually indicates adrenal hyperplasia and excludes adrenal tumor as the etiology. Although small adenomas may not be detected by CT, the adenomas producing Cushing's syndrome usually are large enough to be

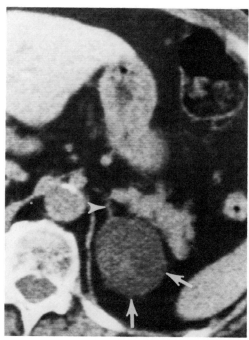

FIG. 13. Cushing's syndrome due to cortical adenoma. A 4-cm low density (−4 HU) inhomogeneous mass (arrows) can be seen originating from the left adrenal (arrowhead).

detected by CT. The abundant retroperitoneal fat in Cushingoid patients ensures an adequate CT examination, and the accuracy of CT in diagnosing or excluding an adrenal neoplasm as the cause of excess corticosteroid production should approach 100%. In rare cases when CT examination is negative but biochemical studies suggest adrenal neoplasm, adrenal venous sampling may be useful for further evaluation.

PRIMARY ALDOSTERONISM

Primary aldosteronism, a rare cause of hypertension, is characterized by hypokalemia, decreased plasma renin activity, and increased plasma aldosterone following sodium loading (7). Primary aldosteronism is most commonly due to adrenal cortical adenoma (75%), but hyperplasia (25%) and rarely adrenal carcinoma also are causes (20). In normal individuals and in patients with aldosteronism secondary to adrenal cortical hyperplasia, plasma aldosterone levels rise with upright activity. Since plasma aldosterone usually falls with upright activity in patients with an aldosterone-producing adenoma, measurement of supine and upright plasma aldosterone levels aids in distinguishing aldosteronism secondary to hyperplasia from an aldosterone-producing adenoma (7). The distinction between an adenoma and hyperplasia and the localization of the tumor are critical to patient management, since adenomas are treated surgically but hyperplasia usually is managed medically.

Aldosteronomas are indistinguishable from other

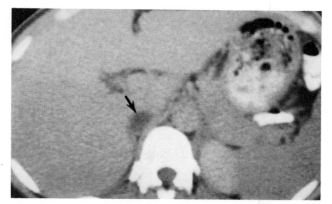

FIG. 14. Aldosteronoma. CT scan following administration of intravenous contrast material shows a 1-cm near-water density mass in the right adrenal (arrow). Despite the paucity of retroperitoneal fat, the mass is easily identified because of its low attenuation.

adenomas on CT scans alone and may have a low density simulating adrenal cyst (Fig. 14). Combining the four largest published series (11,16,25,40), CT detected 70% of aldosteronomas. Poor visualization of the adrenal glands with older scanners and the lack of surrounding fat in thin patients accounted for most of the false negative scans. Although improvements in CT scanners should increase the detection rate (Fig. 9), these tumors can be quite small (5 mm or less) and even optimum CT techniques may not detect some adenomas. In one recent series, the median diameter of surgically excised aldosteronomas was 1.8 cm with only 2 of 21 lesions greater than 2.5 cm in diameter (11). As in Cushing's syndrome, hyperplastic glands may appear enlarged, but most patients with primary aldosteronism due to hyperplasia have normal CT examinations.

Computed tomography is the logical first imaging procedure in patients with biochemical evidence of primary aldosteronism, but a negative result should not be considered conclusive for the absence of an adenoma. Adrenal venous sampling or scintigraphy using I[131]-iodocholesterol preparations may be necessary when CT is negative to exclude a small adenoma definitely.

ADRENAL CARCINOMA

Approximately 50% of adrenal carcinomas present as functioning tumors and patients may have Cushing's syndrome, virilization, feminization, or, rarely, aldosteronism (33). These rapidly growing tumors are usually large masses (4,24) at the time of presentation (greater than 4 cm) and are readily detectable by CT. Low density areas resulting from necrosis or prior hemorrhage often are seen and calcifications sometimes are present (Fig. 15). Lymphatic or hepatic metastases are common (24) at the time of clinical presentation. Examination of the liver (Fig. 16) and ret-

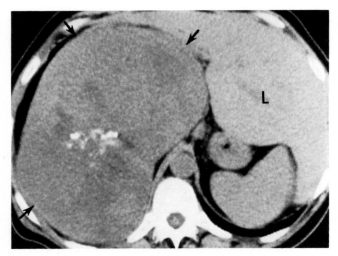

FIG. 15. Adrenal carcinoma. A large right upper quadrant mass (arrows) is demonstrated displacing the liver (L) toward the left. Coarse central calcifications as well as low density areas of necrosis are seen within the mass. (Case courtesy of Dr. Larry Anderson, Everett, Washington.)

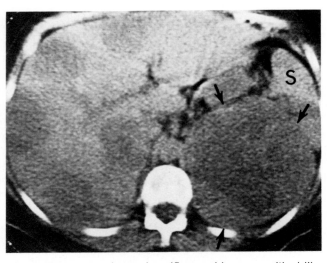

FIG. 16. Adrenal carcinoma in a 45-year-old woman with virilizing syndrome. A large low density mass is seen in the region of the left adrenal gland (arrows) displacing the spleen (S) anteriorly. Multiple low density liver metastases are also present. (From Karstaedt et al., ref. 22, with permission from the publisher.)

roperitoneum should be performed to define the extent of the primary tumor and to detect metastases prior to attempts at resection. Renal vein and vena cava extension of tumor has been described and may be visualized by CT (10), especially with the use of intravenous contrast media by the techniques described for examining patients with renal tumors.

PHEOCHROMOCYTOMA

Pheochromocytomas presenting as episodic or sustained hypertension are responsible for approximately

1 in 200 cases of hypertension (21). In nearly every patient with a symptomatic pheochromocytoma urinary catecholamine, vanillymandelic acid (VMA) and total metanephrine levels are elevated (8). Patients with multiple endocrine adenomatosis type II (MEA-II) may be asymptomatic with normal laboratory studies but still harbor pheochromocytomas (35), which can precipitate a hypertensive crisis at the time of surgery for other lesions. In addition to the MEA-II, there is an increased incidence of pheochromocytomas in patients with neurofibromatosis, von Hippel Lindau disease, and multiple cutaneous neuromas (33). Except in these patients, the search for a pheochromocytoma probably is not warranted in patients with hypertension and normal urinary catecholamines and VMA. Since clinically apparent pheochromocytomas average 5 to 6 cm in diameter (33) and are seldom less than 3 cm, CT has been highly successful in detecting these adrenal tumors. Combining the six largest published series, 83 of 91 (91%) of pheochromocytomas were detected by CT (12,19,25,34,36,37). False negative examinations occurred when the adrenal glands were not clearly visualized in thin patients, a problem that is less frequent with newer scanners, or when extraadrenal tumors were in locations other than the paraaortic regions examined by CT. False positive examinations are rare with only one reported in the above cited series.

The CT findings in pheochromocytoma are not specific but with appropriate history and laboratory findings, the diagnosis usually is apparent. On CT these tumors often appear as homogeneous masses with an attenuation value comparable to other soft tissue such as muscle (Fig. 17). Not infrequently, central necrosis is present, producing a central low density with a thick peripheral rim of soft tissue (Fig. 18). Calcifications within the mass sometimes are noted. The use of glucagon for gastrointestinal paralysis, which is sel-

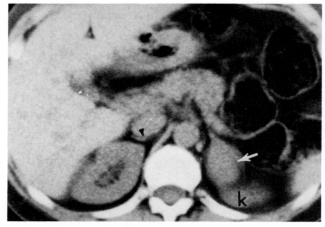

FIG. 17. Pheochromocytoma. A 3-cm mass (arrow) is seen in the left adrenal. Normal right adrenal (arrowhead) is also demonstrated. k, kidney.

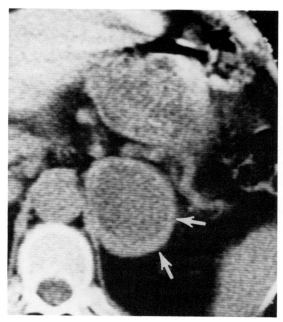

FIG. 18. Pheochromocytoma. A 4-cm mass (arrows) in the left adrenal, with a thick rim and low density center, is seen. This correlated with central necrosis in the resected specimen. (From Karstaedt et al., ref. 22, with permission from the publisher.)

dom necessary with sub 5-sec scanners, should be avoided in patients suspected of having pheochromocytomas, as glucagon causes a release of catecholamines from the tumor and may precipitate a hypertensive crisis.

Pheochromocytomas are bilateral in approximately 10% of cases (21) and a careful evaluation of both adrenal glands should be performed (Fig. 19). Additionally, as many as 10% of pheochromocytomas occur in extraadrenal locations. They are most frequent in the paracaval or paraaortic regions along the course of the sympathetic ganglia (7%) or near the organ of Zuckerkandl. These tumors also occur in the mediastinum

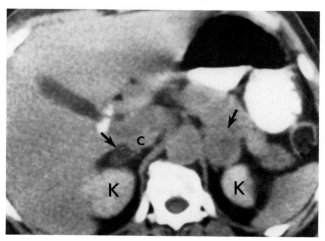

FIG. 19. Bilateral pheochromocytomas. Bilateral adrenal masses (arrows) are seen with central low density. C, inferior vena cava; K, kidney.

(1%) and in the wall of the urinary bladder (1%) (15). Detection of extraadrenal pheochromocytomas in the organ of Zuckerkandl (19,37) and in the wall of the urinary bladder (25) by CT has been reported. In patients with biochemical evidence of pheochromocytoma, a complete CT examination of the retroperitoneum should be performed if the adrenal glands appear normal. In comparison to most pheochromocytomas, which are unilateral, those associated with MEA-II syndrome are more often bilateral (75%) and are rarely extraadrenal (35). Pheochromocytomas are malignant in 6 to 10% of cases (21) and lymph node or liver metastases may be seen by CT providing evidence of malignancy. In patients who develop recurrent hypertension following removal of a pheochromocytoma, CT may demonstrate recurrent or metastatic disease in the abdomen or thorax (36).

NONFUNCTIONING TUMORS

With the exception of adrenal carcinoma, which is nonfunctioning in approximately 50% of cases, most patients with nonfunctioning adrenal tumors are asymptomatic, and these tumors often are incidental findings on CT examinations performed for other indications.

Nonfunctioning Adenomas

The CT appearance of these tumors resembles other adenomas (Fig. 20), but the patients have no clinical or

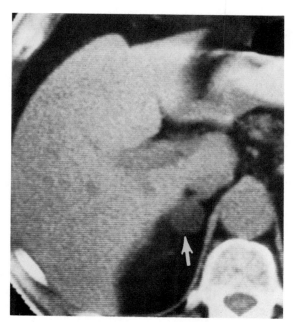

FIG. 20. Incidental nonfunctioning adenoma. CT scan performed because of low back pain demonstrates a 2-cm slightly inhomogeneous low density (−2 HU) mass (arrow) projecting from the posterior aspect of the right adrenal. Biochemical evaluation of adrenal function was normal. Follow-up scan 1 year later demonstrated no interval change. Ultrasound examination confirmed the mass to be solid.

biochemical evidence of adrenal disease. Such lesions have ranged from 1 to 6 cm in diameter with 50% of the lesions 2 cm or less in diameter (17). Small incidental adenomas have been found in 2 to 8% of autopsies and are most common in elderly obese diabetics (30%), elderly women (29%), and hypertensives (20%) (33). They also have been found with increased incidence associated with malignant tumors of the bladder, kidney, and endometrium; in such circumstances they may be indistinguishable from metastases to the adrenal gland by CT or angiography. Confusion with functioning adrenal tumors is also possible, and an adrenal mass in a patient with appropriate clinical symptoms, such as hypertension, should not be considered to represent a functioning adrenal tumor without appropriate biochemical confirmation. Since adrenal carcinomas are rare and are rapidly growing tumors that are seldom found when less than 4 cm in diameter (4,24), these small relatively common nonfunctioning lesions are statistically unlikely to represent malignant lesions. If carcinoma is a clinical consideration, follow-up CT scans in 6 to 8 weeks may be helpful to exclude such a rapidly growing tumor.

Metastatic Disease

Adrenal metastases are demonstrated by CT as soft tissue masses that vary considerably in size; they frequently are bilateral (Fig. 21). In one series all adrenal metastases that produced macroscopic change in the adrenal gland were detected by CT, but microscopic metastases were not detected (6). The most common primary tumors metastasizing to the adrenal gland are lung and breast malignancies, but thyroid, renal, gastric, colon, pancreatic, and esophageal carcinomas as well as melanoma not infrequently metastasize to the adrenals (Fig. 22). Adrenal metastases have been detected by CT in up to 15% of patients with carcinoma

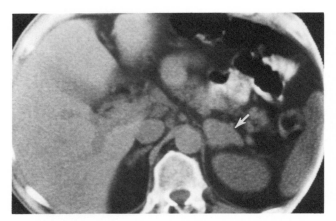

FIG. 22. Left adrenal metastasis (arrow) in patient with esophageal carcinoma.

of the lung (38). In a patient with a solitary adrenal mass as the only evidence of metastatic disease, a nonfunctioning adenoma must also be considered as an alternative diagnostic possibility. If this distinction is critical to patient management, biopsy of the lesions should be considered, and can be performed percutaneously (43) using CT or ultrasound guidance.

Cysts

Cystic lesions of the adrenal are extremely rare and most are asymptomatic. The most common adrenal cysts are endothelial cysts (45% of all adrenal cysts), which are predominantly lymphangiomatous cysts (23). These are usually small (1–15 mm) and asymptomatic. Pseudocysts (39% of all adrenal cysts) are the most common clinically detected cysts and result from hemorrhage into normal adrenal glands or into adrenal neoplasms (14,23). These are usually larger than the endothelial cysts, and pseudocysts containing up to 12 liters of fluid have been reported (14). These large cysts may produce lumbar or flank pain due to compression of adjacent structures or due to rupture of the cyst. Other rare adrenal cystic lesions include parasitic cysts (7%), which usually are echinococcal, and true epithelial cysts, which comprise only 9% of all adrenal cysts. Malignant tumors arising from the wall of adrenal cysts have not been reported (23).

The few reported cases of the CT appearance of benign adrenal cysts have shown well-defined, near-water density masses (Fig. 23). The distinction between a cyst and a low density adenoma can be difficult by CT. If this distinction is not apparent from clinical or biochemical data, ultrasound and/or percutaneous aspiration (43) may be helpful.

Myelolipoma

Myelolipoma of the adrenal gland is a benign nonfunctioning lesion probably arising from reticulum cell

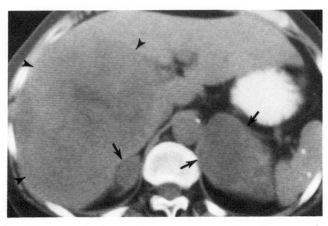

FIG. 21. Bilateral adrenal metatases (arrows) in patient with colonic carcinoma. A large liver metastasis (arrowheads) is also present.

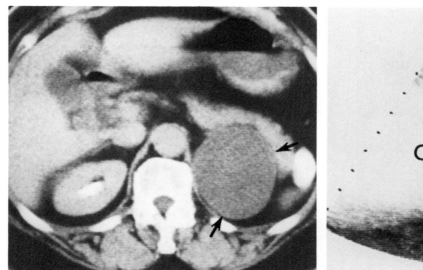 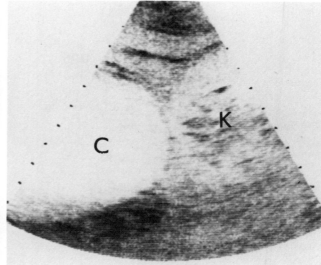

FIG. 23. Adrenal cyst. **Left:** CT scan after intravenous contrast material shows a round, well-marginated, homogeneous noncontrast-enhancing mass of water density in the left adrenal (arrows). **Right:** Ultrasound demonstrates a cleavage plane between the left kidney (K) and cystic mass (C) compatible with adrenal cyst.

metaplasia (29). These masses are composed of abundant fatty tissue but also contain myeloid and erythroid elements. Myelolipomas are usually small masses discovered incidently during the evaluation of other diseases or at autopsy when they have been reported in up to 0.2% of patients (9). Large masses up to 10 to 12 cm in diameter may be seen, and rarely patients present with flank or abdominal pain presumably secondary to hemorrhage or necrosis within the mass (13).

Myelolipomas (Fig. 24) appear as well-defined predominantly fatty masses by CT (3), but because other tissue types are also present, soft tissue components in varying amounts may be seen. Although the presence of fat can be suggested by other techniques, CT permits definitive characterization of the fatty nature of

the mass, a feature not seen with other adrenal lesions. Since these lesions are benign, a definitive CT diagnosis obviates surgery in asymptomatic patients.

OTHER DISEASES

Granulomatous disease involving the adrenal glands may be detected by CT. Diffuse enlargement of the adrenal glands has been seen in patients with acute histoplasmosis (Fig. 25). Following appropriate therapy, the glands have been noted to decrease in size on CT scans. Calcifications in the adrenal secondary to prior granulomatous disease or previous intraadrenal hemorrhage occasionally may be seen (Fig. 26). These should not be confused with calcifications in an adrenal tumor, which are associated with a soft tissue mass.

Acute adrenal hemorrhage is rare in adults but the

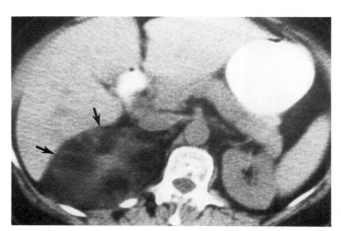

FIG. 24. Myelolipoma. CT scan demonstrates a large inhomogeneous mass (arrows) replacing the right adrenal gland. Much of the mass is of fatty density. Also seen are linear areas of soft tissue density traversing the mass, representing nonfatty components. (Case courtesy of Dr. Avery Brinkley, Pensacola, Florida.)

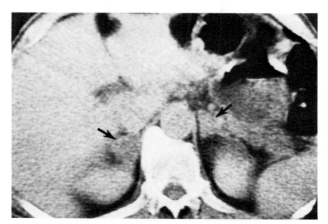

FIG. 25. Bilateral adrenal enlargement (arrows) secondary to disseminated histoplasmosis. (From Karstaedt et al., ref. 22, with permission from the publisher.)

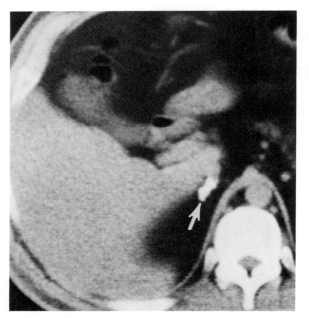

FIG. 26. Adrenal calcification. A calcified right adrenal gland (arrow) was noted on a scan performed for unrelated problems.

CT findings have been reported following venography (26) and in a patient with a coagulopathy and acute hypoadrenalism (25). In these cases, CT demonstrated bilateral soft tissue masses secondary to hemorrhage. As with hematomas in other locations, the density of these masses varies depending on the age of the hematoma.

Computed tomography may also be useful in patients following adrenal surgery to rule out abscess in the adrenal bed. In these cases, CT may demonstrate a mass (Fig. 27) but, as in other locations, it usually is not specific for abscess or hemorrhage. Correlation with laboratory findings and physical examination often is helpful, and CT-guided aspiration may be performed in these cases for a definitive diagnosis.

CT AND OTHER IMAGING TECHNIQUES

With improvements in the resolution obtained by newer CT scanners, CT has assumed the primary imaging role in the evaluation of patients with suspected adrenal disease. Conventional tomography following intravenous infusion of iodinated contrast material has

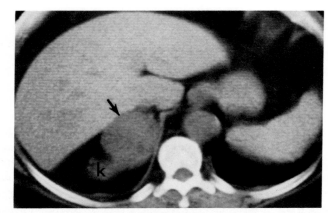

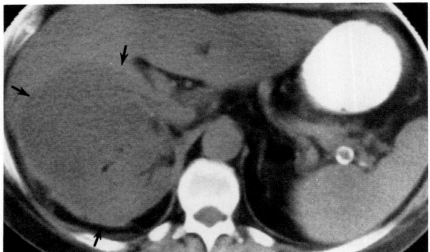

FIG. 27. Hematoma following right adrenalectomy. **Above:** Preoperative CT scan shows a large right adrenal adenoma (arrow) anteromedial to right kidney (k) in this patient with Cushing's syndrome. **Below:** CT scan performed because of fever post adrenalectomy demonstrates a large low density mass (arrows) in the adrenal bed. Needle aspiration under CT guidance yielded sterile reddish brown fluid compatible with postoperative hematoma.

28a,b,c

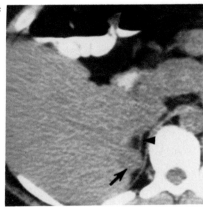
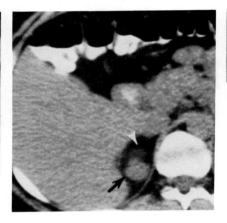
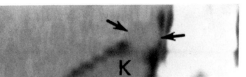

FIG. 28. Cushing's syndrome due to cortical adenoma. **a:** A 2-cm mass measuring 35 HU (arrow) is seen projecting from the posterior aspect of the right adrenal gland (arrowhead). **b:** Scan 4-mm below (a) demonstrates inferior aspect of adrenal mass (arrow) immediately adjacent to upper pole of right kidney (arrowhead). **c:** Coronal reconstruction shows right adrenal mass (arrows) clearly separate from right kidney (K).

been replaced by CT as the preferred screening technique for adrenal tumors. The sensitivity of conventional tomography for detecting adrenal tumors is low, and masses less than 2 cm in diameter are not reliably depicted by this technique (28). There is also a high false positive rate due to adjacent structures such as bowel loops or the spleen. Computed tomography is not infrequently performed to evaluate suspected suprarenal masses diagnosed by conventional tomography and can be useful in differentiating pseudomasses from true adrenal masses (Fig. 7).

Although similar sensitivity has been achieved with ultrasound and CT in detecting adrenal masses in some series (31,42), adrenal sonography is more difficult to perform and interpret (31). A higher false positive rate and lower specificity also have been reported for ultrasound as compared to CT (1). Due to the location of the adrenal glands, ultrasound (US) may be compromised by bowel gas or overlying ribs, especially on the left side. However, adrenal masses can be detected by US and this technique may be useful in some patients such as very thin individuals or children. The primary site of large upper abdominal masses or small masses adjacent to the upper pole of the kidney also may be more easily determined by US due to the ability to define organ boundaries and interfaces in coronal, sagittal, and oblique planes (Fig. 23) when transverse cross-sectional relationships are obscured. However, this advantage has been diminished by newer CT scanners with improved resolution and with the capability of coronal and sagittal reconstruction (Fig. 28). In some patients with low density masses detected by CT, US is helpful in distinguishing low density adenomas that appear solid on sonography from cysts that are sonolucent.

Adrenal scintigraphy using I¹³¹-iodocholesterol preparations (NP-59, NM-145) has an accuracy of 95%

in distinguishing adrenal cortical adenomas from hyperplasia in Cushing's syndrome (18). The accuracy in distinguishing aldosterone-producing adenomas from hyperplasia in primary aldosteronism has been reported to be 90% when dexamethasone suppression is used prior to and during the examination (18). Compared to CT, adrenal scintigraphy has several disadvantages. Iodocholesterol imaging requires multiple imaging sessions over a 4- to 6-day period, and in primary aldosteronism an additional 7 days of dexamethasone suppression may be required prior to the examination. Radiation doses to the adrenals are high with radionuclide imaging (25-60 rad) (18) as compared to a dose on the order of 1 rad for modern CT equipment. In addition to the more rapid diagnosis and lower radiation dose, CT is more readily available due to the investigational status and limited availability of the iodocholesterol scanning agents. However, adrenal scintigraphy may be valuable as a noninvasive test in selected patients with aldosteronism, when CT is normal and the distinction between hyperplasia and a small adenoma is critical to patient management. It probably has little clinical utility in the patient with Cushing's syndrome in whom an adrenal neoplasm can be distinguished from hyperplasia accurately by CT.

Adrenal angiography or venography and venous sampling have been used extensively in the diagnosis of adrenal disease. Although angiographic abnormalities are present in most patients with pheochromocytomas, the angiographic findings may be subtle and these tumors may be avascular. This more invasive examination is seldom indicated in view of the excellent results with CT in diagnosing pheochromocytomas. Angiography should be reserved for patients with definite biochemical abnormalities but a normal or equivocal CT examination. Although angiography is less reliable for adenomas, the diagnostic accuracy of adrenal venous sampling and venography approaches 100% in aldosteronism (20). This examination is more invasive than CT and is relatively difficult to perform. The right adrenal vein cannot be catheterized in up to 20% of patients, and the complications of adrenal infarction and hemorrhage are well documented (2). Venography and venous sampling should, therefore, be reserved for patients with strong clinical and biochemical evidence of a functioning adenoma but a normal CT examination, and where radionuclide imaging is not readily available.

REFERENCES

1. Abrams HI, Siegelman SS, Adams DF, Sanders R, Finberg HJ, Hessel SJ, McNeil BJ: Computed tomography versus ultrasound of the adrenal gland: a prospective study. *Radiology* 143: 121–128, 1982

2. Bayliss RI, Edwards OM, Starer F: Complications of adrenal venography. *Br J Radiol* 43:531–533, 1970

3. Behan M, Martin EC, Muecke EC, Kazam E: Myelolipoma of the adrenal: Two cases with ultrasound and CT findings. *AJR* 129:993–996, 1977

4. Bennett AH, Harrison JH, Thorn GW: Neoplasms of the adrenal gland. *J Urol* 106:607–614, 1971

5. Brownlie K, Kreel L: Computer assisted tomography of normal suprarenal glands. *J Comput Assist Tomogr* 2:1–10, 1978

6. Cedermark BJ, Ohlsen H: Computed tomography in the diagnosis of metastases of the adrenal glands. *Surg Gynecol Obstet* 152:13–16, 1981

7. Cryer PE: The adrenal cortex. In: *Diagnostic Endocrinology,* 2nd ed, ed. by PE Cryer, New York, Oxford University Press, 1979, pp 55–94

8. Cryer PE: The adrenergic nervous system. In: *Diagnostic Endocrinology,* 2nd ed, ed. by PE Cryer, New York, Oxford University Press, 1979, pp 117–134

9. Desai SB, Dourmashkin L, Kabakow BR, Leiter E: Myelolipoma of the adrenal gland: Case report, literature review and analysis of diagnostic features. *Mt Sinai J Med (NY)* 46:155–159, 1979

10. Dunnick NR, Doppman JL, Geelhoed GW: Intravenous extension of endocrine tumors. *AJR* 135:471–476, 1980

11. Dunnick NR, Doppman JL, Gill JR, Strott CA, Keiser HR, Brennan MF: Localization of functional adrenal tumors by computed tomography and venous sampling. *Radiology* 142:429–433, 1982

12. Eghrari M, McLoughlin MJ, Rosen IE, St. Louis EL, Wilson SR, Wise DJ, Yeung HPH: The role of computed tomography in assessment of tumoral pathology of the adrenal glands. *J Comput Assist Tomogr* 4:71–77, 1980

13. Fink DW, Wurtzebach LR: Symptomatic myelolipoma of the adrenal. *Radiology* 134:451–452, 1980

14. Foster DG: Adrenal cysts. *Arch Surg* 92:131–143, 1966

15. Fries JG, Chamberlin JA: Extra-adrenal pheochromocytoma: Literature review and report of a cervical pheochromocytoma. *Surgery* 63:268–279, 1968

16. Ganguly A, Pratt JH, Yune HY, Grim CE, Weinberger MH: Detection of adrenal tumors by computerized tomographic scan in endocrine hypertension. *Arch Intern Med* 139:589–590, 1979

17. Glazer HS, Weyman PJ, Sagel SS, Levitt RG, McClennan BL: Nonfunctioning adrenal masses: Incidental discovery on computed tomography. *AJR* 139:81–85, 1982

18. Gross MD, Thrall JH, Beierwaltes WH: The adrenal scan: A current status report on radiotracers, dosimetry and clinical utility. In: *Nuclear Medicine Annual, 1980,* ed. by LM Freeman and HS Weissmann, New York, Raven Press, 1980, pp 127–175

19. Hattery RR, Sheedy PF II, Stephens DH, Van Heerden JA: Computed tomography of the adrenal gland. *Semin Roentgenol* 16:290–300, 1981

20. Horton R, Finck E: Diagnosis and localization in primary aldosteronism. *Ann Intern Med* 76:885–890, 1972

21. Hume DM: Pheochromocytoma in the adult and in the child. *Am J Surg* 99:458–496, 1960

22. Karstaedt N, Sagel SS, Stanley RJ, Melson GL, Levitt RG: Computed tomography of the adrenal gland. *Radiology* 129:723–730, 1978

23. Kearney GP, Mahoney EM, Maher E, Harrison JH: Functioning and nonfunctioning cysts of the adrenal cortex and medulla. *Am J Surg* 134:363–368, 1977

24. King DR, Lack EE: Adrenal cortical carcinoma. A clinical and pathologic study of 49 cases. *Cancer* 44:239–244, 1979

25. Korobkin M, White EA, Kressel HY, Moss AA, Montagne JP: Computed tomography in the diagnosis of adrenal disease. *AJR* 132:231–238, 1979

26. Laursen K, Damgaard-Pedersen K: CT for pheochromocytoma diagnosis. *AJR* 134:277–280, 1980

27. Montagne JP, Kressel HY, Korobkin M, Moss AA: Computed tomography of the normal adrenal glands. *AJR* 130:963–966, 1978

28. Pickering RS, Hartman GW, Week RE, Sheps SG, Hattery RR: Excretory urographic localization of adrenal cortical tumors and pheochromocytomas. *Radiology* 114:345–349, 1975

29. Plaut A: Myelolipoma in the adrenal cortex. *Am J Pathol* 34:487–515, 1958

30. Reynes CJ, Churchill R, Moncada R, Love L: Computed tomography of adrenal glands. *Radiol Clin North Am* 17:91–104, 1979

31. Sample WF, Sarti DA: Computed tomography and gray scale ultrasonography of the adrenal gland: A comparative study. *Radiology* 128:377–383, 1978

32. Schaner EG, Dunnick NR, Doppman JL, Strott CA, Gill JR, Javadpour N: Adrenal cortical tumors with low attenuation coefficients: A pitfall in computed tomography diagnosis. *J Comput Assist Tomogr* 2:11–15, 1978

33. Sommers SC: Adrenal glands. *In: Pathology, Vol. 2,* ed. by WAD Anderson and JM Kissane, St. Louis, Mosby, 1977, pp 1658–1679

34. Stewart BH, Bravo EL, Haaga J, Meaney TF, Tarazi R: Localization of pheochromocytoma by computed tomography. *N Engl J Med* 299:460–461, 1978

35. Thomas JL, Bernardino ME: Pheochromocytoma in multiple endocrine adenomatosis. Efficacy of computed tomography. *JAMA* 245:1467–1469, 1981

36. Thomas JL, Bernardino ME, Samaan NA, Hickey RC: CT of pheochromocytoma. *AJR* 135:477–482, 1980

37. Tisnado J, Amendola MA, Konerding KF, Shirazi KK, Beachley MC: Computed tomography versus angiography in the localization of pheochromocytoma. *J Comput Assist Tomogr* 4:853–859, 1980

38. Vas W, Zylak CJ, Mather D, Figueredo A: The value of abdominal computed tomography in the pre-treatment assessment of small cell carcinoma of the lung. *Radiology* 138:417–418, 1981

39. Vermess M, Bernardino ME, Doppman JL, Fisher RI, Thomas JL, Velasquez WS, Fuller LM, Russo A: Use of intravenous liposoluble contrast material for the examination of the liver and spleen in lymphoma. *J Comput Assist Tomogr* 5:709–713, 1981

40. White EA, Schambelan M, Rost CR, Birlieri EG, Moss AA, Korobkin M: Use of computed tomography in diagnosing the cause of primary aldosteronism. *N Engl J Med* 303:1503–1507, 1980

41. Wilms G, Baert A, Marchal G, Goddeeris P: Computed tomography of the normal adrenal glands: Correlative study with autopsy specimens. *J Comput Assist Tomogr* 3:467–469, 1979

42. Yeh HC: Sonography of the adrenal glands: Normal glands and small masses. *AJR* 135:1167–1177, 1980

43. Zornoza J, Ordonez N, Bernardino ME, Cohen MA: Percutaneous biopsy of adrenal tumors. *Urology* 18:412–416, 1981

Chapter 15

Pelvis

Joseph K. T. Lee and Dennis M. Balfe

The pelvis is a complex structure that is made of an osseous ring formed by the innominate bones and sacrum with numerous attached muscles for support and ambulation. Within this musculo-osseous skeleton reside various internal organs and major blood vessels, lymphatics, and nerves. Computed tomography is well suited for evaluation of pelvic pathology because the genitourinary organs, pelvic muscle groups, blood vessels, and lymph nodes are either midline or bilaterally symmetrical structures within this framework (5,41,50,51,58). Furthermore, tissue planes and organs generally are well defined by normal accumulations of pelvic fat, and the quality of CT scans, even with units having slower scanning times, is not degraded by respiratory motion. Despite these advantages, a successful CT examination of the pelvis still depends on meticulous patient preparation as in other parts of the body. Because multiple small bowel loops reside in the pelvis, complete opacification of the alimentary tract is essential lest they be misinterpreted as mass lesions. Scanning when the urinary bladder is distended is often helpful since some bowel loops can be displaced out of the pelvis, thus making identification of other pelvic structures easier. As dense contrast material in the bladder sometimes results in scan artifact and obscures adjacent structures, it is generally best to obtain scans when the bladder is filled with unopacified urine. A vaginal tampon is often useful in female patients to facilitate the identification of the vaginal canal (9). Rectosigmoid opacification frequently can be achieved by giving oral contrast material several hours before the examination; a contrast material enema occasionally may be necessary to expedite opacification of this region. Intravenous contrast medium is used in cases where there are uncertainties about the soft tissue densities on precontrast scans in order to identify blood vessels and ureters positively. Although transaxial scans are used as the routine scanning format, direct coronal scans obtained with the patient sitting on a specially designed support device may provide a unique view of the pelvic floor (33,46,60) (see Fig. 5 in Chapter 2). This technique can generate remarkably clear images of the urogenital diaphragm, the levator ani muscles, the interface between the superior surface of the prostate gland and the floor of the bladder, and other structures in close apposition to the bladder, uterus, and the rectum (see Fig. 5 in Chapter 2). Such an ability to obtain direct coronal scans rapidly, rather than a computer-reconstruction requiring multiple contiguous transverse images, may enhance our capability in staging pelvic neoplasms.

Although moderately enlarged pelvic lymph nodes are easily identified on CT scans, as is the case in the upper retroperitoneum or mediastinum, recognition of normal or mildly enlarged pelvic lymph nodes (smaller than 2 cm) is more difficult in the pelvis. This is largely due to the great variability in location, diameter, and transaxial CT plane orientation of the pelvic arteries and veins (Fig. 1). Although asymmetry of the pelvic neurovascular bundles often is used as a clue to the presence of lymph node enlargement, slight degrees of assymetry should not be overinterpreted. The normal anatomical details of the pelvis are illustrated in Chapter 6.

Although indications for staging neoplasms of male and female genitourinary organs are still evolving, the contributions of CT in the follow-up of patients with documented advanced disease, as well as clarification of suspected pelvic abnormality shown on other radiologic studies, are well established.

In this chapter, pathologic conditions affecting the urinary bladder, the reproductive organs, and the pelvic lymph nodes will be described and the current indications for pelvic CT discussed. Disease processes involving the musculoskeletal system are covered in Chapter 17. With the exception of a brief discussion on the CT appearance of the pelvis in patients with prior abdominoperineal (AP) resection of the rectum, abnormalities of the colon and the rectum will also be included in Chapter 12 on the gastrointestinal tract.

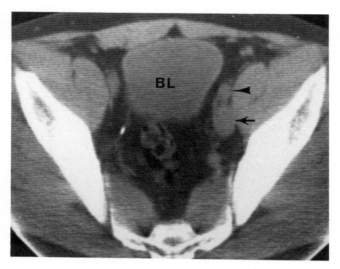

FIG. 1. Enlarged left external iliac vein (arrow), prospectively misinterpreted as an enlarged lymph node. This interpretive error probably could have been avoided if intravenous contrast media had been administered, preferably via an infusion into a left pedal vein. BL, bladder; arrowhead, external iliac artery.

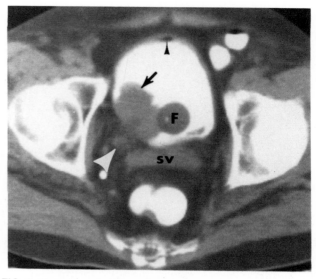

FIG. 2. Transitional cell carcinoma of the bladder. An irregular, sessile soft tissue mass (arrow) is noted projecting into the bladder lumen. The tumor was confined to the bladder wall at surgery. The scan was obtained after cystoscopy accounting for air (black arrowhead) within the bladder. White arrowhead, dilated right ureter; F, Foley catheter; sv, seminal vesicles.

STAGING OF PELVIC NEOPLASMS

Urinary Bladder

Most neoplasms of the urinary bladder are of uroepithelial origin, with transitional cell carcinoma much more common than the squamous cell variety. Although the prognosis depends on the extent of the tumor involvement at presentation, the degree of cellular differentiation affects the rate of bladder wall invasion.

In general, there is a higher tendency for the poorly differentiated tumors to infiltrate the bladder wall than the well-differentiated types (1,14).

On CT scans, a bladder neoplasm appears as a sessile or pedunculated soft tissue mass projecting into the bladder lumen (21,24,45,52,53) (Fig. 2). It can also present as a focal or diffuse thickening of the bladder wall (Fig. 3). When neoplasm causes diffuse thickening of the bladder wall, it can be confused with cystitis, although the thickening is often more uniform in the latter entity (Fig. 4). The density of a bladder neoplasm is similar to muscle, including that of normal bladder

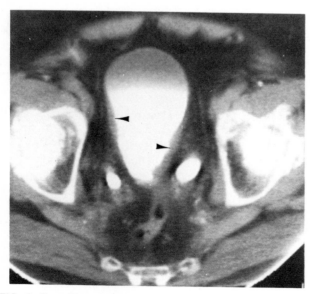

FIG. 3. Transitional cell carcinoma of the bladder. Irregular, focal thickening (arrowheads) is noted along both lateral walls of the bladder. There is no tumor extension into the perivesicle fat.

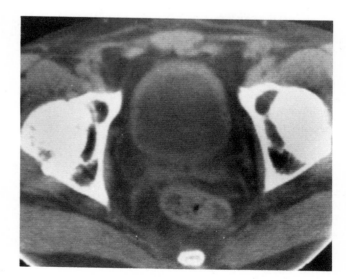

FIG. 4. Cytoxan-induced cystitis, producing diffuse thickening of the bladder wall.

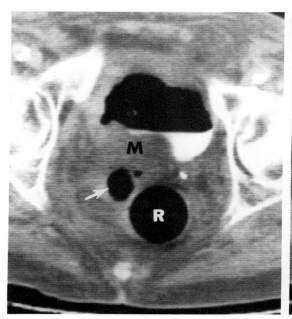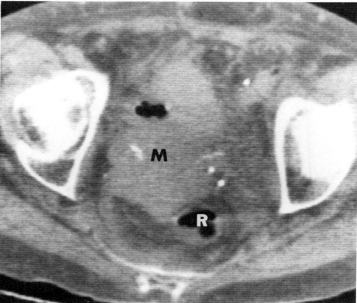

FIG. 5. Far advanced bladder cancer. **Left:** A large fungating mass (M) is present along the right posterolateral wall of the bladder. The tumor has extended posteriorly to encircle the tampon-filled vaginal canal (arrow). R, rectum. **Right:** At a slightly more cephalad level, the tumor mass (M) obliterates the entire cervix and involves the anterior wall of the rectum (R). Because of the marked extent of the disease, the patient was started on palliative radiation.

wall; calcification within the tumor may be seen on rare occasions.

Because cystoscopy is very sensitive in detecting small bladder neoplasms and biopsy of these lesions at cystoscopy quite adequately defines the depth of tumor extension into the submucosa and deep muscular layers, these methods remain the primary diagnostic procedures in patients with suspected bladder carcinomas. The clinical role of CT in bladder cancer is, therefore, to determine the presence or absence of invasion into the surrounding perivesicle fat, adjacent viscera, and pelvic lymph nodes. Accurate determination of the extent of a bladder tumor is important because it dictates the treatment and prognosis of such a patient (14,28).

On CT scans, extravesicle extension of the tumor is recognized as blurring or obscuration of the perivesicle fat planes. In more advanced cases, a soft tissue mass can be seen extending from the bladder into adjacent viscera (Fig. 5) or muscles (e.g., obturator internus). However, it is often difficult to determine whether actual tumor invasion is present or whether the tumor is merely contiguous with the pelvic wall muscle. When invasion of the pelvic bone is present, the diagnosis can be readily made by CT. Invasion of the seminal vesicles can be predicted when the normal angle between the seminal vesicle and the posterior wall of the bladder is obliterated (52,53). Caution must be taken not to overuse this sign, as the normal seminal vesicle angle can be distorted by a distended rectum (52,53). The normal seminal vesicle angle can

similarly be obscured when the patient is prone. Because no distinct fat plane is present between the urinary bladder and the vagina or prostate in normal subjects, a confident CT diagnosis of early invasion into the neighboring structures is difficult. Metastases to the pelvic lymph nodes can be diagnosed only when the involved nodes are enlarged (38). In the lymphatic spread from bladder cancer, the medial (obturator) and middle groups of the external iliac nodes are often affected first, followed by the internal iliac and the common iliac nodes (1). Obturator node metastases are best seen on slices obtained 1 to 3 cm superior to the acetabula.

Computed tomography is capable of differentiating bladder neoplasms with extravesical extension from those confined to the wall but is incapable of distinguishing tumors in the latter group (stages 0, A, B_1, and B_2) (Table 1) from each other (12,21,24,31,45, 52,53). The overall accuracy in detecting perivesicle

TABLE 1. *Staging of bladder tumors according to the Marshall system*

O: Epithelial
A: Lamina propria
B_1: Superficial muscle
B_2: Deep muscle
C: Perivesicle fat
D_1: Adjacent organs, lymph nodes
D_2: Distant metastases

From Marshall (43), with permission.

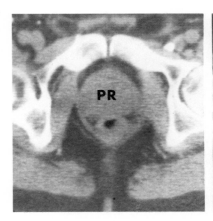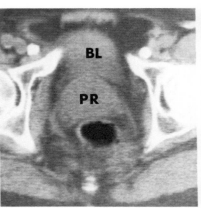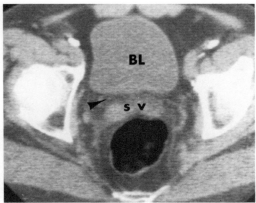

FIG. 6. Intracapsular prostatic cancer. CT scans at 1-cm serial intervals in cephalad direction demonstrate an enlarged prostate (PR). The periprostatic tissue is clearly delineated and the seminal vesicle angle (arrowhead) is well maintained. BL, bladder; sv, seminal vesicle.

and seminal vesicle involvement is in the range of 65 to 85% (12,21); the accuracy in detecting lymph node metastases ranges from 70 to 90%, with a false negative rate of 25 to 40% (21,31,38,45,63). The major limitation of CT in staging bladder cancer lies in its inability to detect microscopic invasion of the perivesicle fat and to recognize normal-sized but neoplastically involved lymph nodes as abnormal. False positive cases are mostly due to confusion produced by normal contiguous extravesicle structures mimicking tumor spread or asymmetrical perivesicle fat planes.

Although disagreement exists among disparate groups as to the best contrast agents suitable for bladder distention in staging bladder cancer, results from different investigators do not differ significantly from one another. Although some advocate instillation of 150 cc of carbon dioxide via a Foley catheter followed by intravenous administration of 50 cc of iodinated contrast medium (52), others recommend intravenous injection of 30 cc of iodinated contrast medium without gas insufflation (21). We have found that scanning through a bladder filled with urine or dilute iodinated contrast media instilled via a Foley catheter (10 cc of

Conray 60 mixed with 500 cc of water) provides an adequate contrast between the bladder tumor and the normal bladder wall/lumen. Dense opacification of the bladder should be avoided since the resultant artifacts may obscure the perivesicle space.

Arteriography, triple contrast cystography, and lymphangiography have all been used in the past in the preoperative staging of bladder neoplasms (27,32,61). The first two procedures are invasive and have produced variable results (27,32); lymphangiography only evaluates the status of the pelvic and retroperitoneal lymph nodes and not the visceral organs (61). None of these procedures has been routinely applied. Computed tomography provides a noninvasive method of differentiating early from advanced stages of bladder neoplasms and, therefore, helps avoid needless radical surgery in advanced cancers. In patients in whom the CT study is negative or indeterminate for nodal metastasis or extramural extension of the bladder cancer, a lymphangiogram may be helpful in detecting normal-sized lymph nodes that are involved with metastatic disease. When combined with percutaneous thin-walled needle biopsy of the suspicious-appearing nodes (70),

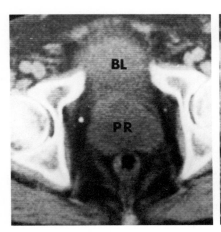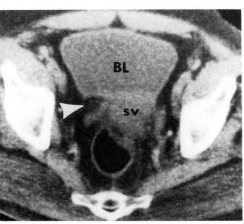

FIG. 7. Prostatic cancer invading a seminal vesicle. **Left:** The prostate gland (PR) is enlarged but the periprostatic fat is clear. **Right:** Three centimeters cephalad, the left seminal vesicle (sv) is markedly enlarged. In addition, the left seminal vesicular angle is obliterated by the tumor invasion. Note that the right seminal vesicular angle (arrowhead) is sharply delineated with fatty tissue. BL, bladder.

TABLE 2. *Clinical staging classification*
for prostatic carcinoma

A: Occult cancer
B: Cancer nodule confined within prostatic capsule
C: Cancer with extracapsular extension into surrounding
structures or confined within capsule with elevation
of serum acid phosphatase. Pelvic nodes may be
involved
D: Bone or extrapelvic involvement

From Jewett (25), with permission.

lymphangiography also can help patients with nodal metastases avoid unnecessary radical cystectomy.

Prostate

Adenocarcinomas comprise more than 95% of prostatic malignancies with the rest being transitional or squamous cell carcinoma or sarcomas (6). Computed tomography is not used as a screening procedure for detection of prostatic carcinoma because of its inability to differentiate among normal, hyperplastic, and cancerous glands (49,56,59). Nevertheless, CT does provide useful information as to the extent of the tumor once a histological diagnosis of malignancy is established. Computed tomography is capable of differentiating patients with stage A and B diseases from those with stage C and D diseases (Figs. 6 and 7) (Table 2). The criteria used to diagnose extracapsular extension from prostatic carcinomas are essentially the same as those used in the staging of bladder carcinomas, namely, symmetry of peripelvic fat planes and seminal vesicle angles. Metastases to pelvic lymph nodes can also be detected if they cause nodal enlargement (Fig. 8). As with urinary bladder neoplasms, lymphatic drainage of the prostate is mainly into external and internal iliac nodal groups. Similarly, understaging by CT occurs in cases where there is microscopic invasion into periprostatic fat or involved but normal-sized pelvic lymph nodes. The overall accuracy of CT in detecting pelvic lymph node metastases from prostatic cancers is in the range of 70 to 80% (16,39,45). Although the sensitivity in detecting extracapsular extension is low, the specificity is high, with no false positive CT interpretations reported in one series (16). Due to its low sensitivity in detecting extracapsular extension of the prostatic carcinoma, especially in early clinical stages, it seems reasonable to reserve CT for cases in which there is high clinical suspicion of advanced disease (stages C and D). In patients who are scheduled to receive radiation therapy for prostatic carcinoma, CT can also be used to help design radiation ports because of its high accuracy in assessing the size and precise location of the prostate gland (47). Computed tomography is also valuable in the evaluation of patients with suspected recurrent disease (Fig. 9).

Cervix

Carcinoma of the cervix is the second most common form of cancer in American women. The incidence rises after the age of 20 years, reaching its maximum for the group 65 to 69 years of age. The overwhelming majority of carcinomas of the cervix are epidermoid. In general, grading (degree of histological differentiation) of epidermoid carcinoma is of little prognostic value (1). After the histological diagnosis of cervical carcinoma is established, assessment of actual extent of the disease will dictate the method of treatment. Whereas surgery is recommended for patients with early stage disease (stages 0, 1, 2A) (Table 3), those with advanced disease are often treated with pelvic and abdominal radiation. Clinical staging procedures involve bimanual pelvic examination and conventional radiologic methods, such as excretory urography, barium enema, and lymphangiography. Cystoscopy and proctoscopy are also used in cases where there is a clinical suspicion of direct invasion into the bladder and rectum.

Computed tomography is capable of detecting tumor

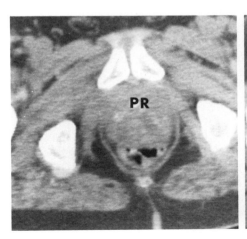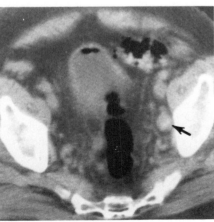

FIG. 8. Prostatic cancer with nodal metastasis. **Left:** The prostate gland (PR) is slightly enlarged. **Right:** Three centimeters cephalad, a 1.5-cm left obturator lymph node (arrow) is seen. Percutaneous needle biopsy confirmed metastatic disease.

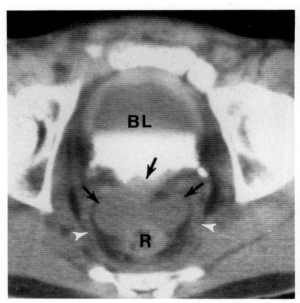 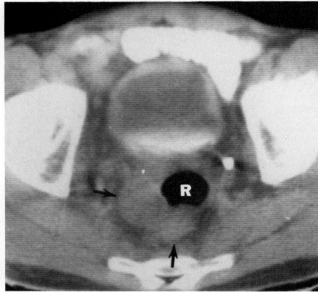

FIG. 9. Recurrent prostatic carcinoma. **Left:** An irregular soft tissue mass (arrows) is noted between the bladder (BL) and rectum (R). Biopsy confirmed recurrent prostatic carcinoma. The thickened perirectal fascia (arrowheads) are due to previous pelvic radiation. **Right:** One centimeter cephalad, the tumor mass (arrows) extends posterior to the rectum (R), an occurrence not uncommonly seen in prostatic carcinoma.

extension into the perineum, parametrium, or pelvic side wall (30,58,64,68). It can also detect metastases to lymph nodes if they are enlarged (Fig. 10). Computed tomography is slightly more accurate than pelvic examination and other radiographic studies (e.g., IVP, barium enema) in detecting tumor extension into the parametrium and the pelvic side wall. The reported accuracy for CT ranges from 66 to 80% (30,64,68), whereas the accuracy of clinical staging is generally cited at 60 to 70% (26). In some cases, CT is incapable of determining whether invasion of a structure is present or whether the tumor is just contiguous, especially in the rectal area.

Besides local invasion, carcinoma of the cervix metastasizes primarily by the lymphatic system. Initial metastases are found in the external and internal iliac lymph nodes. With more extensive primary neo-

plasms, metastases to the paraaortic nodes in addition to the pelvic nodes will be present at the time of initial evaluation. Documentation of such lymph node metastasis precludes surgical salvage. The overall accuracy for CT in detecting pelvic nodal metastases from cervical carcinoma is in the range of 70 to 80% (13,30,63,68). As in other pelvic malignancies, false negative cases are mostly due to microscopic disease or metastases less than 1 cm in size; false positive cases are largely secondary to misinterpretation of hyperplastic lymph nodes as metastatic disease. Because metastases from cervical carcinoma often replace a portion of a lymph node without enlarging it, the reported false negative rate for CT has been as high as 40% (38). Since lymphangiography is capable of delineating intranodal architecture, and hyperplastic changes usually can be differentiated from metastatic disease, lymphangiography is more accurate than CT in diagnosing lymph node involvement from cervical carcinoma (13).

Computed tomography is not indicated in patients with carcinoma *in situ;* the role of CT in early (stages I and IIA) invasive cervical carcinoma is less well defined. Whereas some use CT to evaluate the pelvis and retroperitoneum in all patients having more than microinvasive disease (30), others, including ourselves, continue to use conventional radiologic procedures (barium enema, excretory urography, and lymphangiography) to stage patients with clinical evidence of low stage disease (13). A definitive role of CT in evaluation of this group of patients must await further clinical studies.

TABLE 3. *Staging classification for cervical carcinoma*

O: Carcinoma *in situ*
I: Carcinoma strictly confined to cervix
   IA—lesions less than 2 cm; IB—lesions greater than 2 cm
II: Carcinoma extends beyond cervix but has not reached pelvic wall or involves vagina but not lower third
   IIA: Medial parametrial extension
   IIB: Lateral parametrial involvement
III: Carcinoma has extended on to pelvic wall or lower third of vagina
IV: Carcinoma involves mucosa of bladder or rectum or has extended beyond limits of true pelvis

From International Federation of Gynecology and Obstetrics (23), with permission.

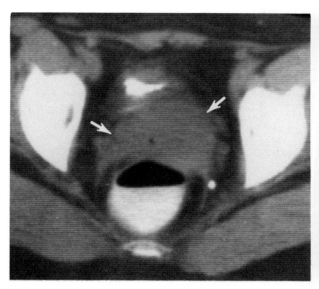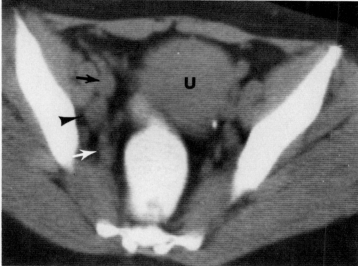

FIG. 10. Cervical carcinoma with nodal metastasis. **Left:** The cervix (arrows) is enlarged and irregular in this patient with clinical stage IB disease. **Right:** A right obturator lymph node (arrowhead) is enlarged and measures 2 cm in diameter. U, uterus; black arrow, external iliac vessels; white arrow, internal iliac vessels.

Computed tomography should be used as the initial staging procedure in patients in whom there is a clinical suspicion of advanced disease (stages III and IV). Not only is CT more accurate than other available imaging methods in detecting pelvic side wall invasion, it also provides direct delineation of the tumor mass, thereby assisting in the design of radiation ports. Cystoscopy and sigmoidoscopy should be reserved for patients with hematuria or guaiac positive stool. In patients with documented advanced disease, CT can be used to monitor tumor response to treatment. Computed tomography is also the procedure of choice in patients with suspected recurrence (62,64) (Fig. 11).

Uterus

The predominant neoplasm of the uterine body is adenocarcinoma of the endometrium. The prognosis of this neoplasm, which usually affects older women, depends on the histology, the grade (degree of cellular differentiation), and the stage (anatomical extent) of the tumor. Whereas the well-differentiated adenocarcinomas of the endometrium are often localized on initial presentation, poorly differentiated adenocarcinomas and endometrial sarcomas tend to metastasize widely. In the lymphatic spread from neoplasms of the uterine body, the paraaortic and paracaval nodal groups are most frequently involved, followed by external iliac and inguinal nodes (1). Metastases to the omentum also may occur.

On CT scans, focal or diffuse enlargement of the uterine body can be seen (Fig. 12). The degree of

uterine wall involvement is better appreciated on postcontrast scans (19). As with cervical carcinoma, CT is more valuable in delineating the actual tumor mass in patients with suspected advanced lesions than in patients with early disease. Computed tomography is especially useful in detecting clinically unsuspected omental and nodal metastases in patients with sar-

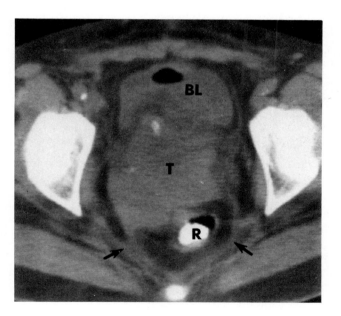

FIG. 11. Recurrent cervical carcinoma. A large soft tissue mass (T) is present in the cervical area in this patient with new onset of vaginal bleeding. The mass involves the posterior wall of the bladder (BL) and the anterior wall of the rectum (R). The perirectal fascia (arrows) is thickened secondary to prior radiation. Air in the bladder is the result of a preceding cystoscopy.

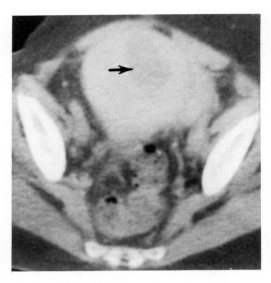

FIG. 12. Carcinoma of the uterus. The uterus is markedly enlarged with an area of necrosis (arrow) noted in its center. No metastatic disease is found.

TABLE 4. *Staging classification for ovarian carcinoma*

Stage I: Growth limited to the ovaries
   Stage IA: one ovary; no ascites
   Stage IB: both ovaries; no ascites
   Stage IC: one or both ovaries; ascites present with malignant cells in the fluid
Stage II: Growth involving one or both ovaries with pelvic extension
   Stage IIA: Extension and/or metastases to the uterus and/or tubes only
   Stage IIB: Extension to other pelvic tissues
Stage III: Growth involving one or both ovaries with widespread intraperitoneal metastases (the omentum, the small intestine, and its mesentery), limited to the abdomen
Stage IV: Growth involving one or both ovaries with distant metastases outside the peritoneal cavity

From International Federation of Gynecology and Obstetrics (23), with permission.

comas and high-grade endometrial carcinomas. Computed tomography is also valuable in evaluating patients with suspected neoplastic recurrence and in following the response to chemotherapy or radiation treatment.

Ovary

Ovarian cancer is the most lethal of all gynecologic malignancies. The peak incidence is in women between 40 and 65 years of age. The prognosis depends on the clinical stage, the degree of cellular differentiation, and the histologic type of ovarian cancer. Because of a paucity of symptoms in early stages, most patients present with advanced disease. Approximately 85 to 90% of ovarian cancers are epithelial in origin, with the remaining 10 to 15% derived from germ or stromal cells (1). In patients with epithelial ovarian carcinomas, the great majority (90%) have either serous or mucinous cystadenocarcinoma, with the rest being endometrial or solid carcinomas. Stage for stage (Table 4), the prognosis for patients with solid carcinomas is worse than that for either serous or mucinous tumors.

Ovarian carcinomas usually spread by implanting widely on the omental and peritoneal surfaces. Although not pathognomonic, demonstration of an "omental cake," which manifests as an irregular sheet of nodular soft tissue densities beneath the anterior abdominal wall, is highly suggestive of an ovarian malignancy (40) (Fig. 13). Although intraperitoneal seeding is the almost exclusive metastatic mode in mucinous carcinomas, lymphatic metastases to the paraaortic lymph nodes and occasionally to the ingui-

nal nodes do occur in serous and other types of ovarian carcinomas.

In our medical center, CT does not play a primary role in the initial evaluation of ovarian carcinoma. When the diagnosis of an ovarian carcinoma is suspected, based on physical examination or sonographic findings, exploratory laparotomy should follow. Computed tomography is unable to demonstrate intraperitoneal implants less than 2 cm (2) and surgical exploration is necessary to document the exact stage of the disease in all cases; surgical debulking of the neoplasm is particularly helpful in patients with stages III or IV ovarian cancer (18). Cytoreductive surgery not only allows for greater drug exposure and penetration, it may also favorably affect tumor cell kinetics allowing for greater cell kill with chemotherapeutic agents (18). Computed tomography is especially valuable in

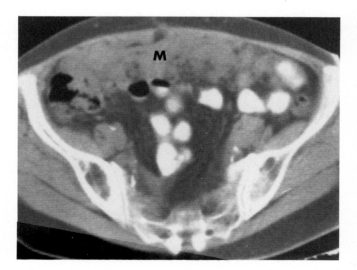

FIG. 13. Omental metastases (M) secondary to a serous cystadenocarcinoma of the ovary. Note the posterior displacement of adjacent bowel loops.

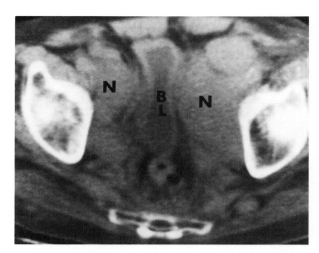

FIG. 14. Enlarged pelvic lymph nodes (N) causing compression of the urinary bladder (BL).

the evaluation of treatment response in patients with ovarian malignancy (2), and is useful in patients with suspected recurrent disease.

CLARIFICATION OF KNOWN AND SUSPECTED PELVIC ABNORMALITIES

Evaluation of Urinary Bladder Deformity

When the lateral aspect of the urinary bladder is noted to be compressed on an excretory urogram, either unilaterally or on both sides, the differential diagnosis usually includes pelvic lipomatosis, pelvic lymph node enlargement (Fig. 14), hypertrophic iliopsoas muscles (7), lymphocele, urinoma, hematoma, or pelvic venous thrombosis. Documentation of a

urinoma/hematoma or pelvic lymphadenopathy can be accomplished quickly with sonography (44). Pelvic lipomatosis is often suspected from apparent increased lucency on the plain radiograph. A diagnosis of venous thrombosis and pelvic collateral venous congestion causing bladder deformity usually required venography previously. Because of its superior contrast sensitivity, CT is capable of differentiating among fat, water, and soft tissues. Since neutral fat has a characteristic CT density, a definitive diagnosis of pelvic lipomatosis can be made by CT and surgical exploration or percutaneous biopsy obviated (8,20,57,67). The true nature of venous collaterals can be established on CT scans by administering contrast medium intravenously. In cases where the bladder deformity is on the basis of compression by enlarged pelvic lymph nodes, CT may be valuable to assess the status of the retroperitoneal and mesenteric lymph nodes as well.

Characterization of Presacral Masses

Ultrasound is not as accurate in detecting presacral masses as in diagnosing gynecological masses. Sonographic studies are often suboptimal in obese patients because of marked attenuation of the sound beam by abundant subcutaneous fat. Furthermore, ultrasound is incapable of evaluating bony abnormalities, which are often associated with presacral masses. Computed tomography is useful in these circumstances in confirming the presence of a pelvic mass when one is suspected either by physical examination or by other radiologic tests (e.g., barium enema) (41,51). When a mass is detected, CT can characterize many lesions by virtue of their attenuation values (Fig. 15), and give an

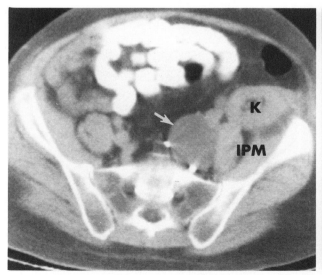

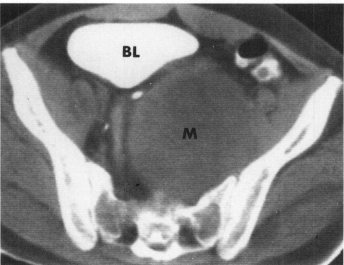

FIG. 15. Presacral masses. **Left:** A 4-cm mass (arrow) is seen medial to the left iliopsoas muscle (IPM) in this patient who received a kidney transplant (K) several weeks ago. The attenuation value of this mass approaches that of water and is compatible with a lymphocele. **Right:** A large presacral mass (M) is present in this patient with left leg pain. The attenuation value of this mass is only slightly less than that of adjacent psoas muscle. Surgical biopsy showed myxoliposarcoma. BL, urinary bladder.

accurate assessment of possible bony involvement.
Air, fat, fluid, and soft tissue are easily differentiated.
An air-containing mass suggests an abscess cavity (4)
(Fig. 16), whereas a mass with the density of neutral
fat is compatible with a benign lipoma. Masses with
near-water density include seroma, urinoma, and cystic teratoma, although the latter often contains areas of
fatty and calcific elements and usually has a thick wall.
When a mass is of soft tissue density, definitive histologic diagnosis by CT is not possible. Although CT is
capable of delineating the size and shape of the mass as
well as its effect on neighboring viscera, differentiation
between a benign and a malignant tumor may be difficult unless secondary findings such as lymph node
metastases and bony destruction are also present. The
attenuation value of abscess, hematoma, and a necrotic tumor also may overlap and distinction among
these entities often depends on the clinical history and
physical findings.

Evaluation of Gynecologic Masses

Because of its nonionizing radiation and ease in obtaining longitudinal and transverse scans, ultrasound is
used as the primary imaging method in the evaluation
of patients with suspected gynecologic pathology. Ultrasound can accurately differentiate cystic from solid
lesions and uterine from ovarian masses (65). Also,
ultrasound is probably superior to CT in detecting
internal septations within a cystic mass (11). However,
CT can be helpful when ultrasound is suboptimal
either because of abundant intestinal gas or because of

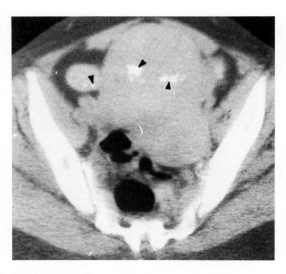

FIG. 17. Calcified uterine leiomyomata. The uterus is markedly enlarged and lobulated. Clusters of calcification (arrowheads) are noted in several areas.

marked obesity. Since a successful pelvic sonogram is
dependent on the presence of a distended urinary
bladder, CT also can be beneficial in patients with a
small irritable bladder and in patients with prior cystectomy.

On CT scans, malignant and benign uterine neoplasms appear as diffuse or focal enlargement of the
uterus. Unless calcified, a uterine myoma cannot be
distinguished from a malignant uterine neoplasm based
on CT density alone (Fig. 17). Necrosis within a neoplasm can be recognized because it has a lower CT
value and is nonenhancing after administration of intravenous contrast material.

Although normal ovaries cannot be confidently
identified on CT scans, both benign and malignant

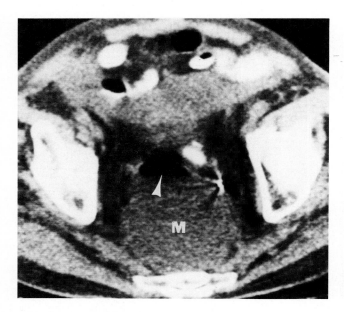

FIG. 16. Presacral abscess. A large mass (M) containing an air-fluid level (arrowhead) is present in presacral area in this patient with recent anterior resection of the rectum. The abscess was successfully drained percutaneously.

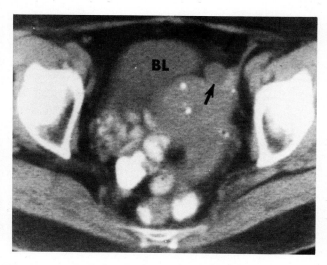

FIG. 18. Ovarian cyst. The attenuation value of the ovarian cyst (arrow) is similar to that of the urinary bladder (BL). A calcified uterine leiomyoma is present posteriorly.

19a,b

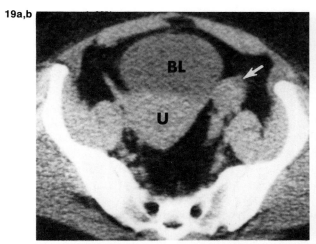
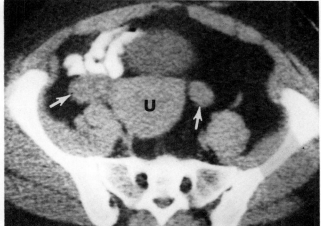

19c

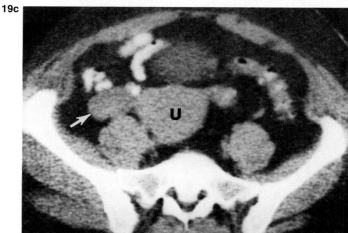

FIG. 19. Stein-Leventhal syndrome. Scans at 1-cm serial intervals in a cephalad direction demonstrate bilaterally enlarged ovaries (arrows). The ovaries are of soft tissue density without discernible cysts. BL, bladder; U, uterus.

ovarian tumors have been diagnosed by CT. A benign ovarian cyst appears as a well-circumscribed, round, near-water density structure with an almost imperceptible wall (Fig. 18). It does not enhance after intravenous administration of water-soluble iodinated contrast medium. The CT appearance of an ovarian cyst is quite similar to cysts in other organs (e.g., renal cysts, hepatic cysts). A follicular cyst cannot be differentiated from a corpus luteum cyst based on CT appearances alone. In patients with the Stein-Leventhal syndrome, both ovaries are enlarged and contain numerous cysts. The diagnosis usually can be made by CT. On occasion, the cysts are too small to be discernible by CT and the ovaries may simply appear as two enlarged soft tissue masses (Fig. 19). Under these circumstances, polycystic ovarian disease cannot be differentiated from other solid ovarian neoplasms.

Dermoid cysts occur in young females and are bilateral in 25% of patients. They are composed of ectodermal, mesodermal, and endodermal elements. When calcific (or bony) and fatty elements are present within the tumor, its diagnosis by CT is quite easy (Fig. 20).

Ovarian cystadenomas often are quite large when they first present. They appear as well-defined, low

density masses with thick, irregular walls and multiple internal septae (65) (Fig. 21). Papillary projections of soft tissue density are not infrequently seen within the tumor. Whereas serous cystadenoma has a central CT

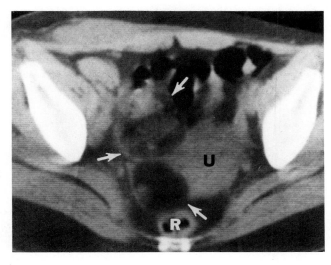

FIG. 20. Ovarian dermoid. A large, septated mass (arrows) is present in right adnexal area. The mass has a mixture of soft tissue and fatty components. R, rectum; U, uterus.

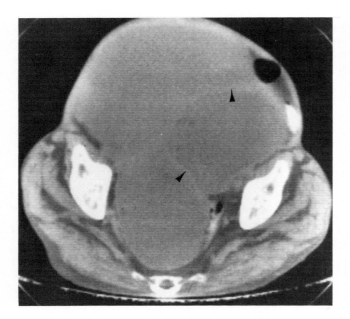

FIG. 21. Ovarian cystadenoma. A large, low-density mass occupies almost the entire pelvis and lower abdomen. Note the presence of several internal septae (arrowheads).

The CT appearance of a tubo-ovarian abscess is similar to abscesses occurring in other parts of the body. It appears as a soft tissue mass with central areas of lower density and a thick irregular wall (Fig. 23). If it contains air, a precise diagnosis can be provided. In the absence of gas bubbles, a tubo-ovarian abscess cannot be differentiated from a necrotic tumor or a hematoma based on the CT findings alone. Pelvic inflammatory disease that does not present as a discrete abscess also has a nonspecific CT appearance. The normal pelvic structures are poorly defined because of obliteration of fat planes by the inflammatory process.

Congenital uterine anomalies, such as bicornate uterus and hydrometrocolpos, may also be diagnosed on CT scans, but the experience in this area is quite limited and ultrasonography usually suffices as a diagnostic technique.

density approaching that of water, mucinous cystadenoma has a density slightly less than that of soft tissue. Amorphous, coarse calcifications sometimes can be seen in the wall or within the soft tissue component of a serous cystadenoma. Malignant ovarian cystadenocarcinomas cannot be reliably distinguished from benign cystadenomas unless metastases are present (Fig. 22).

The CT appearances of primary solid ovarian carcinomas are similar to their benign counterparts. Concomitant metastases to the lymph nodes, other organs, and omentum may be detected on CT scans.

LOCALIZATION OF UNDESCENDED TESTES

Gray scale sonography is the procedure of choice in evaluation of patients with suspected testicular pathology when the testis lies within the scrotal sac. However, CT can almost always accurately depict the presence and location of the testis when it is not palpable on physical examination.

The testis develops from the elongated embryonic gonad lying ventral to the mesonephric ridge. It migrates from its intraabdominal position to the scrotal sac during the latter third of gestation (3). Interruption of this normal migratory process results in ectopic positioning of the testis. Because malignancy occurs 12 to 40 times more commonly in the undescended (intraabdominal) than in the descended testis, it is widely agreed that orchiopexy be performed in patients

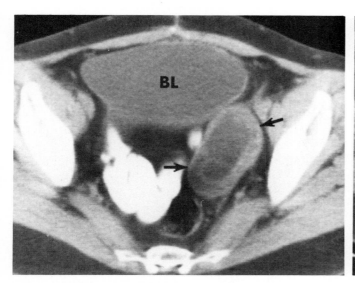

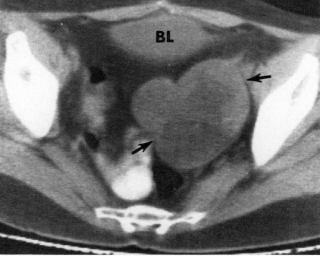

FIG. 22. Ovarian cystadenocarcinoma. A lobulated, cystic mass with an irregular, thick wall and internal septae is present in the left lower quadrant (arrows). A benign cystadenoma can have a similar CT appearance. BL, urinary bladder.

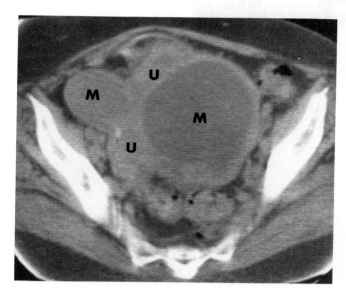

FIG. 23. Bilateral tubo-ovarian abscesses. Low-density masses (M) with thick, irregular walls are seen on both sides of the grossly distorted uterus (U). Culture grew out *E. coli.*

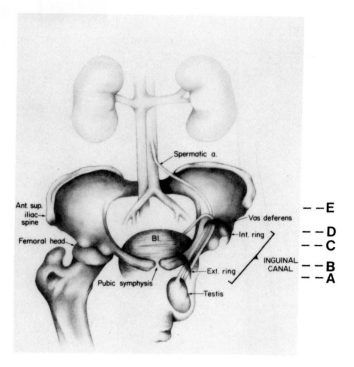

FIG. 24. A schematic drawing showing the relationship between the inguinal canal, the spermatic cord (containing spermatic artery and vas deferens), and adjacent bony landmarks. The inguinal canal is a superficial structure that runs parallel to the iliac wing. The internal inguinal ring is located half-way between the pubic symphysis and anterior superior iliac spine, i.e., approximately 5 to 6 cm caudad to the anterior superior iliac spine. The external inguinal ring is just cephalad to the pubic ramus. Letters **A–E** correspond to plane of imaging in Fig. 25. (Reproduced from Lee et al., ref. 36, with permission.)

younger than 10 years of age and orchiectomy be performed in patients who are seen after puberty (48). Preoperative localization of a nonpalpable testis by radiologic methods often helps in planning the surgical approach and shortens the anesthesia time.

Detection of an undescended testis by CT is based on recognition of a mass, which is of soft tissue density and oval in shape, along the expected course of testicular descent (34,36,69) (Figs. 24–27). When the undescended testis is unusually large, it may be due to malignant transformation (Fig. 28). Usually it is easier to detect an undescended testis in the inguinal canal or in the lower pelvis where structures are usually symmetrical. An undescended testis as small as 1 cm has been accurately located in these areas. Detection of such an atrophic testis and differentiation from adjacent structures are more difficult in the upper pelvis and lower abdomen because bowel loops, vascular structures, and lymph nodes are more abundant. Despite these limitations, CT has proven accurate in localization of nonpalpable testes (34).

Other radiologic methods that have been used to localize an undescended testis include testicular arteriography, venography, and gray scale ultrasound (15,29,42). Testicular arteriography is not only technically difficult but also painful. Although testicular venography is less traumatic than arteriography, it is also associated with a high radiation dose and some morbidity, although the false negative rate is relatively low. Selective catheterization of the right testicular vein is technically difficult; selective venography of either testicular vein can be unsuccessful due to the presence of venous valves. Although ultrasound is useful in localizing an undescended testis within the

inguinal canal, it is usually not reliable in the pelvis or abdomen (42). Because of its ease of performance and noninvasive nature, we believe CT is the procedure of choice in the preoperative localization of a nonpalpable testis. In cases where CT cannot resolve the problem, testicular venography or arteriography can still be employed for further evaluation.

ASSESSMENT OF THE POSTOPERATIVE PELVIS

Postcystectomy

The detection of possible surgical complications and local neoplastic recurrences has been difficult by conventional radiologic methods in patients with prior cystectomy for bladder cancers. Barium gastrointestinal studies are insensitive in detecting masses not closely related to the bowel; gallium radionuclide imaging is of little help in the immediate postoperative period. Since the ability to detect pelvic pathology by sonography is highly dependent on the presence of a distended urinary bladder, sonography also is of lim-

25a,b

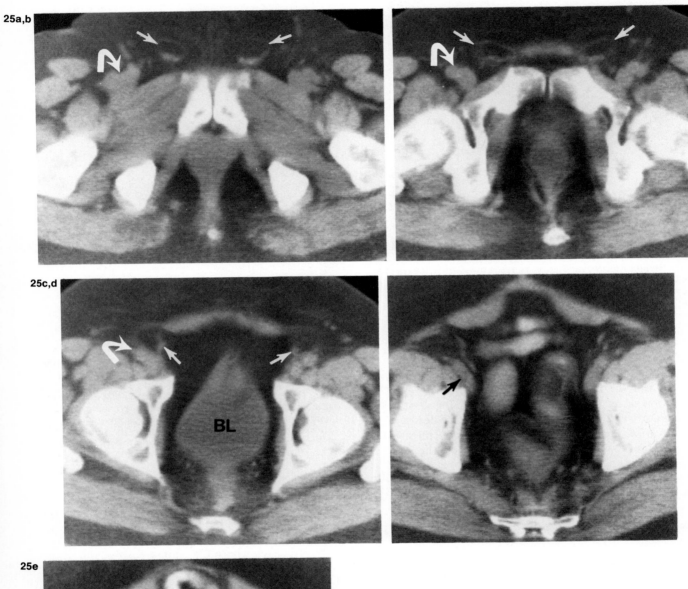

25c,d

BL

25e

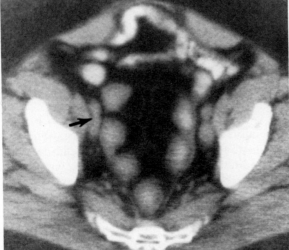

FIG. 25. Serial CT scans showing some of the normal structures as outlined in Fig. 24. Note that the spermatic cords (straight white arrows) move laterally as they ascend along the inguinal canal. BL, bladder; curved white arrows, femoral vessels; black arrows, iliac vessels.

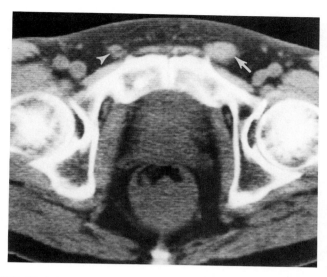

FIG. 26. Intracanalicular testis. A 2-cm atrophic testis (arrow) is seen anterolateral to the pubic symphysis on the left. This corresponds to the level of distal inguinal canal near the external inguinal ring. Note a normal size spermatic cord (arrowhead) on the right.

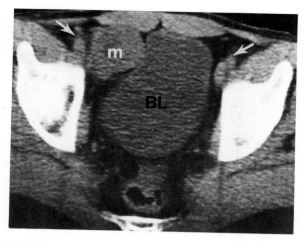

FIG. 28. Malignant transformation in an intraabdominal testis. A soft tissue mass (m), with an area of lower density representing necrosis, is seen indenting the superolateral border of the bladder (BL). At surgery, a partially necrotic intraabdominal testicular neoplasm was found. Arrows, iliac vessels. (Reproduced from Lee et al., ref. 36, with permission.)

ited use in postcystectomy patients. Furthermore, the presence of surgical wounds, with or without drains, further constrains its usefulness.

Computed tomography is well suited for evaluation of such patients (35). The ileal bladder can be imaged on CT scans (Fig. 29). Normal surrounding anatomy and pathologic alterations likewise can be delineated in patients with prior cystectomy. In male patients after radical cystectomy, the bladder, the prostate, and the seminal vesicles are absent (Fig. 30). In female patients, the uterus and both fallopian tubes as well as the urinary bladder are absent. Small bowel loops and, rarely, a loop of sigmoid colon fill in the space previ-

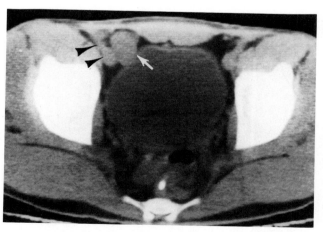

FIG. 27. Intraabdominal testis. A 3 × 2 cm oval-shaped soft tissue density (arrow) is seen medial to the right external iliac vessels (arrowheads) and posterior to the anterior abdominal wall. On occasion, a segment of spermatic cord can be seen within the inguinal canal in patients with an intraabdominal testis.

ously occupied by these structures. Although the perivesicle fat plane often is disrupted in postcystectomy patients, the muscle groups lining the pelvic side wall, namely the obturator internus in the lower pelvis and the iliopsoas in the upper pelvis, remain symmetrical. Recognition of alterations in the symmetry of the remaining structures enables diagnosis of pathologic conditions at a much earlier stage than formerly possible (Fig. 31). Local recurrences, surgical complications (i.e., urinoma, lymphoceles, abscesses), and distant metastases all can be recognized on postoperative CT examinations. A recurrent tumor often appears as a mass of soft tissue density, separate from bowel, with or without central necrosis. Although unopacified bowel loops and other normal pelvic structures may masquerade as recurrent disease, routine use of orally and rectally administered contrast medium, intravenous contrast agents, and a vaginal tampon has largely eliminated this potential problem. An abscess cavity can be confidently diagnosed if an extraalimentary tract mass containing gas is shown on CT scans (4). However, in the absence of gas bubbles, an abscess cavity may be confused with a necrotic tumor based on the CT findings alone. Correlation with clinical history and physical examination, or biopsy of the lesion directly at surgery or via a percutaneous needle, is often required. A urinoma is seen as a low density mass with an imperceptible wall located outside the genitourinary tract. Although the density of a urinoma is close to that of water in most cases, it varies with the specific gravity of the urine (54); enhancement may occur after intravenous contrast medium administration. A urinoma could be confused with a seroma, lymphocele, or even an abscess on CT. Correlation

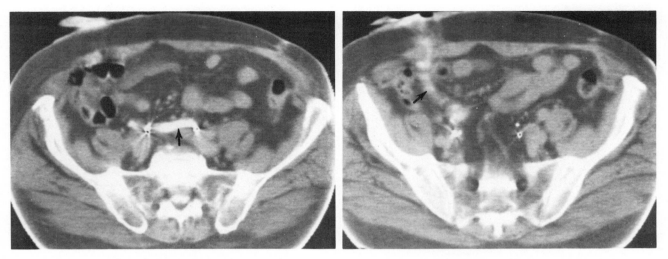

FIG. 29. Ileal bladder. **Left:** A horizontal segment of a contrast material-filled ileal bladder (arrow) is shown at this level. **Right:** Two centimeters caudad, the ileal bladder (arrow) can be traced from the intraabdominal location to its cutaneous site.

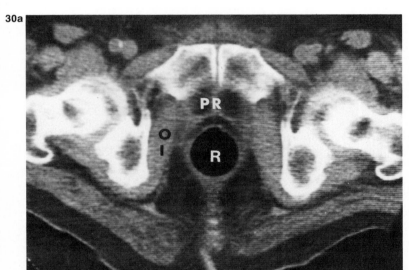

FIG. 30. Normal male pelvic anatomy after total cystectomy. The prostatic bed (PR) is empty. Bowel loops now reside in the empty bladder fossa. Note that the pelvic side wall muscle groups and vascular bundles remain bilaterally symmetrical. OI, obturator internus muscle; R, rectum; arrows, external iliac vessels.

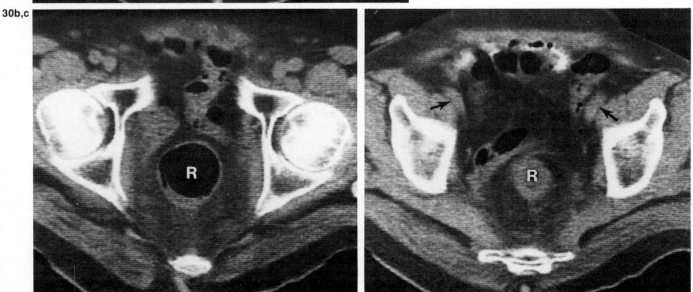

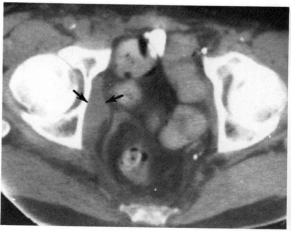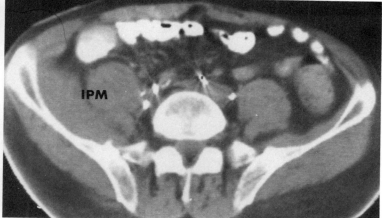

FIG. 31. Pelvic recurrence 7 months after radical cystectomy for transitional cell carcinoma of bladder. The right obturator internus (arrows) and iliopsoas (IPM) muscles are much larger than their counterparts on the left side. The presence of such asymmetry in pelvic muscles in a patient with prior cystectomy suggests tumor recurrence.

again, with clinical information and sometimes chemical analysis of the aspirated fluid, is needed for such a differentiation.

Postabdominoperineal Resection

Abdominoperineal (AP) resection of the rectum and distal sigmoid colon is the standard surgical procedure in treating patients with mid to distal rectal carcinoma. The incidence of tumor recurrence following AP resection is high in patients initially presenting with advanced stage disease. In one study (66), more than half of the patients with Dukes B and C rectal carcinoma (Table 5) developed recurrent disease within 5 years. Approximately 50% of the patients with recurrence manifested only distant metastases; the rest had local recurrence either alone or in conjunction with distant metastases.

Since conventional radiologic methods, including contrast gastrointestinal studies, are insensitive in detecting pelvic recurrence, the ability to detect local recurrence has relied largely on the presence of a palpable mass on physical examination or the development of severe pelvic pain. Knowledge of the size of the recurrent tumor is essential in designing radiation ports so that maximal dose can be given to the tumor with sparing of adjacent normal structures.

Because of its ability to provide detailed cross-sectional images of the pelvic anatomy easily, CT has

become the imaging method of choice in following these patients for possible recurrence. In the immediate postoperative period, amorphous soft tissue densities, felt to represent edema or hemorrhage, can be seen in the surgical bed (Fig. 32). The normal fascial planes and contour of the remaining pelvic organs are often obscured. Although the exact duration of the postoperative changes probably varies from patient to patient, such changes resolve within several months in most cases (37).

Several months after AP resection, the urinary bladder can be seen on CT scan to occupy a presacral (precoccygeal) location. Although the prostate gland remains fixed in its preoperative position, the seminal vesicles in men (Fig. 33) and the uterus in women move with the bladder and can be seen in a presacral location (37). In addition, loops of small bowel also may be seen in the previous rectal fossa (Fig. 34) if the surgical procedure does not include restoration of the peritoneal floor or if the surgical sutures are disrupted.

On CT scans, recurrent tumor appears as an irregular soft tissue mass with or without central necrosis. When the recurrence is large or is associated with metastases to other organs such as lymph nodes, the bones, and the liver, the diagnosis can be confidently made. When the local recurrent tumor is small (less than 2 cm), difficulty in the differentiation between recurrent tumor and postoperative fibrosis has been reported (17,22,55). However, our own studies showed that pelvic CT scans in patients without local recurrence usually contained no detectable abnormality or minimal streaky densities located anterior to the sacrococcygeal bone (37). Thus, postoperative changes usually are quite distinct and can be confidently distinguished from a local recurrent tumor, which often appears as a mass-like lesion (Fig. 35). Since our patients had uncomplicated postoperative courses, it is conceiv-

TABLE 5. *Dukes' classification of colon cancer*

A: Confined to the bowel wall
B: Tumor invasion through the muscularis into the serosa
   or into the mesenteric fat
C: Tumor distant from the bowel

From Dukes (10), with permission.

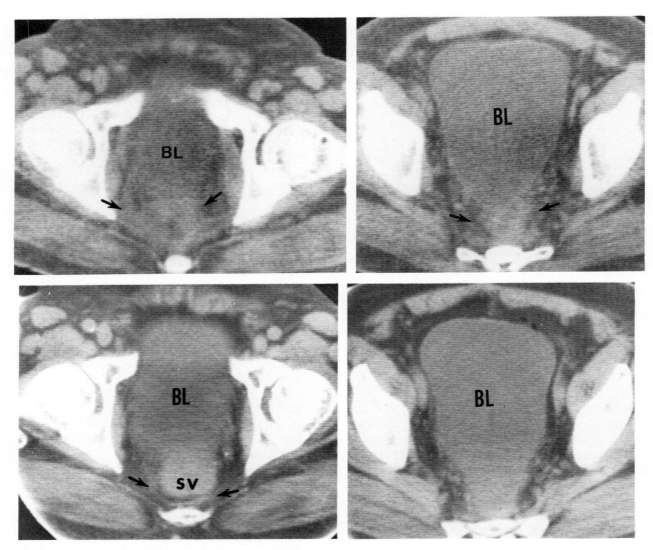

FIG. 32. Resolution of postsurgical changes following AP resection of the rectum. **Above:** CT scans obtained 1 month after AP resection show amorphous soft tissue densities (arrows) obliterating normal fascial planes in the operative bed. **Below:** Follow-up scans obtained 8 months after surgery demonstrate much clearer delineation of the seminal vesicles (SV), with only minimal streaky densities (arrows) in the postsurgical space in front of the coccyx. BL, urinary bladder. (Reproduced from Lee et al., ref. 37, with permission.)

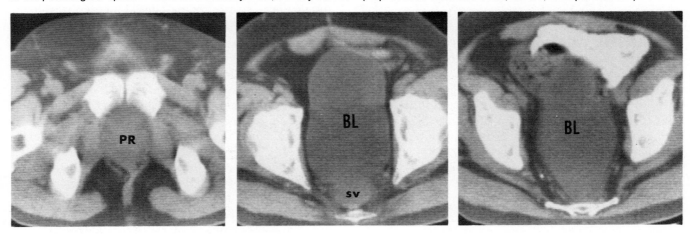

FIG. 33. Normal male pelvic anatomy following AP resection of the rectum. The prostate gland (PR) remains fixed in its anterior position; the seminal vesicles (SV) and the posterior wall of the bladder both fall posteriorly to occupy the empty rectal fossa. Other than these relocated pelvic structures, the operative bed contains no soft tissue masses. BL, urinary bladder.

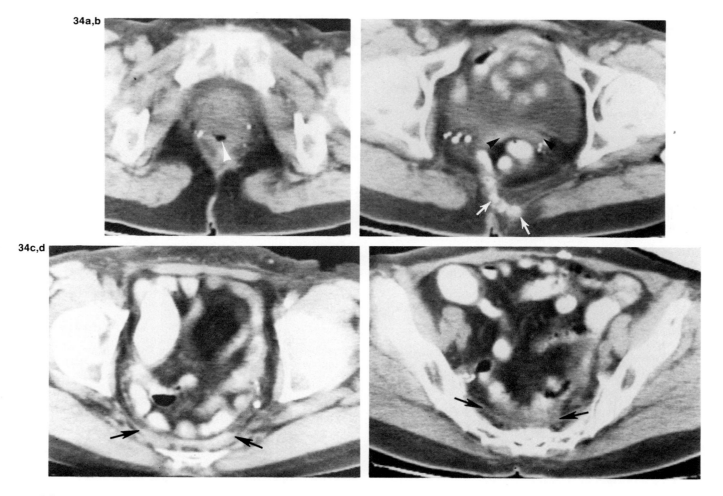

FIG. 34. Normal female pelvic anatomy following AP resection. Serial scans in cephalad direction show a few streaky densities (black arrows) in the operative bed parallel to the sacrococcygeal bone. In addition, a single loop of small bowel (white arrows) herniates into the perineum, presumably through a surgical defect in the reconstructed peritoneal floor. White arrowhead, air in the vagina; black arrowheads, cervical stump. (Reproduced from Lee et al., ref. 37, with permission.)

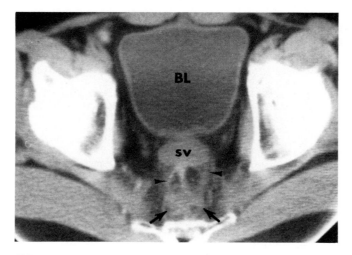

FIG. 35. Small pelvic recurrence 2 years after AP resection of rectal carcinoma. A 2-cm irregular soft tissue mass (arrows) is present in the presacral location. In addition, strands of soft tissue densities (arrowheads) are seen between the presacral mass and the seminal vesicles (sv), suggesting tumor extension toward the latter organ. BL, urinary bladder.

able that surgical complications, including prolonged wound infection, may lead to extensive scar formation and, therefore, result in a mass-like lesion on CT scans. Since postoperative changes could theoretically simulate recurrent neoplasm, a base-line CT study several months following the AP resection may be beneficial. Changes detected on subsequent CT evaluations will then be more readily identified as recurrent tumor or as evolving postoperative tissue alterations. Percutaneous biopsy of any visible mass lesion in the operative bed is valuable to confirm recurrent neoplasm.

REFERENCES

1. Ackerman LV, delRegato JA: *Cancer. Diagnosis, Treatment and Prognosis.* 4th ed. St. Louis, Mosby, 1970
2. Amendola MC, Walsh JW, Amendola BE, Tisnado J, Hall DJ, Goplerud DR: Computed tomography in the evaluation of carcinoma of the ovary. *J Comput Assist Tomogr* 5:179–186, 1981
3. Arey LB: *Developmental Anatomy.* 7th ed. Philadelphia, Saunders, 1965, pp 315–341
4. Aronberg DJ, Stanley RJ, Levitt RG, Sagel SS: Evaluation of

abdominal abscess with computed tomography. *J Comput Assist Tomogr* 2:384–387, 1978

5. Bonney WW, Chiu LC, Culp DA: Computed tomography of the pelvis. *J Urol* 120:457–464, 1978

6. Catalona WJ, Scott WW: Carcinoma of the prostate: A review. *J Urol* 119:1–8, 1978

7. Chang SF: Pear-shaped bladder caused by large iliopsoas muscles. *Radiology* 128:349–350, 1978

8. Church PA, Kazam E: Computed tomography and ultrasound in diagnosis of pelvic lipomatosis. *Urology* 14:631–633, 1979

9. Cohen WN, Seidelmann FE, Bryan PJ: Use of a tampon to enhance vaginal localization in computed tomography. *AJR* 128:1064–1065, 1977

10. Dukes CE: The classification of cancer of the rectum. *J Pathol Bacteriol* 35:323–332, 1932

11. Federle MP, Filly RA, Moss AA: Cystic hepatic neoplasms: Complementary roles of CT and sonography. *AJR* 136:345–348, 1981

12. Frodin L, Hemmingsson A, Johansson A, Wicklund H: Computed tomography in staging of bladder carcinoma. *Acta Radiol [Diagn] (Stockh)* 21:763–767, 1980

13. Ginaldi S, Wallace S, Jing BS, Bernardino ME: Carcinoma of the cervix: Lymphangiography and computed tomography. *AJR* 136:1087–1091, 1981

14. Gittes RF: Tumors of the bladder. In: *Urology,* ed. by JH Harrison, RF Gittes, AD Perlmutter, TA Stamey, and PC Walsh, Philadelphia, Saunders, 1970, pp 1033–1070

15. Glickman MG, Weiss RM, Itzchalk Y: Testicular venography for undescended testes. *AJR* 129:71–75, 1977

16. Golimbu M, Morales P, Al-Askari S, Shulman Y: CAT scanning in staging of prostatic cancer. *Urology* 18:305–308, 1981

17. Grabbe VE, Buurman R, Winkler R, Bucheler E, Schreiber H-W: Computer-tomographische befunde nach rektumamputation. *ROEFO* 131:135–139, 1979

18. Griffiths CT, Parker LM, Fuller AF Jr: Role of cytoreductive surgical treatment in the management of advanced ovarian carcinoma. *Cancer Treat Rep* 63:235–240, 1979

19. Hamlin DJ, Burgener FA, Beecham JB: CT of intramural endometrial carcinoma: Contrast enhancement is essential. *AJR* 137:551–554, 1981

20. Harris RD, Bendon JA, Robinson CA, Seat SG, Herwig KR: Computed tomographic evaluation of pear-shaped bladder. *Urology* 14:528–530, 1979

21. Hodson NJ, Husband JE, Macdonald JS: The role of computed tomography in the staging of bladder cancer. *Clin Radiol* 30:389–395, 1979

22. Husband JE, Hodson NJ, Parsons CA: The use of computed tomography in recurrent rectal tumors. *Radiology* 134:677–682, 1980

23. International Federation of Gynecology and Obstetrics: Classification and staging of malignant tumors in the female pelvis. *J Int Fed Gynecol Obstet* 3:204, 1965

24. Jeffrey RB, Palubinskas AJ, Federle MP: CT evaluation of invasive lesions of the bladder. *J Comput Assist Tomogr* 5:22–26, 1981

25. Jewett JH: The present status of radical prostatectomy for stages A and B prostatic cancer. *Urol Clin North Am* 2:105–124, 1975

26. Kademian MT, Bosch A: Staging laparotomy and survival in carcinoma of the uterine cervix. *Acta Radiol (Ther) [Stockh]* 16:314–324, 1977

27. Kafkas M: Study and diagnosis of bladder tumors by triple contrast cystography. *J Urol* 109:32–34, 1973

28. Kenny GM, Hardner GJ, Moore RM, Murphy GP: Current results from treatment of stages C and D bladder tumors at Roswell Park Memorial Institute. *J Urol* 107:56–59, 1972

29. Khademi M, Seebode JJ, Falla A: Selective spermatic arteriography for localization of impalpable undescended testis. *Radiology* 136:627–634, 1980

30. Kilcheski TS, Arger PH, Mulhern CB, Coleman BG, Kressel HY, Mikuta JI: Role of computed tomography in the presurgical evaluation of carcinoma of the cervix. *J Comput Assist Tomogr* 5:378–383, 1981

31. Koss JC, Arger PH, Coleman BG, Mulhern CB, Pollack HM, Wein AJ: CT staging of bladder carcinoma. *AJR* 137:359–362, 1981

32. Lang EK: The use of arteriography in the demonstration of staging of bladder tumors. *Radiology* 80:62–68, 1963

33. Lee JKT, Barbier JY, McClennan BL, Stanley RJ: Technical note: A support device for obtaining direct coronal CT images of the pelvis and lower abdomen. *Radiology* (in press)

34. Lee JKT, Glazer HG: CT in the localization of the nonpalpable testis. *Urol Clin North Am* (in press)

35. Lee JKT, McClennan BL, Stanley RJ, Levitt RG, Sagel SS: Use of CT in evaluation of postcystectomy patients. *AJR* 136:483–487, 1981

36. Lee JKT, McClennan BL, Stanley RJ, Sagel SS: Utility of computed tomography in the localization of the undescended testis. *Radiology* 135:121–125, 1980

37. Lee JKT, Stanley RJ, Sagel SS, Levitt RG, McClennan BL: CT appearance of the pelvis after abdomino-perineal resection for rectal carcinoma. *Radiology* 141:737–741, 1981

38. Lee JKT, Stanley RJ, Sagel SS, McClennan BL: Accuracy of CT in detecting intraabdominal and pelvic lymph node metastases from pelvic cancers. *AJR* 131:675–679, 1978

39. Levine MS, Arger PH, Coleman BG, Mulhern CB, Pollack HM, Wein AJ: Detecting lymphatic metastases from prostatic carcinoma: Superiority of CT. *AJR* 137:207–211, 1981

40. Levitt RG, Sagel SS, Stanley RJ: Detection of neoplastic involvement of the mesentery and omentum by computed tomography. *AJR* 131:835–838, 1978

41. Levitt RG, Sagel SS, Stanley RJ, Evens RG: Computed tomography of the pelvis. *Semin Roentgenol* 13:193–200, 1978

42. Madrazo BL, Klugo RC, Parks JA, DiLoreto R: Ultrasonographic demonstration of undescended testis. *Radiology* 133:181–183, 1979

43. Marshall VF: The relation of the preoperative estimate to the pathologic demonstration of the extent of vesical neoplasms. *J Urol* 68:714–723, 1952

44. Mittelstaedt CA, Gosink BB, Leopold GR: Gray scale patterns of pelvic disease in the male. *Radiology* 123:727–732, 1977

45. Morgan CL, Calkins RF, Cavalcanti EJ: Computed tomography in the evaluation, staging, and therapy of carcinoma of the bladder and prostate. *Radiology* 140:751–761, 1981

46. Osborn AG, Koehler PR, Gibbs FA, Leavitt DD, Anderson RE, Lee TG, Ferris DT: Direct sagittal computed tomographic scans in the radiologic evaluation of the pelvis. *Radiology* 134:255–257, 1980

47. Pilepich MV, Perez CA, Prasad S: Computed tomography in definitive radiotherapy of prostatic carcinoma. *Int J Radiat Oncol Biol Phys* 6:923–926, 1980

48. Pinch L, Aceta T, Meyer-Bahlburg HFL: Cryptorchidism. A pediatric review. *Urol Clin North Am* 1:573–592, 1974

49. Price JM, Davidson AJ: Computed tomography in the evaluation of the suspected carcinomatous prostate. *Urol Radiol* 1:38–42, 1979

50. Redman HC; Computed tomography of the pelvis. *Radiol Clin North Am* 15:441–448, 1977

51. Seidelmann FE, Cohen WN: Pelvis In: *Computed Tomography of Abdominal Abnormalities,* ed. by J Haaga and NE Reich, St. Louis, Mosby, 1978, Chapter 7, pp 221–276

52. Seidelmann FE, Cohen WN, Bryan PJ: Computed tomographic staging of bladder neoplasms. *Radiol Clin North Am* 15:419–440, 1977

53. Seidelmann FE, Cohen WN, Bryan PJ, Temes SP, Kraus D, Schoenrock G: Accuracy of CT staging of bladder neoplasms using the gas-filled method: Report of 21 patients with surgical confirmation. *AJR* 130:735–739, 1978

54. Stanley RJ: Fluid characterization with computed tomography. In: *Computed Tomography, Ultrasound and X-ray: An Integrated Approach,* ed. by AA Moss and HI Goldberg. San Francisco, San Francisco University of California, Department of Radiology, pp 65–66, 1980

55. Steinbrich VW, Modder U, Rosenberger J, Friedmann G: Computer-tomographische diagnostik jokaler rezidive nach operationen von rektumkarzinomen. *ROEFO* 131:499–503, 1979

56. Sukov RJ, Scardino PT, Sample WF, Winter J, Confer DJ:

Computed tomography and transabdominal ultrasound in the evaluation of the prostate. *J Comput Assist Tomogr* 1:281–289, 1977

57. Susmano DE, Dolin EH: Computed tomography in diagnosis of pelvic lipomatosis. *Urology* 13:215–220, 1979

58. Tisnado J, Amendola MA, Walsh JW, Jordan RL, Turner MA, Krempa J: Computed tomography of the perineum. *AJR* 136:475–481, 1981

59. Van Engelshoven JMA, Kreel L: Computed tomography of the prostate. *J Comput Assist Tomogr* 3:45–51, 1979

60. VanWaes PFGM, Zonneveld FW: Direct coronal body computed tomography. *J Comput Assist Tomogr* 6:58–66, 1982

61. Wajsman Z, Baumgartner G, Murphy GP, Merrin C: Evaluation of lymphangiography for clinical staging of bladder tumors. *J Urol* 114:714–724, 1975

62. Walsh JW, Amendola MA, Hall DJ, Tisnado J, Goplerud DR: Recurrent carcinoma of the cervix: CT diagnosis. *AJR* 136:117–122, 1981

63. Walsh JW, Amendola MA, Konerding KF, Tisnado J, Hazra TA: Computed tomographic detection of pelvic and inguinal lymph node metastases from primary and recurrent pelvic malignant disease. *Radiology* 137:157–166, 1980

64. Walsh JW, Goplerud DR: Prospective comparison between clinical and CT staging in primary cervical carcinoma. *AJR* 137:997–1003, 1981

65. Walsh JW, Rosenfield AT, Jaffe CC, Schwartz PE, Simeone J, Dembner AG, Taylor KJW: Prospective comparison of ultrasound and computed tomography in the evaluation of gynecologic pelvic masses. *AJR* 131:955–960, 1978

66. Walz BJ, Lindstrom ER, Butcher HR, Baglan RJ: Natural history of patients after abdominal-perineal resection implications for radiation therapy. *Cancer* 39:2437–2442, 1977

67. Werboff LH, Korobkin M, Klein RS: Pelvic lipomatosis: Diagnosis using computed tomography. *Urology* 122:257–259, 1979

68. Whitley NO, Brenner DE, Francis A, Villa Santa U, Aisner J, Wiernik PH, Whitley J: CT evaluation of carcinoma of the cervix. *Radiology* 142:439–446, 1982

69. Wolverson MK, Jagannadharao B, Sundaram M, Riaz A, Nalesnik WJ, Houttuin E: CT in localization of impalpable cryptochid testes. *AJR* 134:725–729, 1980

70. Zornoza J, Wallace S, Goldstein HM, Lukeman JM, Jing B-S: Transperitoneal percutaneous retroperitoneal lymph node aspiration biopsy. *Radiology* 122:111–115, 1977

Chapter 16

Spine

Mokhtar H. Gado, Fred J. Hodges, III, and Jash I. Patel

DEGENERATIVE DISEASE OF THE LUMBAR SPINE

Degenerative processes in the lumbar spine may affect the intervertebral disc space and both posterior articular joints. Any or all of these three joints may be involved. Moreover, degeneration of the intervertebral disc may be the primary condition and result in subsequent posterior articular joint degeneration. Likewise, the degenerative disease in the posterior articular joints may be the primary change with resultant secondary disc degeneration (58).

The ability of computed tomography to demonstrate degenerative conditions of the lumbar spine, particularly herniation of the nucleus pulposus, has stimulated its recent widespread application since the major alternative diagnostic method—myelography—is an invasive technique with a definite associated morbidity.

Technique

Computed tomographic examination of the lumbar spine for the purpose of diagnosis of degenerative disc disease requires a higher spatial resolution than that ordinarily used with "standard" examinations of the body or the brain, i.e., a pixel size of less than 1 mm. A slice thickness of 4 or 5 mm usually is adequate for visualization of the disc material and the dural sac and its contents with an acceptable degree of volume averaging. The use of thicker slices (e.g., 8 to 10 mm) results in more volume averaging and unacceptable degradation of the resolution in the axis perpendicular to the plane of the slice. Thinner slices of 1.5 or 2 mm should be reserved for unique problem cases because of the much larger number of slices and therefore longer examination time required. In addition, the decrease in photon flux with the use of thin slices degrades the statistical quality of the image and the contrast discrimination possible.

The examination of one intervertebral disc space should cover the region from the pedicle of the vertebra above to the pedicle of the vertebra below. Thus, the entire extent of the intervertebral foramen as well as the intervertebral disc spaces are included.

We believe that the slices should be oriented parallel to the plane of the intervertebral space. Thus, the orientation of the set of slices may be changed from one disc level to another (Fig. 1). With such a technique, reformatting of images in either a sagittal or coronal plane, if required, will be obtainable only for each set of parallel slices obtained. The majority of interpretations is rendered from the transverse images oriented in the plane of the disc, and reformatting is not used routinely. Some radiologists, however, do advocate examination of the entire region of interest with contiguous and often overlapping parallel slices in order to enable reformatting in every case (27). In those instances, it is still advisable to obtain one or two additional slices through each disc space (34).

Selection of the proper location and orientation of the slices requires first obtaining a "scannogram" or "scout view." This preliminary digital radiograph is got by moving the patient couch through the X-ray beam while the tube and detectors are kept stationary. Through software interaction, the level and orientation of the slice are selected for each set of parallel slices (74).

Normal CT Anatomy

The anatomy, from the pedicle of the vertebra above the disc (the superior vertebra) to the pedicle of the vertebra below the disc (the inferior vertebra), can be described from above downward in the following sequence:

1. The superior pedicle (Fig. 2). At this level, the vertebral body, pedicle, and laminae of the superior vertebra form a complete bony ring. When a lordotic angle exists between two vertebrae, the most cephalad slice of the series may run through the interlaminar space above the upper vertebra. The next lower slice, however, will then demonstrate the complete bony ring. The configuration of the bony ring is more or less triangular and the dural sac occupies the entire contained space in the upper lumbar region. More caudad, particularly at the lumbosacral junction, the

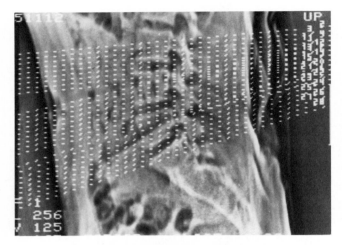

FIG. 1. A scout lateral view of the lumbosacral spine. The dotted lines are entered on the digital radiograph (scout view or scannogram) by software interaction between the operator and the computer of the CT scanner. These lines determine the level and plane of orientation of each individual slice. Note that this examination consisted of three groups or subsets of parallel slices. Each subset covers one intervertebral disc space and extends from one pedicle to the other. The change in orientation from one subset to the other is dictated by the lordosis of the lumbosacral spine.

dural sac is significantly smaller in size, and occupies only a fraction of the area of the bony spinal canal. Epidural fat fills the space around the dural sac. Below the lower end of the "cul-de-sac," the sacral and coccygeal nerve roots as seen in cross section appear as a series of small rounded soft tissue structures amid the low-density fat.

2. The upper part of the intervertebral foramen (Fig. 3). Just below the pedicle, the intervertebral foramen appears as a "gap" separating the posterior

aspect of the body of the superior vertebra and the laminae at the base of the inferior articular process of that vertebra. In at least one cephalad slice in this series the ganglion of the lumbar nerve root and its surrounding fat occupy the entire "gap" (foramen) with no sharing of the space by the superior articular process of the vertebra below. It is normal, however, to visualize the capsule of the posterior articular joint behind the nerve ganglion, covering the anterior aspect of the inferior articular process of the vertebra above. Immediately below, the superior vertebra is represented by its inferior disc plate which differs in texture from the vertebral body; this plate consists of compact bone with no cancellous components. It therefore appears denser and more homogeneous and also tends to have a rounded rather than a square shape.

3. The lower part of the intervertebral foramen (Fig. 4). At this level, the intervertebral disc replaces the vertebral body if the slice was oriented exactly in the plane of the disc and if the thickness of the slice was less than the thickness of the disc. Behind the disc and separated from it by the intervertebral foramen is the posterior articular joint. Both the inferior articular process of the vertebra above and the superior process of the vertebra below are visualized in this slice. As a result, the foramen itself might appear small in its anteroposterior diameter; this should not be considered a pathological stenosis since the nerve is now already lateral to the foramen which is occupied only by fat. The capsule of the posterior articular joint gives origin to the ligamentum flavum, which also arises in part from the superior border of the lamina. Since the lamina is slanting downward and posteriorly, the thickness of the ligamentum flavum increases in a

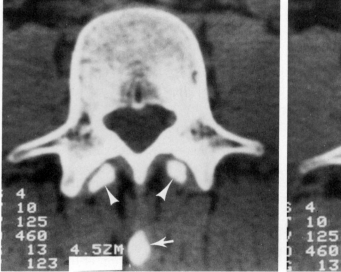

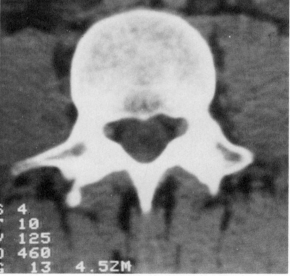

FIG. 2. Normal anatomy through the pedicle of the superior vertebra. **Left:** The vertebral body, pedicle, and laminae form a complete bony ring at this level. The tip of the inferior articular processes (arrowheads) and spinous process (arrow) of the preceding vertebra also can be seen. **Right:** Four millimeters caudal, only the bony structures which belong to this vertebra are shown.

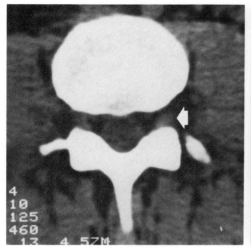 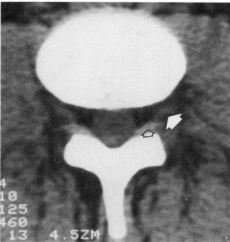

FIG. 3. Normal anatomy through the upper part of the intervertebral foramen. **Left:** The nerve ganglion (arrow) occupies the intervertebral foramen which appears as a gap in the bony ring on each side. A portion of the transverse process also can be seen at this level. **Right:** Four millimeters caudal, the nerve (closed arrow) distal to the ganglion can be identified. Posteromedial to the nerve root lies the capsule of the posterior articular joint (open arrow), an attachment site for the ligamentum flavum.

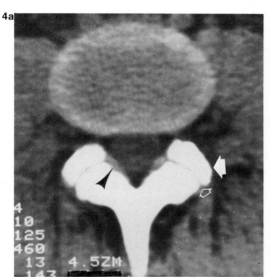

FIG. 4. Normal anatomy through the lower part of the intervertebral foramen. **a:** At this level, the posterior aspect of the intervertebral disc, which has a higher density than the adjacent dural sac, forms the anterior border of the foramen. The superior articular process of the inferior vertebra (closed arrow) lies anterior to, and articulates with, the inferior articular process of the superior vertebra (open arrow). The laminae of the superior vertebra are continuous with the inferior articular process and the spinous process of the same vertebra. The ligamentum flavum (arrowhead) lies anteromedial to the lamina and the joint. **b:** Four millimeters caudal, the upper disc plate of the inferior vertebra, together with the intervertebral disc, form the anterior border of the foramen. The foramen appears smaller in size; the nerve (arrow) has migrated farther lateral to the foramen. The superior articular process of the inferior vertebra is larger in size than in the previous slice, while the laminae of the superior vertebra are no longer in continuity with the spinous process. The ligamentum flavum (arrowhead) can again be seen. **c:** Twelve millimeters caudal, a complete bony ring of the inferior vertebra is established. The upper border of the laminae and the superior articular process of the inferior vertebra are now seen. The nerve root sheath (arrow) for the next intervertebral foramen lies medial to the pedicle.

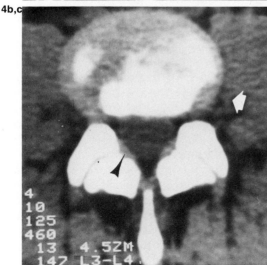 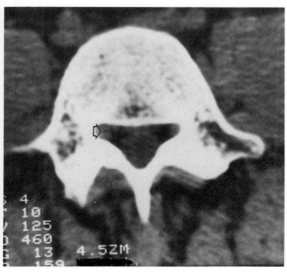

cephalo−caudad direction on the sequential slices toward the lamina of the inferior vertebra.

The nerve that has crossed the intervertebral foramen appears more laterally. The fat-filled foramen at this level often is very small in its anteroposterior diameter. The nerve root sheath that originates from the dural sac close to the posterior disc border later leaves the spinal canal just below the lower border of the pedicle of the next inferior vertebra. This is in contradistinction to the nerve that has already left through the more cephalad intervertebral foramen and is lying close to the lateral aspect of the disc rather than its posterior border.

The superior articular processes of the inferior vertebra increase gradually in size in the caudal direction while the inferior aspect of the laminae and the spinous process of the superior vertebra diminish in size and finally disappear. Eventually, at the lowest slice of the set, the base of the superior articular process connects with the upper border of the pedicle, the upper disc plate, and the laminae. The complete bony ring of the inferior vertebra below is thus formed. At this level the root sheath that will ultimately exit in the foramen below appears close to the medial aspect of the pedicle. Since the amount of epidural fat at the level of the pedicle is much less than at the level of the foramen, visualization of the root sheath at this level may be difficult; in the lower lumbar region, at L4/5 and L5/S1, sufficient fat generally is present so that the sheaths are visible (Fig. 5).

Pathology

Degeneration of the Intervertebral Disc

Pathogenesis.

Because the process of intervertebral disc degeneration occurs in different stages, variable radiologic findings can result. The earliest change is the occurrence of radiating "tears" in the annulus. Since there is no disruption of the annulus, the nucleus pulposus remains contained within the annulus. Prior to potential herniation, tears in the annulus may lead to its thinning and weakening at one point. The nucleus pulposus can extend peripherally in that region, and although still contained within the posterior border of the disc, may protrude at the particular weakened spot. This protrusion consists of the thinned annulus and the nucleus within. When one or more of these tears involve the posterior border of the disc, actual "rupture" of the annulus can occur and the nucleus pulposus may herniate through it. The herniated fragment is still retained by fibers of the posterior longitudinal ligament. On CT, protrusion of the annulus with

the nucleus contained within is identical in appearance to the herniated nucleus retained within the fibers of the posterior longitudinal ligament. Both conditions may cause compression of the nerve root that happens to lie close to the protrusion or herniation. Most commonly, protrusion or rupture occurs at the posterior border of the disc just off the midline (posterolateral protrusion of herniation) or in the midline (central protrusion or herniation). Lateral disc rupture is uncommon.

Should the herniated fragment pierce through a hole in the posterior longitudinal ligament, the fragment will lie free in the epidural space. This stage is called extrusion. Such a position of the fragment allows migration away from the site of the ruptured annulus and potential loss of continuity between the ruptured fragment and the rest of the disc material within the disc space. Migration of the fragment is usually caudad and less commonly cephalad. When it occurs caudad, the extruded disc lies dorsal to the upper part of the vertebral body below. Similarly, when it occurs cephalad, the fragment lies behind the lower part of the vertebral body above. When the rupture occurs laterally, cephalad migration of the fragment causes it to lie within the intervertebral foramen, contacting and compressing the nerve root in that foramen just above the level of the disc. Caudad migration, with the fragment lying behind the body of the vertebra below, causes compression of the nerve root that exits below the pedicle of the inferior vertebra, i.e., in the foramen below the level of the disc. Such potential migrations must be considered when correlating the radiologic findings and the clinical level of the neurologic deficit.

Clinical considerations.

Two clinical syndromes must be clearly distinguished. The first, compression of the cauda equina, presents with back pain that radiates into both lower extremities. Pain usually is described as being more severe in the standing position and may be worse with walking. The neurologic examination may be surprisingly negative. When weakness occurs, it occurs bilaterally and symmetrically. When the deep tendon reflexes are involved, they are also depressed bilaterally.

The second syndrome, compression of a root by herniation of the nucleus pulposus, results in sciatica which may be associated with backache. Pain radiates along the distribution of the root involved and may persist in spite of bedrest. Associated with this may be loss of sensation, motor power, or the deep tendon reflexes in the distribution of the involved nerve root. A positive straight-leg raising sign and a positive Lasègue test also suggest nerve root compression.

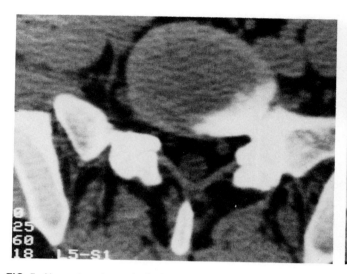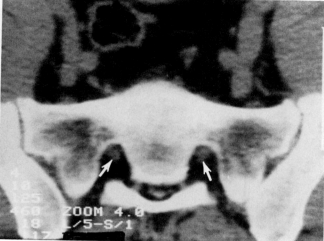

FIG. 5. Normal anatomy. **Left:** At the level of the lumbosacral junction, the dural sac is small and is surrounded by a large amount of the epidural fat. **Right:** Inferior to the lower end of the cul-de-sac, the sacral and coccygeal root sheaths appear as rounded soft tissue structures surrounded by far (arrows).

Herniation of the nucleus pulposus most commonly involves the nerve root that exits in the foramen below the level of the ruptured disc; it is not generally at the same level as the disc. In only a small fraction of cases, in which rupture occurs laterally and the fragment migrates cephalad in the foramen, do the clinical symptoms and signs direct attention to the nerve root that exits at the same level as the disc; these findings may erroneously be interpreted as due to rupture of the disc at the level above.

In those patients with herniation of a very large disc fragment, the cauda equina may be compressed and the clinical picture may show features of a combination of the two syndromes. Similarly, disc herniation can occur in association with spinal stenosis, and the clinical presentation also may exhibit features of a combination of both syndromes.

CT findings (refs. 29,48,74; Figs. 6–12).

1. Deformity of the posterior border of the disc. The posterior border of the intervertebral disc normally appears parallel to the border of the bony disc plate. In cases of disc herniation, there is focal projection from the posterior border of the disc (Figs. 6 and 11a). The focal nature of the deformity distinguishes disc rupture from diffuse bulging which is a sign of early degenerative change.

2. Displacement of the epidural fat. There is usually abundant epidural fat in the lower lumbar region, especially at the L4/5 and L5/S1 levels where the dural sac is smaller (Fig. 5). The lucent epidural space normally is symmetrical in shape and size. When rupture of the annulus occurs, the herniated nucleus pulposus which has a soft tissue density replaces the lower den-

sity epidural fat, resulting in asymmetry of the lucent area at the level of disc rupture compared to the other side (Figs. 9 and 12a).

3. Soft tissue density in the extradural space. The herniated nucleus pulposus has a higher density than the dural sac and epidural fat. The soft tissue density in the epidural space represents the size and location of the herniated fragment (Fig. 9). When the fragment is small and has been retained by the posterior longitudinal ligament, the soft tissue mass appears continuous with the density of the intervertebral disc and can only be seen on scans which show the disc itself (Fig. 12a). When the herniated fragment is large, a soft tissue density may appear on slices other than at the level of the disc (Fig. 11). A similar appearance can occur when the fragment has ruptured through the posterior longitudinal ligament, has lost continuity with the intervertebral disc, and has migrated away from the site of rupture in the annulus (Fig. 7). Depending upon the site of the disc rupture, the soft tissue density may appear in the midline or posterolaterally. When true lateral disc rupture occurs the soft tissue density appears within the intervertebral foramen. Depending on the direction of migration in cases of extrusion, the fragment may appear behind the body of the vertebra below the disc (Fig. 11c) or it may lie in the lateral gutter against the pedicle of the vertebra (Figs. 7b and d). It may also be situated in the intervertebral foramen resembling an enlarged ganglion (Fig. 8).

4. Deformity of the dural sac. The dural sac and its contents have a lower density than the intervertebral disc. In the upper lumbar region the dural sac normally occupies the entire area of the bony spinal canal. An interface between the border of the sac and the border of the disc can be identified by the density difference

6a,b

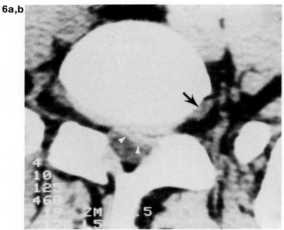
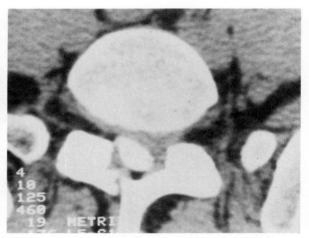

6c

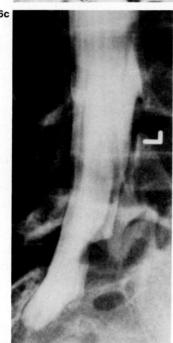

FIG. 6. Herniated disc at L5/S1 level. **a:** Plain CT. There is loss of parallelism between the posterior border of the high density disc and the disc plate on the left. The herniated disc fragment (arrowheads) has completely replaced the epidural fat and deformed the anterior aspect of the dural sac. Since the nerve root (arrow) that exits at this level lies farther laterally to the intervertebral foramen, it may not be affected by the disc herniation. **b:** Repeat scan after a metrizamide myelogram again demonstrates the distorted dural sac. Notice that the herniated disc material intimately contacts the origin of the root sheath of the nerve at the corner of the metrizamide column; this nerve root eventually exits at the foramen below the level of the disc. **c:** Oblique view of the metrizamide myelogram confirms the CT findings but offers no additional information.

(Fig. 4a). This interface has the configuration of the posterior border of the bony disc plate. It is usually concave in the upper lumbar region, a straight line at the level L4, and a slightly convex border at the L5/S1 level. When there is herniation of an intervertebral disc, the posterior border of the disc is deformed as previously described. The dural sac also may be likewise deformed (Figs. 6a and b and 7b and d). In the lower lumbar region, where the dural sac does not fill the entire area of the bony spinal canal and does not abut on the posterior border of the intervertebral disc, deformity of the smooth rounded contour of the dural sac occurs only when the disc herniation is large enough to obliterate the epidural fat and impinge upon the wall of the dural sac (Fig. 11a). A herniated fragment thus may be of sufficient size to compress the nerve root and yet cause little or no deformity of the

dural sac (Figs. 9 and 12). Rarely, in cases of large disc herniation, the shape of the dural sac may be severely distorted and reduced to a crescentic slit when a large central disc fragment occupies the greater part of the bony spinal canal.

5. Compression and displacement of the root sheath. The root sheath normally appears as a soft tissue density in the epidural fat in the lateral aspect of the bony spinal canal medial to the pedicle and in the intervertebral foramen just below the pedicle. When the herniated fragment lies in the lateral aspect of the bony spinal canal, the root sheath may be displaced posterior to the fragment. In many cases, the root sheath cannot be identified separately from the herniated fragment. This in itself is a sign of compression of the root by the fragment (Figs. 9, 11b, and 12a).

6. Calcification of the herniated nucleus pulposus.

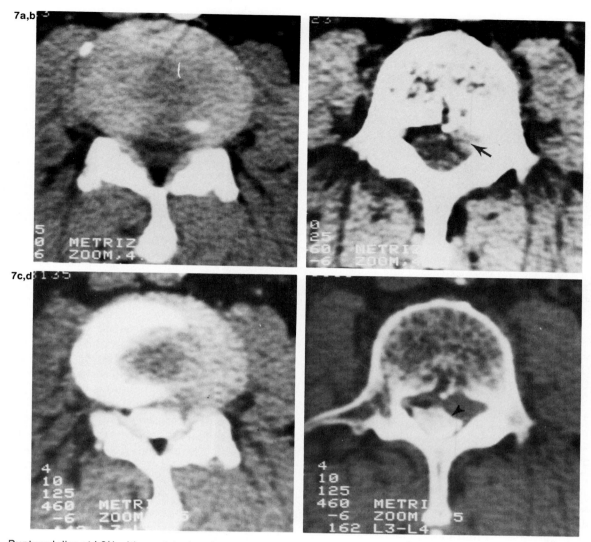

FIG. 7. Ruptured disc at L3/4 with caudal migration of the fragment. **a:** Plain CT at the level of the intervertebral disc is normal. **b:** In a scan taken 1.5 cm below, the herniated fragment appears as a dense soft tissue mass (arrow) against the medial border of the pedicle of L4. The fragment has lost continuity with the ruptured disc. **c:** CT scan taken after the administration of metrizamide confirms the dural sac to be uninvolved at the level of the intervertebral disc. **d:** Scan at the same level as (b) shows indentation of the contrast-filled dural sac (arrowhead) by the caudally displaced herniated disc fragment.

Such an area of increased attenuation within the otherwise soft tissue density of the herniated material tends to occur in long-standing herniation (Fig. 10); the fragments may be continuous with the border of the disc plate.

7. Vacuum phenomenon in the bony spinal canal. Degenerative dessicative changes which occur in the nucleus pulposus itself may be recognizable on radiologic examination. The accumulation of gas, particularly nitrogen, within the nucleus pulposus creates the so-called "vacuum" appearance. Very minute amounts of gas within a degenerated nucleus pulposus may be recognized on CT. The accumulation of a small amount of gas at the posterior border of the disc indicates extreme thinning of the annulus (23).

The presence of gas in the intervertebral disc mate-

rial is a sign of degeneration, not of herniation. It is only when gas appears beyond the posterior border of the disc plate that disc herniation should be diagnosed (Fig. 11). This can be a helpful finding when the fragment itself is not demonstrable; this can occur when the degenerated disc material has a density similar to that of the dural sac and the epidural fat is scanty on both sides.

Differential diagnosis.

Pathologic conditions that lead to the formation of a soft tissue mass in the epidural space may mimic the appearance of a herniated nucleus pulposus on CT.

1. Primary neoplasm. A neurofibroma of the nerve root or ganglion can present as a soft tissue mass in the

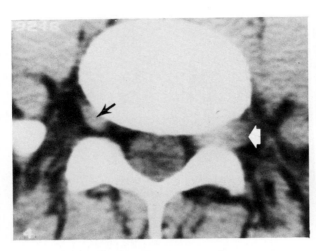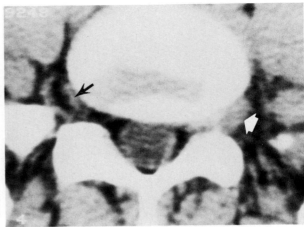

FIG. 8. Lateral disc herniation. **Left:** A herniated disc fragment, shown here as an oblong-shaped mass (white arrow), fills the left intervertebral foramen. This can be confused with an enlarged ganglion. The black arrow points to a normal nerve ganglion on the right. **Right:** Four millimeters caudal, the nerve root distal to the ganglion is also obscured by the herniated disc fragment (white arrow). A normal nerve root (black arrow) can be seen on the opposite side.

lateral gutter of the bony spinal canal medial to the pedicle or in the intervertebral foramen just below the pedicle (Fig. 13). Generally, such a mass appears less dense than disc herniation. After intravenous contrast injection, however, there is frequently an increase in the density of the neoplasm; a normal ganglion usually does not enhance. When long-standing, the neoplasm may cause enlargement of the intervertebral foramen. In neurofibromatosis, the lesions may be multiple, a feature that should suggest the correct diagnosis.

2. Metastatic neoplasm. A metastatic lesion may appear as a soft tissue mass in the epidural space. The mass may extend to the intervertebral foramen (Fig. 14). Unlike a neurofibroma, a metastatic lesion usually has an ill-defined margin and infiltrates the

paravertebral fat causing an increase in the thickness of the normal paravertebral tissue. Most important, the hallmark of malignancy is the presence of bony destruction, which usually is recognizable on CT. An additional very helpful feature is the clinical history of a known primary or metastatic neoplasm elsewhere.

3. Conjoined sheath anomaly. This anomaly, which is usually unilateral, involves the fifth lumbar and first sacral roots. The anomaly consists of a common origin of two root sheaths. While each root sheath has its own arachnoid space, they share the same dural sheath (5). Consequently, this results in an asymmetric appearance of the root sheaths on CT (Fig. 15). On the side of the conjoint sheath, the root sheath is large and may resemble a soft tissue mass in the lateral gutter medial to the pedicle. Just caudad, no root sheath comes off the lateral aspect of the dural sac since the

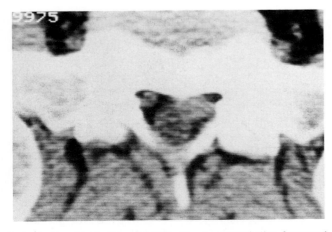

FIG. 9. Herniated disc at L5/S1. The herniated disc fragment, shown as a soft tissue mass, obliterates the epidural fat and obscures the root sheath on the left. The latter finding is indicative of nerve root compression. The dural sac is only minimally deformed due to the normally large epidural space at this level.

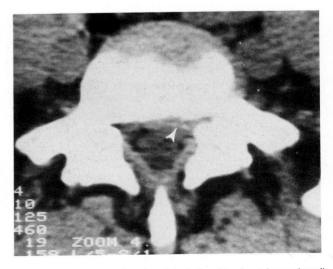

FIG. 10. Calcification in a herniated disc fragment (arrowhead).

11a,b

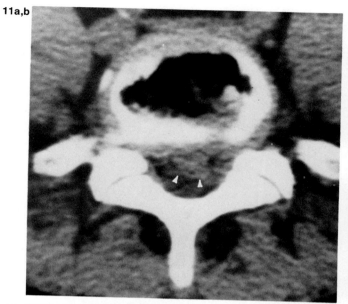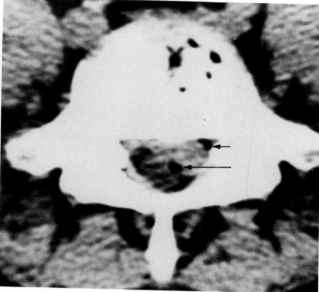

11c

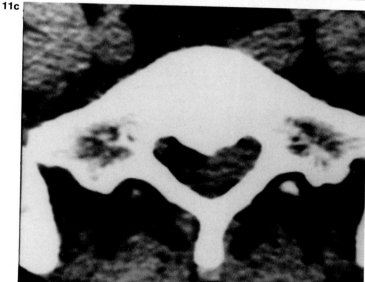

FIG. 11. Gas associated with herniated disc. **a:** CT scan at the level of the disc space. Gas appears as a lucency within the intervertebral disc. The presence of gas in this location alone is not a sign of disc herniation. Also of note is a herniated soft tissue fragment (arrowheads) encroaching upon the dural sac. **b:** CT scan below the level of the disc space demonstrates collections of gas bubbles within the herniated disc fragment (arrows). The fragment is denser than the dural sac. The nerve root is indistinct from the herniated fragment indicative of nerve root compression. **c:** The lower border of the herniated fragment is still present on this scan obtained more than 2 cm below the disc space. This is seen when the herniated material is large in size or when part of the herniated material has been extruded from the disc.

lower root sheath is a branch of the upper root sheath. The clue to the diagnosis is that the "mass" has a uniform density similar to the dural sac. The mass does not enhance after intravenous contrast medium injection. A definitive diagnosis can be achieved on CT following intrathecal metrizamide administration; this shows filling with contrast material of the very same structure which appeared as a mass on the plain CT scans.

This anomaly has been reported in association with disc rupture and spinal stenosis. Failure to recognize this anomaly may result in inadvertent damage to the nerve roots and contribute to poor surgical results.

4. Epidural and subdural collections of blood and pus (see discussion on pp. 435–436).

Relative roles of CT and myelography.

Using the criteria described above, several investigators compared CT with myelography in the diagnosis of disc herniation (25,32,62). The results of these studies indicate that in the majority of the cases CT should replace myelography and patients be spared the morbidity and risks of myelography (Fig. 6). When CT findings are inconclusive or do not explain the clinical features, a myelogram should be performed.

In the studies cited, not only was CT adequate for making the diagnosis in the majority of patients, but it was sometimes better than myelography in detecting disc herniation. This was particularly true when the lesion was at one of the lower disc levels, such as

12a,b

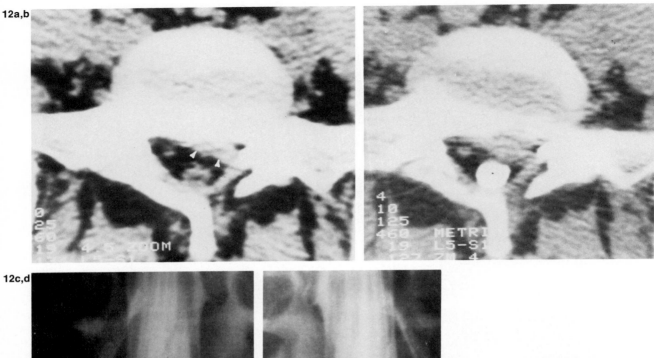

12c,d

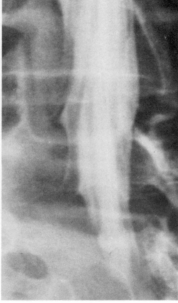

FIG. 12. Herniated disc at L5/S1 level. **a:** Plain CT shows a herniated disc fragment (arrowheads) in the epidural space. The dural sac itself is small and there is no contact between the herniated disc material and the dural sac. The root sheath, however, is indistinct from the fragment, indicative of nerve root compression. **b:** CT after a metrizamide myelogram. Note the lack of deformity of the contrast column due to the small size of the dural sac. **c and d:** Both oblique views of a metrizamide myelogram show no deformity of the dural sac. Other than a slight thickening of a left nerve root within its sheath, the myelogram is normal.

L5/S1, or when the disc herniation was lateral (Figs. 9 and 12). As emphasized before, the herniated fragment may cause little or no deformity of the dural sac in these locations. In such cases, a diagnosis of disc herniation by myelography depends upon recognition of asymmetry in filling or widening of the root sheath. These findings may be difficult to recognize with certainty in comparison to the much more readily appreciated demonstration by CT of the dense herniated fragment within the lucent epidural fat. The presence of disc rupture with negative myelographic findings is not surprising; surgical exploration and disc removal have been repeatedly performed in the past in patients with a negative myelogram.

Computed tomography may fail to provide a defini-

tive diagnosis of disc herniation for several reasons. A paucity or absence of epidural fat, such as in the patient with associated hypertrophic changes in the dorsal elements, can cause failure to outline the deformed contour of the posterior border of the disc or of the disc fragment itself (Fig. 16). The lack of epidural fat may eliminate the possibility of comparing the two sides for asymmetry. In addition, on rare occasion the herniated fragment may have a lower density, which makes differentiation from the adjacent spinal fluid difficult. In these cases, myelography usually can demonstrate deformity of the dural sac and root sheath (Fig. 16). It should be emphasized that a clinical picture suggestive of disc herniation may be due to another pathologic condition, such as an intradural tumor or

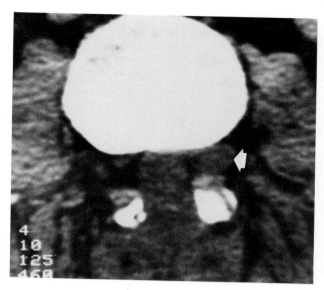

FIG. 13. Neurofibroma of the nerve root sheath within the foramen. A soft tissue mass (arrow) is present in the left intervertebral foramen in this patient with a prior laminectomy for removal of an intradural neurofibroma in the cauda equina. Although slightly lower in density than a disc fragment, this mass can easily be confused with a lateral herniated disc.

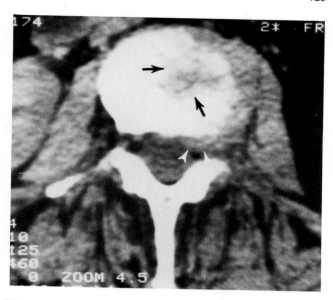

FIG. 14. Metastases from a renal cell carcinoma. A soft tissue mass (arrowheads) is present in the left intervertebral foramen. In addition, there is a left paraspinal soft tissue mass associated with vertebral destruction (arrows). These findings are most compatible with metastatic bone disease with intraspinal extension.

arachnoid adhesions within the dural sac; neither is demonstrable by plain CT. Thus, even if the CT examination is unequivocally normal in appearance, if the clinical history and physical examination strongly suggest a spinal abnormality, a myelogram should be performed to evaluate for a possible intradural lesion. Those patients who do require a myelogram should

have it performed with metrizamide unless contraindicated. This allows repeating the CT study after the myelogram if necessary. The unique cross-sectional display of the contour of the contrast column provided by CT may be particularly helpful in patients with central disc herniation. Another advantage of the post-myelogram CT is to confirm and define dorsolateral

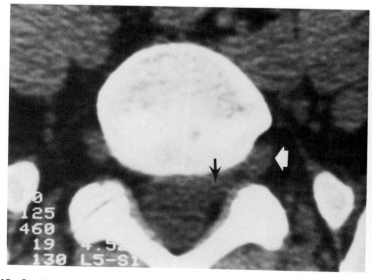

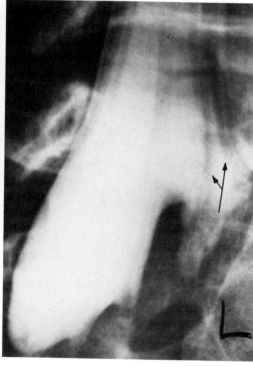

FIG. 15. Conjoint root sheath of L5 and S1 on the left side. **Left:** Plain CT. The conjoint root sheath (black arrow), which has a density identical to that of the dural sac, obliterates the epidural fat. The nerve ganglion (white arrow) is continuous with, and to the lateral side of, the conjoint sheath. **Right:** Myelogram of the same case shows the two roots to appear within a large conjoint sheath (arrows), thus firmly establishing the diagnosis.

16a,b,c

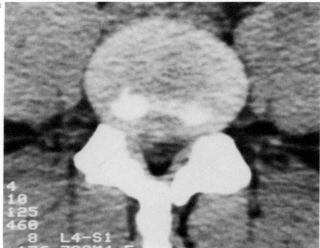

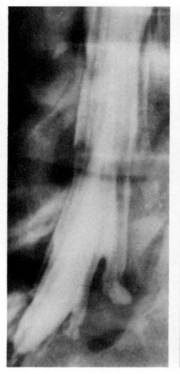

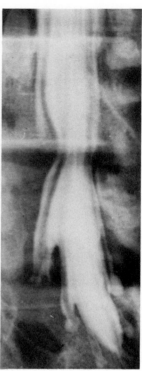

FIG. 16. Herniated disc; value of myelography. **a:** Plain CT. Very little epidural fat is present in the spinal canal due to diffuse bulging of the disc margin and hypertrophic changes of the articular processes. Lack of epidural fat makes the diagnosis of disc herniation by CT difficult. **b and c:** Both oblique views of a myelogram of the same patient. The asymmetry on the right of the contour of the contrast column is unequivocal.

compression of the contrast column due to hypertrophy of the dorsal elements; such a diagnosis can be made more readily on the cross-sectional CT images than with the conventional views of the myelogram.

Recurrent disc herniation.

The recrudescence of symptoms after removal of the herniated disc material may be due to recurrence of disc herniation or to the formation of hypertrophic scar tissue. Differentiation between these two conditions has been difficult with myelography. In patients with prior surgery, both a bony defect (the size of which depends upon whether or not partial or complete hemilaminectomy and a medial partial facetectomy were performed) and a defect in the ligamentum flavum can be seen on CT (Fig. 17). The dural sac is displaced toward the side of surgery. A fibrous tissue band, higher in density than the dural sac, is seen obliterating the space between the sac and the site of surgery. This band extends from the disc border anteriorly, hugs the lateral aspect of the dural sac, and extends to the laminectomy defect. If the exploration involved the intervertebral foramen, the fibrous tissue also extends there. The lucent epidural fat is obliterated on the side of surgery and the nerve roots cannot be distinguished.

The density of scar tissue is not sufficiently different from the density of disc material to reliably distinguish disc herniation from an accumulation of abundant scar tissue at the site of the previous disc removal. How-

ever, some investigators contend that scar tissue usually has a lower density than herniated disc material (49). Additional controversy exists. Some report that the appearance of a "mass" is a sign of disc rupture and not of fibrous tissue (49). Others (65) suggest that a mass of fibrous tissue resembling disc herniation can be differentiated only by the use of intravenous contrast material, with fibrous tissue showing intense enhancement while disc recurrence does not. Therefore, how helpful the presence of a "mass," contrast enhancement, or density differential is in differentiating disc recurrence from scarring remains to be settled.

Degeneration of the Posterior Articular Joints

Degenerative changes in the posterior articular facets include narrowing of the joint space, "vacuum" phenomenon within the joint space, osteosclerosis of the articular margin, and subarticular "cyst-like" formations (42,57,58). In addition, changes in the articular processes themselves may occur. Hypertrophy of the bone can result in large osteophytes. Hypertrophic changes in the synovial membrane may cause a mass in the intervertebral foramen. Hypertrophy of the capsule of the posterior articular joints may be associated with hypertrophy of the ligamentum flavum.

Osteophyte formation of the posterior articular bony processes can extend medially, superiorly, and laterally. Medial extension of the hypertrophic process may produce impingement upon the root sheath which

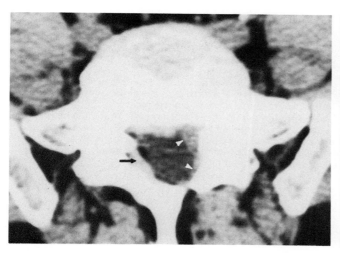 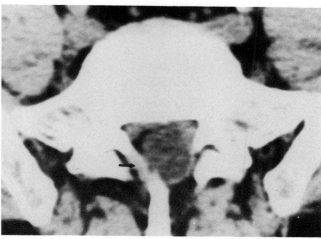

FIG. 17. Normal postoperative changes after left partial hemi-laminectomy for removal of a herniated disc at L5/S1 level. **Left:** There is a small bony defect in the left lamina associated with an absent left ligamentum flavum. In addition, a soft tissue band (arrowheads), felt to represent postoperative scar, can be seen extending along the left lateral aspect of the spinal canal. The normal right ligamentum flavum is clearly seen (arrow).

Right: Four millimeters caudal, the ligamentum flavum is again seen on the right side (arrow) but not on the left. Note the ec-centric position of the dural sac which has extended into the space created by removal of bone and ligamentum flavum, and the replacement of epidural fat by a band of soft tissue (scar) on the left. Asymmetric epidural fat is a normal postoperative find-ing and cannot be used as a sign for recurrent disc herniation.

is heading toward the inferior aspect of the pedicle below. The base of an enlarged superior articular process can encroach upon the lateral aspect of the bony spinal canal. The combination of these two factors results in what is termed lateral spinal stenosis (alternatively root canal stenosis or subarticular compression of the nerve root). Superior extension of the osseous hypertrophy results in elongation of the superior articular process, which may impinge upon the nerve ganglion and compress it against the inferior aspect of the pedicle above. Lateral extension of the osseous hypertrophy alone is not clinically significant.

Idiopathic Developmental Stenosis

This developmental abnormality of unknown cause is due to a growth disturbance of the bony wall of the vertebral canal which results in narrowing of the bony spinal canal at one or more vertebral levels. If sufficient, the narrowing may cause compression of the cauda equina with resultant back pain radiating into both lower extremities. The most consistent measurable abnormality in this condition is the midline sagittal diameter of the bony spinal canal. Absolute stenosis can be diagnosed when the measurement is 10 mm or less. A measurement of 10–12 mm has been termed relative stenosis; additional slight degenerative changes may produce symptomatic stenosis (73).

Attempts to measure the mid-sagittal diameter of the bony spinal canal on plain radiographs often have been disappointing due to the obscuration of the correct landmark by superimposed bony structures on both sides. Even on sagittal tomograms of the lumbar spine

it may be difficult to define the posterior bony wall of the spinal canal. Computed tomography provides an excellent delineation of the borders of the bony vertebral canal in the axial projection, and it is possible to precisely measure the mid-sagittal diameter (Fig. 18). For this measurement, a wide window width should be used and the window level should be set midway between the density of the dural sac and the density of the bone. An additional precaution, in order to achieve an exact measurement, requires that the plane of the slice be perpendicular to the plane of the anterior bony wall of the canal, which is the posterior border of the vertebral body. In the upper and mid-lumbar regions, it is possible to obtain such an image without difficulty by tilting the gantry, by flexion of the patient's hips and knees, or by examining the patient in the prone position. At the lumbosacral junction, however, it might be impossible to orient the slice to the desired plane. In such cases, reformatting scans obtained in the transverse plane to sagittal images, or projections in the plane of the disc, is required (42,73). The best results with reconstructed images are achieved using a 2 mm slice thickness and table increments of 2 mm.

The laminae normally slope posteriorly in a caudal direction in relation to the anterior wall of the vertebral canal. Therefore, the mid-sagittal diameter taken at the upper border of the lamina will be shorter than that measured at the lower border of the lamina. Both measurements should be considered. In patients with idiopathic developmental bony spinal stenosis, the slope of the laminae may be obliterated, i.e., there is verticalization of the laminae. As a result, the lower border of the laminae will lie at the same distance

18a

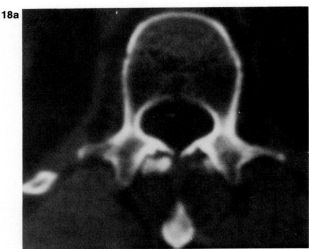

FIG. 18. Idiopathic developmental stenosis of the bony spinal canal. **a:** The bony spinal canal at L1 appears normal. **b:** At L3, there is marked decrease in both the anteroposterior and transverse diameters of the spinal canal. **c:** CT scan through the L3/4 level shows superimposed degenerative changes with bulging of the disc as well as hypertrophy of the posterior articular joints, resulting in further narrowing of the already small spinal canal.

18b,c

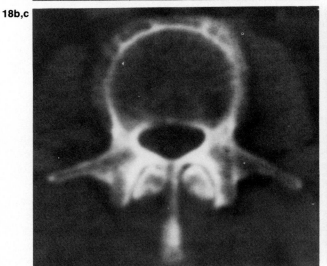 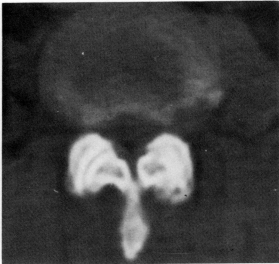

from the posterior surface of the vertebral body as the upper border. Normally, the ligamentum flavum occupies the space in front of the sloping anterior surface of the laminae, and the posterior wall of the epidural space is parallel to its anterior wall. When the laminae have lost this normal slope, the ligamentum flavum will further compromise the space available to the dural sac and cauda equina (73).

Degenerative Spinal Stenosis

In this condition the cauda equina and nerve roots can be encroached upon at three locations: the spinal canal, the lateral recess (gutter), and the neural foramina. The encroachment may be due to the hypertrophied articular processes, osteophytes at the borders of the vertebral bodies, or subluxation of the posterior articular joints (42,47,57).

1. Central spinal stenosis is caused by hypertrophy of the inferior articular process and the lamina, resulting in a decrease in the anteroposterior diameter of the

bony spinal canal (Fig. 19, left). The condition may be complicated by bulging of the posterior border of the disc or associated osteophyte formation at the posterior border of the disc plates at the level involved. A puacity of epidural fat is almost always present.

2. Lateral spinal stenosis or stenosis of the lateral recess (or gutter) is caused by hypertrophy of the superior articular process which forms the posterior wall of the bony nerve root canal (Fig. 19, right). This hypertrophy results in narrowing of the space available to the nerve root within the bony canal. The anterior wall of the nerve root canal is formed by the border of the vertebral body and the disc, while the lateral wall is formed by the pedicle. The posterior wall is formed by the superior articular process of the vertebra below, the pars interarticularis of the vertebra above, and the ligamentum flavum, which arises from the capsule of the posterior articular joint. It is the hypertrophy of the sweep of the superior articular process behind the nerve root that causes narrowing of the space available to the nerve root. In lateral spinal stenosis, the bony

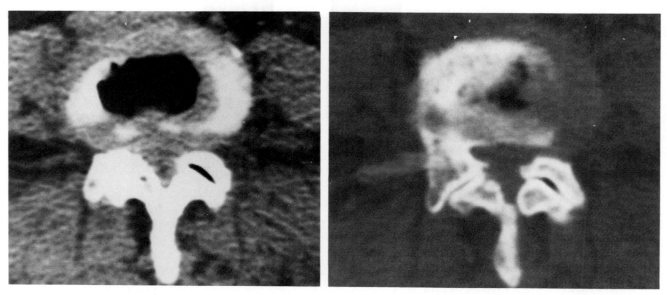

FIG. 19. Central and lateral degenerative spinal stenosis at L4/5 level. **Left:** The posterior bulging of the intervertebral disc coupled with the hypertrophy of the lamina and the inferior articular processes leave very little space in the mid-sagittal plane for the cauda equina and the ligamenta flava. Gas in the disc space is present. **Right:** Four millimeters caudal, using a wide window setting to demonstrate the bony structures, hypertrophy of the superior articular processes can be seen. It is the medial extension of the hypertrophic process, which encroaches upon the lateral part of the bony spinal canal, that causes lateral stenosis.

spinal canal has a trefoil configuration rather than being open and triangular. It should be emphasized, however, that a trefoil configuration is a normal variant at the L4 and L5 levels (Fig. 4c). Here, the distinction between a narrow lateral recess (or gutter) and a normal one is simply a matter of subjective impression based upon experience. No reliable quantitative measurements establishing the patency of the lateral recess (or gutter) exist. Recognition of lateral stenosis is extremely important in surgical planning. Poor results from laminectomy for decompression of the cauda

equina have often been due to failure to appreciate the lateral extent of the stenosis and subsequent failure to extend the decompression laterally to include the apophyseal joints.

A particularly incapacitating type of lateral stenosis can result from spondylolisthesis (Fig. 20). Although spondylolisthesis is usually the result of a defect in the pars interarticularis, it may also occur in association with degenerative changes. Forward slipping of the posterior elements of the vertebra above results in compression of the spinal nerve in the lateral recess

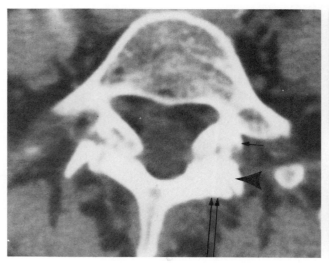
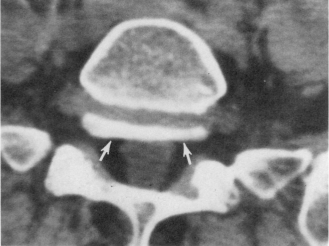

FIG. 20. Spondylolisthesis at L5/S1. **Left:** Bilateral defects in the pars interarticularis of L5 are seen between the base of the superior articular process anteriorly (arrow) and the inferior articular process (double arrow). In the gap between the two components of the neural arch of L5, the tip of the superior articular process of S1 (arrowhead) can be seen. **Right:** The posterior borders of S1 (arrows) and L5 are seen on the same slice, creating the so-called "double margin" sign.

against the posterior margin of the body of the vertebra below. This generally can be readily appreciated on CT, which shows what has been described as the "double margin sign" because the posterior borders of adjacent vertebrae appear as two separate lines in the same slice.

3. Foraminal stenosis can be caused by several abnormalities (Fig. 21). The boundaries of the foraminal space include the pedicle above, the posterior border of the body of the vertebra in front, and the pars interarticularis of the superior vertebra posteriorly. Normally, there is enough space between the tip of the superior articular process of the inferior vertebra and the pedicle of the superior vertebra at each intervertebral foramen to accomodate the nerve root and its ganglion. If the superior articular process of the inferior vertebra is elongated by hypertrophic osteophyte formation, or if the process is displaced upward due to severe narrowing of the intervertebral disc space caused by disc degeneration, the tip of the superior articular process can approximate the inferior border of the pedicle and compress the nerve root and ganglion in that foramen. In addition, hypertrophic changes including osteophyte formation at the posterolateral border of the disc plate or the disc itself might lead to encroachment upon the foramen. Again, a CT diagnosis of foraminal stenosis relies on a subjective impression based upon experience because no documented measurements exist for the normality of the intervertebral foramen. Sagittal reformatted images in the plane of either the lateral gutter or the foramen may add to the appreciation of the degree of severity of stenosis in these areas.

In the past, the diagnosis of degenerative spinal stenosis, which can involve one or more levels, usually required myelography. Characteristic findings include hourglass constriction of the contrast column and poor filling of the root sheaths. In severe cases, the contrast column may be interrupted at the site of the severe compression, which would even be complete. Important limitations of myelography, however, are the inability to visualize the dural sac beyond the point of a block and the failure to demonstrate the condition of the nerve root in the foramen.

INTRASPINAL TUMORS

Intraspinal disorders classically are divided into three groups according to the compartment which they occupy. The tissue within each section determines the type of tumor that can originate within them (Table 1). Most intraspinal tumors have X-ray attenuation values not notably different from the spinal cord, roots, dura, and the combined density of the cauda equina bathed in the cerebrospinal fluid (CSF). Some tumors are of visibly lower density and a few of higher density.

Except in the cervical and lumbar regions, CT without metrizamide should not be used as a screening procedure and even with metrizamide, it should be reserved for regional examination dictated by clinical findings, plain spine radiographs, myelography, or nuclear scanning. Recognition of the compartment occupied by an intraspinal tumor frequently depends upon examination after the intrathecal administration of metrizamide. The relationship between an intraspinal neoplasm, the spinal cord, and the subarachnoid space is optimally shown in cross-section without superimposition. In some circumstances, the CSF is visible without contrast agent administration, but in

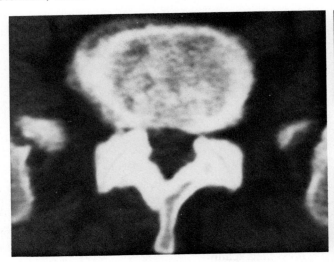 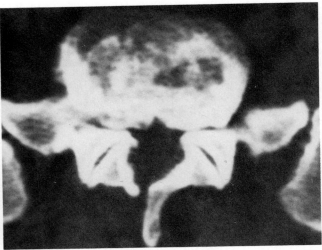

FIG. 21. Severe foraminal and lateral stenosis. **Left:** The intervertebral foramen is markedly narrowed due to approximation of the tip of the superior articular process of the inferior vertebra and the lower disc plate of the superior vertebra. Bony hypertrophy of the superior articular process of S1 close to the underface of the pedicle of L5 leaves insufficient space for the fifth lumbar root that is exiting at this location; the root is therefore compressed between the elongated process and the inferior surface of the pedicle. **Right:** Scan 4 mm lower shows the medial extent of the superior articular process to be encroaching upon the lateral gutter.

TABLE 1. *Primary intraspinal neoplasm and cyst*

Intramedullary

Glial cells	Astrocytoma
Ependymal cells	Ependymoma
Neurons	Neuroblastoma, ganglial tumors
Neurilemma	Neurilemmoma (Schwannoma)
Vascular structures	Hemangioblastoma
Ectopic tissue	Neurenteric cyst
	Lipoma
	Dermoid-epidermoid tumor/cyst

Intradural, extramedullary

Arachnoid, dura	Meningioma
Neurilemma	Neurilemmoma (Schwannoma)
Nerve root	Neurofibroma
Filum terminale	Ependymoma, glioma
Vascular structures	Hemangiopericytoma
Ectopic tissue	Dermoid-epidermoid tumor/cyst
	Lipoma
	Neurenteric cyst

Extradural, intraspinal

Connective tissue	
Fibrous	Sarcoma, fibroma
	Synovial cyst
Vascular	Hemangiopericytoma
	Extramedullary hematopoietic tissue
Lymphoid	Lymphoma, chloroma
Adipose	Lipoma, liposarcoma, angiolipoma
Nerve root	Neurofibroma, neurilemmoma
	Neuroblastoma
	Paraganglioma
Ectopic tissue	Dysraphic conditions
	Neurenteric cyst
	Ependymoma
	Chordoma

others, it is too sparse to be detected (Fig. 22). In complete block, the subarachnoid space may be so compromised that the above relationships cannot be determined even with metrizamide.

Intravenous contrast medium, unlike its value in the diagnosis of intracranial abnormalities, is of limited help in spinal CT and is not routinely used (18). It may be selectively utilized to enhance certain neoplasms and vascular lesions, as well as such extramedullary tissues as the dura and blood vessels. Determination of the attenuation values (Hounsfield numbers) also is of limited use in differentiating neoplasm from non-neoplastic disease, as well as in distinguishing different types of neoplasm, and sometimes even differentiating between neoplasm and normal tissue. However, visible differences in density do constitute an important aid in recognizing cysts, lucent tumors, and hyperdense lesions or calcifications.

Calcification and ossification within intraspinal tumors are rare, but the state of the vertebral bone is quite useful in diagnosis. Bone destruction is common in metastatic disease, while bone erosion and excavation can occur with slowly expanding lesions (Fig. 23). Congenital dysraphic deformities have characteristic bony abnormalities.

While the value of CT in the identification of intraspinal masses is tremendous, its use is considerably more limited in differentiating among the many causes and types of morphologic abnormality. Differential diagnosis still depends to a large extent upon the age, sex, history, physical features, laboratory findings, and precise location of the abnormality.

Computed tomography has already replaced myelography as the initial radiologic procedure for suspected intervertebral disc disease and spinal stenosis. No doubt, CT with or without dilute metrizamide will replace myelography in the evaluation of suspected intraspinal tumors. It already has largely displaced isophendylate (Pantopaque®) myelography because of the potentially greater information available from the cross-sectional view and recognition of masses with slight density differences. Only the smallest and finest of morphologic details will be shown by Pantopaque and not by CT with metrizamide.

Technical Factors

Certain physical limitations of CT or interfering structures can compromise intraspinal tumor evaluation. These include:

1. Restrictions on using CT for overall survey of an area. Computed tomographic assessment of intraspinal neoplasm usually follows metrizamide myelography and, therefore, the examination is limited or directed by the results of that study. Occasionally, CT is the first procedure, carried out without metrizamide, though usually restricted to a region as suggested by the clinical findings. It is not practical to use CT as a method of surveying the entire vertebral column and canal.

2. The relatively small size of the spinal canal (especially in large patients) compared to the surrounding structures, which limits the spatial resolution and contrast sensitivity achievable at even maximal photon flux.

3. Small size of the spinal canal relative to the artifacts produced by the large surrounding tissues, especially the complex and dense vertebrae and shoulder girdle or structures that are in biologic motion, including the heart, ribs, and diaphragm.

4. High density materials such as clips, Harrington rods, or Pantopaque, or subdural and epidural placement or leakage of metrizamide, in addition to layering of metrizamide.

5. Severe scoliosis or kyphosis or other conditions which limit or compromise placement of the patient within the scanner.

Some of these problems can be minimized.

To maximize spatial resolution, it is desirable to use the smallest field of reconstruction practicable to ensure the smallest size possible represented by each

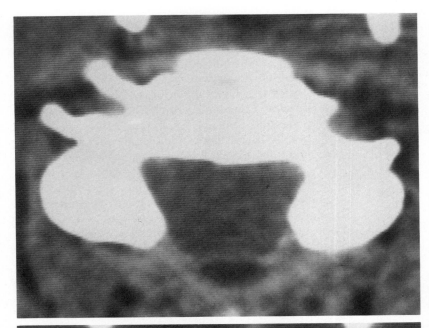

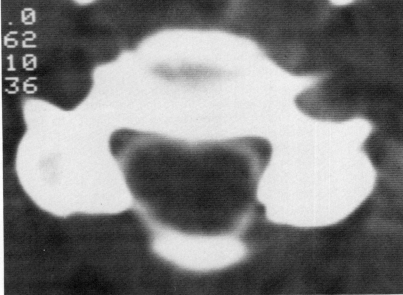

FIG. 22. Recurrent astrocytoma. **Above:** The entire spinal canal is filled with a homogeneous soft tissue mass. Neither the spinal cord nor the subarachnoid space can be distinguished from the tumor mass. **Below:** After the administration of metrizamide, CT scan demonstrates marked narrowing of the subarachnoid space by the tumor.

pixel, not simply to expand the image after it has been fully processed, in which case the pixels will simply be enlarged. Images must be viewed at an appropriate window level and width to allow good contrast differentiation between CSF, fat, and soft tissue density, even though bone is generally rendered completely white at this setting. To study the bony texture in detail, the same image must be reexamined with a wider (bone) window. Similarly, when metrizamide is used, a wide enough window setting should be used to differentiate bone, metrizamide, and soft tissue components.

A relatively short scan time should be used, generally in the range of 10 s. Shorter times, though desirable, usually result in inadequate photon flux, and longer times increase the severity and likelihood of motion artifacts. If possible, large patients should be examined at the maximal milliamperage setting or by increasing scan time to overcome the greater absorption of photons.

Thin (2 mm) sections, although increasing spatial resolution and allowing smoother image reformation, reduce photon flux and, therefore, contrast resolution. Scans 4–5 mm in thickness generally are used, at least in the initial survey.

Occasionally, the lateral decubitus position may be used with gantry tilt to compensate for lateral scoliosis. The prone position may be helpful to counteract the effect of metrizamide layering or pooling. Attempts to mix the CSF and metrizamide by rotating

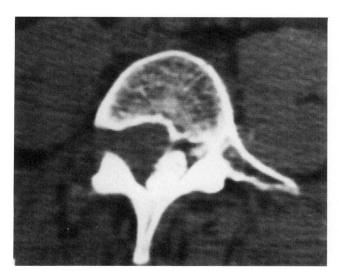

FIG. 23. Fibrolipoma. A homogeneous low density extradural mass markedly deforms the metrizamide-filled canal and accounts for smooth focal excavation along the right posterior surface of L4. The smooth bony deformity with a cortical margin that appears normal, usually implies a slow growing lesion of benign nature.

the patient before and during scanning may be useful. The ideal concentration of metrizamide for CT has not been established; dilutions less than those appropriate for direct radiographic myelography are desirable.

It is always desirable to have conventional radiographs of the spine performed prior to the CT examination. The familiar widening of the interpedicular space and flattening of the medial margins of the pedicles caused by an expanding intraspinal mass, seen on plain films, are frequently not evident on the cross-sectional CT scans unless rather gross. Of course, some bone changes will be shown better, or exclusively, by CT.

Intramedullary Compartment

The spinal cord is regularly shown by plain CT at the level of C1 and C2, and variably below that level; it is demonstrated relatively infrequently or incompletely in the thoracic region (71). Assessment of the spinal cord in the thoracic region nearly always requires intrathecal contrast. Artifacts produced at the level of the pectoral girdle commonly seriously impair scanning at the levels of C7, T1, and T2, even after metrizamide administration.

Recognition of widening or increased caliber of the cord produced by an intramedullary tumor presupposes knowing the normal range, size, and shape of the cord at various levels, but such values have not been established as yet with certainty, either anatomically or by CT (17,53,72). The normal range, especially in the cervical region, is fairly broad. In order to obtain the most accurate measurements, the window level

should be set one-halfway between the attenuation value of CSF (or CSF stained with metrizamide) and the value of the cord substance (66). Some useful generalizations regarding measurements by CT in adults include the following.

1. The cervical cord is fairly constant in its anteroposterior diameter from C1 to C7, measuring 6−8 mm, slightly smaller in the mid-cervical region. The transverse measurement is 8−12 mm at the level of C1 and 7−10 mm at C7, widening gradually to a maximum of 12−15 mm at C5.

2. The thoracic cord is slightly ovoid, its anteroposterior diameter slightly smaller than the transverse diameter. It gently narrows from T1 to T7 and then becomes gradually wider from T9 to the conus medullaris. From T1 to T9 it measures 5−7 mm in its anteroposterior dimension and 7−9 mm in its transverse dimension. Normal limits are probably not much more than 1 mm on either side of these average dimensions.

A precise determination of abnormal cord enlargement (or cord diminution) is not possible. While distortion may result from dural impingement by disc, ligament, or bone, gross enlargement is nevertheless easily detected as it is with standard myelography. Focal or non-symmetric enlargements are even more readily appreciated. Asymmetric or unilateral focal deformity and enlargement of the cord may indicate exophytic growth of an intramedullary lesion or could be due to an abnormality adjacent to its surface, actually an extramedullary lesion.

The largest group of intramedullary neoplasms is the gliomas (astrocytoma, oligodendroglioma, ependymoma, and glioblastoma). Most of these neoplasms are not demonstrably different in density from surrounding structures and are detected only by virtue of enlargement or deformity of the cord. Some of them, however, are less dense than the surrounding cord because of their inherent cellular composition or due to edema, microcysts or macrocysts, and decreased blood content (2,59). A low-density glioma tends to have a serrated border while a cyst or syrinx has a smooth margin (18). Rarely, ependymomas or hemangioblastomas may cause a hyperdense lesion (2), but they are virtually never calcified within the spinal canal. After intravenous contrast material administration, this group of neoplasms generally does not exhibit selective enhancement or differing iodine content.

Lipomas, dermoid cysts, and neurenteric cysts theoretically should be less dense than cord, but they may contain sufficient connective or epithelial tissue to render them as dense as the cord or lumbar dural contents (41) (Fig. 23). Cystic development usually results in a density comparable to CSF, but such spaces containing large amounts of protein or desquamated

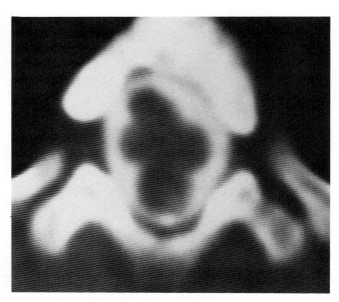

FIG. 24. Neurenteric cyst. The metrizamide-outlined cord is shaped like a 4-leaf clover in the high dorsal region of a two-year-old boy. The attenuation values were the same for all four lobes. At the time of surgery, the posterior and anterior lobes were composed of a large, thin-walled cyst, filled with jelly-like contents, covered by the pia mater of the cord (therefore intramedullary), splitting the spinal cord represented by the two lateral lobules.

material may transform their attenuation value upward. In addition, a cystic lesion may have a spuriously high attenuation value because of the diffusion of metrizamide into it. The spinal cord, like the brain, is known to increase in density when bathed in metrizamide, although the relationship between concentration, duration of exposure, and increased attenuation value has not been established. Similarly, intraspinal cystic lesions also increase in density with time when exposed to metrizamide. As a result, a simple neurenteric cyst may have a much higher CT number than

would be expected from its intrinsic contents (Fig. 24). Awareness of this potential occurrence may help prevent misinterpreting a cyst as a solid neoplasm. At times, this diffusion phenomenon can provide useful diagnostic information. An intramedullary, low-density syrinx also will become denser with the passage of time after the intrathecal administration of metrizamide due to the migration of the contrast agent into the cyst. This may occur either directly via the central canal, as in hydromyelia, or over a longer duration, as in non-communicating syringomyelia and arachnoid cysts, from diffusion across tissue barriers (3) (Figs. 25 and 26). Metrizamide also may accumulate slowly within a neoplasm or parasitic cyst (44).

Primary cord tumors occasionally undergo greater enhancement than the normal cord after intravenous contrast injection, but not often enough to make its administration worthwhile as a routine procedure. However, if a hemangioblastoma is clinically suspected, because of the rich blood supply and enhancing characteristics of this neoplasm, it is worthwhile to administer intravenous contrast material (Fig. 27). Certain other vascular neoplasms such as choriocarcinoma, hemangiosarcoma, and renal cell carcinoma, as well as the non-neoplastic arteriovenous malformations, logically should be seen better after administration of intravenous contrast material. Other non-neoplastic intramedullary lesions tend to resemble true neoplasms. Tuberculous or sarcoid granulomas (37), abscesses, hematomas, and the swollen cord caused by viral transverse myelitis, multiple sclerosis (12), and contusion or infarction may be impossible to differentiate from neoplasm. Clinical features and sometimes follow-up scanning may be helpful in their distinction. A relatively high-density determination should suggest a hematoma, but such an attenuation value does not exclude neoplasm. If an immediate de-

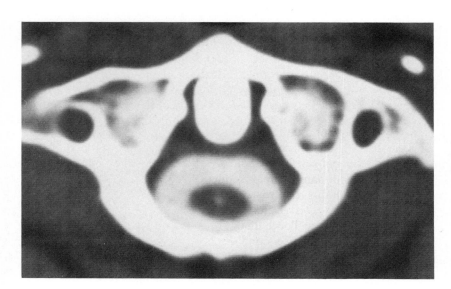

FIG. 25. Hydromyelia. Transverse CT scan through C1 shows a narrow column of metrizamide centrally in the cervical cord, compatible with hydromyelia.

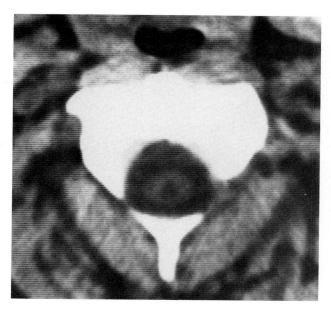

FIG. 26. Syrinx. A low-density (the same as CSF) cavity is seen in the center of the normal diameter cervical cord at C2.

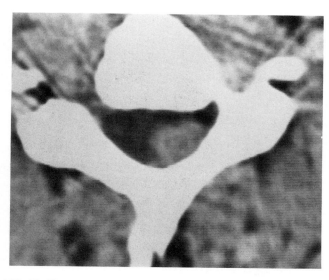

FIG. 27. Hemangioblastoma. The cord itself at the C3 level is not seen in this scan after intravenous contrast injection. An eccentric intramedullary hemangioblastoma is readily shown.

cision is not needed, follow-up CT study is indicated since hematomas should diminish in volume and density over a 2- or 3-week interval.

Intramedullary metastatic disease (Fig. 28), presumably hematogenously spread and formerly considered extremely rare, is now being recognized more frequently (50,68).

Extramedullary, Intradural Compartment

The intradural nerve roots and filum terminale are considered as extramedullary structures.

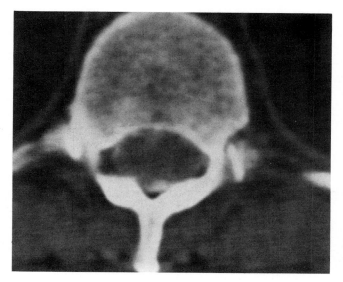

FIG. 28. Intramedullary metastasis from bronchogenic carcinoma. The cord in the conus region is markedly enlarged and metrizamide is barely visible surrounding it. There was a total block by myelography.

Most tumors in this space are either meningiomas or Schwannomas. The familiar features shown by myelography and radiography also are depicted by CT, including an enlarged intervertebral foramen, smooth bone erosion, and usually both intra- and extradural involvement (Fig. 29). At times, multiple lesions may be recognized with Schwannomas, and occasionally calcification seen with meningiomas (Fig. 30); intravenous contrast material injection may cause selective enhancement of meningiomas (33).

Other intradural neoplasms include the dermoid and epidermoid tumor (33) and lipomas (64). Glial tumors may arise from the filum terminale, notably ependymoma, and neuronal tumors rarely may arise from the nerve roots. Both "drop metastases" and blood-borne metastases, such as melanomas, carcinomas, and lymphomas may also present as intradural lesions (Fig. 31).

Non-neoplastic conditions are not infrequent, especially cysts, usually nonspecific arachnoid cysts but rarely neurenteric or parasitic. The tethered cord syndrome, which includes a variety of intradural deformities, is a developmental abnormality. The granulomas, the abscesses, and hematomas can likewise present as extramedullary, intradural masses (10,24).

Other non-neoplastic conditions include arteriovenous malformation, which may be shown specifically by dynamic rapid sequence scanning after intravenous bolus contrast medium injection (51), hypertrophic neuritis (Déjérine Sottas disease) (Fig. 32), Charcot Marie Tooth disease, and a variety of neurofibromatosis. These conditions may be confused, at least by myelography, with the markedly redundant roots not infrequently accompanying severe lumbar stenosis.

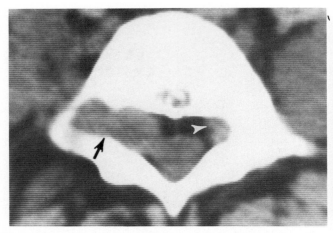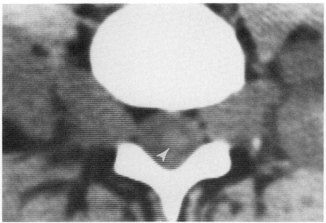

FIG. 29. Neurofibromatosis. **Left:** Scan at the L5/S1 level in a 13-year-old boy demonstrates multiple intraspinal and paraspinal tumors. The large tumor on the right has resulted in a markedly enlarged intervertebral foramen (arrow). A smaller lesion fills the left lateral recess (arrowhead). **Right:** At the L4/5 level, large tumors fill the foramina bilaterally. In addition, an intradural lesion is also seen (arrowhead), outlined by CSF.

Arachnoiditis, with its variable disruption and distortion of the subarachnoid space, may produce an appearance suggesting either an intra- or extramedullary tumor. On myelography, it can be confused with a subdural injection of Pantopaque or drop metastases. Subdural metrizamide, either as the result of subdural injection or leakage from the hole created after needle withdrawal, may cause similar confusion on CT.

Extradural Compartment

Part of the extradural space is normally occupied by normal fat. The amount and extent are variable but deformity or absence in the anticipated locations or asymmetric contour is a valuable sign of pathologic alteration.

The commonest extradural lesions relate to degenerative disease of the intervertebral discs and posterior articular joints, and have been discussed previously. The next most frequent lesions are metastatic neoplasms and lymphomas (Fig. 33), and rarely chloromas (16), usually part of already recognized systemic disease. Primary intraspinal extradural neoplasms are uncommon. The tissues in this compartment are varied and potentially can give rise to a spectrum of tumors including those of lymphoid, vascular, adipose, and primitive notochord origin. Neural tissue may generate neurilemmoma (76), neurofibroma, ependymoma (67), or paraganglioma (52); connective tissue can give rise to firbroma and synovioma. Tumors arising outside the spinal cord, including those from bone and cartilage, can invade this space (Fig. 34).

Non-neoplastic, non-osseous processes which can involve the extradural compartment include abscess (Fig. 35), granuloma, synovial cyst (6), hydatid cyst

(26), hematoma (56), extramedullary hematopoiesis, and excessive fat resulting from hypercorticism (11).

SPINE TRAUMA

The prognosis and management of a patient with spinal trauma depends on accurate determination of the anatomic type and precise level of the injury. Accurate radiographic demonstration of the traumatic bony and soft tissue abnormalities is crucial in their proper management. Failure to recognize a specific type of injury may lead to permanent neurologic damage.

Optimal plain radiographs are often difficult to obtain in severely traumatized patients, either because of a reluctance or inability to move the patient in order to get different projections, sometimes due to multiple associated injuries. Certain regions of the spine, such as the craniocervical junction and cervical thoracic junction, are difficult to evaluate because of the overlapping structures. Plain radiographs may appear normal in the presence of spinal fractures (46).

Because of numerous limitations of plain radiography, thin-section conventional tomography has been widely used to supplement the evaluation of spinal trauma (46). Thin-section tomography has been shown to be superior to plain radiography, particularly in evaluation of the craniocervical junction and the dorsal spine. Again, as with plain roentgenography, it is frequently necessary to move the traumatized patient for optimal tomographic assessment. Furthermore, soft tissue and spinal cord injuries are inadequately evaluated by conventional tomography.

Computed tomography, with the newer generation body scanners which allow production of high resolution scans along with the ability to reformat images in sagittal, coronal, and oblique projections, has in recent

30a,b

30c,d

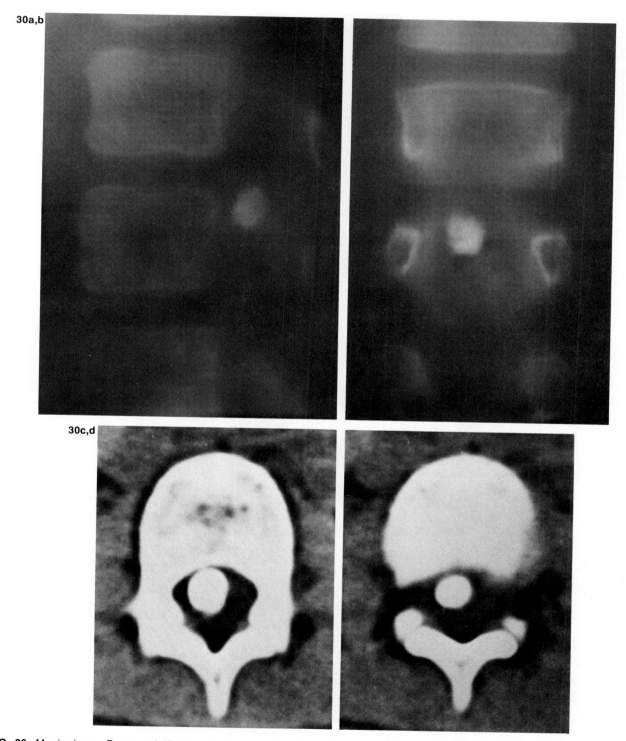

FIG. 30. Meningioma. Dense calcification is shown within the spinal canal by AP and lateral tomograms **(a,b)** and also by the transverse CT scan **(c,d)** in a 10-year-old girl. At operation, an intradural meningioma was removed from within the filaments of the cauda equina.

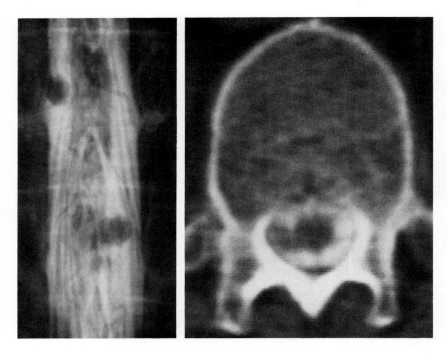

FIG. 31. Metastatic melanoma to the roots of the cauda equina. These multiple nodular lesions shown by the metrizamide lumbar myelogram **(left)** are also recognized on the transverse CT examination **(right).**

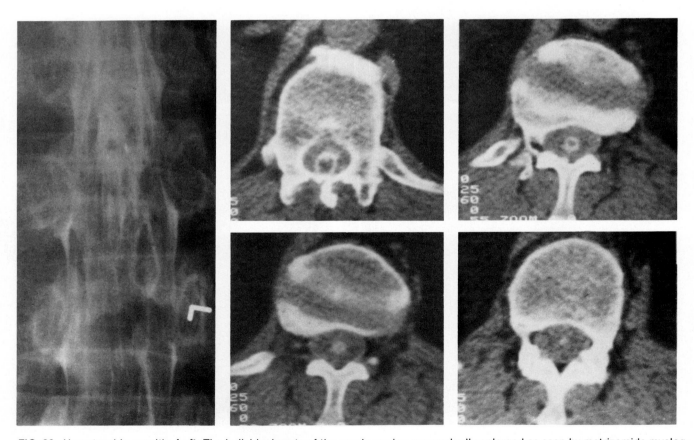

FIG. 32. Hypertrophic neuritis. **Left:** The individual roots of the cauda equina are markedly enlarged as seen by metrizamide myelography. **Right:** Four scans from a CT study taken after the administration of metrizamide demonstrate that the contrast-filled subarachnoid space can only be seen around the conus and filum terminale. At the more inferior levels, the subarachnoid space is obliterated by the thickened roots of the cauda.

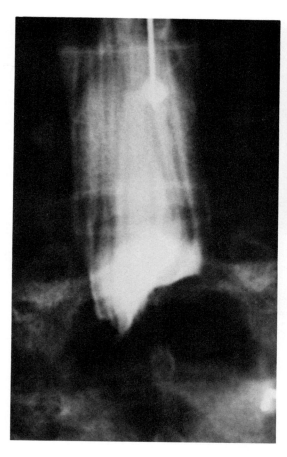

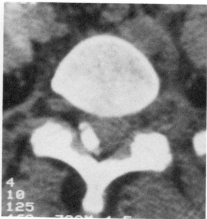

FIG. 33. Extradural metastasis. **Left:** There is a smooth extradural mass at L5 producing a complete myelographic block. **Above:** CT scan through L5 shows marked displacement and distortion of the subarachnoid canal by a soft tissue mass. In the absence of any bone destruction, several other entities would have to be considered, including benign tumor and herniated disc.

years dramatically changed the approach to the evaluation of spine trauma (19,30).

Advantages of CT

Patients with spine trauma, especially those with unstable fractures, are at a high risk of developing permanent neurologic deficit if they are moved. Computed tomography can be obtained with the patient in one position.

The actual CT examination can be performed in a relatively short time since the study is performed in only one plane. Later, sagittal, coronal, or oblique planes can be reformatted without any further scanning or manipulation of the patient. An additional minor advantage is that radiation doses in CT are much lower than in conventional thin-section tomography (8).

The axial plane of the CT scan is optimal for assessing cord compression, determining spinal canal size, and for determining whether intraspinal body fragments are present (19). Unlike plain radiography, CT has the ability to distinguish subtle soft tissue density differences. The intervertebral disc, ligaments, and the spinal cord can all be demonstrated by CT. Hematomas in the epidural space and in the spinal cord

may be detected (33,56). In penetrating injuries such as gunshot wounds, the position of foreign body fragments relative to the spinal canal and cord can be easily determined by the transaxial scans. Fresh or healing fracture lines, especially those in the rostro-

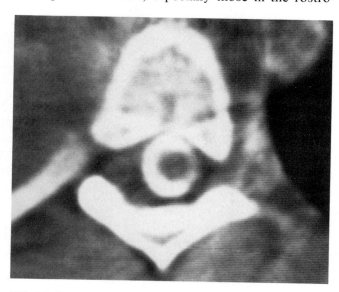

FIG. 34. Neuroblastoma in a 10-year-old boy. The tumor mass enters the dorsal spinal canal through an intervertebral foramen and displaces the metrizamide-filled subarachnoid canal and spinal cord to the left.

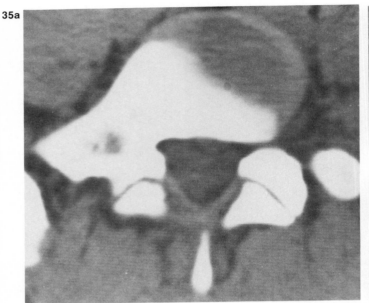

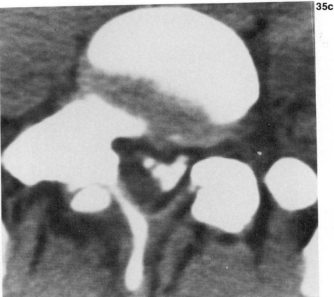

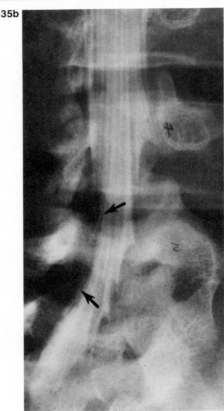

FIG. 35. Epidural empyema. Twelve-year-old boy with back pain, one month after treatment for an abdominal infection. **a:** Plain CT study was prospectively interpreted as normal. In retrospect, blurring of the epidural fat can be seen on the right side, presumably due to infiltration of the fat by inflammatory cells. No diagnosis was made. **b:** Metrizamide myelogram shows a posterolateral extradural defect on the right (arrows). **c:** Post-myelogram CT through the level of the myelographic abnormality demonstrates a soft tissue mass deviating the contrast-filled subarachnoid space to the left. An extradural empyema was drained surgically.

caudal plane, and subluxations generally are effectively demonstrated. Fractures of the demineralized spine that are difficult to evaluate by conventional radiography and tomography are easily demonstrated by CT (30). The ability to reformat images in coronal, sagittal, and oblique projections facilitates the diagnosis of dislocation and facet locking. The use of intrathecal metrizamide allows demonstration of swollen cord or a tear in the dura.

Limitations of CT

Non-displaced fractures that are oriented in the transaxial plane can be completely missed on the standard CT scans. Reformatting the images may help, but the clarity of these images depends on the thickness of the original slices. A change in the position of the patient between two consecutive scans may lead to missing a fracture altogether. Alternatively, the partial

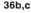

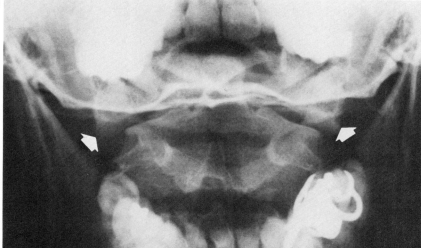

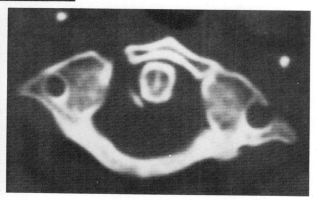

FIG. 36. Jefferson's fracture. **a:** Open mouth anteroposterior radiograph of the cranio-cervical junction shows lateral displacement of the lateral masses of the atlas (arrows). **b:** CT demonstrates fractures of the anterior and posterior arches (arrows) of the atlas. **c:** Follow-up CT scan of the same patient 8 months later shows healing with bony fusion at three of the four fracture sites.

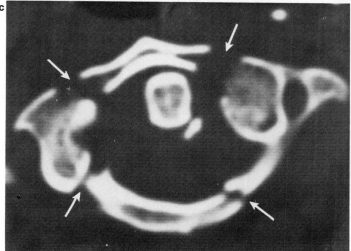

volume averaging phenomenon with CT may produce appearances simulating fractures. Narrowing or widening of the intervertebral disc spaces and subluxations also may be overlooked on the transaxial images. To demonstrate the stability of the spine, radiologic examination is required in both extension and flexion. Such manipulations are difficult to accomplish with CT. They are better done with fluoroscopy or thin-section tomography. Artifacts caused by postoperative metallic clips or fixation devices (e.g., Harrington rod placement) may jeopardize evaluation in the postoperative stage.

Survey of the entire spinal column by CT would be time-consuming and cumbersome. By obtaining a conventional radiograph as the primary examination, the region of trauma to the spine can be localized. A digital radiograph (''scannogram'') obtained by the CT machine is an alternative technique to limit the area subsequently to be studied in detail (8). A CT study in the region of interest then greatly enhances the information about the type and extent of the injury and generally obviates thin-section tomography.

Cervical Spine Injury

Craniocervical Junction

Fractures of the atlas result from either hyperextension or axial compression injury. The posterior arch of the atlas is trapped between the occipital squama and the posterior arch of the axis. In these cases, the usual break involves at least two points. In the axial compression type of injury (the classical fracture described by Jefferson), injury to the atlas causes a break of both the anterior and posterior arches (Fig. 36). Fractures of the atlas which involve the atlanto-axial joint are important to recognize, since the stability of the region depends on this joint as well. Neurologic deficits are uncommon in fractures of the atlas and axis due to the large subarachnoid space around the cord (60).

37a,b

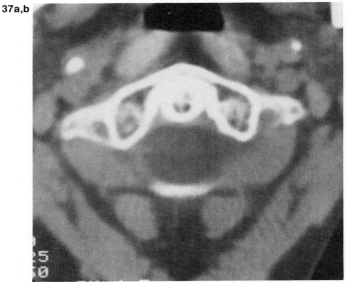
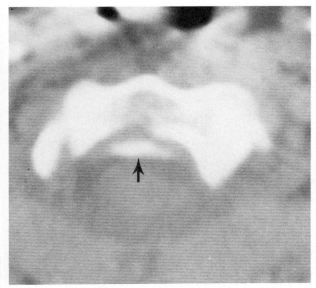

37c

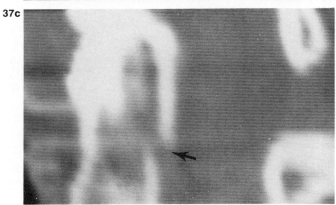

FIG. 37. Fracture at the base of the dens. **a:** At the level of the anterior arch of atlas the relationship of the odontoid and anterior arch is normal. **b:** At the level of the body of the axis, the inferior posterior border of the factured dens (arrow) is seen posterior to the body of C2. **c:** Reformatted image in the sagittal plane provides better demonstration of the fracture (arrow).

The ring-shaped structure of the atlas makes it difficult to evaluate by plain radiography or thin-section tomography. Computed tomography in the axial projection can better assess the complete ring of the atlas for the presence of fractures and involvement of the atlanto-axial joint (38,39). Repeat CT may be valuable in appraising healing of fractures in this region.

The relationship of the dens and the atlas is easily evaluated by CT (20,60,70), thus facilitating the detection of atlanto-axial subluxation. Another type of injury, atlanto-axial fixation, involves rotatory trauma to this area and can similarly be imaged with CT.

Fractures of the axis can affect the dens or the body. The horizontally oriented nondisplaced fracture of the base of dens, usually caused by a forward movement of the head in relation to the rest of the cervical spine, is difficult to evaluate by CT, but sagittal images reformatted from the transaxial scans may help (Fig. 37).

The classic hangman's fracture of the axis, caused by hyperflexion injury, involves the lateral masses bilaterally. The fracture lines are oriented in the rostrocaudal plane and are easily demonstrated by CT. "Pseudo-hangman's" fractures (Fig. 38) affect the

body of the axis rather than the lateral masses. In both types, the integrity of the posterior arch of axis is best evaluated with CT.

Lower Cervical Spine

Trauma of the lower cervical region deserves particular attention since the subarachnoid space around the cord in this region is small and any substantial impingement on the spinal canal is likely to produce cord compression. Injuries here may be caused by hyperflexion, hyperextension, hyperrotation, or axial compression. Wedge fractures (Fig. 39) and "burst fractures" (Fig. 40) are most commonly seen with diving type injuries. A wedge fracture is caused by hyperflexion while the burst fracture results from a combination of hyperflexion and axial compression. Both types of fracture tend to produce neurologic deficits, with subluxation compromising the spinal canal in the former variety and by displacement of a fragment into the spinal canal in the latter type. The presence of free bony fragments within the canal is easily detected

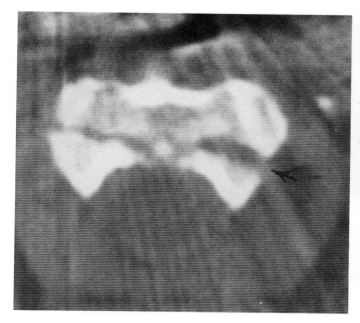

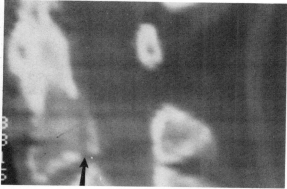

FIG. 38. Psuedo-hangman's fracture. **Left:** The transverse fracture through the body of axis (arrow) is oriented in the rostrocaudal plane and easy to demonstrate by CT. **Above:** Reformatted image in the sagittal plane shows the rostrocaudal orientation of the fracture line (arrow).

by transaxial CT (13), while in subluxation sagittal reformatted images may be required.

Hyperextension injuries may result in only a chip fracture of an anterior vertebral body or fractures of the neural arch including the pedicles, articular pillars, laminae, and spinous process.

A combination of flexion and rotation injuries may lead to subluxation or dislocations of the facet joints, and possible resultant facet locking. The superior articular facet of the lower vertebra is locked posterior to the inferior facet of the upper vertebra. Although this type of injury can be diagnosed on a plain radiograph, associated fractures of the facet joints, which usually require open reduction, may be difficult to see. Computed tomographic scans can show both the locked facet and the presence or absence of a fracture of the facet (Fig. 41). Reformatted images in the plane of the facet joints can be very helpful.

Thoracolumbar Spine Injury

Fractures of the upper thoracic spine are not as common as in the cervical or lumbar region. Hyperflexion injuries which cause only compression fractures of the mid- and upper thoracic spine usually result in no neurologic damage. In contradistinction,

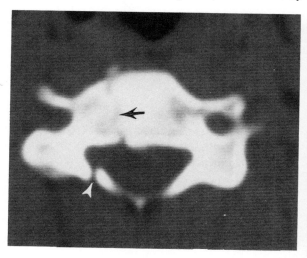

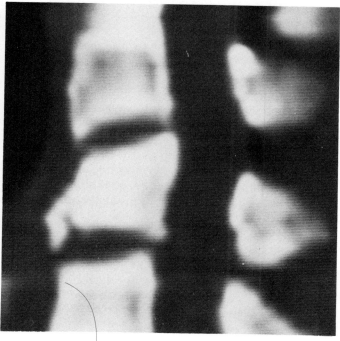

FIG. 39. Compression fracture. **Above:** Transaxial CT shows fracture through the body of the fourth cervical vertebra (arrow) and the right lamina (arrowhead). There is no encroachment upon the spinal canal by bony fragments. **Right:** Sagittally reformatted image also demonstrates the wedged compression fracture and a small chip fracture at the anterior inferior border of the body, and an intact spinal canal.

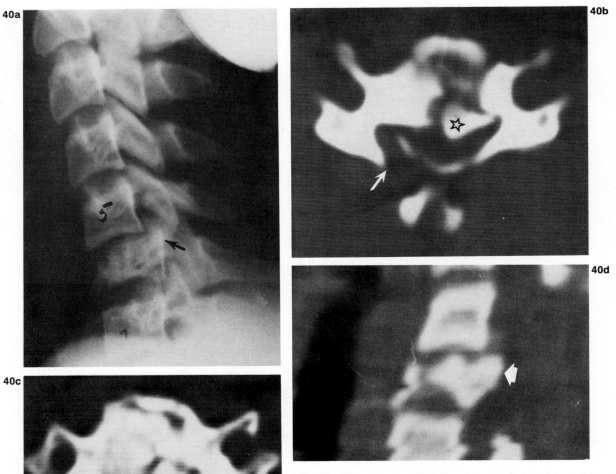

FIG. 40. "Burst fracture" of the sixth cervical vertebra with posterior subluxation. **a:** Lateral radiograph demonstrates that the posterior border of the body of the sixth cervical vertebra is displaced into the spinal canal (arrow). **b:** Transaxial CT shows a comminuted fracture with fragmentation. A large fragment (star) impinges upon the spinal canal. There is also a fracture of the right lamina (arrow). **c and d:** Postoperative axial CT (c) and a sagitally reformatted image (d) show marked posterior displacement of the fractured body (arrow). The neural arch has been removed.

vertical compression and hyperflexion injuries may cause severe deficits (61). The absence of a fracture of the dorsal elements usually presages a good prognosis. Plain radiographs in the anterioposterior and lateral projections are of limited value in detecting neural arch fractures. Computed tomography, including image reformation, is vastly superior in evaluating thoracic spine injuries.

Fracture-dislocations at the thoracolumbar junction are the most common spine fractures (40%). Hyperflexion injuries can result in different types of fractures (55). In the more common type, a wedge compression fracture results from compressive forces on the anterior half of the vertebral body, and the neural arch structures usually are not disturbed. In severe deacceleration injuries associated with seat belts, if the vector force passes through the vertebral body, a horizontal (Chance) fracture of the vertebral body with distraction of the dorsal elements will occur (Fig. 42). If the vector force occurs in the plane of the disc space, there is usually disruption of the neural arch and "naked" distracted facets (14) (Fig. 43).

Bursting fracture (14,54) of the vertebral body in the lumbar region usually results from a vertical compressive force. Computed tomography most reliably demonstrates any encroachment upon the spinal canal by a fracture fragment or a displaced dorsal element (Fig. 44).

Neurologic damage or deficit can result from trauma to the spinal cord without any detectable fracture. In such cases, an intraspinal hematoma (Fig. 45) or swell-

41a,b

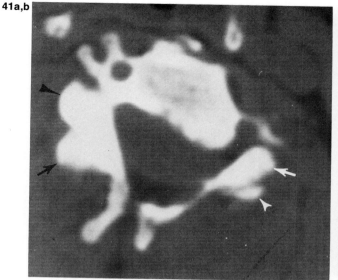

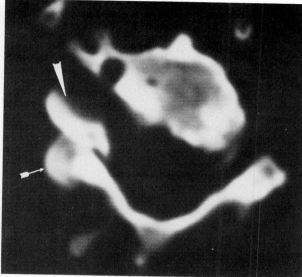

41c

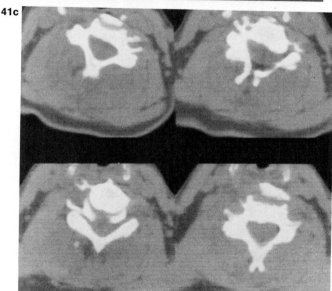

FIG. 41. Fracture dislocation at C5/6 with locked facet on the right side. **a:** Scan through the articulation between C5/6 shows that the superior articular process of C6 (white arrow) lies in front of the inferior articular process of C5 (white arrowhead) on the normal left side. On the right side, the superior articular process of C6 (black arrow) lies behind the inferior articular process of C5 (black arrowhead). **b:** Same level, at bone window setting. Note the concave anterior surface of the inferior articular process of C5 on the right side (arrowhead), which is supposed to articulate with the posterior surface of the superior articular process of C6 (arrow). In addition, a fracture of the right superior articular process is present. **c:** Composite illustration of four slices through C5, C5/6 articulation, and C6 in the same patient. Compare the orientation of the mid-sagittal plane of C5 (upper left corner) with that of C6 (lower right corner). This malalignment is an expression of the rotatory nature of the injury, and is maintained by the locking of the facets.

ing of the cord (33) usually is present. Such cord swelling can be detected on CT after the intrathecal administration of metrizamide (Fig. 46).

Localization of bullet fragments in relation to the spinal canal and vertebral bodies is best provided by transaxial CT images (Fig. 47).

CONGENITAL ANOMALIES

The term spinal dysraphism includes various developmental anomalies that arise from cutaneous, mesodermal, or neural derivatives of the median dorsal region of the embryo. It comprises a tethered cord, diastematomyelia, and neurenteric cysts; meningoceles and myelomeningoceles are also part of this entity although at times described separately. Myelographic findings of the tethered cord include low posi-

tion of the conus medullaris, dorsally located filum terminale (which is greater than 2 mm in width), abnormal position of the spinal arterial supply, and translucent defects in the contrast column due to traction bands from the dura to the cord (28). Tethered cord may also be associated with Arnold–Chiari malformation (21). Most of these findings can be demonstrated by CT (36), although the use of metrizamide may be necessary for precise definition of the abnormal anatomic structures (Figs. 48 and 49). Computed tomography may be helpful in demonstrating the small size of the subarachnoid space around the cord in the lumbar region and craniocervical junction prior to lumbar or cisternal puncture.

In diastematomyelia (Fig. 50), the spinal canal is divided by a bony septum, spicule, or fibrous septum in approximately 70% of the cases (1). More importantly,

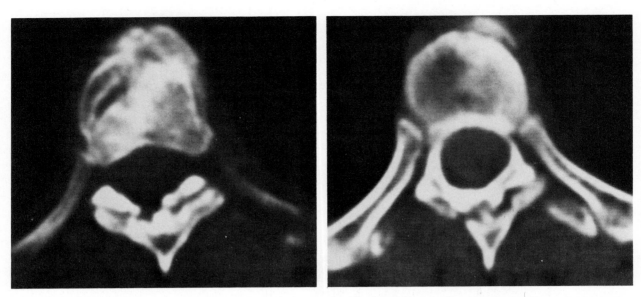

FIG. 42. Chance fracture. **Left:** An oblique fracture through the vertebral body is noted on this scan. **Right:** Four millimeters caudal, a transverse fracture of the neural arch is present.

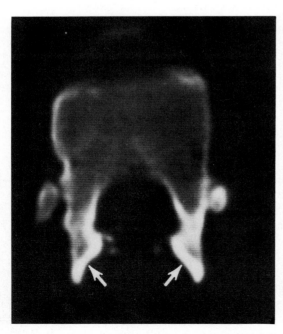

FIG. 43. The naked facet. The superior articular processes of the twelfth thoracic vertebra (arrows) are not in contact with any articular process of T11. There has been soft tissue distraction that caused wide separation of the elements of the posterior articulation.

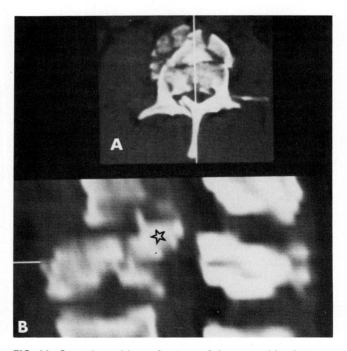

FIG. 44. Comminuted burst fracture of the second lumbar vertebra with encroachment upon the spinal cord. **A:** Severe comminution of the body. The size of the spinal canal has been greatly reduced by displacement of fragments of the comminuted vertebral body into the bony spinal canal. **B:** Sagittal reformatted image shows marked reduction of the anteroposterior diameter of the bony spinal canal by a displaced fragment (star).

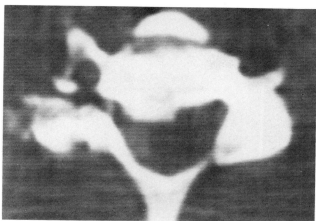

FIG. 45. Fracture of a vertebra complicated with hematoma. Fracture of the body of a cervical vertebra, as well as the right lateral mass, can be seen. An intraspinal hematoma is also present medial to the right lamina.

the spinal cord may be divided into two hemicords. Diplomyelia is a rare condition of segmental duplication of the entire cord including gray and white matter (1,63). The nerve roots arise laterally only in diastematomyelia in comparison to diplomyelia where the spinal nerve roots arise from both sides of each cord. Computed tomographic findings in diastematomyelia (1,45,69,75) include the demonstration of the septum and the two hemicords. The enlarged subarachnoid space generally allows identification of the hemicords or fibrous septum on noncontrast images, but their visualization is greatly enhanced by use of intrathecal metrizamide (1,15), which also can be helpful in demonstrating an associated meningocele or myelomeningocele.

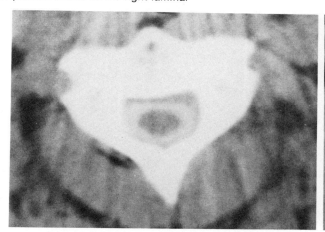

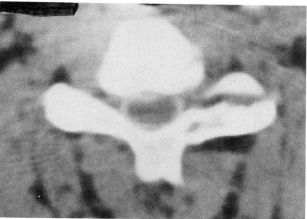

FIG. 46. Traumatic swelling of the cord. CT scan of the cervical region after intrathecal injection of metrizamide. **Left:** The metrizamide outlines the normal size of the cord at the level of the second cervical vertebra. **Right:** At the level of the third cervical vertebra, the metrizamide around the cord is reduced due to encroachment upon the subarachnoid space by the swollen cord. Note asymmetry in the configuration of the cord due to uneven swelling.

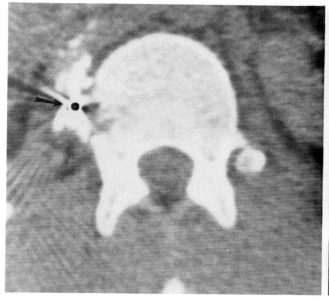

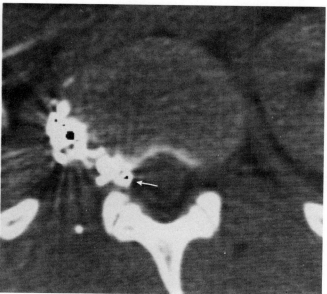

FIG. 47. Gunshot injury of the spine. **Left:** The missile fragment (arrow) lies against the body of the vertebra. It does not encroach upon the cauda equina or the nerve root. **Right:** Another fragment within the intervertebral foramen (arrow). At this location, injury to the nerve root and ganglion is expected.

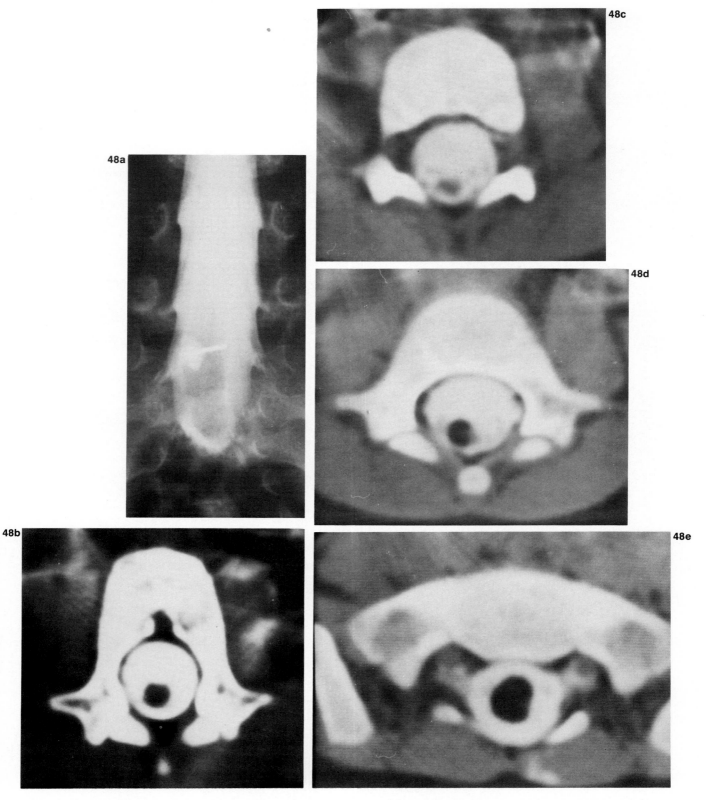

FIG. 48. Tethered cord in conjunction with a lipoma. **a:** Metrizamide myelogram shows a defect in the lower end of the dural sac. The exact location of the cord cannot be determined. **b:** At the L3 level, the conus medullaris can be seen. **c:** The tip of the conus is shown at the level of the lower disc plate of L3 with several nerve roots around it. **d:** A lipoma, which has a much lower density than the conus, is seen in the subarachnoid space below the tip of the conus lying among the roots of the cauda equina. **e:** The thicker part of the lipoma lies at the level of the sacral segments.

49a,b

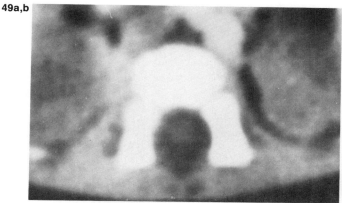 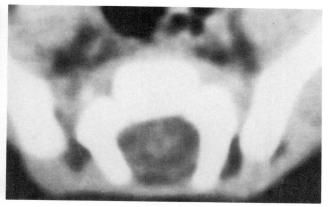

49c

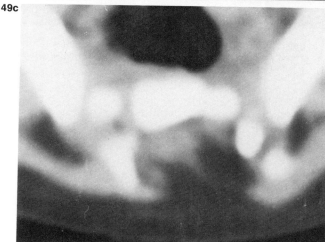

FIG. 49. Lipomeningocele with tethered cord. **a and b:** The tethered cord is surrounded with CSF and demonstrated on plain CT at the level of L3 and S1. There is a defect in the neural arch at both levels. **c:** A larger defect in the neural arch is seen at the level of the upper sacral segments. A lipoma fills the spinal canal at this level.

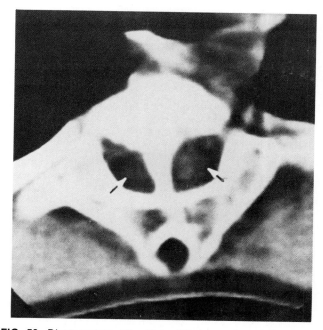

FIG. 50. Diastematomyelia. Plain CT shows the midline osseous spicule. The hemicords (arrows) can be identified on either side of the spicule. (Reproduced with permission from ref. 34.)

Congenital malformations of the neural arch of the vertebral body with protrusion of the meninges through the congenital defect outside the confines of the spinal canal are termed a meningocele when the contents of the herniated sac consist only of CSF, a myelomeningocele when neural elements are included, and a lipo-meningocele when fat and CSF are present. Meningoceles are most common in the sacral region and at the lumbo-sacral junction, but may also occur in the cervical region. The anomaly may be associated with a tethered cord. In anterior meningoceles, plain CT accurately demonstrates the relationship of the lesion and the soft tissue contents of the pelvic cavity (4). The sac of the meningocele and the bony defect in the neural arch of the lumbar vertebra or sacrum are easily seen. The fibrous band connecting the meningocele to the skin, and the low-density fatty component of a lipomeningocele, are also usually well depicted. The use of metrizamide with CT can outline the soft tissue contents of the sac, especially a tethered cord (Fig. 48).

Syringomyelia occurs when cavitation develops in the spinal cord extending over many segments. When the cavity is a distended central canal, the condition is known as hydromyelia; it is a congenital anomaly usu-

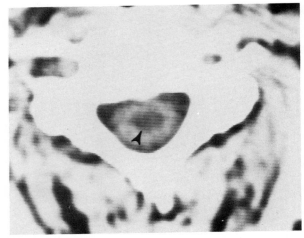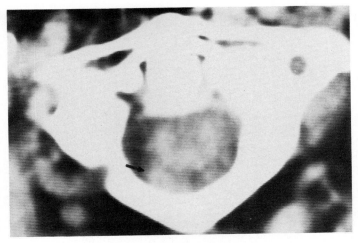

FIG. 51. Syringohydromyelia with associated Chiari type I malformation. **Left:** At the C2 level, an enlarged cord is seen surrounded by cerebral spinal fluid. The central low-density cavity within the cord is enlarged (arrowhead). **Right:** At the C1 level, the cerebellar tonsils (arrow) are seen behind the cord.

ally associated with Chiari type I malformation (22). These two conditions may be difficult to differentiate even at necropsy (35), and the term syringohydromyelia is used to encompass the entire entity. In this disorder, expansion and swelling of the spinal cord may occur (Fig. 51). Flattening and consequent atrophy of the cord, rather than expansion, may be present when the cavity is decompressed by communication with the subarachnoid space (7). Both the cavity within the cord, the surrounding CSF in the subarachnoid space, and the ectopia of the cerebellar tonsils may be shown by plain CT (Fig. 51). The cord containing the cavity may appear enlarged, normal in size, flattened, or atrophic. Opacification of the subarachnoid space with metrizamide in conjunction with CT may show filling of the cavity either immediately or after a few hours (Fig. 25). The contrast material completely clears from the cavity within 24 hours.

Neurenteric cysts are a form of spinal dysraphism in which the spinal defect is anterior. The cord anomaly, intraspinal cyst, and anterior spinal dysraphia can be demonstrated by plain CT (31). As mentioned previously, the fluid of the intraspinal cyst may contain high protein (mucinous) material and be indistinguishable from the cord itself on the noncontrast CT images. Introduction of metrizamide will show the change in cord configuration or diffusion of contrast into the cyst.

Bony spinal anomalies, such as hemivertebrae and block vertebrae, can be identified on CT, but it is easier to demonstrate them by plain radiography or thin-section tomography. At times, the posterior arch anomalies, such as absent cervical pedicle, can be better evaluated by CT (9,43). Computed tomography can differentiate this condition from a metastatic tumor, neurofibroma, or trauma by demonstrating malformation and displacement of the lateral mass, abnormal transverse process, intact cortex at the site of the missing pedicle, and normal density of the soft tissue in the foramen.

REFERENCES

1. Arrendondo F, Haughton VM, Hemmy DC, Zelaya B, Williams AL: Computed tomographic appearance of spinal cord in diastematomyelia. *Radiology* 136:685–688, 1980
2. Aubin ML, Jardin C, Bar D, Vignaud J: Computerized tomography in 32 cases of intraspinal tumor. *J Neuroradiol* 6:81–92, 1979
3. Aubin ML, Vignaud J, Jardin C, Bar D: Computed tomography in 75 clinical cases of syringomyelia. *AJNR* 2:199–204, 1981
4. Baleriaux-Waha D, Osteaux M, Terwinghe G, de Meeus A, Jeanmart L: The management of anterior sacral meningocele with CT. *Neuroradiology* 14:45–46, 1977
5. Bernini PM, Wiesel SW, Rothman RH: Metrizamide myelography and the identification of anomalous lumbosacral nerve roots. *J Bone Joint Surg* 62-A:1203–1208, 1980
6. Bhushan C, Hodges FJ III, Wityk JJ: Synovial cyst (ganglion) of the lumbar spine simulating extradural mass. *Neuroradiology* 18:263–268, 1979
7. Bonafe A, Ethier R, Melancon D, Belanger G, Peters T: High resolution computed tomography in cervical syringomyelia. *J Comput Assist Tomogr* 4:42–47, 1980
8. Brant-Zawadzki M, Miller EM, Federle MP: CT in the evaluation of spine trauma. *AJR* 136:369–375, 1981
9. Brugman E, Palmer Y, Staelens B: Congenital absence of a pedicle in the cervical spine: A new Approach with CT scan. *Neuroradiology* 17:121–125, 1979
10. Campbell JN, Black P, Ostrow PT: Sarcoid of the cauda equina: Case report. *J Neurosurg* 47:109–112, 1977
11. Chapman PH, Martuza RL, Poletti CE, Karchmer AW: Symptomatic spinal epidural lipomatosis associated with Cushing's syndrome. *Neurosurgery* 8:724–727, 1981
12. Coin CG, Hucks-Folliss A: Cervical computed tomography in multiple sclerosis with spinal cord involvement. *J Comput Assist Tomogr* 3:421–422, 1979
13. Coin CG, Pennick M, Ahmad WD, Keranen VJ: Diving-type injury of the cervical spine: Contribution of computed tomography to management. *J Comput Assist Tomogr* 3:362–372, 1979
14. Colley DP, Dunsker SB: Traumatic narrowing of the dorsolumbar spinal canal demonstrated by computed tomography. *Radiology* 129:95–98, 1978
15. Di Chiro G, Schellinger D: Computed tomography of spinal cord

after intrathecal introduction of metrizamide (computer assisted myelography). *Radiology* 120:101–104, 1976
16. Dunnick NR, Heaston DK: Computed tomography of extracranial chloroma. *J Comput Assist Tomogr* 6:83–85, 1982
17. Elliot HC: Cross-sectional diameters and areas of the human spinal cord. *Anat Rec* 93:287–293, 1945
18. Ethier R, King DG, Melancon D, Belanger G, Thompson C: Diagnosis of intra- and extramedullary lesions by CT without contrast achieved through modifications applied to the EMI CT 5005 Body Scanner. In: *Radiographic Evaluation of the Spine: Current Advances with Emphasis on Computed Tomography,* ed. by M Judith Donovan Post, New York, Masson Publishing USA, 1980, pp 377–393
19. Faerber EN, Wolpert SM, Scott RM, Belkin SC, Carter BL: Computed tomography of spinal fractures. *J Comput Assist Tomogr* 3:657–661, 1979
20. Fielding JW, Stillwell WT, Chynn KY, Spyropoulos EC: Use of computed tomography for the diagnosis of atlanto-axial rotatory fixation. A case report. *J Bone Joint Surg* 6-A:1102–1104, 1978
21. Fitz CR, Harwood-Nash DC: The tethered conus. *Am J Roentgenol Radium Ther Nucl Med* 125:515–523, 1975
22. Forbes WSC, Isherwood I: Computed tomography in syringomyelia and the associated Arnold-Chiari Type I malformation. *Neuroradiology* 15:73–78, 1978
23. Ford LT, Gilula LA, Murphy WA, Gado M: Analysis of gas in vacuum lumbar disc. *AJR* 128:1056–1057, 1977
24. Frager D, Zimmerman RD, Wisoff HS, Leeds NE: Spinal subarachnoid hematoma. *ANJR* 3:77–79, 1982
25. Gado MH, Patel J, Chandra-Sekar B, Kapila A, Hodges FJ: An integrative approach to the diagnosis of lumbar disc disease by CT and myelography. Presented at the 67th Scientific Assembly and Annual Meeting of Radiological Society of North America, Chicago, IL, Nov. 15–20, 1981
26. Giordano BG, Cerisoli M, Bernardi B: Hydatid cysts of the spine. *J Comput Assist Tomogr* 6:408–409, 1982
27. Glenn WV, Rhodes ML, Altschuler EM, Wiltse LL, Kostanek C, Kuo YM: Multiplanar display computerized body tomography applications in the lumbar spine. *Spine* 4:282–294, 1979
28. Gryspeerdi GL: Myelographic assessment of occult forms of spinal dysraphism. *Acta Radiol [Diagn](Stockh)* 1:702–717, 1963
29. Gulati AN, Weinstein ZR: Gas in the spinal canal in association with the lumbosacral vacuum phenomenon: CT findings. *Neuroradiology* 20:191–192, 1980
30. Handel SF, Lee Y: Computed tomography of spinal fractures. *Radiol Clin North Am* 19:69–89, 1981
31. Harwood-Nash DCF, Fitz CR, Rasjo IM, Chuang S: Congenital spinal and cord lesions in children and computed tomographic metrizamide myelography. *Neuroradiology* 16:69–70, 1978
32. Haughton VM, Eldevik OP, Magnaes B, Amundsen P: A prospective comparison of computed tomography and myelography in the diagnosis of herniated lumbar disks. *Radiology* 142:103–110, 1982
33. Haughton VM, Williams AL: *Computed Tomography of the Spine,* St. Louis, CV Mosby, 1982
34. Hirschy JC, Leue WM, Berninger WH, Hamilton RH, Abbott GF: CT of the lumbosacral spine: Importance of tomographic planes parallel to vertebral end plate. *AJR* 136:47–52, 1981
35. Hughes JT: Diseases of the spine and spinal cord. In: *Greenfield's Neuropathology,* 3rd ed, ed. by W Blackwood, JAN Corsellis, London, Edward Arnold, 1976, pp 668–670
36. James HE, Oliff M: Computed tomography in spinal dysraphism. *J Comput Assist Tomogr* 1:391–397, 1977
37. Kanoff RB, Rubert R: Sarcoidosis presenting as a dorsal spinal cord tumor: Report of a case. *J Am Osteopath Assoc* 79:765–767, 1980
38. Keene GCR, Hone MR, Sage MR: Atlas fracture: Demonstration using computerized tomography. A case report. *J Bone Joint Surg* 60-A:1106–1107, 1978
39. Kershner MS, Goodman GA, Perlmutter GS: Computed tomography in the diagnosis of an atlas fracture. *AJR* 128:688–689, 1977
40. Kim KS, Weinberg PE, Hemmati M: Spinal pachymeningeal carcinomatosis: Myelographic features. *ANJR* 1:199–200, 1980
41. Kwok DMF, Jeffreys RV: Intramedullary enterogeneous cyst of the spinal cord. *J Neurosurg* 56:270–274, 1982
42. Lancourt JE, Glenn WV, Viltse LL: Multiplanar computerized tomography in the normal spine and in the diagnosis of spinal stenosis: A gross anatomic-computerized tomographic correlation. *Spine* 4:379–390, 1979
43. Lauten GJ, Wehunt WP: Computed tomography in absent cervical pedicle. *AJNR* 1:201–203, 1980
44. Ley A, Marti A: Intramedullary hydatid cyst: Case report. *J Neurosurg* 33:457–459, 1970
45. Lohkamp F, Claussen C, Schuhmacher G: CT demonstration of pathologic changes of the spinal cord accompanying spina bifida and diastematomyelia. *Prog Pediatr Radiol* 6:200–227, 1978
46. Maravilla KR, Cooper PR, Sklar FH: The influence of thin-section tomography on the treatment of cervical spine injuries. *Radiology* 127:131–139, 1978
47. McAfee PC, Ullrich CG, Yuan HA, Sherry RG, Lockwood RC: Computed tomography in degenerative spinal stenosis. *Clin Orthop* 161:221–234, 1981
48. Meyer GA, Haughton VM, Williams AL: Diagnosis of herniated lumbar disk with computed tomography. *N Engl J Med* 301:1166–1167, 1979
49. Meyer JD, Latchaw RE, Poppolo HM, Choshhajra K, Deeb ZL: Computed tomography and myelography of the postoperative lumbar spine. *AJNR* 3:223–228, 1982
50. Moffie D, Stefanko SZ: Intramedullary metastasis. *Clin Neurol* 82:199–202, 1980
51. Nagashima C, Yamaguchi T, Tsuji R: Arteriovenous malformation of the spinal cord: Computed tomography with intraarterial enhancement. *J Comput Assist Tomogr* 5:586–587, 1981
52. Nakagawa H, Mallis LI, Huang YP: Computed tomography of soft tissue masses related to the spinal column. In: *Radiographic Evaluation of the Spine: Current Advances with Emphasis on Computed Tomography,* ed. by M. Judith Donavan Post, New York, Masson Publishers USA, 1980, pp 320–352
53. Nordqvist L: The sagittal diameter of the spinal cord and subarachnoid space in different age groups. *Acta Radiol* 227(Suppl):1–96, 1964
54. Nykamp PW, Levy JM, Christensen F, Dunn R, Hubbard J: Computed tomography for a bursting fracture of the lumbar spine. Report of a case. *J Bone Joint Surg* 60-A:1108–1109, 1978
55. O'Callaghan JP, Ullrich CG, Yuan HA, Kieffer SA: CT of facet distraction in flexion injuries of the thoracolumbar spine: The "naked" facet. *AJR* 134:563–568, 1980
56. Post MJD, Seminer DS, Quencer RM: CT diagnosis of spinal epidural hematoma. *AJNR* 3:190–192, 1982
57. Postacchini F, Pezzeri G, Montanaro A, Natali G: Computerized tomography in lumbar stenosis. *J Bone Joint Surg* 62-B:78–82, 1980
58. Reilly J, Yong-Hing K, MacKay RW, Kirkaldy-Willis WH: Pathological anatomy of the lumbar spine. In: *Disorders of the Lumbar Spine,* ed. by AJ Helfet, DM Lee, Philadelphia, J.B. Lippincott, 1978, pp 26–50
59. Resjo MI, Harwood-Nash DC, Fitz CR, Chuang S: CT metrizamide myelography for intraspinal and paraspinal neoplasms in infants and children. *AJR* 132:367–372, 1979
60. Rinaldi I, Mullins WJ, Delaney WF, Fitzer PM, Tornberg DN: Computerized tomographic demonstration of rotational atlanto-axial fixation. Case report. *J Neurosurg* 50:115–119, 1979
61. Rogers LF, Thayer C, Weinberg PE, Kim KS: Acute injuries of the upper thoracic spine associated with paraplegia. *AJR* 134:67–73, 1980
62. Sachsenheimer W, Hamer J, Muller HA: The value of spinal computed tomography in diagnosis of herniated lumbar discs. *Acta Neurochir (Wien)* 60:107–114, 1982
63. Scatliff JH, Bidgood WD, Killebrew K, Staab EV: Computed tomography and spinal dysraphism: Clinical and phantom studies. *Neuroradiology* 17:71–75, 1979
64. Schroeder S, Lackner K, Weiand G: Lumbosacral intradural lipoma. *J Comput Assist Tomogr* 5:274, 1981
65. Schubiger O, Valavanis A: CT differentiation between recurrent

disc herniation and postoperative scar formation: The value of contrast enhancement. *Neuroradiology* 22:251−254, 1982

66. Siebert CE, Barnes JE, Dreisbach JN, Swanson WB, Heck RJ: Accurate CT measurement of the spinal cord using metrizamide: Physical factors. *AJNR* 2:75−78, 1981

67. Siegel RS, William AG, Mettler FA Jr, Wicks JD: Intraspinal extradural ependymoma. Case report. *J Comput Assist Tomogr* 6:189−192, 1982

68. Smaltino F, Bernini FP, Santoro S: Computerized tomography in the diagnosis of intramedullary metastases. *Acta Neurochir* 52:299−303, 1980

69. Tadmor R, Davis KR, Roberson GH, Chapman PH: The diagnosis of diastematomyelia by computed tomography. *Surg Neurol* 8:434−436, 1977

70. Tadmor R, Davis KR, Roberson GH, New PFJ, Taveras JM: Computed tomographic evaluation of the traumatic spinal injuries. *Radiology* 127:825−827, 1978

71. Taylor AJ, Haughton VM, Doust BD: CT imaging of the thoracic spinal cord without intrathecal contrast medium. *J Comput Assist Tomogr* 4:223−224, 1980

72. Thijsson HOM, Keyser A, Horstink MWM, Meijer E: Morphology of the cervical spinal cord on computed tomography. *Neuroradiology* 18:57−62, 1979

73. Verbiest H: The significance and principles of computerized axial tomography in idiopathic developmental stenosis of the bony lumbar vertebral canal. *Spine* 4:369−378, 1979

74. Williams AL, Haughton VM, Syvertsen A: Computed tomography in the diagnosis of herniated nucleus pulposus. *Radiology* 135:95−99, 1980

75. Wolpert SM, Scott RM, Carter BL: Computed tomography in spinal dysraphism. *Surg Neurol* 8:199−206, 1977

76. Yang WC, Zappulla R, Malis L: Neurilemmoma in lumbar intervertebral foramen. *J Comput Assist Tomogr* 5:904−906, 1981

Chapter 17

Musculoskeletal System

William A. Murphy, Louis A. Gilula, Judy M. Destouet, Barbara S. Monsees, Chandrakant C. Tailor, and William G. Totty

Application of CT to the study of musculoskeletal anatomy and disease has developed slowly (82,84). Reasons for this are complex, but relate to the information gain provided by CT compared with those imaging examinations already in use. Conventional radiography, radionuclide bone scans, and ultrasonography are generally effective for confirmation and localization of musculoskeletal disease, as well as providing information regarding diagnosis, treatment planning, and prognosis.

In general, the purpose of musculoskeletal imaging is to gain the maximum information via the fewest studies, to achieve the highest possible diagnostic accuracy, and to do both at the lowest cost and radiation dose to the patient. Each musculoskeletal imaging procedure contributes information with relatively different sensitivity and specificity. Our job, as a diagnostic radiologist, is to apply each wisely for the purposes of learning if a lesion exists, localizing a position of origin, estimating its seriousness or aggressiveness, defining the local and distant relationships or extent, and, finally, refining the data into a diagnosis.

Initially, most potential musculoskeletal lesions are evaluated by conventional films, which contribute a great deal of information concerning presence of a skeletal lesion and estimation of aggressiveness and diagnosis. Conventional films have intermediate sensitivity, but high specificity. Variations of conventional radiography (magnification, xeroradiography, conventional tomography) are sometimes employed to confirm a lesion, but they are only slightly more sensitive. If a skeletal lesion is suspected but conventional studies are nonconfirmatory, or if lesion multiplicity is to be determined, radionuclide bone scanning is often the second study. It contributes greatly to confirmation of skeletal lesion presence and establishment of local extent, distant spread, or multiplicity, and does so with the highest sensitivity of any skeletal imaging examination, but at a low specificity. If a soft tissue problem is to be studied, particularly in thin, lean extremities, ultrasonography may be the first or second

musculoskeletal imaging test. Although sensitive, it is relatively nonspecific.

Computed tomography has many advantages as a musculoskeletal imaging technique (4,41,43,44,82–84,90,96,110,125). Among these are display of cross-sectional anatomy and spatial relationships, simultaneous optimal display of both bone and soft tissue, exhibition of both sides for comparison purposes, enhancement of density discrimination, and provision for image manipulation and reformation. These gains, beyond what is possible by conventional radiography, bone scanning, and ultrasonography, are accomplished at levels of sensitivity and specificity that are generally equal to or greater than each of the other imaging procedures. Computed tomography can usually confirm the presence of either skeletal or soft tissue disease, and, once confirmed, can show local extent and relationships to various structures.

In our practice, CT is used as a problem-solving examination. It is usually the second imaging procedure following conventional films or a bone scan, but may be the initial study of extremity soft tissue masses and regions of complex skeletal anatomy. In individual cases, CT has often replaced other secondary imaging procedures (e.g., conventional tomography and arteriography) formerly used to determine disease extent and anatomic relationships.

Since the information gained by musculoskeletal CT is generally additive and a refinement of that provided by radiographs and bone scans, rather than being unique, the estimation of efficacy for musculoskeletal CT is difficult. There have been several attempts to do this accurately and meaningfully (41,125,126). One study showed that the CT information (mostly of primary bone tumors) improved diagnostic understanding in 45% of cases and led to an improved treatment plan in 52% (126). A more recent study of 140 musculoskeletal cases indicated that CT was helpful in the categories of diagnosis (44%), extent of disease (71%), and treatment planning (69%) (41). Our own experience is in general agreement with these findings.

TECHNIQUE

Since the musculoskeletal system is so variable from one region of human anatomy to another, and since CT of musculoskeletal disease is most successful if applied as a problem-solving procedure, the technique for each patient or problem should be tailored to the individual. The approach that follows is meant only as a guideline. Each technical variable should be individually considered and optimized.

Scout views prior to CT should include a radiograph of the region to be studied or a computed radiograph (scanogram) if the CT unit has that capability. Fortunately, most CT units can obtain computed radiographs in frontal and lateral projections (Fig. 1). These are useful for confirmation of osseous pathology, localization for the initial scan, determination of angles for gantry position, and definition of planes for image reconstruction.

Less optimally, a conventional radiograph may be used as the scout film; an anatomic landmark or some type of device will be necessary to localize the appropriate anatomic level. This may be a multiple catheter system or an air-groove system (116). Whatever system is chosen, it must be positioned so as to keep parallax and resultant positioning inaccuracy to a minimum. It must be positioned identically for both the scout film and the CT scan. Otherwise, scans will be obtained at incorrect anatomic levels.

Precise patient or limb positioning is important to ensure symmetric display of both sides. Many observations are facilitated if the opposite side is normal and positioned identically to the abnormal side; this is par-

ticularly true in the extremities. Usually, the plane of CT section should be perpendicular to the region of interest. In our experience, this may be facilitated by use of bolsters, pillows, or sponges to elevate one portion of anatomy relative to another, or by gantry angulation. Variations of positioning have been described for the shoulder and upper extremities (44), pelvis (94), sacroiliac joints (18), cruciate ligaments (98), ankle (79), femoral anteversion or torsion (49,58), and tibial torsion (62). It may be necessary to surround extremities with packing material to avoid computer overrange artifacts.

Beam collimation may be varied according to the type and size of the lesion studied, as well as the need to reformat the data. For example, 1.0-cm slices are suitable for most soft tissue and bone tumors; 0.5-cm slices may be necessary for small skeletal lesions, fractures, and confirmation of bone scan abnormalities; 0.2-cm slices may be necessary for certain fractures (e.g., cervical spine or wrist), when detail is needed and when reformation is anticipated.

Section sequencing should be tailored for the problem undergoing evaluation. Soft tissue and bone tumors may be evaluated with slices at every other centimeter. Smaller lesions, joints, and fractures may require contiguous slices. A decision should be made each time whether to survey an area or to study it thoroughly.

Once the images are obtained and available for review, they should be displayed at several window settings. The usual soft tissue window settings should be followed by skeletal window settings (high window level and wide window width). Since there are no spe-

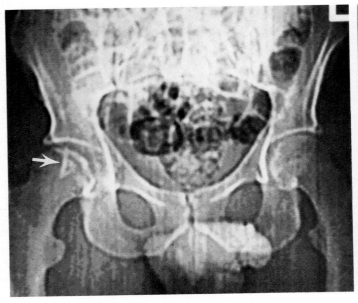

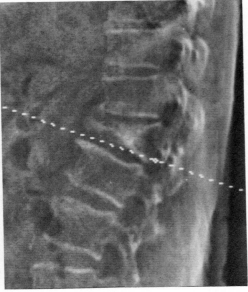

FIG. 1. Scanogram images. **Left:** Frontal scanogram shows a rotated fracture fragment separated from the right posterior acetabulum (arrow). **Right:** Lateral scanogram shows the angle selected to ensure scans perpendicular to a collapsed vertebral body in a region where the spine is not parallel to the examination table.

cific numbers for these window settings, it is important for the reviewer to select settings optimal for the individual case. Measure mode analysis with a narrow window width may be useful for rapid assessment of a lesion's average attenuation coefficient. Those units that have appropriate software programs can provide average attenuation values for regions of interest. If long bone medullary metastasis or infection is suspected, the attenuation coefficients of diaphyseal medullary canals should be measured and compared with the opposite side (56,57,67).

Administration of contrast agents should be considered according to the problem under evaluation. If it is necessary to evaluate the degree of vascularity of a tumor, appropriate CT sections may be obtained during the rapid intravenous infusion of a contrast agent (30). If a peripheral vascular aneurysm is to be studied for location, configuration, and thrombus thickness, CT sections may be obtained following the intravenous injection of a contrast bolus or during a rapid intravenous infusion (127) (Fig. 2). Similar techniques are valuable in showing the relationship of major arteries or veins to musculoskeletal masses (41,44) (Fig. 3). Veins in the extremities may be studied during the continuous slow infusion of a contrast agent into a peripheral vein (117). Joints may also be studied following intraarticular instillation of air or iodinated contrast agents.

Candidates for musculoskeletal CT need not be excluded on the basis of plaster casts or orthopedic slings and traction devices. Plaster does not degrade a CT image (82). In fact, CT displays casted musculoskeletal anatomy better than does conventional radiography (Fig. 4). If handled with care and approached with ingenuity, almost any patient in orthopedic traction can be imaged by CT.

SKELETAL NEOPLASIA

Application of CT to the study of skeletal tumors is still evolving. Since there are relatively few primary bone tumors seen at most institutions, it is too soon to

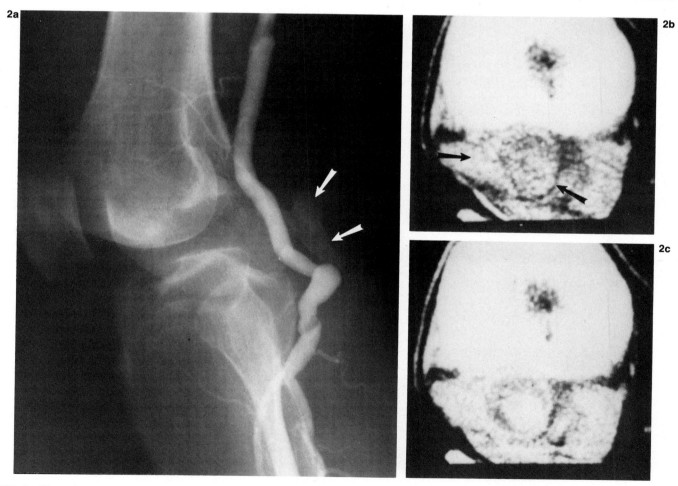

FIG. 2. CT angiogram. **a:** Lateral film from a femoral angiogram in a patient with a painful, pulsatile popliteal mass shows a tortuous popliteal artery next to a dystrophic calcification (arrows). **b:** CT through the tibial plateau confirms a mass posterior to the tibia (arrows). **c:** CT angiogram several seconds following intravenous injection of 50 cc Conray® 400 establishes the diagnosis of a partially thrombosed popliteal artery aneurysm. Note that the lumen opacifies, thus outlining the inner margin of the thrombus.

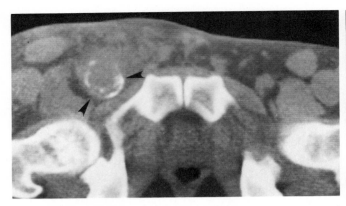 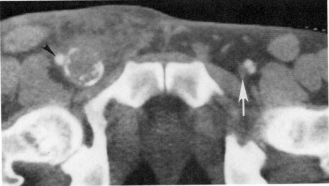

FIG. 3. CT angiogram. **Left:** Precontrast scan shows a mass with shell-like peripheral calcification located in the region of the neurovascular bundle at the base of the femoral triangle (arrowheads). The mass displaces, but does not invade, adjacent muscles. **Right:** CT after intravenous contrast material administration shows the femoral artery (arrowhead) lateral to the mass. At surgery, the mass proved to be a wholly intravenous tumor. Compare the abnormal right femoral vein with the normal unopacified vein on the left side (arrow) just adjacent to the juxtaposed opacified superficial and deep femoral arteries.

formulate final conclusions concerning the role of CT in their detection, characterization, treatment, and follow-up. However, there seems to be a concensus that CT does and will have an influence on these factors in both adults and children (3,5,24,41,45,55,57, 73,74,105,112,122).

It has been well demonstrated that the major advantage of CT in the evaluation of skeletal neoplasia is its ability to provide a unique cross-sectional display of both the neoplasm and surrounding anatomy. This results in images that show the radial spread of tumor in a manner not possible by combining radiography, conventional tomography, and radionuclide scanning. In our experience, CT is the best imaging examination to show the location of a tumor in the bone, to evaluate cortical integrity, to quantify the intramedullary component, and to define extraosseous extent (Fig. 5). It has also helped in the assessment of articular surface

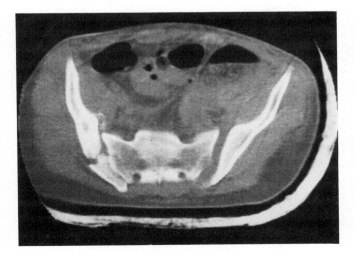

FIG. 4. Body plaster cast, seen here only partially in the image posteriorly and to the left, causes no degradation of CT image quality.

involvement (Fig. 6). Computed tomography is particularly useful to show tumor relationship to vital structures such as vessels, to quantify the number of muscle layers involved, and to provide spatial relationships in areas of complex anatomy. Even through plaster casts, tumor characteristics can be determined by CT (Fig. 7).

Computed tomography may be less effective in showing the soft tissues of lean, small diameter distal extremities. Furthermore, several authors have warned that CT may lead to under- or overestimation of the radial distribution of tumor, both within and outside of bone (64,92). Focal osteopenia about a tumor may not indicate tumor spread (92) and both edema and postbiopsy hemorrhage may mimic tumor spread into soft tissue (64). However, our experience with CT regarding its ability to show the radial distribution of tumor is overwhelmingly favorable. Both surgical and gross pathologic (Figs. 5–7) correlations support reliance on CT for estimation of radial tumor spread.

Conventional radiography is the first study of a skeletal tumor, and it usually provides sufficient information to estimate both the aggressiveness of a lesion and its probable histopathologic diagnosis. If the information clearly indicates that amputation is the treatment of choice, and the level of amputation has been decided, no further imaging tests of the primary tumor are usually necessary. However, current approaches to most tumors emphasize a combination treatment plan aimed at both tumor eradication and maintenance of functional anatomy. Thus, fewer amputations are being performed. When tumor resection is considered, CT is indicated to provide images that precisely show radial tumor spread and other anatomic relationships. The information gained is useful if it either confirms feasibility of resection or shows that amputation is necessary. In many cases, CT will be the second imaging test of a primary skeletal tumor.

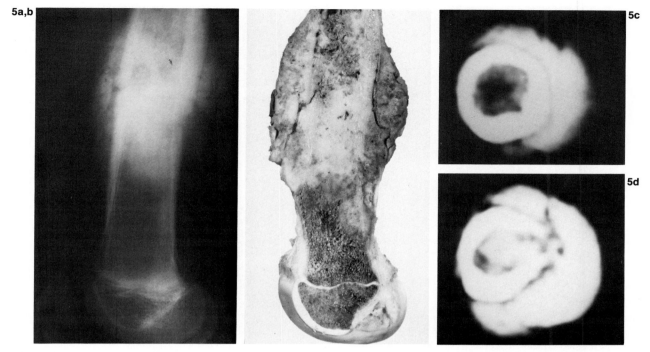

FIG. 5. Intraosseous and extraosseous tumor extent. **a:** Lateral radiograph shows central osteosarcoma of the femur with mineralized tumor encircling the diaphysis. **b:** Sagittally sectioned gross specimen shows close correlation with CT display of intra- and extraosseous tumor distribution. **c:** CT section through the proximal portion of the tumor shows mineralized tumor within the medullary canal and surrounding the medial half. Soft tissue window settings showed that the mineralized mass displaced normal muscles. **d:** CT section through a distal portion of the tumor showed the sarcoma perforating the medial cortex, nearly filling the medullary canal and surrounding most of the shaft. (Gross photograph courtesy of Dr. Michael Kyriakos, St. Louis, Missouri.) (Figures 5a and c reproduced from Destouet et al., ref. 26, with permission.)

Benign Neoplasms

Benign skeletal tumors are usually identified easily by conventional radiography. This information is generally sufficient for both probable diagnosis and treatment planning. Because conventional radiography is so successful, only a few examples of CT images of benign tumors have been reported (5,9,24,25,30,47, 74,105). Other than CT usefulness in the evaluation of some cartilage tumors (60,66), most reports confirm reliance on conventional radiography.

In our experience, CT may provide limited useful information for selected benign skeletal tumors. In general, the information gained influences management or treatment decisions rather than improving the accuracy of a preoperative diagnosis. In several cases, particularly in regions of complex skeletal anatomy, the CT display of spatial relationships provided information that was pivotal in a treatment choice. This is particularly true in the pelvis (Fig. 8). When conventional radiographs fail to provide sufficient information about a tumor's characteristics to facilitate a decision whether or not a biopsy is indicated, CT is usually decisive (Figs. 9–11).

Benign cartilaginous lesions may be the one group of benign bone tumors for which CT will have more frequent usefulness (47,60,66). They occur fairly frequently in most age groups and may present a diagnostic problem (66). Computed tomography can show their pattern of mineralization in cross-section, an important advantage compared with radiography (Fig. 12). Computed tomography of most osteochondromata shows a bony mass with a sharply defined periphery, a lucent organized central matrix, a medullary cavity continuous with the bone from which it arises, and a thin cartilaginous cap (Figs. 13 and 14). The spatial and vascular relationships of pedunculated exostoses are easily shown (Fig. 13). When it is difficult to characterize, localize, and differentiate confidently more sessile osteocartilaginous lesions from chondrosarcoma, CT is usually very helpful (Fig. 14). However, occasionally even the ability of CT to display cross-sectional anatomy and to define the amount of unmineralized cartilage present may not be sufficient to provide a confident preoperative diagnosis (Fig. 15).

As yet, not much is known about CT of the less common benign cartilaginous tumors. Computed tomography may be useful for characterization and preoperative decision making, particularly of atypical or recurrent chondroblastomas (60). Computed tomography may also show the cross-sectional features of juxtacortical (periosteal) chondromas (Fig. 16).

Giant cell tumors of bone may present a spectrum of radiological appearance and clinical aggressiveness.

![6a]
![6b]
![6c]
![6d]

FIG. 6. Tumor invasion of articular surface. **a:** Frontal radiograph shows chondrosarcoma (T) of the proximal tibia adjacent to a zone of sclerosis from a previous bone graft (G). **b:** CT of the tibial plateau shows mineralized tumor at the articular surface and perforating the cortex in several areas medially and anteriorly. **c:** Specimen radiograph of the tibial plateau is virtual- ly identical to the preoperative CT section. **d:** Gross specimen shows tumor extending into the joint anterior to the tibial spines (black arrowheads), through the medial articular cartilage, and around the periphery of the medial plateau (white arrowheads). (Gross photograph courtesy of Dr. Michael Kyriakos, St. Louis, Missouri.)

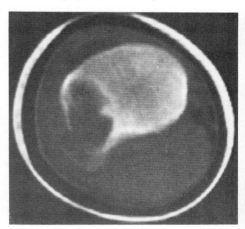

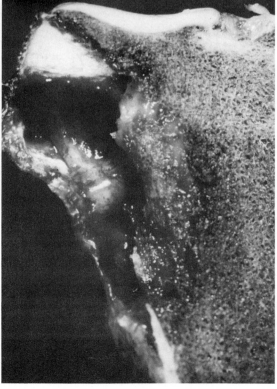

FIG. 7. Tumor character and extent unobscured by plaster cast. **Left:** CT section through proximal tibial metaphysis shows a lytic, moderately well-marginated lesion of the lateral tibial plateau. The tumor has perforated the posterolateral cotex and extended into the soft tissues. **Right:** Correlation with the gross specimen of this telangiectatic os-teosarcoma shows the blood filled cavity and re-gion of cortical destruction. (Gross photography courtesy of Dr. Michael Kyriakos, St. Louis, Mis-souri.)

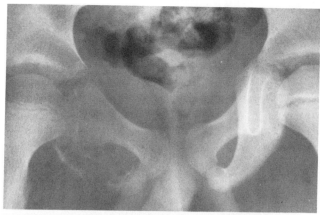

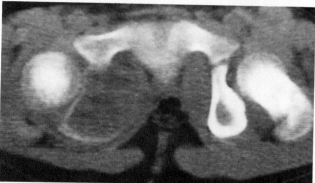

FIG. 8. Aneurysmal bone cyst. **Above:** Frontal radiograph shows an expansile lesion of the right ischium with destruction of the ischial teardrop and ischial portion of the acetabulum. A soft tissue mass pushes into the pelvis. **Below:** CT section through the ischial component of the acetabulum shows tumor expansion, which impinges on the hip joint and displaces rather than invades pelvic soft tissue. CT demonstration that the aneurysmal bone cyst involved such a large percentage of the acetabulum convinced the orthopedic surgeon that transcatheter embolization was preferable to surgery (see also Fig. 28).

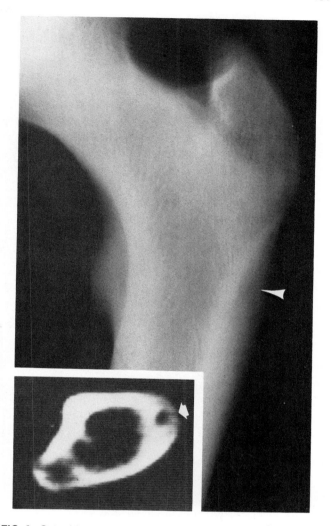

FIG. 9. Osteoid osteoma. Tomography of femur in a 13-year-old boy with hip pain suggested a lucent nidus (arrowhead) in the lateral cortex opposite the lesser trochanter. Inset: CT section through the lesser trochanter convincingly showed the nidus (arrow) and its location.

The most effective therapy is initial complete surgical excision. One report indicated that CT was helpful in preoperative definition of intraosseous and extraskeletal tumor extent (25). Computed tomography was superior to angiography in assessment of preoperative disease extent, and superior to conventional films in demonstrating the volume of residual tumor postoperatively.

Malignant Neoplasms

Malignant skeletal sarcomas, including chondrosarcoma, osteosarcoma, and fibrosarcoma, have been studied by CT and reported from various institutions (41,45,73). There is general agreement that CT provides more information about tumor location, intramedullary extent, extraosseous extent, and local relationships than do conventional radiographs or other specialized imaging studies. Likewise, there is agreement that such information has a positive effect on therapeutic decision making.

Computed tomography is generally reliable when it is difficult to distinguish an osteochondroma from a chondrosarcoma by the tumor characteristics shown on conventional radiographs (66). Computed tomography of most chondrosarcomata shows a mass that is predominantly unmineralized, and when mineralized, is heterogeneous (Fig. 17). Like others, we have found the information provided by CT to be helpful in planning surgical removal of the chondrosarcoma.

Computed tomography of osteosarcoma has shown a spectrum of characteristics parallel to the various descriptive clinical and pathologic subtypes. Lytic, sclerotic, and mixed lytic-sclerotic central (medullary) osteosarcomata are most common. Computed tomography of parosteal, periosteal, and cortical osteosarcomata has also been reported (23,26).

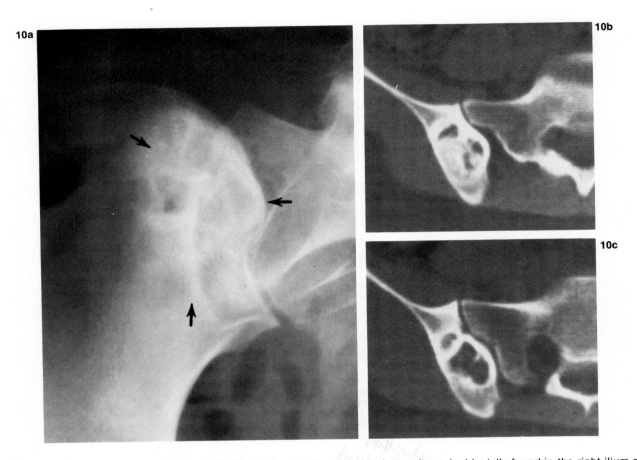

FIG. 10. Unconfirmed fibrous dysplasia. **a:** A mixed lytic and sclerotic lesion (arrows) was incidentally found in the right ilium of an 18-year-old girl with no musculoskeletal symptoms. The radiographs were insufficient for confident assignment of a diagnosis. **b** and **c:** CT sections through the lesion confirmed its mixed lytic and sclerotic nature, but also showed that the lesion was both confined to the ilium and circumscribed by a thick sclerotic rim. The summated features were sufficient for a presumptive diagnosis of fibrous dysplasia, and no surgery was performed.

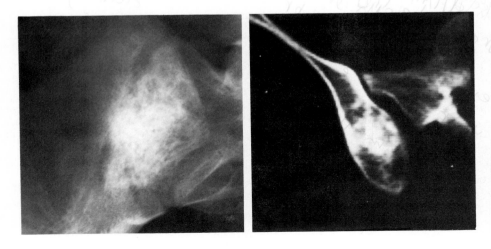

FIG. 11. Confirmed nonspecific benign fibro-osseous lesion. **Left:** A primarily sclerotic lesion was found in the right ilium of a 15-year-old girl with "low back pain." The radiographs were insufficient for confident assignment of diagnosis, but suggested a tumor of osteogenic orgin. **Right:** CT section through the lesion confirmed its primarily sclerotic nature and showed that it was confined to the ilium. Open biopsy proved that it was benign. (Case courtesy of Dr. Ken Elson, Omaha, Nebraska.)

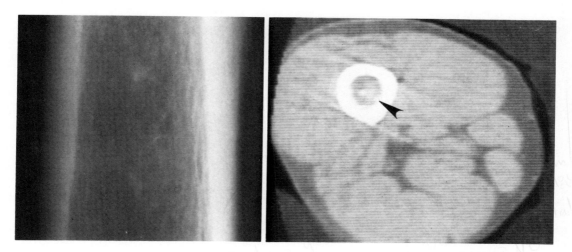

FIG. 12. Enchondroma. **Left:** Following a positive bone scan, radiographs confirmed faint calcifications of the femur in the region of the focal radionuclide accumulation. **Right:** CT of this region showed medullary location of the calcifications (arrowhead) and a biopsy was performed.

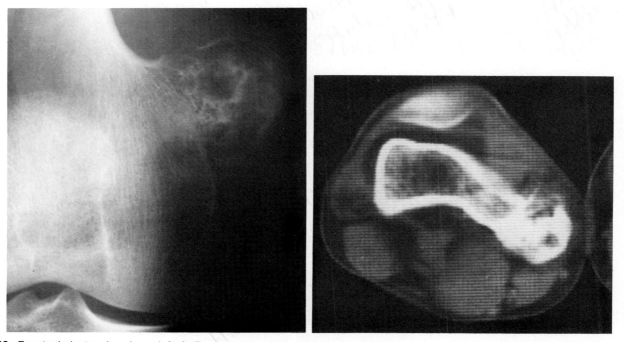

FIG. 13. Exostosis (osteochondroma). **Left:** Frontal radiograph shows a characteristic pedunculated exostosis arising from the medial femoral condyle. The periphery of the lesion is indistinct. **Right:** CT section through the stalk shows how the spongiosa and cortex of the metaphysis and the stalk are continuous. CT also excluded a soft tissue mass or thick cartilage cap, and showed that the exostosis did not compromise the popliteal artery.

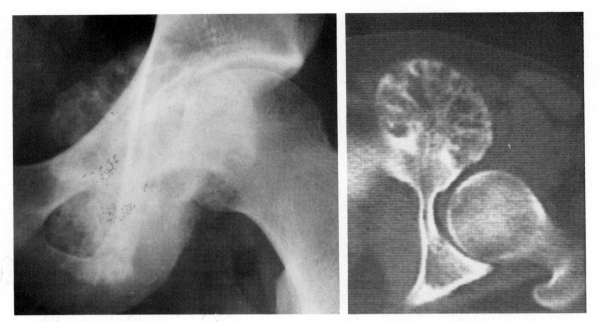

FIG. 14. Exostosis (osteochondroma). **Left:** Frontal radiograph shows a large cartilaginous tumor superimposed on the left hip. Multiple special projections failed to demonstrate adequately its relationship to the pubis or to provide sufficient information to differentiate an exostosis from a chondrosarcoma. **Right:** CT showed its origin from the superior pubic ramus, excluded any soft tissue component, correctly indicated its benign nature, and provided anatomic information that helped in surgical planning. (Reproduced from Kenney, ref. 66, with permission.)

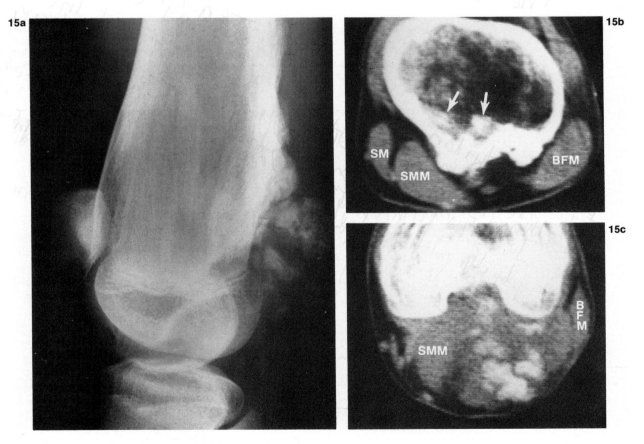

FIG. 15. Sessile exostosis (osteochondroma). **a:** Lateral radiograph shows an improperly modeled distal femoral metaphysis with a broad based posterior lesion having cortical thickening proximally and osteocartilaginous masses distally (compare with Fig. 21). **b:** CT of the proximal region shows no cartilage cap. The muscle bundles, although slightly displaced, are normal. The posterior cortex is nodular and irregular. Several densities (arrows) in the adjacent spongiosa raise the possibility of medullary tumor spread. **c:** CT of the distal region shows an osteocartilaginous mass insinuated between the biceps femoris (BFM) and semimembranosus (SMM) muscles. Because the amount of unmineralized cartilage present seemed too great, malignancy was suspected and the lesion was resected. SM, sartorius muscle.

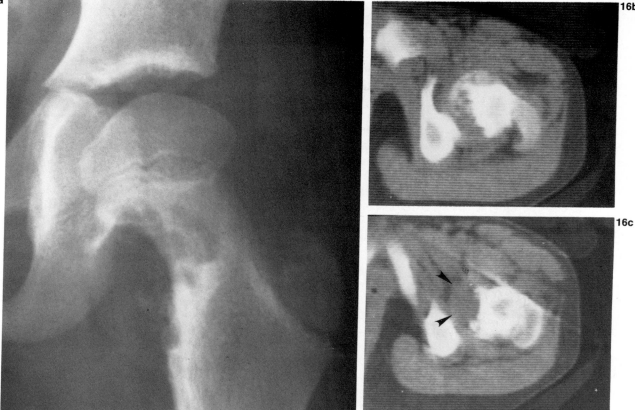

FIG. 16. Juxtacortical chondroma. a: Found incidentally in a 7-year-old girl, during an excretory urogram, this lesion was radiologically characterized as a destructive process in the femoral neck. b: CT through the proximal margin of the lesion shows a productive bone reaction with irregularity of the posteromedial aspect of the femoral neck. c: A section through the middle of the lesion shows an oval soft tissue mass (arrowheads) next to the femoral neck medially with reactive bone forming a rim around the mass anteriorly and posteriorly. CT correctly identified the lesion as bone reaction to the adjacent soft tissue mass rather than a destructive lesion of the bone itself.

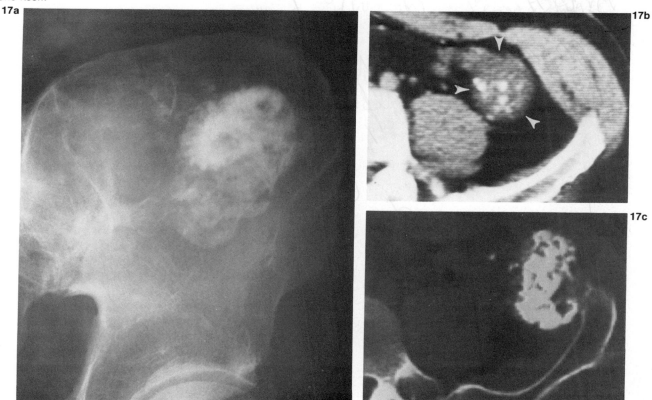

FIG. 17. Chondrosarcoma. a: In a 30-year-old man with multiple hereditary exostoses, a new calcified mass was discovered. b: CT section at a soft tissue window just proximal to the densely mineralized mass shows a large, round soft tissue mass (arrowheads) with a few small internal calcifications. This large cartilaginous component strongly suggested chondrosarcoma. c: A section at a bone window through the mineralized mass shows that it arises and projects medially from the anterior iliac crest. (Figure 17a reproduced from Kenney et al., ref. 66, with permission.)

Currently, it is acceptable to consider either local resection or amputation as the surgical component of a treatment plan for central (medullary) osteosarcoma. The cross-sectional display of radial tumor spread provides information that makes such a decision more anatomically certain than ever before. If the tumor is purely intraosseous (Fig. 18), local resection may be strongly considered (23). If the osteosarcoma has spread through the cortex, but is still confined within the first fascial plane, an en bloc or monobloc resection may still be considered (73). If the osteosarcoma has spread far enough into the soft tissues so that vessels and nerves cannot be salvaged (Fig. 19), then amputation may be the only surgical choice.

Another manifestation of osteosarcoma that may cause a diagnostic problem is the possibility of skip metastases (23,73). Fortunately, the number of medullary metastases seems to be few. There are now recommendations both for (23) and against (73) the use of CT as a routine method for studying medullary regions both proximal and distal to the primary tumor. It may be too early in our combined experience to say that CT should not be used to survey for skip metas-

tases in osteosarcoma. The potential presence of skip metastases is important enough that, as a minimum, conventional films and the radionuclide bone scan should be closely scrutinized. Data are accumulating that show how sensitive CT is at evaluating the marrow cavity in osteomyelitis and some metastases (56). Computed tomography could have a limited role in the detection of confirmation of osteosarcoma skip metastases.

Parosteal osteosarcoma is the second important subtype of osteosarcoma and is treated differently because it has a much less aggressive clinical course. For years, the accepted treatment has been local resection with a sufficient margin of normal tissue. Many local recurrences seem to be related to insufficient resection of the tumor at both medullary and cortical margins. In addition to tumor characterization in a cross-sectional plane, CT can more precisely define the depth that parosteal osteosarcoma has spread into the medullary cavity and along the cortex (Fig. 20). Computed tomography can also show radial tumor spread into the soft tissues and the tumor's relationship to muscles, vessels, and nerves (Fig. 21). This information is use-

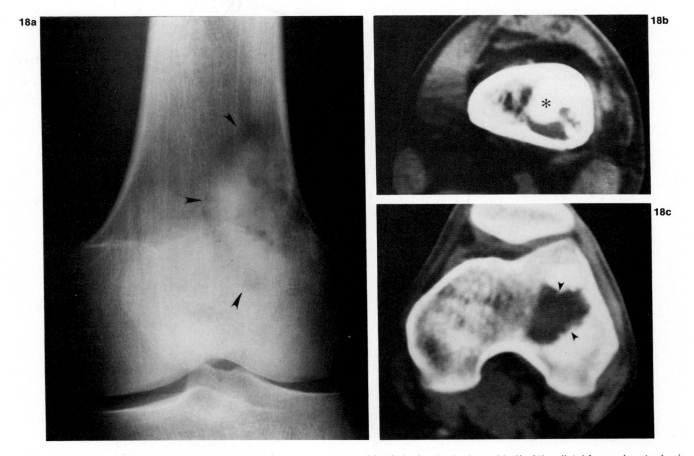

FIG. 18. Central osteosarcoma. **a:** Frontal radiograph shows an osteoblastic lesion in the lateral half of the distal femoral metaphysis (arrowheads). **b:** CT section through the proximal portion of the lesion shows its blastic component (∗). **c:** A section through the distal portion shows a more lytic zone in the lateral condyle (arrowheads). Contiguous CT sections showed that the osteosarcoma was confined to the medullary cavity, that no cortical disruption had occurred, and that the surrounding soft tissues were normal.

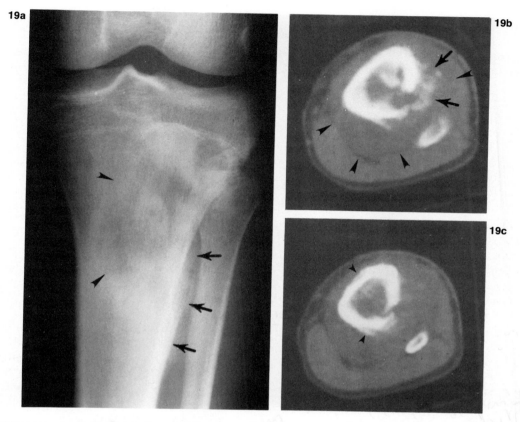

FIG. 19. Central osteosarcoma. **a:** Frontal radiograph shows a predominantly lytic lesion (arrowheads) in the lateral aspect of the proximal tibia. Periosteal reaction is present (arrows). **b:** CT section through the metaphysis shows posterolateral cortical disruption, mineralizing tumor outside of bone (arrows), and a soft tissue mass (tumor) surrounding the tibia (arrowheads). The fibular cortex adjacent to the soft tissue mass is destroyed. **c:** A section distally shows the periosteal reaction (arrowheads). (Figures 19a and b reproduced from Destouet et al., ref. 26, with permission.)

ful when it is necessary to decide between local resection and amputation. Furthermore, the CT definition of tumor extent should help surgical planning such that adequate tumor-free margins are more frequently obtained. In the interpretation of CT images, under- and overestimation of tumor extent may occur (92). However, CT seems better at estimating the extent of parosteal osteosarcoma than our previous imaging techniques, and our estimates should improve as we gain more experience with these uncommon tumors.

Periosteal and intracortical osteosarcomata are rare, and our experience with CT studies of them are limited to a few examples (26). Although CT can provide cross-sectional images of these tumors, there is insufficient experience to finalize a CT role in their work-up and management.

Beyond the initial evaluation of osteosarcomata, CT has an important role in assessing the tumor's response to therapy and detecting local or distant recurrence. If the tumor is not removed, comparison of follow-up CT images with the base-line study will show the success or failure of the treatment plan as gauged by tumor size. If the tumor is resected, a postoperative base-line CT is optimal for later comparison.

Experience with CT of the small round cell tumors of bone is limited. Computed tomography has been reported to be useful, especially in Ewing's sarcoma, in detecting these tumors in sites of complex skeletal anatomy, in evaluating the radial extent of the tumor, in planning radiation ports, in planning surgery, and in evaluating therapeutic response (48).

In the evaluation of adult leukemia (Fig. 22) and lymphoma (Fig. 23), CT images display patterns of bony abnormality that parallel those seen on conventional radiographs. These patterns include skeletal permeation, destruction, and sclerosis. Soft tissue may be normal, displaced, or invaded by large or small masses. The cross-sectional display of these changes may be helpful in particular problem cases. A common problem is whether or not to do a biopsy, followed by a decision of where or what to biopsy. In this regard, CT has been helpful in both the initial work-up and in the evaluation of patients with possible recurrence. Computed tomography is generally useful in the follow-up of patients with skeletal lymphoma to evaluate response to therapy and detect early recurrence. We believe that CT is more sensitive than conventional radiography in this setting.

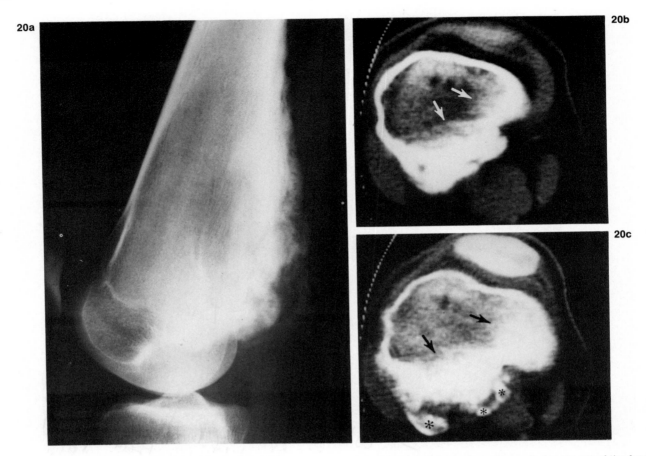

FIG. 20. Parosteal osteosarcoma. **a:** Lateral radiograph shows a long, dense, knobby tumor along the posterior aspect of the femur. **b** and **c:** CT sections show the tumor arising from the posterior cortex, and extending into the medullary trabecular bone (arrows). Other than small juxtaosseous mineralized nodules (*), the tumor was confined to bone. On the basis of this information, a local resection was performed. (Reproduced from Destouet, ref. 26, with permission.)

Experience with CT evaluation of myeloma, and particularly plasmacytoma, is similar to that with Ewing's sarcoma and lymphoma. Computed tomography has individual uses in detecting and confirming lesions, for showing the radial spread, in choosing biopsy and surgical procedures, and in evaluation of tumor response and recurrence. Many of the patterns shown by radiography are also shown by CT, but in cross-section and with the advantage of visualizing the soft tissue component (Fig. 24).

Metastases to the skeleton from any tumor of soft tissue or bone are usually detected or confirmed by radiography or radionuclide bone scan. Sometimes, skeletal metastases are displayed on CT images obtained in the evaluation of another clinical problem, and some of these "incidental" metastases are unexpected. The CT images of any patient undergoing a scan for known or possible malignancy should have all sections viewed at a bone window, as well as the optimized window for the primary problem. Such "thoroughness" does not require a great deal of time, and, for a few patients, may have importance in the management of their primary tumor.

Computed tomography patterns of metastasis are similar to those seen by conventional radiography (Fig. 25). However, in addition to confirmation of a lytic or sclerotic lesion, the radial extent of the metastasis is more easily defined. This may be important in the planning of radiation therapy ports. Computed tomography may be the only imaging test to detect and localize a metastasis convincingly. Computed tomography can be particularly useful in the detection of metastases that are suspected because of bone scan abnormalities, but not confirmed by standard films or special radiographic projections. When it has been necessary to obtain tissue for histopathologic confirmation, CT has helped us plan an approach for fluoroscopic percutaneous biopsy, or has been the imaging technique used to guide the biopsy procedure (53).

For all malignancies involving the skeleton, CT is very helpful in the evaluation of therapeutic response and detection of tumor recurrence (5,23,41,48,73) (Fig. 26). It is even more helpful to solve problems that arise during the follow-up of these patients when they are not resolved by our other imaging procedures (Figs. 27 and 28). For CT to be most useful during follow-up of

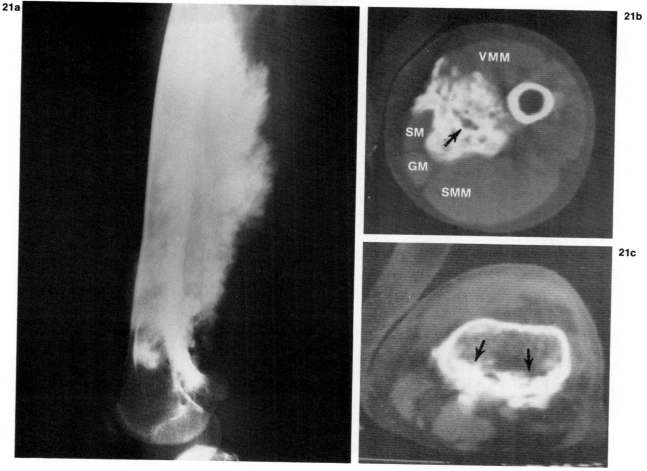

FIG. 21. Parosteal osteosarcoma. **a:** Lateral radiograph shows a huge mineralized mass in the thigh. **b:** CT of the proximal portion of the mass shows the tumor insinuated among the vastus medialis (VMM), sartorius (SM), gracilis (GM), and semimembranosus (SMM) muscles and extending from the bone surface to the subcutaneous fat. Furthermore, the mineralized mass encases the femoral artery, vein, and nerve (arrow). **c:** Distally, CT shows the tumor arising from the posterior femoral cortex and invading the medullary trabecular bone (arrows). On the basis of this information, a hip disarticulation was performed.

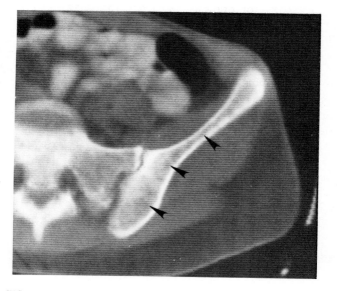

FIG. 22. Leukemia. CT of pelvis in 26-year-old woman with chronic myelogeneous leukemia in blastic crisis shows numerous small foci of trabecular destruction (arrowheads).

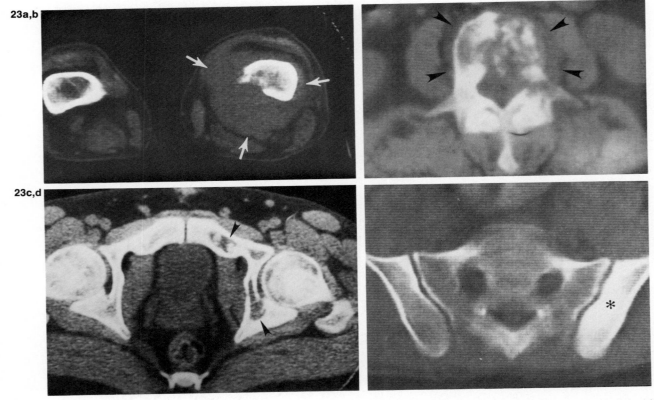

FIG. 23. Lymphoma. **a:** Lymphocytic lymphoma of distal left femur fills the medullary cavity, destroys the posteromedial cortex, and surrounds the entire metaphysis (arrows). **b:** Histiocytic lymphoma has partially destroyed T₁₁ vertebral body, but only a small paravertebral soft tissue mass is present (arrowheads). **c:** Histiocytic lymphoma has completely replaced the marrow of the left superior pubic ramus and ischium (arrowheads). The marrow space is imaged as lucent except for several round calcifications. At no site was there cortical disruption or a soft tissue mass. **d:** Histiocytic lymphoma has stimulated a diffuse sclerosis (*) of the left ilium. No bone destruction or soft tissue mass was identified.

malignancies, it is best to have a base-line pretreatment or postsurgical CT study.

Pseudotumors of the skeleton are occasionally encountered. This is particularly true in hemophilic patients who develop intraosseous hemorrhages that may expand bone (50,68). Just as with a true neoplasm, CT can display the radial extent of these lesions and define their spatial relationships with other important structures (Fig. 29). Such information can be of importance in their management, particularly if surgery becomes necessary. Neurofibromatosis is sometimes associated with dysplastic bone that must be differentiated from bone changes due to benign and malignant neural tumors. Because of its soft tissue density resolution and cross-sectional display, CT can resolve the difference between osseous dysplasia mimicking tumor and the true presence of a tumor (Fig. 30).

Clinical Application

Conventional radiography is the imaging procedure of choice in the initial work-up of bone tumors. For benign tumors, that is usually sufficient for both diag-

nosis and treatment. Computed tomography can be used to help solve problems related to detection, characterization, or treatment management. For malignant neoplasms, again conventional radiography is utilized for detection and diagnosis. We very seldom use conventional tomography or arteriography in the evaluation of such patients. When further information is needed for detection or diagnosis, we use CT to solve the problem. If further characterization is necessary for the treatment plan, we use CT to estimate radial spread and anatomic spatial relationships. Radionuclide scans are used to survey for axial spread, multiplicity of the primary tumor, and for distant skeletal metastases. Computed tomography may be used to help solve any diagnostic problems that may arise.

In most instances, CT is not useful in the detection, diagnosis, or characterization of tumors if it has already been decided to amputate and at what level to amputate. However, CT is useful in the initial work-up to characterize tumors in regions of complex anatomy and to show radial spread if resection is considered. Posttherapy, CT is useful to detect early recurrence if

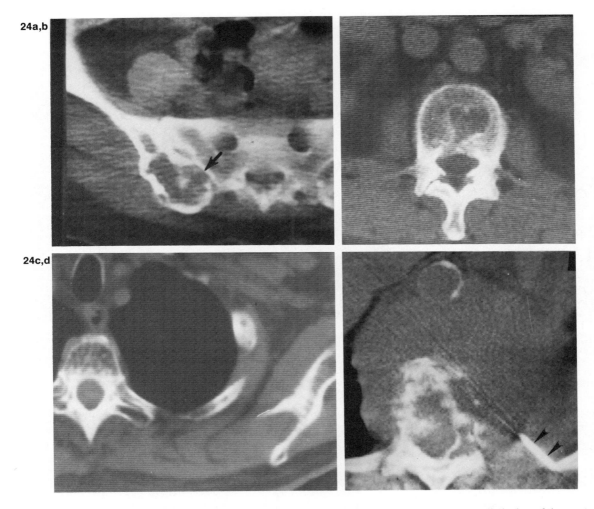

FIG. 24. Multiple myeloma. **a:** Plasmacytoma in a 45-year-old woman is characterized by an expansile lesion of the posterior iliac spine that has irregular margins, and focal cortical destruction adjacent to the sacroiliac joint (arrow). **b:** Plasmacytoma in a 71-year-old man incidentally found in L_2 vertebral body is a sharply marginated, heart-shaped zone of trabecular lysis. **c:** Myelomatosis in a 65-year-old woman is manifested as many small holes in the vertebral body, ribs, and scapula. **d:** Myeloma with a large paravertebral soft tissue mass, as well as vertebral body dissolution in an 81-year-old woman. Note the needle (arrowheads) in position for percutaneous biopsy of the paraspinal mass.

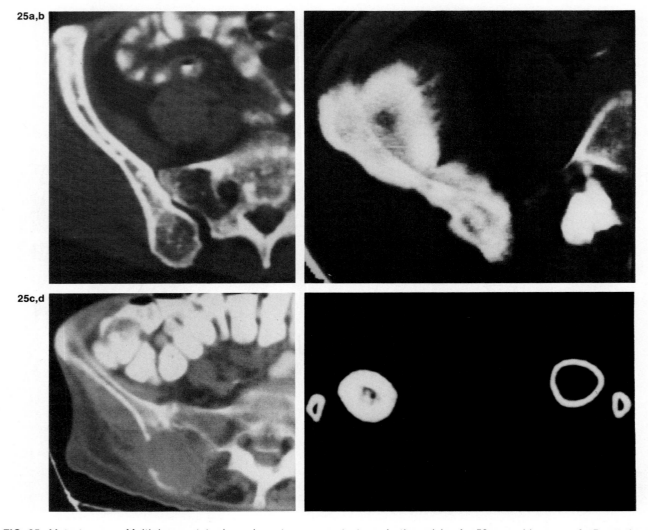

FIG. 25. Metastases. **a:** Multiple punctate dense breast cancer metastases in the pelvis of a 52-year-old woman. **b:** Prostatic cancer metastasis completely permeates the ilium and pushes into the pelvis of this 70-year-old man. Note the "sunburst" orientation of the mineralized metastatic tumor as shown at this bone window. **c:** Metastatic carcinoma from an unknown primary tumor has replaced the entire posterior iliac spine of this 69-year-old woman. **d:** Breast cancer metastasis nearly fills the right tibial diaphysis of this 61-year-old woman.

26a,b

26c,d

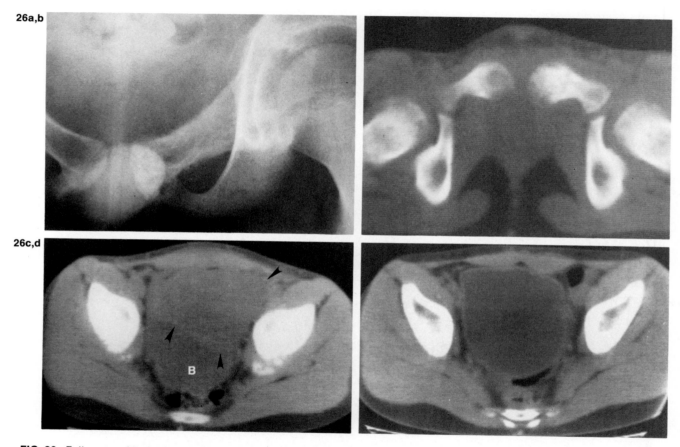

FIG. 26. Follow-up of Ewing's sarcoma, treated with chemotherapy. **a:** Frontal radiograph at initial presentation shows a moth-eaten, slightly sclerotic left superior pubic ramus. **b:** CT of the superior pubic ramus shows slight expansion and sclerosis of the bone. **c:** CT through the pelvis, just proximal to the hips, shows a large tumor mass (arrowheads) anterior to the bladder (B). **d:** Following chemotherapy, the mass has disappeared. The entire pelvis is now occupied by the fluid filled bladder.

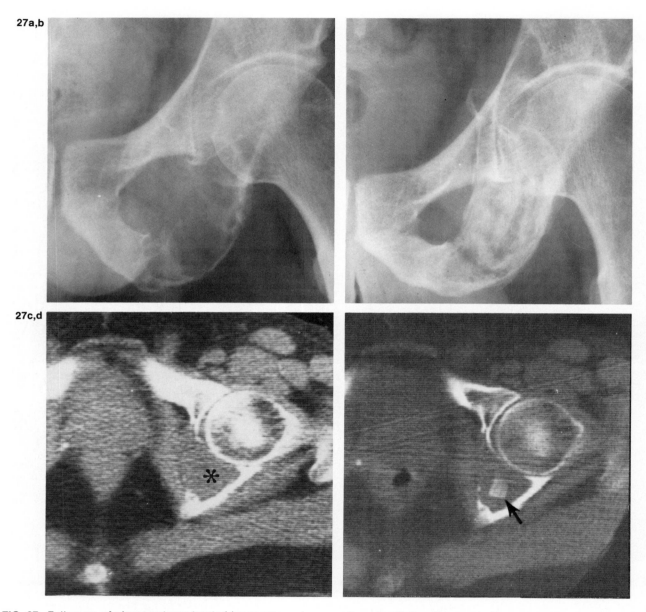

FIG. 27. Follow-up of plasmacytoma treated by curettage, bone graft, and radiation therapy. **a:** Frontal radiograph before treatment shows a lytic lesion of the ischium. **b:** A similar radiograph following therapy seems to show incorporation of the bone graft and healing. **c:** The pretherapy CT through the ischial contribution to the posterior acetabulum confirms the plasmacytoma (*). **d:** Following treatment, CT performed at the same time as the radiograph in (b) shows the bone graft fragment (arrow) surrounded by a persistent soft tissue mass. On the basis of this finding, further diagnosis and therapy were instituted.

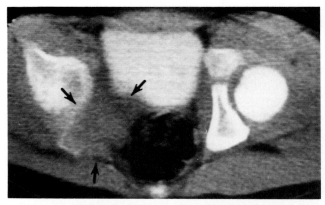

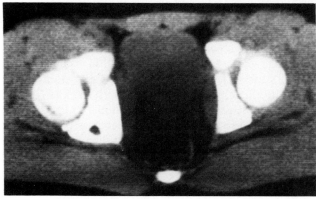

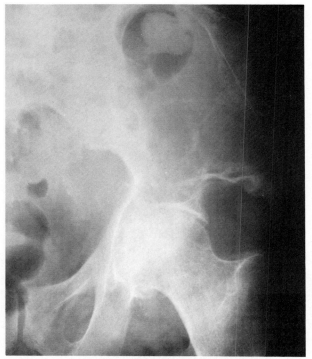

FIG. 28. Follow-up of an ischial aneurysmal bone cyst (see Fig. 8) treated by transcatheter embolization. **Above:** Pretherapy CT section shows nearly complete lysis of the right ischium (arrows). **Below:** Approximately 2 years following therapy, the ischium has almost completely reconstituted. CT showed these changes better than did conventional radiographs.

a pretherapy base-line CT was obtained, and is otherwise useful to determine therapeutic response. Furthermore, CT as a problem-solving tool is useful to confirm subtle metastases and to provide biopsy guidance.

SOFT TISSUE DISEASES AND MASSES

The basis of CT diagnosis of muscle disease and evaluation of soft tissue masses is a knowledge of normal anatomy. Since human body habitus and CT machinery configuration make positioning and study of the lean upper extremities technically difficult, and since a majority of soft tissue diseases and masses involve the lower extremities, analysis of normal anatomy will be limited to the lower extremities. Similar principles apply to study of the upper extremities.

Prior to a discussion of normal anatomy, a few technical details should be emphasized. The examiner should take full advantage of human symmetry by careful patient positioning. The part to be imaged should be centered within the gantry so that right and left anatomic levels are as identical as possible. Le-

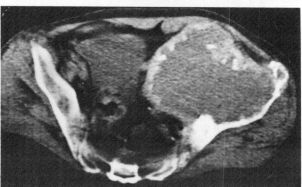

FIG. 29. Pseudotumor of hemophilia. **Above:** Frontal radiograph shows a lytic, expansile lesion of the left ilium. Its true extent cannot be determined. **Below:** CT section through midportion of the lesion shows its size, location, and homogeneous matrix.

sions should be surveyed from one end to the other, and normal tissue included at each extreme. A mass's relationship to both bone and neurovascular structures must be determined and intravenous contrast agents used as necessary to assure documentation of vascular relationships. Measurement of tumor area and muscle or lesion average attenuation value may be necessary.

Normal Anatomy

Figure 31 is a lower extremity diagram that localizes sequential regions of soft tissue anatomy that correspond to Fig. 32. The limbs are divided into flexor and

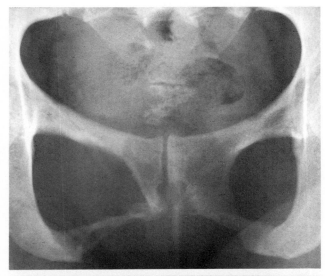

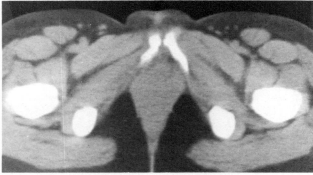

FIG. 30. Pseudotumor of neurofibromatosis. **Above:** Frontal radiograph shows an enlarged right obturator foramen, as well as what appear to be pressure erosions of the pubic bones. **Below:** CT section through the obturator foramina shows normal muscles and no tumor. Bone "erosions" were then attributed to the osseous dysplasia that sometimes accompanies neurofibromatosis.

extensor compartments. The chief hip flexors are the iliacus and psoas major muscles that, having crossed anterior to the hip joint, insert on the lesser trochanter via a common tendon (Fig. 32a–c). The rectus femoris muscle also crosses the hip joint, but is a knee extensor and part of the quadriceps mechanism. The adductor group, the pectineus and sartorius, also contribute to hip flexion (Fig. 32b–e). The most powerful hip extensor is the gluteus maximus, but in normal gait, hip extension is achieved by the hamstring muscles. The hamstrings, which attach to the ischial tuberosity, include the semimembranosus, semitendinosus, long head of the biceps femoris, and a portion of adductor magnus muscles and make up the muscle mass of the posterior thigh (Fig. 32e–i). With the exception of the adductor magnus, they insert distal to the knee and are also knee flexors. Hip abductors are the gluteus medius and gluteus minimus muscles. The adductor longus, brevis, and magnus muscles are the hip adductors (Fig. 32d–f). The lateral rotators of the

hip include the piriformis, obturator internus, quadratus femoris, and obturator externus muscles (Fig. 32b–d).

The midportion of the thigh may be divided into three compartments—the extensor, adductor, and flexor (Fig. 32f). The extensor muscles (vastus group) almost surround the anterolateral aspect of the femur. The bulky adductors comprise a medial compartment and insert into the femur distally. The knee flexor muscles (hamstrings) make up a posterior compartment. The adductor canal, a division between the flexor and adductor groups, spirals down the medial aspect of the thigh and is bordered medially by the sartorius muscle. Within the adductor canal descend the femoral vessels and saphenous nerve (Fig. 32f). The sciatic nerve is sandwiched between the hamstring and adductor magnus muscles.

The knee is a synovial joint that primarily functions as a hinge joint. The quadriceps tendon attaches to the patella superiorly (Fig. 32g). The patella then articulates with the femur, and, at this point, the knee joint is reinforced on each side of the patella by medial and lateral aponeurotic expansions known as patellar retinaculae (Fig. 32h and i). The patellar tendon arises from the inferior pole of the patella (Fig. 32i) and inserts at the tibial tubercle (Fig. 32j). In normal knees, the joint space including the suprapatellar bursa is not visualized because the potential intraarticular space is collapsed (Fig. 32g–i).

The thigh muscle, in addition to moving the hip, also moves the knee. The quadriceps muscles are its extensors and the hamstrings its flexors. Leg muscles that attach to the femur assist in knee flexion. They include the gastrocnemius, popliteus, and plantaris muscles (Fig. 32h–i). The popliteal artery and vein are located centrally, just posterior to the distal femur.

The calf muscles that move the ankle and tarsus are divided into three compartments—anterior, posterior, and lateral (Fig. 32i–l). The anterior or extensor compartment contains the three dorsiflexors, the tibialis anterior, the extensor hallucis longus, and the extensor digitorum longus. In the posterior or plantar flexor compartment are the gastrocnemius, soleus, flexor hallucis longus, flexor digitorium longus, and tibialis posterior muscles. The peroneus longus and brevis muscles form the lateral or peroneal compartment and act to evert the foot. The principal inverter of the foot is the tibialis posterior, which is assisted by the tibialis anterior muscle.

The paraspinal muscles including the retroperitoneal psoas compartment and the dorsal sacrospinalis muscles have always been difficult to image and evaluate by conventional radiography (29,52). Because of the difficulty in their evaluation, and the ability for disease to extend their length before discovery, diagnosis has often been delayed and morbidity or mortality increased (29,102). Whereas in the past radiological signs were indirect, CT can now readily image abnormal iliopsoas and sacrospinalis muscles.

MUSCLE DISEASES

The study of primary muscle diseases relies heavily on a knowledge of normal anatomy in its purest sense. Because of CT density and spatial resolution capability, there is renewed interest in the anatomic study of muscle and its diseases (14,51,75,91,114,118). Computed tomography provides the first real opportunity to image muscle, and it does so at a level of sophistication that has not yet been totally evaluated. Computed tomography can do more than document muscular hypertrophy or atrophy (Fig. 33). In particular, it has a potential future in the evaluation of a broad range of neuromuscular diseases.

Until the advent of CT, there was no way to image the muscular dystrophies. Now it is possible to make diagnoses prior to complete clinical presentation and to analyze the dystrophies both qualitatively and quantitatively (14,91,114). Muscular dystrophies are invariably accompanied by some degree of muscle destruction with replacement of muscle fibers by fat cells and connective tissue. The fascial planes remain intact, and the replacement of muscle tissue may maintain muscle volume such that the decreased muscle mass cannot be clinically detected.

Computed tomography of normal muscle has shown variations that seem to depend on age, sex, and cerebral dominance factors (14). In the muscular dystrophies, the fatty replacement of muscle is manifested on CT images as lower density muscle groups. This decreased density may be seen as either patchy or homogeneous replacement of muscle (91). By surveying the muscular system of the body, it is possible to show selective involvement and sparing of individual muscle groups (14,91,114). Thus, the localization, distribution, and extent of muscular involvement can be described. Perhaps of greater importance is the potential ability to quantitate muscle disease by measurements of muscle density and cross-sectional area (14,51,114).

Soft Tissue Masses

Soft tissue masses of many etiologies may be studied best by CT (24,32,41,55,61,73,74,81,113,119). Its density and spatial resolution capabilities give CT many advantages and few disadvantages. Because of the density differences between fat and soft tissue, CT can display vessels that are usually surrounded by fat. This high inherent contrast difference also allows separation of one muscle from another and provides a cross-sectional image of limb compartments. Based on these imaging abilities, CT is sensitive and informative for

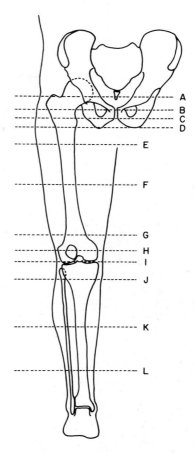

FIG. 31. Lower extremity diagram; each level indicated by a letter corresponds to a CT section displayed in Fig. 32.

exclusion or confirmation of soft tissue masses (24,73–75,81) for localization of neurovascular bundles and determination of their relationship to a mass (24,55,113) and for definition of the radial distribution of a mass within the soft tissue (32,41,55,61,113,119) or adjacent to bone (32).

The major disadvantage of CT is in lean parts of the anatomy where there is insufficient fat to permit separation of normal and pathologic anatomy (7,24,36, 45,81). It has a relative disadvantage when the mass is quite small (32), when the mass is isodense compared with muscle (7,81), or when there is no asymmetry between sides (7). There is a risk that the size of a soft tissue mass might be overestimated because of adjacent edema or hemorrhage.

Although it is not often necessary to study benign cystic masses related to joints, CT can easily confirm their origin and suggest their liquid or cystic nature. Knee joint effusions may be encountered incidentally or as a manifestation of a particular disease process under evaluation (Fig. 34). While most popliteal cysts arise from the posterior aspect of the knee, CT may be useful in the localization and characterization of unusual cysts (56) (Fig. 35).

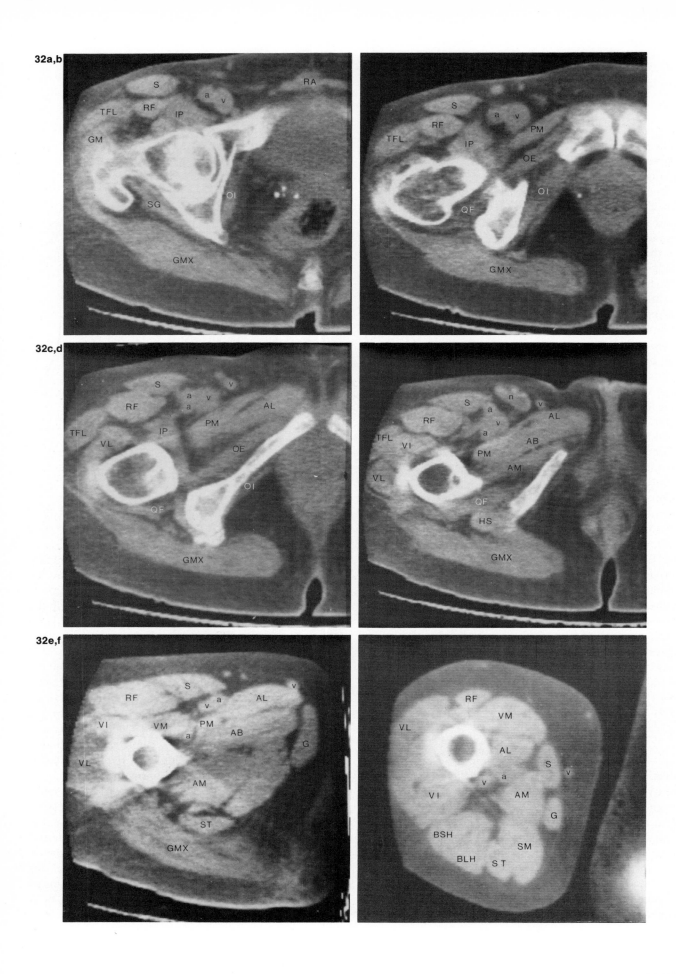

FIG. 32. Normal soft tissue anatomy of the lower extremity; each section is 1 cm thick and identified according to the characteristic skeletal feature(s).

a: Mid portion of hip.

b: Femoral neck and symphysis pubis.

c: Intertrochanteric femur and inferior pubic ramus.

d: Lesser trochanter of femur and ischial tuberosity.

e: Proximal femoral shaft.

f: Mid femoral shaft.

g: Distal femoral metadiaphyseal junction.

h: Distal femoral metaphysis and patella.

i: Femoral condyles and patellar tendon.

j: Proximal tibial metaphysis and tibiofibular joint.

k: Junction of tibial proximal and mid-thirds.

l: Junction of tibial mid and distal thirds.

The importance of discrete knowledge of soft tissue anatomy is in the precision that it gives to confirmation, localization, and characterization of abnormal processes. All images are of the right side. a, artery; v, vein; n, lymph node; AB, adductor brevis muscle; AL, adductor longus muscle; AM, adductor magnus muscle; BF(T), biceps femoris muscles (tendon); BLH, long head of biceps femoris muscle; BSH, short head of biceps femoris muscle; EDL, extensor digitorum longus muscle; EHL, extensor hallucis longus muscle; FDL, flexor digitorum longus muscle; FHL, flexor hallucis longus muscle; G(T), gracilis muscle (tendon); GM, gluteus medius muscle; GML, gastrocnemius muscle lateral head; GMM, gastrocnemius muscle medial head; GMT, gastrocnemius tendon; GMX, gluteus maximus muscle; HS, hamstring muscles; IP, iliopsoas muscle; OE, obturator externus muscle; OI, obturator internus muscle; P, plantaris muscle; PLB, peroneus longus and brevis muscles; PM, pectineus muscle; PO, popliteus muscle; PT, patellar tendon; QF,

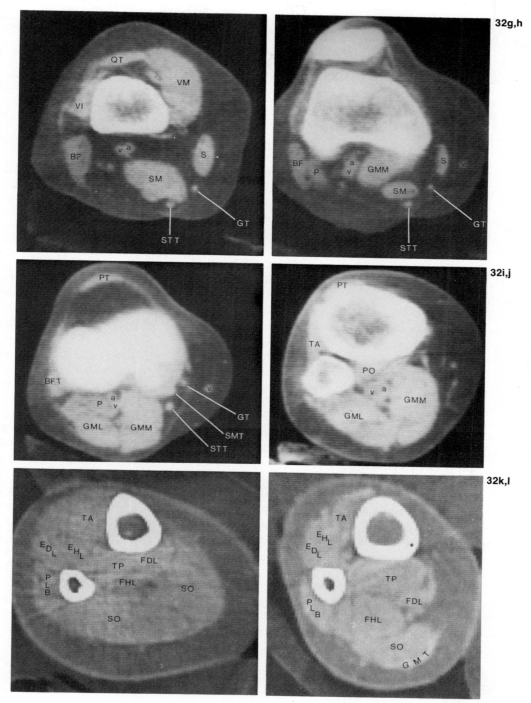

32g,h

32i,j

32k,l

quadratus femoris muscle; QT, quadriceps tendon; RA, rectus abdominis muscle; RF, rectus femoris muscle; S, sartorius muscle; SG, superior gemellus muscle; SM(T), semimembranosus muscle (tendon); SO, soleus muscle; ST(T), semitendinosus muscle (tendon); TA, tibialis anterior muscle; TFL, tensor fascia lata muscle; TP, tibialis posterior muscle; VI, vastus intermedius muscle; VL, vastus lateralis muscle; VM, vastus medialis muscle.

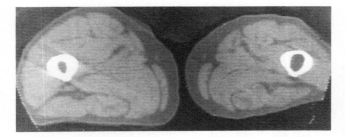

FIG. 33. Muscle atrophy. Due to sciatica, muscles of the left thigh are uniformly smaller than those of the right. Note that the left femoral cortex is thinner than the right. [Reproduced with permission from W. A. Murphy et al. (87).]

It is accepted that CT makes an important preoperative contribution in the evaluation of soft tissue tumors (32,36,55,73,81,113). Since the goal of therapy is complete excision of a tumor with limb salvage and preservation of function, it is best to have as much preoperative definition of normal and tumor anatomy as possible. Computed tomography provides that information. The decision to amputate or remove the tumor en bloc can be determined on the basis of tumor relationships and compartmental localization. Tumors that spare adjacent bone and major vessels and that are limited to one compartment usually can be resected. The aim is to remove the entire tumor, its reactive rim, and a cuff of normal tissue (36). If this can be accomplished, local recurrences are few. If CT shows the tumor to be more extensive, amputation may be necessary for tumor eradication.

In general, CT can help differentiate between benign and aggressive masses. The classic benign mass usually has a well-defined periphery or capsule and a homogeneous matrix. A typical aggressive mass has an ill-defined periphery and a heterogeneous or patchy matrix. Unfortunately, CT may not be capable of differentiation among the various processes that are infiltrating or aggressive. Those that may have similar CT characteristics are hematoma, abscess, and neoplasm.

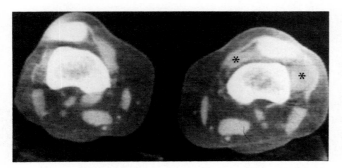

FIG. 34. Knee joint effusion. The medial and lateral recesses (∗) of the left knee are fluid filled and cause the joint capsule to bulge outward.

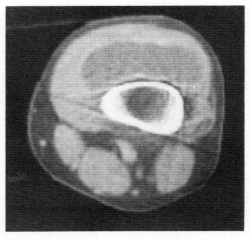

FIG. 35. Noncommunicating suprapatellar bursa. Contrast-enhanced CT through a thigh mass just above the knee shows an encapsulated near-water density collection that wraps around the anterior femur, but is separated from it by a thin layer of fat. The mass displaces the quadriceps femoris muscle.

Tumors usually have an average attenuation value slightly lower than normal muscle. For soft tissue sarcomas, the attenuation value has not been predictive of the histopathologic diagnosis (32,73).

The use of intravenous contrast agents helps define tumor vascularity (41) and the relationship of large vessels to soft tissue tumors (32,74). However, it is not necessary to inject a contrast agent in every case (24). Since it rarely helps establish a diagnosis, we use intravenous contrast material when it is necessary to know more about matrix, tumor margin, pseudocapsule, or large vessel involvement (45).

Tumors of adipose tissue origin are common in the extremities. Lipomas are very common and may be of several types (61). They have a characteristic CT appearance because they are of uniformly low (fat) density and are generally well defined or encapsulated (24,32,61,73). We usually do not evaluate these tumors by CT unless there is a clinical need to know more about their anatomic relationships prior to surgery or the correct diagnosis was not suspected clinically. When they are very large, such as in macrodystrophia lipomatosa, CT may be useful to demonstrate their extent (Fig. 36). Infiltrating angiolipomas are rare, benign, but locally aggressive tumors. By CT, they are primarily low density and may have a characteristic CT pattern (20). Computed tomography can show that they invade and replace skeletal muscle.

Liposarcoma is usually a bulky invasive tumor that may have a pseudocapsule. Margins by CT are often unsharp and the matrix mixed or heterogeneous (24,61). Depending on the amount of fat present, they will vary from soft tissue density (poorly differentiated forms) to something between water density and fat

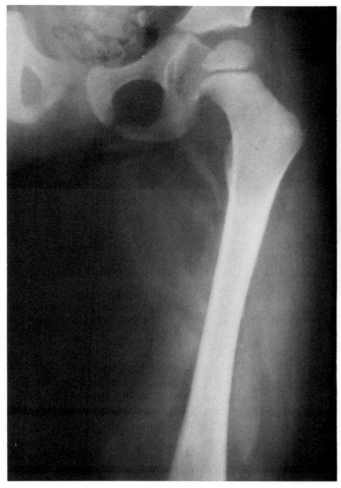

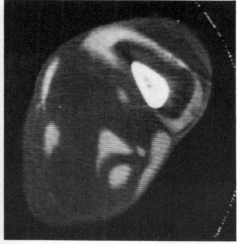

FIG. 36. Macrodystrophia lipomatosa. **Left:** The left lower extremity is larger than the right and normal muscle shadows have been replaced by bizarre fat planes. **Right:** CT section through the distal thigh shows distortion of the femoral shape, as well as overly abundant adipose tissue that has replaced much of the muscle tissue. In this patient, CT localization of remaining musculature helped to plan a surgical debulking procedure.

X-Ray Department
Royal United Hospital
Bath

density (Fig. 37). Even when large portions are near fat density, other areas may be inhomogeneous and have higher attenuation values (Fig. 38).

Fibrosarcoma is a fairly frequent malignant soft tissue tumor of the thigh. In our experience, it is difficult to distinguish it from hemorrhage, infection, or other sarcoma. Various patterns have been observed, in-

cluding tumors that infiltrate soft tissue (Fig. 39), replace muscles (Fig. 40), and invade bone (Fig. 41). The matrix may vary between homogeneous and heterogeneous.

A few neural tumors have been studied including sarcomas, gangliomas, and schwannomas (Fig. 42). Computed tomography has also been used to study

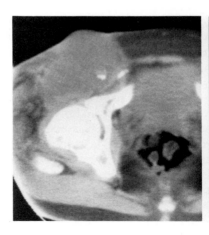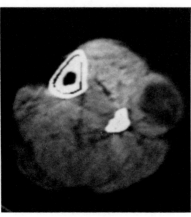

FIG. 37. Liposarcoma compared with fibroxanthosarcoma. **Left:** CT section through the hip of a 60-year-old man shows a large soft tissue mass anterior to the joint. Average attenuation coefficient of the liposarcoma is slightly less than that for muscle. **Right:** CT section through a mass in the leg of a 55-year-old woman localizes the mass to the lateral (peroneal) compartment and shows that although the fibroxanthosarcoma is primarily comprised of lipid, it does have regions of higher attenuation. The black ring within the tibial cortex is a computer overrange artifact.

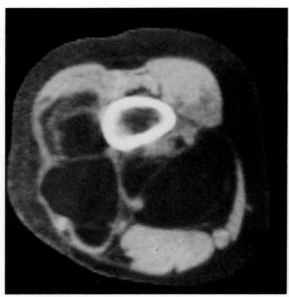 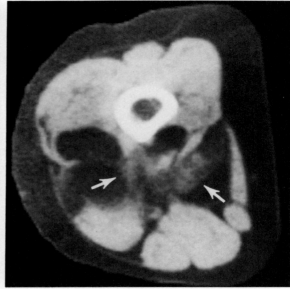

FIG. 38. Intramuscular lipoma with focus of malignant mesenchymoma. This 61-year-old woman presented with a large lipoma of the thigh 12 years following previous resection. **Left:** CT section through midthigh shows adipose tissue replacing many muscles and displacing others. **Right:** A more distal section shows an amorphous tumor infiltrating the lipoma, just posterior to the femur (arrows). This region of malignant mesenchymoma was very small in comparison with the bulky benign lipoma; histologically, it contained areas of osteosarcoma, chondrosarcoma, and liposarcoma.

extraskeletal, extranodal lymphoma (54). It can easily identify and localize subcutaneous metastases (31).

Several soft tissue tumors have presented with a mineralized mass as the primary abnormality (35). On the basis of CT findings alone, it may not be possible to differentiate a benign mineralized lesion from a malig-

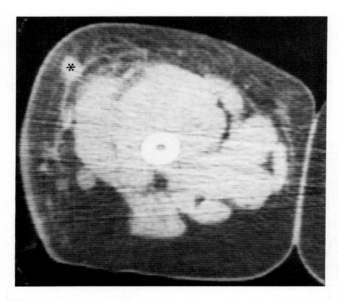

FIG. 39. Fibrosarcoma infiltrating tissue. This 16-year-old girl presented with a short-term history of thigh swelling. No mass was palpable through the indurated skin and subcutaneous fat. CT section through the proximal thigh also shows tumor nodules (·) and infiltration of subcutaneous fat. Note the thickened skin along the lateral aspect of the thigh.

nant one (Fig. 43). However, the CT study is helpful in determining precise location, radial spread of the tumor, and its local anatomic relationships. In each of these cases, CT showed the tumor and its relationships to bone and leg compartments better than did conventional radiographs.

Hemorrhage into soft tissue may have a spectrum of etiology, presentation, localization, and CT appearance. It may occur spontaneously, following trauma, with bleeding diatheses, while a patient is receiving anticoagulants, with inflammatory diseases, into a tumor, and following surgery or percutaneous translumbar arteriography (6,21). Because of the various etiologies and possible presentations, a physician may not always consider the diagnosis. If hemorrhage is considered, the confirmation and precise localization are difficult using conventional imaging tests. However, CT nearly always shows the location and extent of soft tissue hemorrhage, especially in anatomic regions that are difficult to examine physically (Fig. 44). Intramuscular hemorrhage will cause an enlargement of the muscle that is easily recognized when the left and right sides are compared for symmetry. Often, however, the hemorrhage may not be readily differentiated from an abscess or a tumor on the basis of CT findings alone. Any of these may cause swelling of a muscle with an isodense or low density mass. With appropriate clinical history, a diagnosis of hemorrhage may be suggested; in selected cases, CT can be used to guide a percutaneous needle aspiration for confirmation.

In addition to localization of soft tissue hemorrhage,

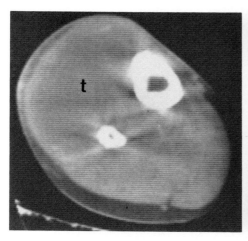 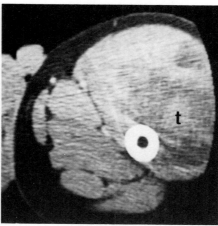

FIG. 40. Fibrosarcoma replacing tissue. **Left:** In this 29-year-old man with a slowly enlarging mass of 1-year duration, CT shows a homogeneous mass (t) of less than muscle density that has replaced the anterior and lateral compartments of the leg. Gross pathologic evaluation showed that much of the tumor was necrotic. **Right:** In this 34-year-old man with a left thigh mass, contrast-enhanced CT shows that an inhomogeneous tumor (t) of less than muscle density has replaced the vastus intermedius and lateralis muscles. Histopathologically, it was a malignant fibrohistiocytoma.

CT can characterize and display the various stages in the natural history of hemorrhage maturation (Fig. 45). Fresh hemorrhage may be of similar or slightly greater density than muscle. If dehydration occurs, it may become even more dense. Initially, the hematoma may be of homogeneous density, and then, as liquefaction begins, it may develop a patchy or heterogeneous appearance. When completely liquefied, the hematoma will have developed a pseudocapsule and homogeneous density lower than that of muscle. If the injury includes muscle necrosis, early mineralization may be detected by CT, indicating ossification of the hematoma or development of myositis ossificans. When associated with hemophilia, CT of soft tissue hemorrhage can accurately localize the pseudotumor before it becomes a clinical mass. Computed tomography follow-up may reduce the time necessary to treat with clotting factor replacement (68). Large hemorrhages resulting in pseudoaneurysms (124) may cause bizarre pressure erosions of bone.

Clinical Application

Computed tomography of soft tissue masses compares very favorably with conventional radiography, angiography, radionuclide bone scans, and ultrasonography. It is generally agreed that CT is far superior to conventional radiography for exclusion, confirmation, and characterization of soft tissue masses (24,45,74,81,113). Computed tomography is superior to angiography and should replace it for lesion localization, definition of boundaries, determination of vascularity and vascular relationships, and estimation of diagnosis (32,73,113). Angiography should be reserved for those few instances when CT does not adequately define vascular invasion. Computed tomogra-

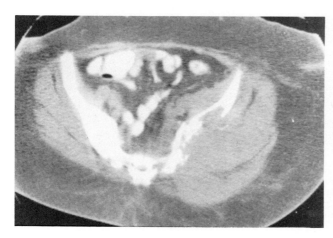

FIG. 41. Soft tissue sarcoma invading bone. This 49-year-old woman had left hip pain for at least 8 months before bone films indicated a destructive lesion in the ilium and this CT scan showed a large soft tissue tumor in the gluteal muscles with destruction of the adjacent iliac wing and sacrum.

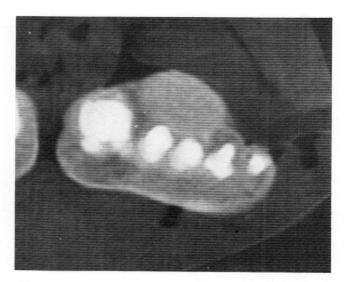

FIG. 42. Malignant schwannoma of foot. This 49-year-old woman returned with a recurrent tumor 4 years following the primary resection. CT clearly demonstrates a circumscribed mass on the dorsum of the foot. It also shows the tumor juxtaposed to the second and third metatarsals and within the intermetatarsal space. This clear demonstration of tumor extent helped the surgeon anticipate anatomic relationships that would be encountered at surgery.

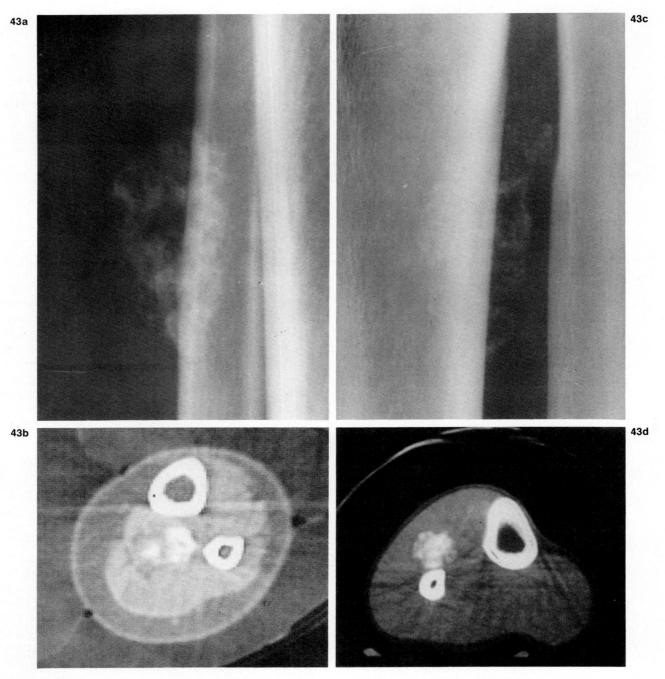

FIG. 43. Mineralized soft tissue tumors. **a:** Lateral radiograph of a 26-year-old woman with leg pain shows a focal area of amorphous calcification posterior to the tibia. **b:** CT section shows the mass located in the posterior (flexor) compartment of the leg. Although much of the mass is mineralized, the medial portion has an attenuation less than muscle. This mineralized tumor is an ossifying hemangioma. **c:** Frontal radiograph of a 31-year-old man with leg pain shows a focus of amorphous calcification similar to that seen in (a). **d:** CT shows the mineralized mass located in the anterior (extensor) compartment. No soft tissue component is apparent. This mineralized mass proved to be a mesenchymal chondrosarcoma. (Figures 43a and b reproduced from Engelstad et al., ref. 35, with permission.)

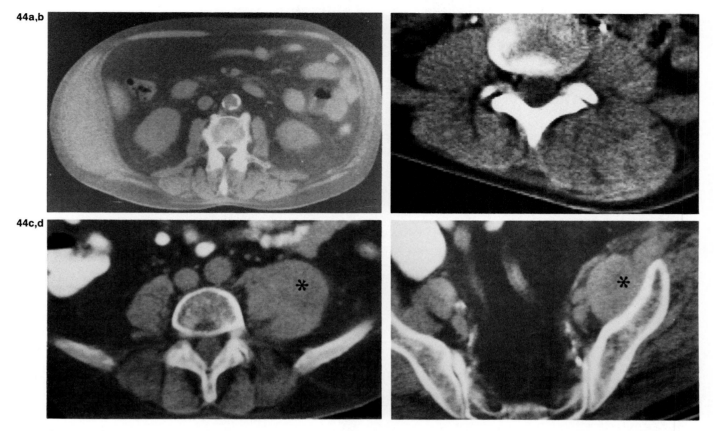

FIG. 44. Hematoma localization. CT has proven useful for localization and definition of extent of musculoskeletal hematomas of the trunk. **a:** Localized to the right internal oblique muscle. **b:** Localized to the left sacrospinalis muscle. **c** and **d:** Localized to the left psoas muscle, where the hematoma (∗) could be followed along the entire course from the paraspinal origin in the abdomen (c) to the confluence of the psoas and iliacus muscles in the pelvis (d).

phy is superior to bone scans for determination of soft tissue position near bone. However, bone scans are complementary because they are more sensitive for early detection of bone involvement due to stimulation by the reactive rim of a tumor (36).

Superiority of CT to ultrasonography as the primary imaging test of a soft tissue mass is less certain. Computed tomography seems to yield better information in most instances, but ultrasonography is usually more valuable in lean portions of the extremities. Although ultrasonography may more accurately define longitudinal extent and total volume (7), CT clearly gives more detailed anatomic information (73) and provides precise definition of radial spread (7). Although ultrasonography can distinguish fluid from a solid mass (13), CT gives more information about tissue density. Furthermore, CT provides a better topographic display of the tumor and its adjacent vascular and bony structures (7,73). Both may provide guidance for percutaneous biopsy procedures (13,32,91) and both may be used to follow patients for tumor recurrence.

REGIONAL COMPLEX MUSCULOSKELETAL ANATOMY

As good as CT is at confirming, localizing, and characterizing neoplastic bone disease and soft tissue masses, it excels at these tasks in regions of complex musculoskeletal anatomy. Formerly, the pelvis, shoulder girdles, sternum, sternoclavicular joints, and accessory vertebral joints were inadequately imaged by the various imaging techniques, either independently or in combination. The skeletal parts of these regions are curved, of variable thickness, and oriented at angles to the major axes of the whole body. Other parts of the skeleton are often adjacent, a situation that may prevent obtaining an image of the desired bone without another superimposed. Overlying densities such as gas, fat, or soft tissue may obscure bone detail. Finally, the soft tissues themselves have never been well imaged. Computed tomography obviates all these problems because of its density resolution and cross-sectional image. It has proven to be the best imaging procedure in each of these regions of complex mus-

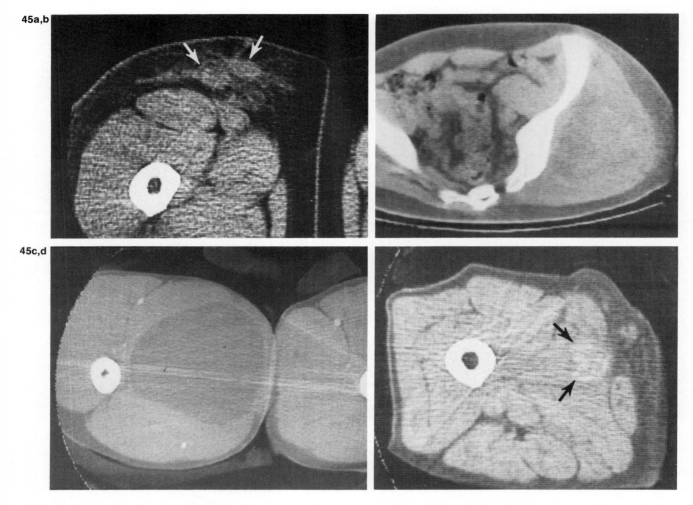

FIG. 45. Hematoma characterization. CT can demonstrate the degree of maturation when a hematoma is imaged. **a:** Early stage of subcutaneous hematoma, shortly after injury when hematoma (arrows) is infiltrating the fat and remains of similar density to muscle. **b:** Intermediate stage of intramuscular hematoma maturation, when the gluteal hemorrhage is partially organized and partially liquefied, and by CT is displayed as an inhomogeneous mass with regions that are less dense than muscle. **c:** Late stage of intramuscular hematoma when the hemorrhage has liquefied and the CT shows a homogeneous mass of density less than muscle. (Contrast media is seen in vessels.) **d:** Late stage of a small intramuscular hematoma or an early state of myositis ossificans when the residual traumatized tissue begins to mineralize (arrows).

culoskeletal anatomy. For tumors, infections, arthritis, and trauma, CT can confirm or exclude the presence of an abnormality, define the lesion's extent, and determine its relationship with adjacent structures. No combination of other medical images can on the average do as well as CT.

Pelvis

The osseous anatomy of the pelvis is a complex union of the sacrum and two hemipelvic bones, each derived from three smaller bones—the ilium, ischium, and pubis. Each of these bones curves, is of variable thickness, and is spatially oriented at a different angle with respect to each other and to the sagittal and coronal axes of the body. Because the pelvis is firmly fixed

at the sacroiliac joints, it moves as a unit. This means it is impossible to project some areas free of overlying osseous structures. Thus, the deeper and more central structures such as the posterior iliac spines, the sacroiliac joints, and most of the sacrum are particularly difficult to image (46,89,115,122). Overlying fecal material and bowel gas further compromise conventional radiologic evaluation of the sacrum (46,115). Computed tomography overcomes these anatomic difficulties and graphically displays both the anatomic location and intraosseous extent of osteolytic lesions of the pelvis (Fig. 46).

Pelvic soft tissue anatomy is as complex as pelvic skeletal anatomy (6,65,89). Muscles, lymph nodes, rectum, and genitourinary organs are present, in addition to nerves and vessels (77). It may be quite difficult to

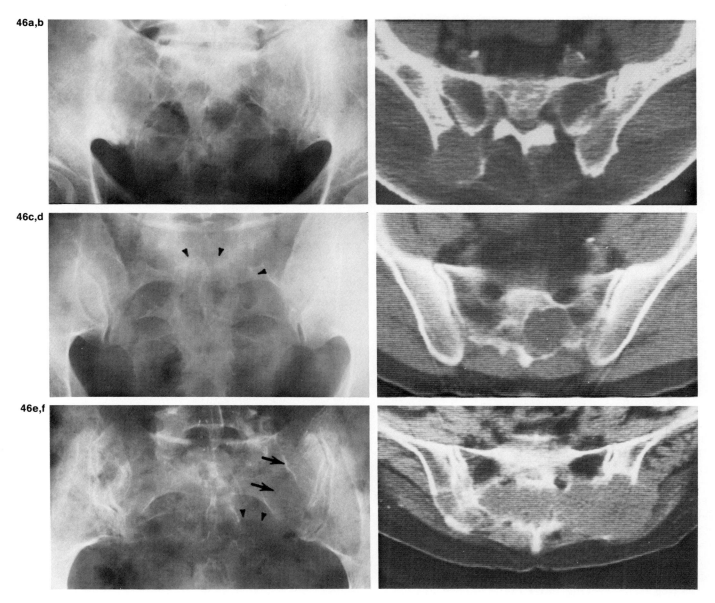

FIG. 46. Complex pelvic skeletal anatomy. CT readily confirms osseous abnormalities in the pelvis when they were previously interpreted as equivocal by conventional radiographic projections. **a** and **b:** Fifty-five-year-old man 4 months following diagnosis of bronchogenic carcinoma developed right hip pain and had a bone scan that was interpreted as having an abnormal right sacroiliac joint. The radiograph (a) confirmed sacroiliac joint osteoarthritis. However, CT (b) showed that a metastasis had destroyed the right posterior iliac spine. **c** and **d:** Fifty-five-year-old man presented with gait disturbance and low back pain. A radiograph (c) showed a subtle curvilinear shadow over the sacrum (arrowheads) that could not be confirmed by other conventional studies. The CT (d) scan clearly showed a well-defined lytic defect in the sacrum. Finally, films from 10 years previously were located, and they showed the same radiologic changes. **e** and **f:** Fifty-five-year-old woman with parotid gland carcinoma presented with incontinence. The radiographs (e) showed destruction of the left posterior iliac spine (arrows) and subtle blurring of the second neural foraminal cortex (arrowheads). CT (f) showed a much more extensive metastasis than was apparent from the radiographs. The tumor extended from the right sacroiliac joint, across the sacrum and left sacroiliac joint, through the left ilium, and into the gluteal muscles. (Figures 46e and f reproduced from Gilula et al., ref. 46, with permission.)

evaluate these structures by physical examination. Likewise, conventional radiography, urography, and barium studies may fail to show a soft tissue abnormality or may show only limited secondary changes. Computed tomography has proven advantages over these other tests in the evaluation of solid tumors (3,112). It more clearly defines the extent of lesions and contributes information necessary for more precise treatment planning. Tumors, hemorrhage, and infections of osseous or soft tissue origin are easily localized to bone, soft tissue, or both (46,88,89). Their intra- or extrapelvic extent is readily defined (Fig. 47).

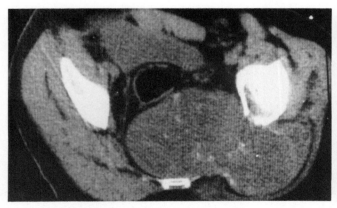
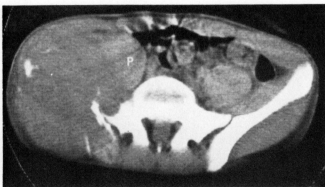

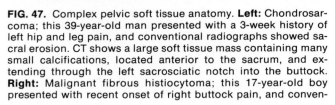

FIG. 47. Complex pelvic soft tissue anatomy. **Left:** Chondrosarcoma; this 39-year-old man presented with a 3-week history of left hip and leg pain, and conventional radiographs showed sacral erosion. CT shows a large soft tissue mass containing many small calcifications, located anterior to the sacrum, and extending through the left sacrosciatic notch into the buttock. **Right:** Malignant fibrous histiocytoma; this 17-year-old boy presented with recent onset of right buttock pain, and conven-tional radiographs showed an expansile lytic lesion of the ilium that appeared to have intact margins. CT confirmed destruction of the ilium, but also showed invasion of the sacrum. The soft tissue component was larger than anticipated, having displaced the gluteal and psoas muscles. Note that the right (P) psoas is rotated and displaced toward the midline. (Figure 43a reproduced from Gilula et al., ref. 46, with permission.)

Sacroiliac Joints

Computed tomography can demonstrate inflammatory, degenerative, neoplastic, and traumatic abnormalities of the sacroiliac joints (SIJs) (28). Criteria for diagnosis are based on a knowledge of normal anatomy, which is different in the sacroiliac joints than in other synovial joints. Each SIJ has two types of articulation—the antero-inferior third, which is synovial, and the postero-superior two-thirds, which is ligamentous. The synovial portion has thinner articular cartilage than other synovial joints, has an undulating surface, and moves minimally. The ligamentous portion is V-shaped, narrowest adjacent to the synovial portion, and widens dorsally. It also undulates and has fairly deep concavities or pits for insertion of the interosseous ligaments (Fig. 48). Criteria of normalcy for the synovial portions of the SIJs are that (a) the cartilage space is uniformly thick, (b) the cortices are uniformly thin and parallel to one another, (c) the left and right sides are symmetrical, and (d) no focal erosion, sclerosis, or fusion is present. Criteria of normalcy for the ligamentous portions are that (a) the cortices are uniformly thin, (b) no erosion, sclerosis, or ligamentous mineralization is present, and (c) the sides are symmetrical (Fig. 48).

Inflammatory sacroiliitis is diagnosed when the criteria of normalcy for the synovial portion of the SIJs are "violated." The articular width will become more wide or narrow depending on the stage of the disease. A combination of erosion and sclerosis may be shown (Fig. 49). Although it is probably unnecessary to obtain a CT scan in patients with a known diagnosis and unequivocally abnormal radiographs (10), we and others (18) believe that CT is useful when a clinical diagnosis has not been established and conventional radiographs are either normal or equivocal. In such cases, CT can probably exclude all but the most subtle anatomic abnormalities, and certainly can show focal sacroiliitis not seen on standard films. Again, CT should be used in a problem-solving sense as a second imaging test. Various manifestations of arthritis may occur and be imaged in both synovial and ligamentous portions of the SIJs as erosion, fusion, sclerosis, and hypertrophic spur formation (Fig. 50).

Hips

The hip is a ball and socket joint with a complex origin of the socket from contributions of three bones joined at the triradiate cartilage. These separate contributions to the acetabulum are seen in pediatric patients (Fig. 51). At this age, it is apparent that the acetabular roof is contributed by the ilium, the small antero-medial portion by the pubic bone, and the major posteromedial portion by the ischium. Application of CT to pediatric hip diseases is in the early stages of evaluation (95). We expect that CT may be shown to have a role in solving selected problems related to congenital hip dislocation. As experience accumulates, CT may be useful in pediatric patients with hip trauma and infection.

In adults, CT of the hip has been useful because of its display of cross-sectional anatomy (Fig. 52). Computed tomography shows that the acetabulum is not merely a socket, but rather is a focal concavity supported at the apex of an arch derived from two sub-

48a,b

48c,d

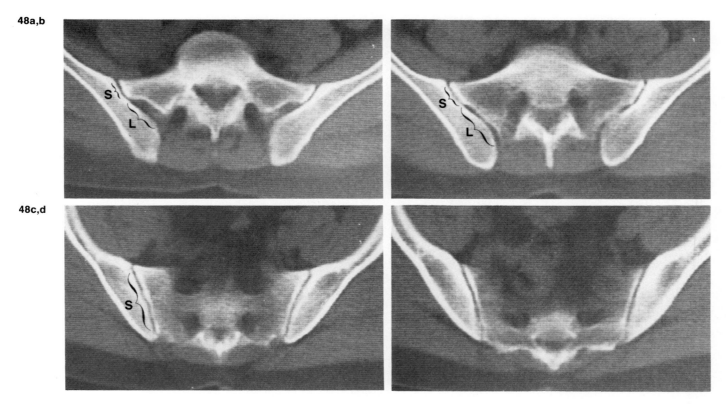

FIG. 48. Normal sacroiliac joints. Examined from cranial to caudal (a–d), CT shows both the synovial (S) and ligamentous (L) portions of the joints, as well as simultaneously demonstrating left and right joints in the same projection. Criteria of normalcy are that the joints be symmetric, with thin uniform cortices, and that the joint spaces be thin and of uniform width throughout. There should be no foci of sclerosis, erosion, or joint ankylosis. Focal unsharpness may occur as the result of partial volume averaging of a curving cortex.

stantial columns of bone. The posterior, or ilioischial, column is large and descends from the sciatic notch to the ischial tuberosity. The anterior, or iliopubic, column runs downward, inward, and forward from the iliac crest to the pubic symphysis. The periphery of the acetabulum narrows into a labrum that is complete except inferiorly, where it meets the acetabular fossa. The posterior acetabular rim is more substantial and extends further laterally than the anterior rim. The femoral head is seated centrally in the acetabulum, but

may not be shown with an equal width of cartilage space around it. When supine and relaxed, the patient, assisted by gravity, will permit the leg to rotate externally. This will cause minimal subluxation of the femoral head so that the anterior joint space is slightly wider than the posterior (Fig. 52d).

Computed tomography of the hip region shows soft tissue as well as skeletal relationships. Thus, CT examination may help elucidate the cause of hip pain due to a soft tissue abnormality. In addition to tumor

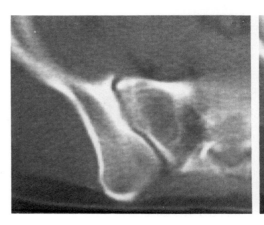
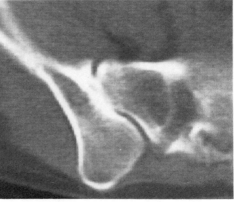

FIG. 49. Ankylosing spondylitis. **Left:** CT shows focal iliac sclerosis adjacent to focal sacral erosion. The joint space and its apposing cortical surfaces are irregular. **Right:** CT shows focal ankylosis of the sacroiliac joint.

50a,b

50c,d

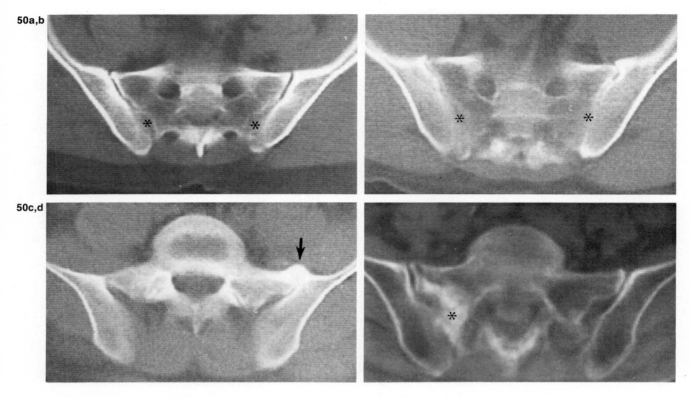

FIG. 50. Arthritis of the sacroiliac joint (SIJ). **a:** Early ankylosis of the ligamentous portions (∗) of the SIJs with sparing of the synovial portion. **b:** Moderately advanced osseous ankylosis of both SIJs (∗) with near obliteration of the posterior two-thirds. **c:** Bridging osteophyte of the left SIJ (arrow). **d:** Osteoarthritis of the ligamentous portion of the right SIJ (∗) manifested as sclerosis and hypertrophy of the dorsal-most region. The joint space is nearly ankylosed by the new bone formation.

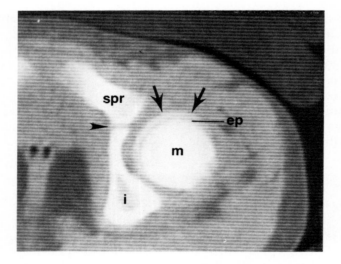

FIG. 51. Normal pediatric hip. CT section through the joint shows the superior pubic ramus (spr), the triradiate cartilage (arrowhead), the ischium (i), and the femoral head. The concentric ring-like appearance of the femoral head is due to simultaneous imaging of the metaphysis (m), the epiphyseal plate (ep), and a small rim of the femoral capital epiphysis (arrows). Note that the medial and posterior portions of the acetabulum are contributed by the ischium.

and infection, CT has helped show iliopsoas bursa abnormalities (99,100). Since the bursa crosses anterior to the hip joint, CT of iliopsoas bursitis will show a fluid-filled mass that displaces the femoral vessels just anterior to the joint. If necessary, the distended bursa can be aspirated, or a hip arthrogram performed for confirmation (100).

Computed tomography of the hip has made its greatest contribution in the evaluation of hip fracture-dislocations (8,69,70,109,111). One reason CT has been successful is that it has few of the disadvantages of conventional radiography. Computed tomography is simple and accurate, whereas radiography now seems cumbersome and less accurate. Standard radiography requires moving the patient into various positions or is limited to a frontal projection. Movement of the patient into various positions can be painful, and there is always concern that further displacement may result. When optimal radiographs are obtained, they still provide only two-dimensional information. Computed tomography is accomplished without moving the patient's leg or pelvis into various positions and provides the third dimension (Fig. 53).

Although it is not within the scope of this chapter to analyze hip fracture-dislocations completely, it is necessary to recognize the importance of classification of hip injuries (37,72). The fracture-dislocation pattern and the complications associated with each determine whether or not the particular injury will be treated closed or be subjected to surgery. Computed tomography has helped with these surgical decisions. For a hip to do well following acetabular fracture, there must be no major intraarticular fragments, the posterior acetabular labrum must be stable, and the fracture fragments must be anatomically reduced so that there is minimal incongruity between the femur and acetabulum (37,72). Because these management decisions have been difficult using conventional radiography, care of acetabular fractures has presented a real management problem. Computed tomography has helped resolve these difficult therapeutic decisions. Formerly, the decision to operate because of intraarticular fragments was based on physical examination, or radiological documentation of an ossified intraarticular fragment or joint space widening. Computed tomography readily confirms and accurately localizes intraarticular fragments first shown radiographically (Fig. 54). More important, CT can show intraarticular fragments not suspected clinically and not shown on radiographs (Fig. 55). However, CT cannot show an intraarticular cartilage fragment if it has no associated cortex (87,109). Computed tomography following reduction of posterior hip dislocations should be used to solve any problem defined clinically or by radiography. It can be expected to show the relationships of fracture fragments, to locate intraarticular osseous fragments, to help estimate stability and congruity, and to show associated soft tissue changes. It may also be useful in the follow-up of certain patients.

Computed tomography may be helpful in certain other orthopedic hip problems. It can show the anatomic orientation of posttraumatic hips prior to total hip replacement (Fig. 56). Such information helps the surgeon plan the procedure for hip replacement by showing the amount of bone stock present in order to seat the acetabular component. Following gunshot wounds, CT may show the radial spread of bullet fragments better than radiographs. The information derived from CT may help the surgeon decide whether or not to explore the hip (Fig. 57). Following total hip replacements, patients may develop painful prosthetic joints. One early study has shown the potential of CT to evaluate such joints with particular emphasis on the femoral component (59). The ability to image the femur with a metallic femoral component in place has potential for both biomechanical and clinical research. However, the artifacts created by the metallic devices degrade CT images so badly that this clinical application has not developed.

Other diseases that affect the hip joint may be imaged by CT, but as yet there is no demonstrated advantage of CT over radiography or radionuclide bone scans. While imaging patients for other reasons, we have encountered many examples of arthritis (Fig. 58) and several examples of femoral head avascular necrosis (Fig. 59).

Shoulder Girdle

A number of muscles unite the scapula and clavicle to the thorax forming a scapulothoracic articulation. This articulation along with the sternoclavicular, acromioclavicular, and glenohumeral joints moves in a synchronized fashion to provide upper extremity mobility. Thus, the shoulder girdle, the most mobile region of the body, is a coordinated balance of muscular function provided by muscles of the neck, back, anterior thorax, and arm. Those muscles directly related to the glenohumeral joint include the supraspinatus, infraspinatus, subscapularis, teres minor, and deltoid (Fig. 60).

Physical examination and standard radiography are usually sufficient to solve clinical problems related to the shoulder joint. However, the density and spatial resolving capabilities that prove advantageous in other regions of complex musculoskeletal anatomy may also be useful in solving selected problems about the shoulder girdle (80) (Fig. 60).

Sternum and Sternoclavicular Joints

The sternum consists of the manubrium, body, and xyphoid. There is a synchondrosis between the man-

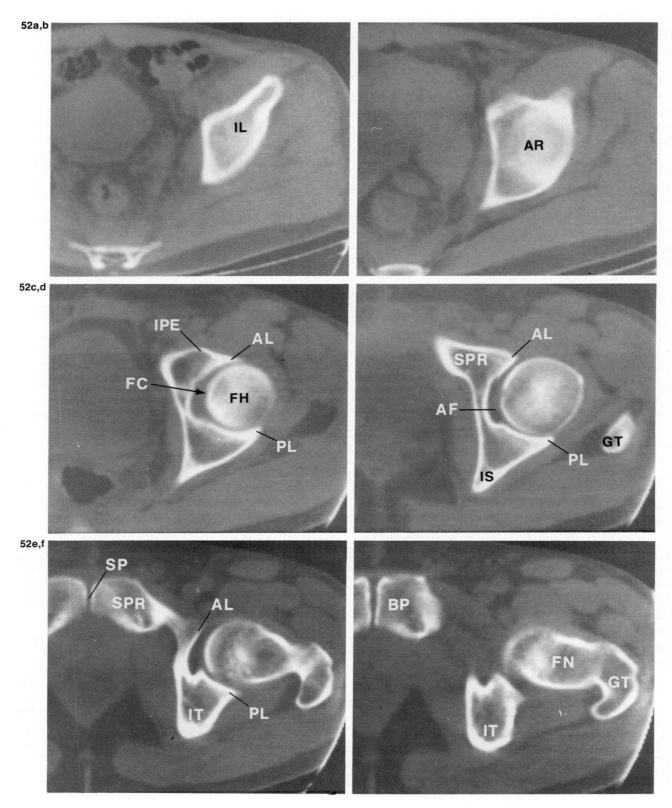

FIG. 52. See facing page for figure legend.

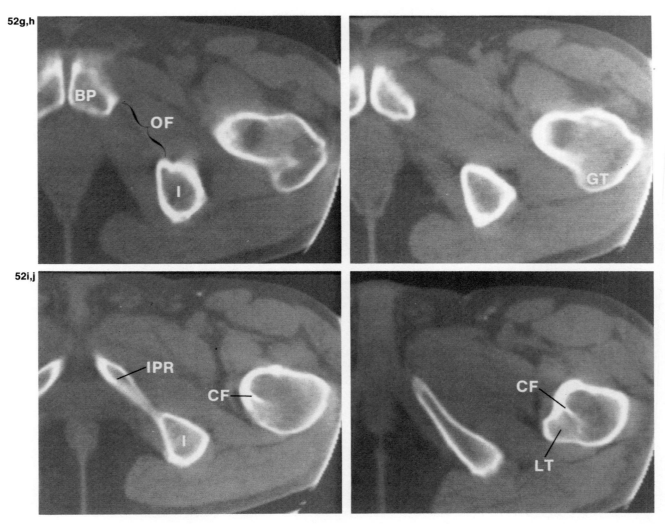

FIG. 52. Normal adult hip. **a:** Supraacetabular ilium. **b:** Ilium broadens into roof of acetabulum. **c:** Cranial aspect of femoral head, maximally surrounded by acetabulum with its anterior and posterior labra. Adjacent to the anterior acetabular rim is the iliopubic eminence, the result of fusion of the triradiate cartilage in this region. The fovea capitis, a shallow depression in the femoral head for the femoral ligament, is just visible. **d:** At mid-section through the femoral head, the lateral aspect of superior pubic ramus and ischial spine are seen. The fat-filled acetabular fossa is maximum size. **e:** Caudal section of the femoral head shows the cranial aspect of the femoral neck, the complete pubic ramus, and the ischial tuberosity. **f:** A section through the femoral neck shows cortical and medullary continuity of the femoral head for the femoral ligament, is just visible. **d:** At mid-symphysis are optimally shown. **g:** Section through the central portion of the obturator foramen between the pubis and ischium. **h:** The greater trochanter is almost incorporated into the femoral shaft. **i:** Just caudal to the greater trochanter the origin of the calcar femoris from the anteromedial cortex is shown. The inferior pubic ramus joins the ischium. **j:** The calcar femoris is still present adjacent to the lesser trochanter. The ischial tuberosity is now shown. Note that the rim of the acetabulum constantly changes contour. Cranially (c), the acetabulum is deepest and the labra longest. Caudally (e), the acetabulum is most shallow and the labra smallest. Throughout, the anterior labrum is always shorter than the posterior, and the ischium makes up the medial and posterior portions of the acetabulum. Also note that when cortices are perpendicular to the cross-sectional tomogram, they are imaged as sharp lines. However, if they pass obliquely through the section, the partial volume effect will cause cortical regions to be represented as broad and unsharp. AF, acetabular fossa; AL, anterior labrum; AR, acetabular roof; BP, body of pubis; CF, calcar femoris; FC, fovea capitis; FH, femoral head; FN, femoral neck; GT, greater trochanter; I, ischium; IL, ilium; IPE, iliopubic (iliopectineal) eminence; IPR, inferior pubic ramus; IS, ischial spine; IT, ischial tuberosity; LT, lesser trochanter; OF, obturator foramen; PL, posterior labrum; SP, symphysis pubis; SPR, superior pubic ramus.

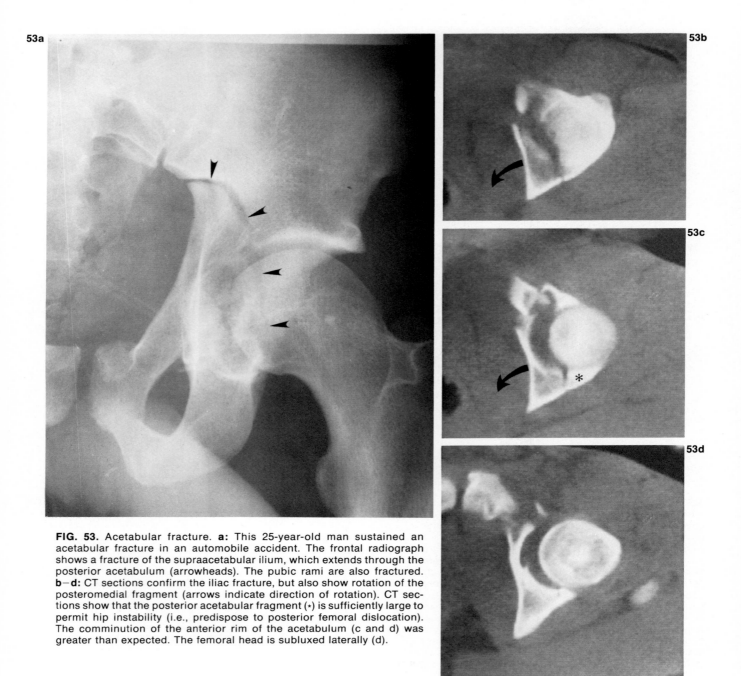

FIG. 53. Acetabular fracture. **a:** This 25-year-old man sustained an acetabular fracture in an automobile accident. The frontal radiograph shows a fracture of the supraacetabular ilium, which extends through the posterior acetabulum (arrowheads). The pubic rami are also fractured. **b–d:** CT sections confirm the iliac fracture, but also show rotation of the posteromedial fragment (arrows indicate direction of rotation). CT sections show that the posterior acetabular fragment (*) is sufficiently large to permit hip instability (i.e., predispose to posterior femoral dislocation). The comminution of the anterior rim of the acetabulum (c and d) was greater than expected. The femoral head is subluxed laterally (d).

54a,b

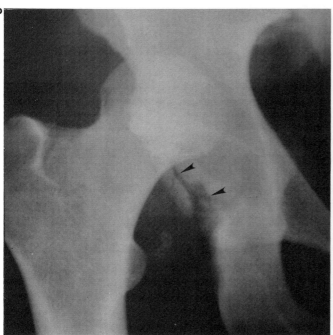

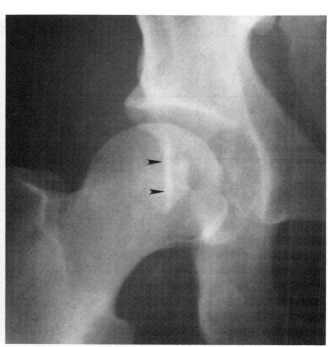

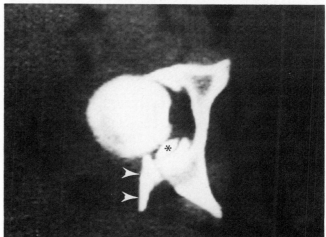

54c

FIG. 54. Intraarticular fracture fragment preventing full reduction. **a:** This 27-year-old man sustained a posterior dislocation of the femoral head in a vehicular accident. The pre-reduction frontal film shows a posterior acetabular fracture (arrowheads). **b:** Following reduction, the femoral head does not resume a centric position in the acetabulum. One of the posterior acetabular rim fragments is now rotated into a sagittal plane (arrowheads). **c:** CT section through the fovea capitis shows anterior displacement of the femoral head due to a posterior intraarticular fragment (*). A posterior rim fracture fragment (arrowheads) is rotated 90° so that its pointed end contacts the femoral head. The intraarticular fragment was surgically removed and the posterior acetabular fragment reduced.

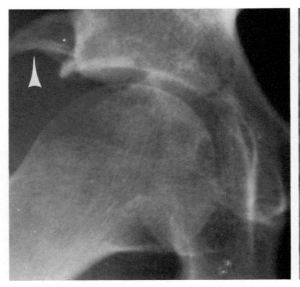 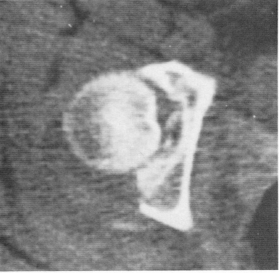

FIG. 55. Intraarticular fracture fragments. **Left:** This 30-year-old woman sustained a posterior dislocation of the femoral head in an automobile accident. Postreduction radiograph shows centric position of the femoral head and a large posterior acetabular fragment displaced cranially (arrowhead). **Right:** CT section through the fovea capitis shows two unsuspected fracture fragments in the acetabular fossa. At surgery, these were in contact with the femoral articular cartilage. Note that the absent posterior acetabulum as shown by CT could predispose the femoral head to recurrent posterior dislocation.

ubrium and body that usually does not fuse until old age. The body segments usually ossify and fuse during childhood, although there are a number of anatomic variations. The xyphoid remains cartilaginous until sometime during adulthood when it ossifies to a variable degree (Fig. 61). The sternoclavicular joints are divided into two articular compartments by a fibrocartilaginous disk (Fig. 62). Each joint is enveloped by a loose fibrous capsule and protected by sternoclavicular, interclavicular, and costoclavicular ligaments. The clavicles articulate with the manubrium laterally, posteriorly, and superiorly. Just posterior to the sternoclavicular joints are major vessels and the trachea (Fig. 61).

Conventional radiography of the sternum and sternoclavicular joints has always been difficult due to the oblique orientation of the joints, the superimposition of other structures, and the relatively low mineral content of the region (27). Computed tomography has eliminated these imaging problems and made it unnecessary to obtain conventional tomograms or specialized radiographic projections. Computed tomography shows soft tissue and bone in the same image, provides similar views of both joints simultaneously, is more comfortable for the patient than special views, and takes less time to perform than conventional tomography (27).

Trauma to the sternoclavicular joint may produce subluxation or dislocation of the clavicle (Fig. 63). Because the posterior sternoclavicular ligament is very strong, anterior malalignments are more frequent than posterior clavicular displacements. Anterior clavicular

malalignment is easier to diagnose clinically, easier to treat, and less serious. Posterior dislocation is less common, more difficult to diagnose both clinically and radiologically, and potentially more serious because of the adjacent vessels and trachea. Fortunately, CT provides all the required information (27,76).

Infection of the sternum and sternoclavicular joints may be difficult to diagnose clinically and radiologically, due primarily to difficulty obtaining detailed images of thin bone. It may be impossible to document normalcy, soft tissue disease, or osteomyelitis. The problem is compounded in the poststernotomy patient where surgical and healing phenomena must be differentiated from infection in undermineralized bone. Computed tomography can usually provide all the necessary information in a few images (Fig. 64). It can help differentiate normal from abnormal and localize the process to soft tissue, bone, joint, or a combination of these sites.

Tumors of the sternum and clavicles are uncommon, and documentation of their presence or location may prove difficult. Computed tomography provides information for localization, determination of radial spread, estimation of local anatomic relationships, and a base-line image for follow-up evaluation of therapeutic response (Fig. 65).

Ribs and Accessory Vertebral Joints

When CT sections are obtained for evaluation of the lungs, hila, or mediastinum, rib abnormalities may be incidentally encountered. Rarely, CT may contribute

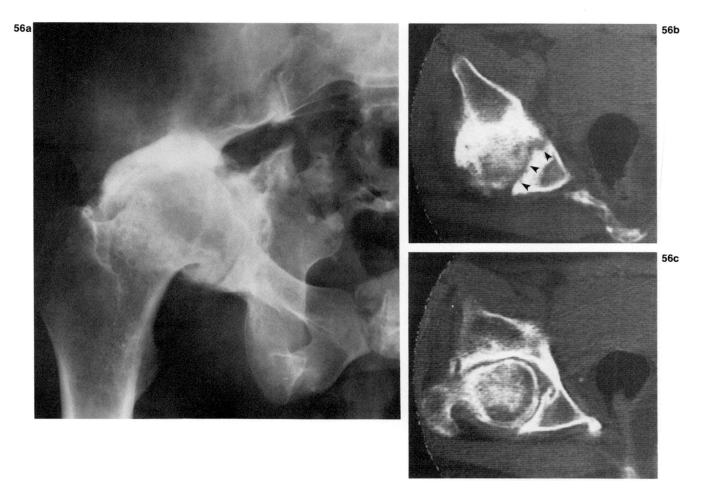

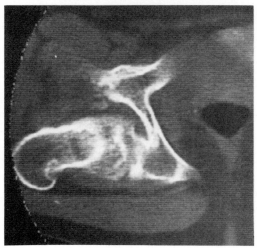

FIG. 56. CT in planning total hip replacement. **a:** A 30-year-old man 6 years following a hemipelvis fracture presented with severe hip pain and limited range of motion for evaluation as a candidate for total hip replacement. Conventional radiographs showed inward rotation of the ischium and advanced secondary osteoarthritis of the hip. **b:** CT sections through the ilium showed incomplete bony bridging of the acetabular roof fracture (arrowheads). **c:** CT section through the hip confirmed osteoarthritis with deformity of the femoral head and acetabulum. **d:** CT section more distally revealed that the inward rotation of the ischium was so severe that there was insufficient posterior bone stock to provide normal anatomic stability for the acetabular component of a total hip replacement. Therefore, the surgical plan would have to include a method to provide posterior stabilization.

57a,b

57c,d

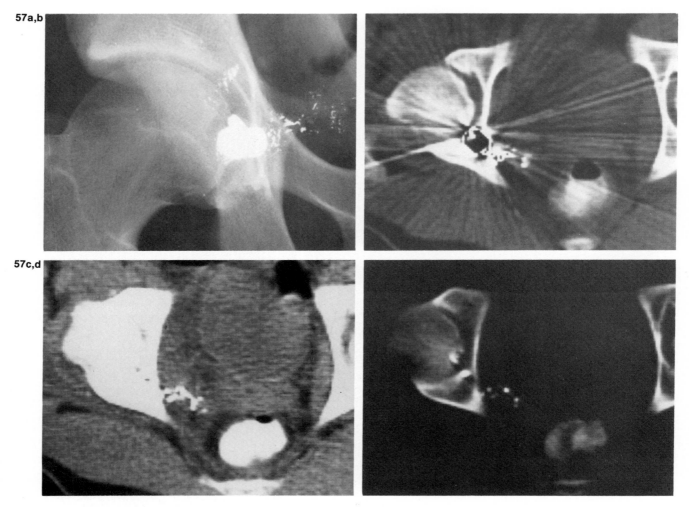

FIG. 57. Localization of intraarticular foreign bodies. **a:** This 20-year-old man had been shot through the left buttock, leaving a bullet lodged near the right hip. Conventional radiographs did not convincingly provide precise localization of the bullet or its fragments. Position of the fragments would determine whether or not surgery was necessary. **b:** CT section through the main bullet fragment showed that it had perforated the acetabulum, but had not contacted the femoral head. **c:** CT section slightly more proximal at a soft tissue window showed several small metallic fragments in the soft tissues. **d:** The same section at a bone window showed one fragment in the ischium and another in the fovea capitis, but none in the joint. Thus, no surgery was done.

FIG. 58. Arthritis of the hip. **Left:** CT of the hip in a young man with ankylosing spondylitis shows diffuse loss of the cartilage space, shallow erosions of the subarticular cortex, and early protrusio acetabulae (arrowheads). **Right:** CT of the hip in a young man with hereditary multiple exostoses unexpectedly showed osteoarthritis of the posterior portion of the joint associated with posterior subluxation of the femoral head.

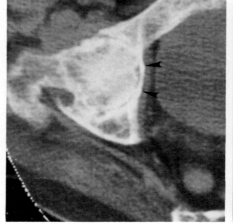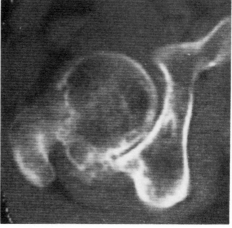

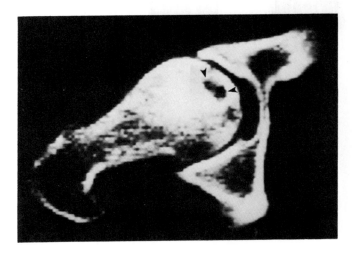

FIG. 59. Avascular necrosis of the femoral head. CT through the mid-femoral head in this moderately advanced stage of avascular necrosis of the femoral head shows an oval lucency (arrowheads) where the necrotic bone is being resorbed, surrounded by a zone of sclerosis from the slow reparative process. Note the slight flattening of the anteromedial aspect of the femoral head.

60a,b

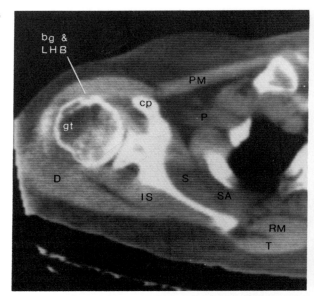

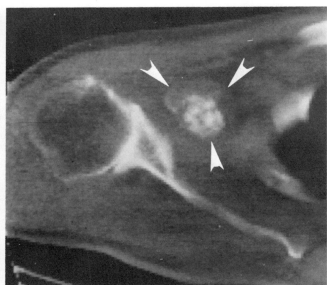

60c

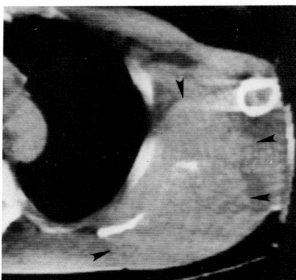

FIG. 60. Shoulder girdle. **a:** CT section through the shoulder joint shows the normal regional anatomy. cp, coracoid process; gt, greater tuberosity of humerus; bg, bicipital groove; LHB, long head biceps tendon; PM, pectoralis major; P, pectoralis minor; S, subscapularis; SA, serratus anterior; RM, rhomboid major; T, trapezius; IS, infraspinatus; D, deltoid. **b:** Osteochondral body. Following conventional radiographs that seemed to show an exostosis arising from the scapula, CT showed that the osteocartilaginous body (arrowheads) was independent of the scapula. This information influenced the surgical procedure for removal. **c:** Metastatic adenocarcinoma of the scapula. CT showed that the metastasis (arrowheads) was more extensive than suspected from examination of the conventional radiographs. This information influenced the field size determination for radiation therapy.

61a

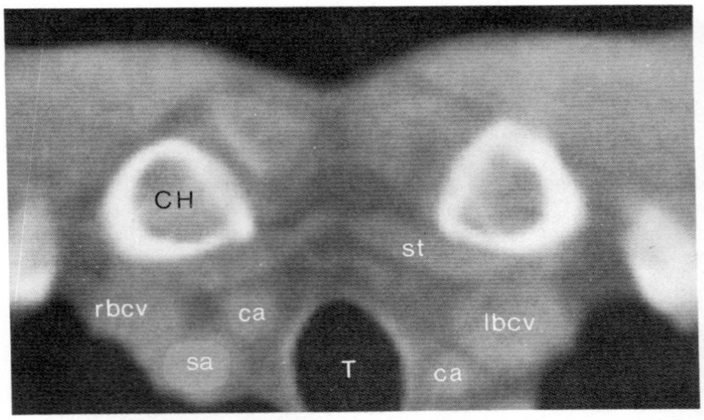

61b

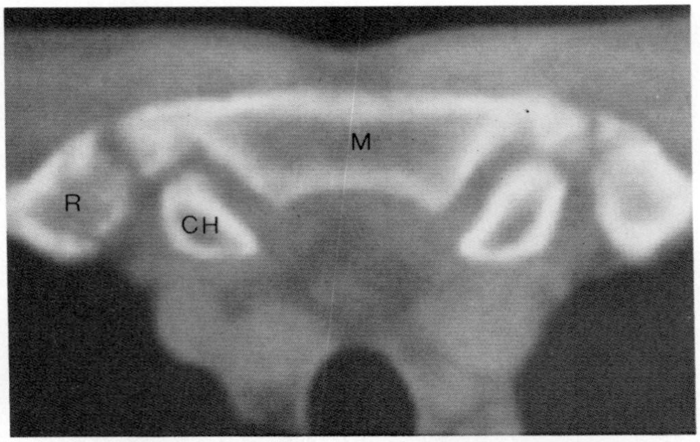

61c

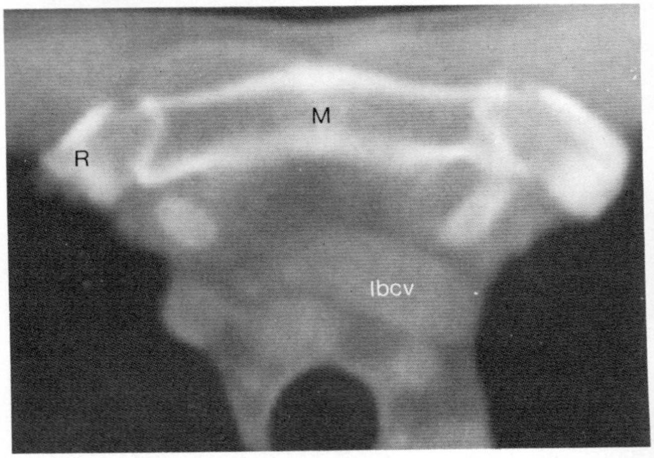

61d

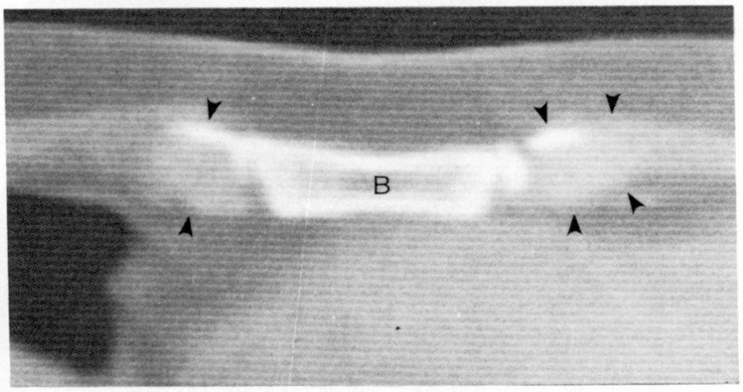

61e

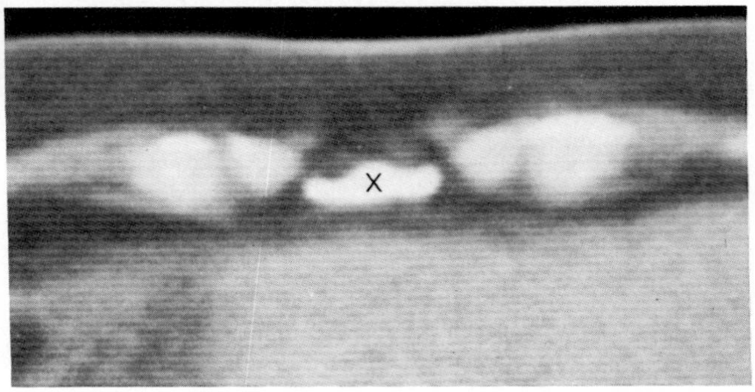

FIG. 61. Normal sternoclavicular joints and sternum. **a:** CT section through medial clavicular heads just cranial to the sternum shows the close proximity of the clavicular heads to vital structures such as the trachea and major vessels for the head and arms. **b:** CT section through the sternoclavicular joints shows the oblique axes of the joints and the posterolateral position of the clavicular heads with respect to the manubrium. It also shows articulation of the first ribs with the manubrium. **c:** CT section just caudal to the sternoclavicular joints shows the well-corticated manubrium and costomanubrial articulation juxtaposed to the left brachiocephalic vein. **d:** CT section through the body of the sternum shows partially calcified costal cartilage (arrowheads). **e:** CT section through the xyphoid process shows the dense bone with adjacent costal cartilages. ca, carotid artery; lbc, left brachiocephalic vein; rbcv, right brachiocephalic vein; sa, subclavian artery; st, sternothyroid muscle; B, body of sternum; CH, clavicular head; M, manubrium; R, rib; T, trachea; X, xyphoid process of sternum.

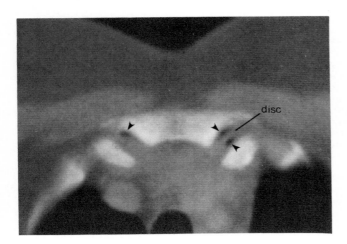

FIG. 62. Vacuum phenomenon in sternoclavicular joints. Gas (arrowheads) released from the adjacent soft tissues is confined to the joint spaces and outlines the left articular disc. (Reproduced from Destouet et al., ref. 27, with permission.)

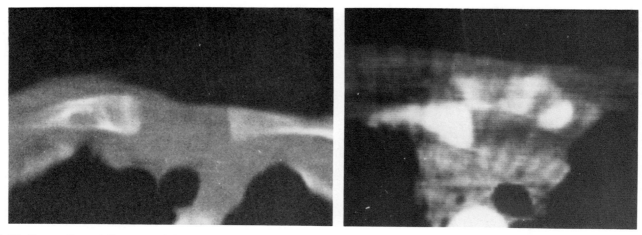

FIG. 63. Traumatic malalignment of the sternoclavicular joint. **Left:** The right clavicle is subluxed ventrally and cranially when compared with the left as shown by a midsection of the right clavicular head while only the superior surface of the left is in the section. Note the chest wall soft tissues adjacent to the subluxed clavicle are swollen and displaced. **Right:** The right clavicle is dislocated posteriorly into the region of the great vessels. The trachea is deviated toward the left. (Case courtesy of Dr. Richard Lynch, Palm Desert, California.) (Fig. 63, right reproduced from Destouet et al., ref. 27, with permission.)

64a,b

64c,d

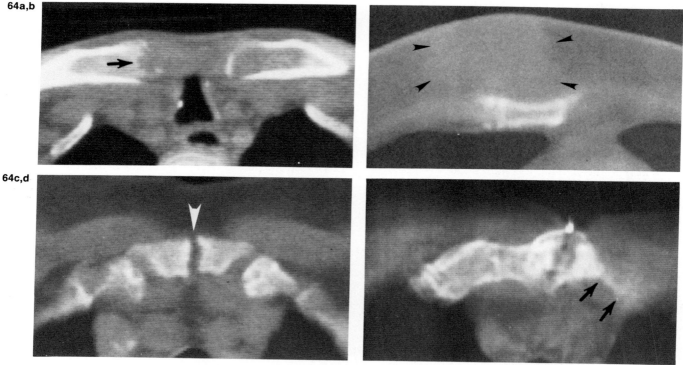

FIG. 64. Infections of the sternoclavicular joint and sternum. **a:** Conventional radiographs of this 49-year-old man with cellulitis were suggestive, but not diagnostic, of clavicular osteomyelitis. CT section clearly shows destruction of the right clavicular head with cortical fragmentation (arrow). **b:** Conventional radiographs of this 71-year-old man with a parasternal chest wall abscess were not diagnostic. CT section shows the soft tissue abscess (arrowheads) separate from a normal sternum. **c:** CT section of the sternum in this 71-year-old woman with persistent sternal pain 6 months following a median sternotomy shows a nonunion of the osteotomy (arrowhead), characterized by smooth cortical surfaces at the osteotomy site and lack of soft tissue swelling. **d:** In another patient, CT section through the region of a sternotomy site that drains purulent material shows a wire suture above an area of bone destruction indicating osteomyelitis. A portion of the sternum to the left of the metallic suture (arrows) is destroyed and the adjacent presternal soft tissues are deficient. (Figure 64d reproduced from Destouet et al., ref. 27, with permission.)

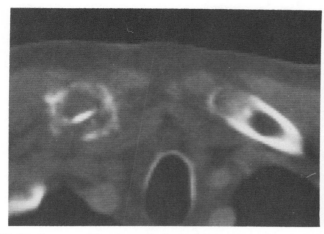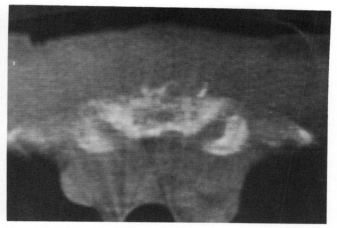

FIG. 65. Tumors of the sternoclavicular joint and sternum. **Left:** Plasmacytoma of the right clavicle has expanded and fragmented the cortex of the medial head. Although the soft tissues are displaced, they are otherwise normal. **Right:** Hodgkin's disease of the manubrium is manifested as permeative destruction associated with infiltration of the presternal and retrosternal soft tissues. (Case courtesy of Dr. Gary Omell, St. Louis, Missouri.) (Figure 65b reproduced from Destouet et al., ref. 27, with permission.)

useful information when a rib lesion is not optimally imaged by other methods. Computed tomography can show the results of trauma, infection, and tumor as they affect ribs (Fig. 66). Similarly, costotransverse and costovertebral joints are imaged each time a CT study is performed on the thorax; CT provides a much better image of these joints than does conventional radiography. Computed tomography may be relied on to solve an occasional imaging problem related to them (Fig. 67).

NONNEOPLASTIC MUSCULOSKELETAL DISEASES

Infection of bone and soft tissue has been considered earlier in this chapter as it related to specific anatomic regions. Computed tomography has not proven generally necessary for documentation, localization, or diagnosis of infection because radiographs are usually adequate for initial differential di-

agnosis. However, there have been a few reports of individual CT findings in certain infections (12,103). Computed tomography analysis of long bone medullary cavities has been proposed as a method to exclude or establish medullary infection (67). The few cases of osteomyelitis that we have studied have been subacute or chronic infections (Fig. 68). In these cases, CT has provided a cross-sectional correlate to the radiological findings. Radiologic intracortical fissuring, which is known to occur in osteomyelitis (106), is nicely shown by CT. Also, CT is generally useful to show the anatomic extent of vertebral column disc space infection and osteomyelitis (Fig. 69). It shows the soft tissue extent much better than conventional radiography, and may be used to follow the course of therapy. The cross-sectional image can be helpful in guiding percutaneous aspiration procedures.

Skeletal trauma is generally well studied by standard radiographic techniques. However, when it is necessary to solve specific orthopedic problems for either

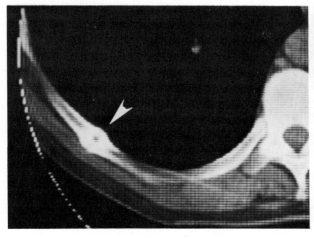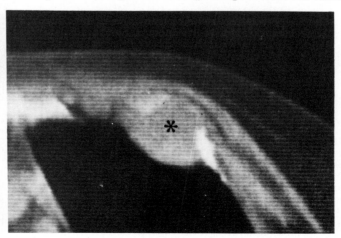

FIG. 66. Rib lesions. **Left:** A healing fracture (arrowhead) of the posterolateral region of this rib was found incidentally while studying the thorax of a 51-year-old man with bronchogenic carcinoma. **Right:** A plasmacytoma (∗) at the costochondral junction of this rib was shown poorly by conventional radiography, but easily defined by CT.

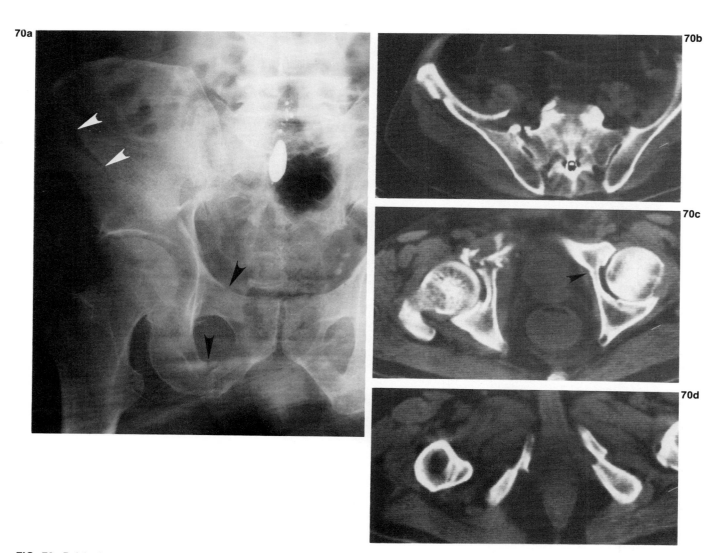

FIG. 70. Pelvic fractures. **a:** After a cement mixer fell on this 54-year-old man, radiographs showed an oblique fracture of the right ilium (white arrowheads) and apparently minimally displaced fractures of the superior and inferior pubic rami (black arrowheads). Since it could not be determined if the fractures constituted a functional hemipelvis injury with potential instability, CT was performed to provide information that would indicate whether the injury should be considered unstable. **b:** CT section through the ilii confirmed the oblique fracture and showed that the sacrum and sacroiliac joints were intact. **c:** CT section through the acetabulae showed an unsuspected shattered right superior pubic ramus and anterior acetabulum, as well as a nondisplaced, buckle fracture of the left ischium (arrowhead). **d:** CT section through the distal ischiopubic junction showed bilateral fractures. On the basis of this information, the injury was judged potentially unstable and the patient carefully mobilized.

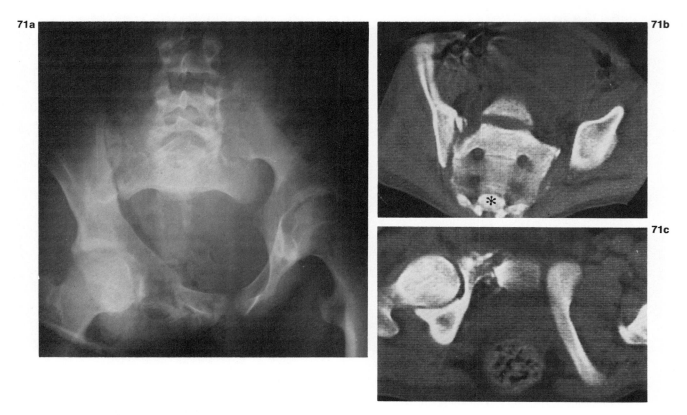

FIG. 71. Unstable pelvic fractures. **a:** Following a vehicular accident, pelvic deformity in this 17-year-old young man became worse. Radiographs showed that the left hemipelvis was disassociated from the sacrum and displaced cranially. The junction of the right superior pubic ramus and ischium was shattered. **b:** CT section through the sacrum and sacroiliac joints showed disruption of both joints. A small fragment of the right first sacral ala remained attached to the subluxed ilium. The craniomedial dislocation of the left ilium was well shown. While the first three sacral segments were imaged frontally, the last segments were viewed end on (*) indicating a transacral fracture between S_3 and S_4. **c:** A more caudal CT section graphically displayed the malalignment and severe deformity by imaging the left ischial tuberosity in the same plane as the right hip. On the basis of information provided by conventional radiographs and CT, a treatment plan was formulated to attempt reduction of this unstable pelvis.

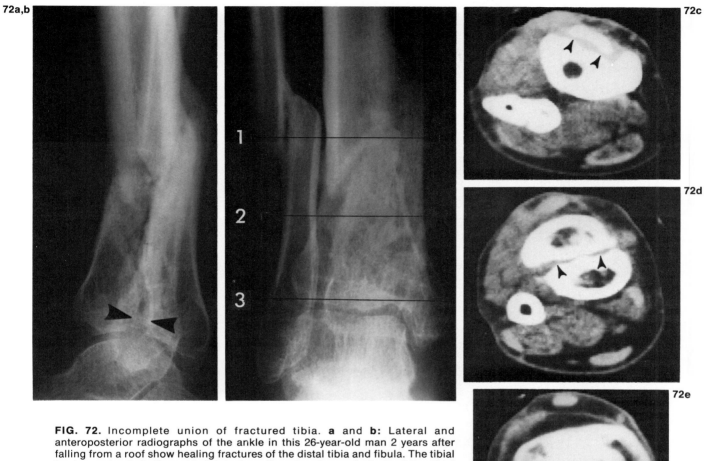

FIG. 72. Incomplete union of fractured tibia. **a** and **b:** Lateral and anteroposterior radiographs of the ankle in this 26-year-old man 2 years after falling from a roof show healing fractures of the distal tibia and fibula. The tibial fracture extends to the ankle joint where there is a 6-mm diastasis of the tibial articular surface (arrowheads). The orthopedic surgeon contemplated doing a distal tibial bone graft and an ankle fusion, but needed to know how well the tibial fracture had healed. Figures **c–e** correspond to levels 1, 2, and 3 as indicated on the AP radiograph. They show that the fibular fracture had healed, but that the majority of the tibial fracture had not (arrowheads). Because of this partial nonunion, the surgeon chose to bone graft the fracture site at the time of ankle arthrodesis. Follow-up CT showed that the bone graft bridged the tibial fracture, and that union was progressing normally.

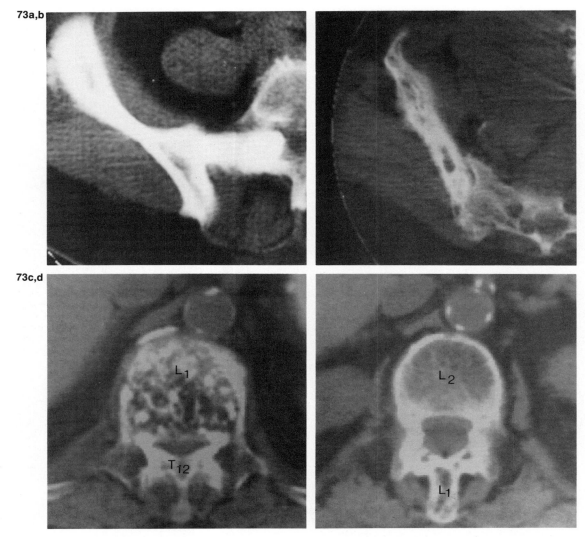

FIG. 73. Paget's disease. **a:** Paget's disease of the right ilium manifested as diffuse cortical thickening and mild focal unsharpness of the bone surface. **b:** Paget's disease of the right ilium manifested as irregular mineralization of a deformed (straightened) iliac wing with diffuse unsharpness of the bone surface. **c** and **d:** Paget's disease of L_1. CT sections show in-volvement of the entire vertebra including the body and pedicles (c), as well as the lamina and spinous process (d). Comparison of images c and d shows the enlarged vertebra with its disorganized trabeculae when compared with the normal spinous process of T_{12} and body of L_2.

no one has demonstrated that CT of cruciate ligaments or menisci has an advantage over conventional arthrography.

Rotational deformities of lower extremity long bones occur developmentally, with certain metabolic bone diseases and following trauma. These are orthopedically important and may require surgical correction. However, measurement of the rotational deformity has always been rather complicated. Computed tomography provides a cross-sectional image of the lower extremities that permits direct measurement of the amount of femoral anteversion (49,58,120,121) or tibial torsion (33,62). Such measurement capability may enhance study and treatment of lower extremity rotational deformities.

Paget's bone disease is best studied by radionuclide bone scans and conventional radiography. However, it

is a common incidental finding when CT studies are obtained of the thorax, abdomen, and pelvis for other reasons. Therefore, it is necessary to be familiar with its manifestations (Fig. 73). Paget's disease is most commonly encountered during the later stages of its natural history. It has usually involved a whole bone, increased the size of the bone, and replaced that bone with abnormal cortex and trabeculae. The cortex is usually thicker than normal and may have a very irregular surface. The trabecular pattern may become globular or chaotic. The pattern seen by CT may be impossible to differentiate from metastasis without the aid of history, laboratory tests, and radiographs. Paget's disease also softens bone such that the bone reshapes according to the mechanical forces across it. This may result in bowing, basilar invagination, and so on (Fig. 74). Anywhere in the natural history, Paget's

74a

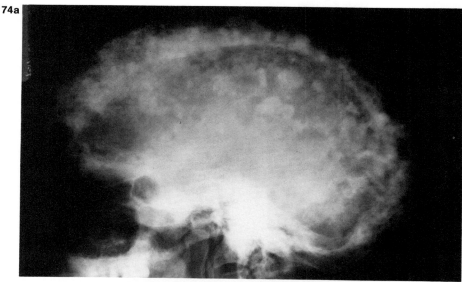

74b,c

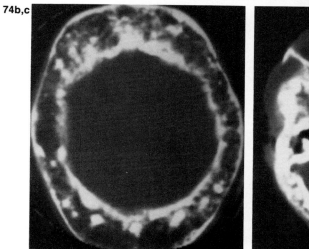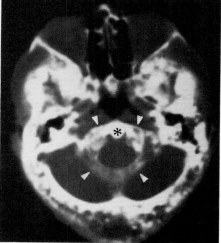

FIG. 74. Paget's disease of the skull with basilar invagination. **a:** Lateral radiograph of this 73-year-old woman's skull shows Paget's disease throughout the skull, manifested as the "cotton wool" pattern. The diploic space is expanded. **b:** CT section through the mid-portion of the skull shows the expanded diploic space with focal dense areas corresponding to the dense areas seen on the radiograph that contribute the "cotton wool" pattern. **c:** CT section through the posterior fossa shows invagination of C_1 vertebra (arrowheads) and the odontoid (*) of C_2.

disease may transform into malignancy, commonly osteosarcoma (Fig. 75). When this happens, CT is helpful in diagnosis, characterization, and treatment planning.

CT CONFIRMATION OF SCINTIGRAPHIC ABNORMALITIES

Many times in the practice of musculoskeletal radiology, we are asked to confirm and decide the importance of an abnormality identified when a patient is surveyed by a radionuclide bone scan. We then obtain conventional or coned-down radiographs of the region of interest and in most cases are able to answer these questions. In the past, when there was no good radiological correlate for a scan abnormality, we had several options: (a) to ignore the scan, (b) to obtain follow-up films at a later date, or (c) to perform a "blind" biopsy. Now, if we decide that the scan abnormality is important, but cannot confirm it by radiographic techniques, we have the additional option

of using CT for confirmation. When used in well-selected cases, this approach has been very rewarding. Computed tomography has proven much more sensitive than radiography at detecting bone density changes (Fig. 76). It has been helpful in confirming a few cases of metastasis to the medullary cavity in long bones (Fig. 77). In many cases, CT has shown convincingly that the focal radionuclide accumulation was caused by a benign process (e.g., dystrophic or degenerative changes). Thus, CT has often clarified bone scan findings, resulting in definitive management decisions.

CT AND PERCUTANEOUS MUSCULOSKELETAL BIOPSY

Percutaneous biopsy of lesions of the musculoskeletal system can be a very valuable diagnostic procedure (85,86). Computed tomography may affect decision making and biopsy performance in several ways (1,53,85). First, CT localizes and characterizes lesions

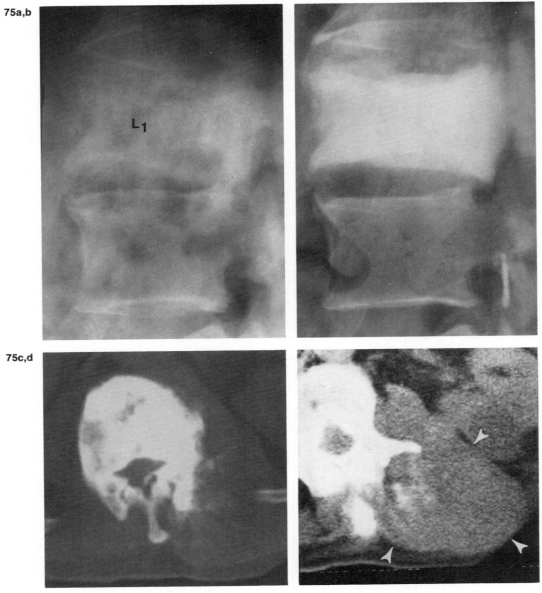

FIG. 75. Malignant transformation of Paget's disease into osteosarcoma. **a:** This 68-year-old man had previously diagnosed Paget's disease of L₁ vertebra. **b:** Within a year, L₁ became densely blastic. **c:** At bone window settings, CT section through L₁ vertebral body shows the blastic lesion with a large left-sided paraspinal mass containing radially oriented tumor mineralization. **d:** At soft tissue window settings, CT section through L₂ vertebral body and L₁ inferior facets and spinous process shows tumor in the L₁ spinous process. Caudal extension of the soft tissue mass is also imaged (arrowheads).

76a

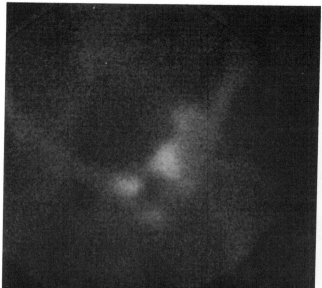

76b

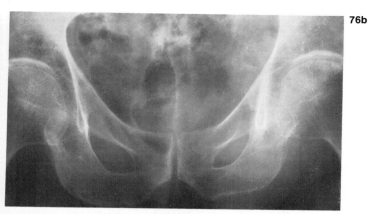

76c

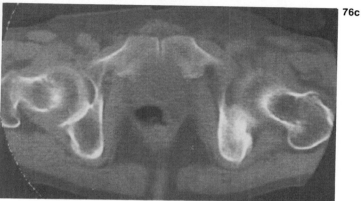

FIG. 76. Confirmation of abnormality shown by bone scan. **a:** ^{99m}Tc bone scan in this 79-year-old man, now 13 years after the diagnosis of prostate cancer, shows focal radionuclide accumulation in the acetabulum. **b:** Although in retrospect, the left "teardrop" is denser than the right, initially the conventional radiographs did not seem to adequately confirm a focal osseous abnormality. **c:** CT sections clearly showed diffuse osteosclerosis of the acetabulum, here seen as sclerosis of the ischial tuberosity and posterior acetabulum.

77a,b

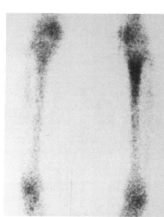

77c

FIG. 77. Confirmation of abnormality shown by bone scan. **a:** ^{99m}Tc bone scan in a 65-year-old woman with newly diagnosed breast cancer shows diffuse radionuclide accumulation in the proximal left tibia. **b:** The conventional radiographs were entirely normal. **c:** CT section through the proximal tibiae with measure mode window settings confirm involvement of the left medullary cavity.

78a,b

78c,d

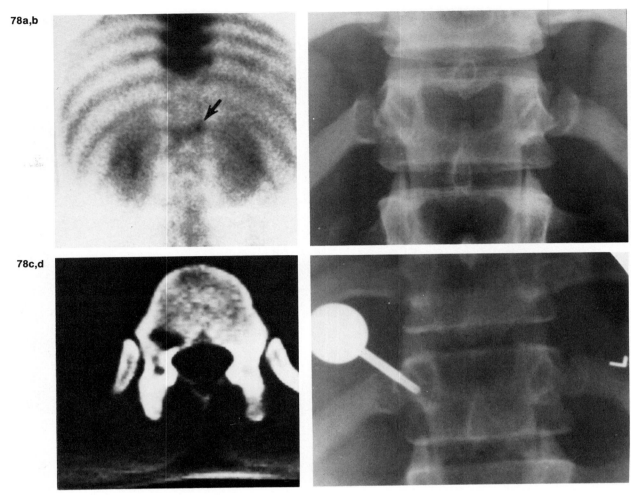

FIG. 78. CT influence on percutaneous bone biopsy. **a:** ⁹⁹ᵐTc bone scan in this 19-year-old man with widely metastatic malignant teratoma of the thorax, now 4 weeks postradiation therapy and with pancytopenia and fever, shows focal radionuclide accumulation in the radiation field and lesser uptake in T_{12} (arrow). **b:** The conventional radiographs were normal. **c:** CT through T_{12} showed focal trabecular destruction at the base of the right pedicle. **d:** Despite a severe coagulation defect and shaking chills, and because of the precise localization of the osseous abnormality, a percutaneous Ackermann needle biopsy was performed under fluoroscopic guidance without complication. A treatment decision would be based on discovery of infection or tumor. The specimen was adequate but showed only necrosis thereby eliminating both infection and tumor.

so that a decision whether or not to perform the biopsy can be made (Fig. 78). Second, it may show radial extent of tumor such that risks of the biopsy procedure are more clear, permitting appropriate decisions to enhance patient safety. Third, CT may provide information that influences choice of biopsy site, needle choice, or needle placement (Figs. 78 and 79). Finally, it may provide the precision and guidance necessary to complete the biopsy itself (Fig. 79). Although we still prefer to perform percutaneous biopsies under fluoroscopic guidance because of experience and convenience, some biopsies are performed using CT guidance, either when the lesion is first identified or sometime later (Fig. 80). Thus, we have found the improved density resolution and anatomic display features of CT important in some patients in whom precise needle placement for percutaneous biopsy is critical.

CT OSTEODENSITOMETRY

Loss of bone mass is a natural occurrence with aging and results as a complication of hormonal changes, many diseases, and some therapeutic medications. Clinical expression of osteopenia—pain, fracture, and deformity—is an important health and socioeconomic problem. Cortical and trabecular bones have different surface areas and consequently different rates of normal and abnormal bone turnover. Axial and peripheral skeletal sites may also turn over at different rates. Thus, the quantitative determination of bone mass at one or more skeletal sites is important for detection of osteopenia, documentation of disease progression, and evaluation of the success or failure of medical intervention.

Until the advent of CT, the only accepted tech-

79a,b

79c,d

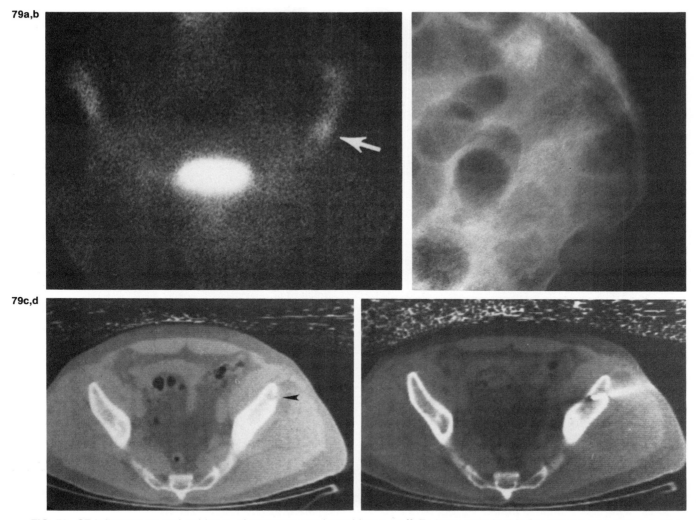

FIG. 79. CT influence on and guidance of percutaneous bone biopsy. **a:** ⁹⁹ᵐTc bone scan in this 64-year-old man with a pulmonary mass, but negative transthoracic biopsy showed multiple areas of focal radionuclide accumulation including one in the left ilium (arrow). **b:** Conventional films did not show the lesion. **c:** CT scan shows a small destructive lesion (arrowhead). **d:** Using the scanner for guidance, a Craig needle percutaneous bone biopsy was performed. Diagnosis: poorly differentiated adenocarcinoma.

niques were those that measured cortical bone in the appendicular skeleton. With the development of CT, several studies showed that CT numbers correlated fairly well with physical measurements of vertebral mineral content (11,71) and with photon absorption measurements of long bones (101). Application of CT to bone mass measurement has progressed along several different technical paths, including single and dual energy techniques for vertebrae (15,16,40,42) and other modifications for cortical or trabecular measurements in long bones (63,78,93,104). One group has developed a unique CT unit based on ¹²⁵I gamma photon transmission for measurement of distal radial cortical and trabecular bone (107,108).

Although the application of CT to mineral mass measurement is a simple concept, translation into a practical system for general clinical use has not been as simple. Early in the development of these tech-

niques, many of the theoretical difficulties that would be encountered were described (123). It was pointed out that processes other than mineral changes might modify bone density, that beam hardening would alter measurement accuracy, and that geometric repositioning of the patient would be difficult. These are, in fact, real problems, but there are more. X-ray beam effective energy varies, requiring a normalization phantom imaged with each study and a mathematical correction for the time related beam energy drift (42). For all methods of CT mineral mass measurement, refinement of the technique to acceptable levels of accuracy and precision has been difficult. Further developmental work will be necessary before any one or several techniques become generally useful.

There have been several clinical research studies performed where these techniques have been evaluated. Computed tomography of vertebral trabecular

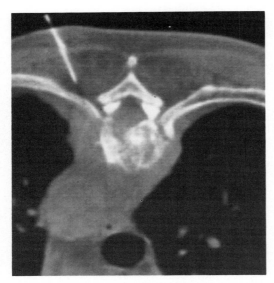

FIG. 80. CT guidance of percutaneous bone biopsy. Aspiration needle headed in direction of T_6 paravertebral mass in 63-year-old woman thought to have lymphoma. Diagnosis: pyogenic disc space infection with vertebral osteomyelitis.

mass measured in women following oophorectomy and compared with conventional appendicular mass measurements showed spinal cancellous bone loss whereas the average peripheral measurements showed no change (17). Using ^{125}I transmission CT of the radius, the Zurich group defined normal parameters of distal radial cortical and trabecular bone (38), used the technique to measure osteosclerosis in patients with chronic renal failure (39), and studied mineral loss following forearm immobilization (34). These early clinical applications of CT osteodensitometry indicate a potential usefulness of the technique.

FUTURE DIRECTIONS

Musculoskeletal CT will continue to be a second imaging procedure to solve many clinical and radiological problems. Many of these will become better defined in the next several years. Computed tomography should be used more as the standard imaging test for soft tissue masses. It should be obtained as a postoperative base-line study in all patients who have local resection of musculoskeletal tumors in order to facilitate early documentation of tumor recurrence.

Computed tomography should prove useful for future studies of normal muscle anatomy and morphology, the natural history of neuromuscular diseases, the effect of intervention in muscular dystrophies, and the results of rehabilitation of various neuromuscular diseases.

Computed tomography will be further developed as an important imaging test for orthopedic surgeons,

particularly in the evaluation and management of complex fractures. It should develop an important role in preoperative planning of major joint replacement for selected problems and has potential research applications in basic biomechanics and orthopedic appliance design.

As certain technical problems are solved and basic research progresses, CT is expected to develop into a standard measurement of bone mineral mass.

REFERENCES

1. Adapon BD, Legada BD, Lim EVA, Silao JV, Dalmacio-Cruz A: CT-guided closed biopsy of the spine. *J Comput Assist Tomogr* 5:73−78, 1981
2. Archer CR, Yeager V: Internal structure of the knee visualized by computed tomography. *J Comput Assist Tomogr* 2:181−183, 1978
3. Arger PH, Mulhern CB, Littman PS, Meadows AT, Coleman BG, Jarrett PT: Management of solid tumors in children: Contribution of computed tomography. *AJR* 137:251−255, 1981
4. Barlow RE, Goldman ML: Computed tomography of the skeletal system. *Comput Tomogr* 2:27−35, 1978
5. Berger PE, Kuhn JP: Computed tomography of tumors of the musculoskeletal system in children. *Radiology* 127:171−175, 1978
6. Bergman AB, Neiman HL: Computed tomography in the detection of retroperitoneal hemorrhage after translumbar aortography. *AJR* 131:831−833, 1978
7. Bernardino ME, Jing BS, Thomas JL, Lindell MM, Zornoza J: The extremity soft-tissue lesion: A comparative study of ultrasound, computed tomography, and xeroradiography. *Radiology* 139:53−59, 1981
8. Blumberg ML: Computed tomography and acetabular trauma. *Comput Tomogr* 4:47−53, 1980
9. Blumberg ML: CT of iliac unicameral bone cysts. *AJR* 136:1231−1232, 1981
10. Borlaza GS, Seigel R, Kuhns LR, Good AE, Rapp R, Martel W: Computed tomography in the evaluation of sacroiliac arthritis. *Radiology* 139:437−440, 1981
11. Bradley JG, Huang HK, Ledley RS: Evaluation of calcium concentration in bones from CT scans. *Radiology* 128:103−107, 1978
12. Braithwaite PA, Lees RF: Vertebral hydatid disease: Radiological assessment. *Radiology* 140:763−766, 1981
13. Braunstein EM, Silver TM, Martel W, Jaffe M: Ultrasonographic diagnosis of extremity masses. *Skeletal Radiol* 6:157−163, 1981
14. Bulcke JA, Termote JL, Palmers Y, Crolla D: Computed tomography of the human skeletal muscular system. *Neuroradiology* 17:127−136, 1979
15. Cann CE: Low-dose CT scanning for quantitative spinal mineral analysis. *Radiology* 140:813−815, 1981
16. Cann CE, Genant HK: Precise measurement of vertebral mineral content using computed tomography. *J Comput Assist Tomogr* 4:493−500, 1980
17. Cann CE, Genant HK, Ettinger B, Gordan GS: Spinal mineral loss in oophorectomized women. *JAMA* 244:2056−2059, 1980
18. Carrera GF, Foley WD, Kozin F, Ryan L, Lawson TL: CT of sacroiliitis. *AJR* 136:41−46, 1981
19. Chafetz N, Mark AS, Helms C, Cann CE, Glick JM, Genant HK: *Computed Tomography (CT) of the Menisci and Cruciate Ligaments.* Presented at 29th Annual Meeting of the Association of University Radiologists, New Orleans, Louisiana, 1981. *Invest Radiol* 16:366, 1981 (abstr.).
20. Chew FS, Hudson TM, Hawkins IF: Radiology of infiltrating angiolipoma. *AJR* 135:781−787, 1980
21. Chuang VP, Fried AM, Chen CQ: Computed tomographic evaluation of para-aortic hematoma following translumbar aortography. *Radiology* 130:711−712, 1979

22. Delgado-Martins H: A study of the position of the patella using computerized tomography. *J Bone Joint Surg [Br]* 61:443–444, 1979

23. deSantos LA, Bernardino ME, Murray JA: Computed tomography in the evaluation of osteosarcoma: Experience with 25 cases. *AJR* 132:535–540, 1979

24. deSantos LA, Goldstein HM, Murray JA, Wallace S: Computed tomography in the evaluation of musculoskeletal neoplasms. *Radiology* 128:89–94, 1978

25. deSantos LA, Murray JA: Evaluation of giant cell tumor by computerized tomography. *Skeletal Radiol* 2:205–212, 1978

26. Destouet JM, Gilula LA, Murphy WA: Computed tomography of long-bone osteosarcoma. *Radiology* 131:439–445, 1979

27. Destouet JM, Gilula LA, Murphy WA, Sagel SS: Computed tomography of the sternoclavicular joint and sternum. *Radiology* 138:123–128, 1981

28. Dihlmann VW, Gürtler KF, Heller M: Sakroiliakale computertomographie. *Fortschr Röntgenstr* 130:659–665, 1979

29. Donovan PJ, Zerhouni EA, Siegelman SS: CT of the psoas compartment of the retroperitoneum. *Semin Roentgenol* 16:241–250, 1981

30. Doppman JL, Marx S, Spiegel A, Brown E, Downs R, Brennan MF, Aurbach G: Differential diagnosis of brown tumor vs cystic osteitis by arteriography and computed tomography. *Radiology* 131:339–340, 1979

31. Dunnick NR, Schaner EG, Doppman JL: Detection of subcutaneous metastases by computed tomography. *J Comput Assist Tomogr* 2:275–279, 1978

32. Egund N, Ekelund L, Sako M, Persson B: CT of soft-tissue tumors. *AJR* 137:725–729, 1981

33. Elgeti H, Grote R, Giebel G: Bestimmung der tibiatorsion mit der axialen computertomographie. *Unfallheikunde* 83:14–19, 1980

34. Elsasser U, Rüegsegger P, Anliker M, Exner GU, Prader A: Loss and recovery of trabecular bone in the distal radius following fracture-immobilization of the upper limb in children. *Klin Wochenschr* 57:763–767, 1979

35. Engelstad BL, Gilula LA, Kyriakos M: Ossified skeletal muscle hemangioma: Radiologic and pathologic features. *Skeletal Radiol* 5:35–40, 1980

36. Enneking WF, Chew FS, Springfield DS, Hudson TM, Spanier SS: The role of radionuclide bone-scanning in determining the resectability of soft-tissue sarcomas. *J Bone Joint Surg [Am]* 63:249–257, 1981

37. Epstein HC: Posterior fracture-dislocations of the hip: Long-term follow up. *J Bone Joint Surg [Am]* 56:1103–1127, 1974

38. Exner GU, Prader A, Elsasser U, Anliker M: Bone densitometry using computed tomography. Part II: Increased trabecular bone density in children with chronic renal failure. *Br J Radiol* 52:24–28, 1979

39. Exner GU, Prader A, Elsasser U, Rüegsegger P, Anliker M: Bone densitometry using computed tomography. Part I: Selective determination of trabecular bone density and other bone mineral parameters. Normal values in children and adults. *Br J Radiol* 52:14–23, 1979

40. Genant HK: Quantitative computed tomography for bone mineral analysis. In: *Computed Tomography, Ultrasound and X-ray: An Integrated Approach,* ed. by AA Moss and HI Goldberg, San Francisco, University of California, 1980, pp 371–377

41. Genant HK: Computed tomography. In: *Diagnosis of Bone and Joint Disorders with Emphasis on Articular Abnormalities,* ed. by D Resnick and G Niwayama, Philadelphia, Saunders, 1981, pp 380–408

42. Genant HK, Boyd D, Rosenfeld D, Abols Y, Cann CE: Computed tomography. In: *Non-invasive Measurements of Bone Mass and Their Clinical Application,* ed. by SH Cohn, Boca Raton, Fla, CRC Press, 1981, pp 121–149

43. Genant HK, Wilson JS, Bovill EG, Brunelle FO, Murray WR, Rodrigo JJ: Computed tomography of the musculoskeletal system. *J Bone Joint Surg [Am]* 62:1088–1101, 1980

44. Gilula LA: An overview of computed tomography of musculoskeletal disease. In: *Computed Tomography, Ultrasound and X-ray: An Integrated Approach,* ed. by AA Moss and HI Goldberg, San Francisco, University of California, 1980, pp 335–352

45. Gilula LA: Computed tomography of musculoskeletal neoplasms. In: *Computed Tomography, Ultrasound and X-ray: An Integrated Approach,* ed. by AA Moss and HI Goldberg, San Francisco, University of California, 1980, pp 353–370

46. Gilula LA, Murphy WA, Tailor CC, Patel RB: Computed tomography of the osseous pelvis. *Radiology* 132:107–114, 1979

47. Ginaldi S: Computed tomography feature of synovial osteochondromatosis. *Skeletal Radiol* 5:219–222, 1980

48. Ginaldi S, deSantos LA: Computed tomography in the evaluation of small round cell tumors of bone. *Radiology* 134:441–446, 1980

49. Grote R, Elgeti H, Saure D: Bestimmung des antetorsionswinkels am femur mit der axialen computertomographie. *Roentgenblaetter* 33:31–42, 1980

50. Guilford WB, Mintz PD, Blatt PM, Staab EV: CT of hemophilic pseudotumors of the pelvis. *AJR* 135:167–169, 1980

51. Häggmark T, Jansson E, Svane B: Cross-sectional area of the thigh muscle in man measured by computed tomography. *Scand J Clin Lab Invest* 38:355–360, 1978

52. Harbin WP: Radiographic anatomy of the sacrospinalis muscle. *Radiology* 140:630, 1981

53. Hardy DC, Murphy WA, Gilula LA: Computed tomography in planning percutaneous bone biopsy. *Radiology* 134:447–450, 1980

54. Hayes DL, McLeod RA, Wiltsie JC: Use of computed tomography in diagnosis of soft-tissue tumors. *Mayo Clin Proc* 54:547–548, 1979

55. Heelan RT, Watson RC, Smith J: Computed tomography of lower extremity tumors. *AJR* 132:933–937, 1979

56. Helms CA, Cann CE, Brunelle FO, Gilula LA, Chafetz N, Genant HK: Detection of bone-marrow metastases using quantitative computed tomography. *Radiology* 140:745–750, 1981

57. Hermann G, Rose JS: Computed tomography in bone and soft tissue pathology of the extremities. *J Comput Assist Tomogr* 3:58–66, 1979

58. Hernandez RJ, Tachdjian MO, Poznanski AK, Dias LS: CT determination of femoral torsion. *AJR* 137:97–101, 1981

59. Hinderling Th, Rüegsegger P, Anliker M, Dietschi C: Computed tomography reconstruction from hollow projections: An application to in vivo evaluation of artificial hip joints. *J Comput Assist Tomogr* 3:52–57, 1979

60. Hudson TM, Hawkins IF: Radiological evaluation of chondroblastoma. *Radiology* 139:1–10, 1981

61. Hunter JC, Johnston WH, Genant HK: Computed tomography evaluation of fatty tumors of the somatic soft tissues: Clinical utility and radiologic-pathologic correlation. *Skeletal Radiol* 4:79–91, 1979

62. Jakob RP, Haertel M, Stüssi E: Tibial torsion calculated by computerised tomography and compared to other methods of measurement. *J Bone Joint Surg [Br]* 62:238–242, 1980

63. Jensen PS, Orphanoudakis SC, Rauschkolb EN, Baron R, Lang R, Rasmussen H: Assessment of bone mass in the radius by computed tomography. *AJR* 134:285–292, 1980

64. Jones ET, Kuhns LR: Pitfalls in the use of computed tomography for musculoskeletal tumors in children. *J Bone Joint Surg [Am]* 63:1297–1304, 1981

65. Kalman MA: Radiologic soft tissue shadows in the pelvis: Another look. *AJR* 130:493–498, 1978

66. Kenney PJ, Gilula LA, Murphy WA: The use of computed tomography to distinguish osteochondroma and chondrosarcoma. *Radiology* 139:129–137, 1981

67. Kuhn JP, Berger PE: Computed tomographic diagnosis of osteomyelitis. *Radiology* 130:503–506, 1979

68. Lackner VK, Hofmann P, Grauthoff H, Brecht G, Thurn P: Computertomographischer nachweis von muskelhämatomen bei hämophilie. *Fortschr Röntgenstr* 129:298–302, 1978

69. Lange TA, Alter AJ: Evaluation of complex acetabular fractures by computed tomography. *J Comp Assist Tomogr* 6:849–852, 1980

70. Lasda NA, Levinsohn EM, Yuan HA, Bunnell WP: Comput-

erized tomography in disorders of the hip. *J Bone Joint Surg [Am]* 60:1099–1102, 1978

71. Laval-Jeantet M, Laval-Jeantet AM, Lamarque JL, Demoulin B: Evaluation de la minéralisation osseuse vertébrale par tomographie computérisée. *J Radiol* 60:87–93, 1979

72. Letournel E: Acetabulum fractures: Classification and management. *Clin Orthop* 151:81–106, 1980

73. Levine E: Computed tomography of musculoskeletal tumors. *CRC Crit Rev Diagn Imaging* 16:279–309, 1981

74. Levine E, Lee KR, Neff JR, Maklad NF, Robinson RG, Preston DF: Comparison of computed tomography and other imaging modalities in the evaluation of musculoskeletal tumors. *Radiology* 131:431–437, 1979

75. Levinsohn EM, Bryan PJ: Computed tomography in unilateral extremity swelling of unusual cause. *J Comput Assist Tomogr* 3:67–70, 1979

76. Levinsohn EM, Bunnell WP, Yuan HA: Computed tomography in the diagnosis of dislocations of the sternoclavicular joint. *Clin Orthop* 140:12–16, 1979

77. Levitt RG, Sagel SS, Stanley RJ, Evens RG: Computed tomography of the pelvis. *Semin Roentgenol* 13:193–200, 1978

78. Liliequist B, Larsson SE, Sjögren I, Wickman G, Wing K: Bone mineral content in the proximal tibia measured by computer tomography. *Acta Radiol Diagn* 20:957–966, 1979

79. Lindsjö U, Hemmingsson A, Sahlstedt B, Danckwardt-Lillieström G: Computed tomography of the ankle. *Acta Orthop Scand* 50:797–801, 1979

80. Lloyd TV, Paul DJ: Erosion of the scapula by a benign lipoma. Computed tomography diagnosis. *J Comput Assist Tomogr* 3:679–680, 1979

81. McLeod RA, Gisvold JJ, Stephens DH, Beabout JW, Sheedy PF: Computed tomography of soft tissues and breast. *Semin Roentgenol* 13:267–275, 1978

82. McLeod RA, Stephens DH, Beabout JW, Sheedy PF, Hattery RR: Computed tomography of the skeletal system. *Semin Roentgenol* 13:235–247, 1978

83. Monsees BS, Danzig LA, Gilula LA, Akeson W: Application of computed tomography to orthopedic surgery. In: *Practice of Surgery*, ed. by H Goldsmith, Hagerstown, Md., Harper & Row, 1981, pp 31–46

84. Murphy WA: Overview of musculoskeletal computed tomography. In: *Computed Tomography, Ultrasound and X-ray: An Integrated Approach*, ed. by AA Moss and HI Goldberg, San Francisco, University of California, 1981, pp 101–111

85. Murphy WA: Percutaneous skeletal biopsy. In: *Computed Tomography, Ultrasound and X-ray: An Integrated Approach*, ed. by AA Moss and HI Goldberg, San Francisco, University of California, 1981, pp 147–156

86. Murphy WA, Destouet JM, Gilula LA: Percutaneous skeletal biopsy 1981: A procedure for radiologists—results, review, and recommendations. *Radiology* 139:545–549, 1981

87. Murphy WA, Siegel MJ, Gilula LA: Arthrography in the diagnosis of unexplained chronic hip pain with regional osteopenia. *AJR* 129:283–287, 1977

88. Naidich DP, Freedman MT, Bowerman JW, Siegelman SS: Computerized tomography in the evaluation of the soft tissue component of bony lesions of the pelvis. *Skeletal Radiol* 3:144–148, 1978

89. Naidich DP, Freedman MT, Bowerman JW, Siegelman SS: Ten section approach to computed tomography of the pelvis. *Skeletal Radiol* 5:213–217, 1980

90. O'Connor JF, Cohen J: Computerized tomography (CAT scan, CT scan) in orthopaedic surgery. *J Bone Joint Surg [Am]* 60:1096–1098, 1978

91. O'Doherty DS, Schellinger D, Raptopoulos V: Computed tomographic patterns of pseudohypertrophic muscular dystrophy: Preliminary results. *J Comput Assist Tomogr* 1:482–486, 1977

92. Orcutt J, Radsdale BD, Curtis DJ, Levine MI: Misleading CT in parosteal osteosarcoma. *AJR* 136:1233–1236, 1981

93. Orphanoudakis SC, Jensen PS, Rauschkolb EN, Lang R, Rasmussen H: Bone mineral analysis using single-energy tomography. *Invest Radiol* 14:122–130, 1979

94. Osborn AG, Koehler PR, Gibbs FA, Leavitt DD, Anderson RE, Lee TG, Ferris DT: Direct sagittal computed tomographic scans in the radiographic evaluation of the pelvis. *Radiology* 134:255–257, 1980

95. Padovani J, Faure F, Devred P, Jacquemier M, Sarrat P: Intérêt et indications de la tomodensitométrie dans le bilan des luxations congénitales de la hanche. *Ann Radiol* 22:188–193, 1979

96. Paul DF, Morrey BF, Helms CA: Computerized tomography in orthopedic surgery. *Clin Orthop* 139:142–149, 1979

97. Pavlov H, Frieberger RH, Deck MF, Marshall JL, Morrissey JK: Computer-assisted tomography of the knee. *Invest Radiol* 13:57–65, 1978

98. Pavlov H, Hirschy JC, Torg JS: Computed tomography of the cruciate ligaments. *Radiology* 132:389–393, 1979

99. Penkava RR: Iliopsoas bursitis demonstrated by computed tomography. *AJR* 135:175–176, 1980

100. Peters JC, Coleman BG, Turner ML, Arger PH, Mulhern CB, Dalinka MK, Allan DA, Schumacher HR: CT evaluation of enlarged iliopsoas bursa. *AJR* 135:392–394, 1980

101. Posner I, Griffiths HJ: Comparison of CT scanning with photon absorptiometric measurement of bone mineral content in the appendicular skeleton. *Invest Radiol* 12:542–544, 1977

102. Ralls PW, Boswell W, Henderson R, Rogers W, Boger D, Halls J: CT of inflammatory disease of the psoas muscle. *AJR* 134:767–770, 1980

103. Ram PC, Martinez S, Korobkin M, Breiman RS, Gallis HR, Harrelson JM: CT detection of intraosseous gas: A new sign of osteomyelitis. *AJR* 137:721–723, 1981

104. Revak CS: Mineral content of cortical bone measured by computed tomography. *J Comput Assist Tomogr* 4:342–350, 1980

105. Rose JS, Hermann G: Computerized tomography of the extremities in children. *Ann Radiol* 22:160–170, 1979

106. Rosen RA, Morehouse HT, Karp HJ, Yu GSM: Intracortical fissuring in osteomyelitis. *Radiology* 141:17–20, 1981

107. Rüegsegger P, Anliker M, Dambacher M: Quantification of trabecular bone with low dose computed tomography. *J Comput Assist Tomogr* 5:384–390, 1981

108. Rüegsegger P, Elsasser U, Anliker M, Gnehm H, Kind H, Prader A: Quantification of bone mineralization using computed tomography. *Radiology* 121:93–97, 1976

109. Sauser DD, Billimoria PE, Rouse GA, Mudge K: CT evaluation of hip trauma. *AJR* 135:269–274, 1980

110. Schumacher TM, Genant HK, Korobkin M, Bovill EG: Computed tomography: Its use in space-occupying lesions of the musculoskeletal system. *J Bone Joint Surg [Am]* 60:600–607, 1978

111. Shirkhoda A, Brashear HR, Staab EV: Computed tomography of acetabular fractures. *Radiology* 134:683–688, 1980

112. Siegel MJ, Glasier CM, Sagel SS: CT of pelvic disorders in children. *AJR* 137:1139–1143, 1981

113. Stephenson TF: Computerized tomography of soft tissue abnormalities. *Comput Tomogr* 4:181–188, 1980

114. Termote JL, Baert A, Crolla D, Palmers Y, Bulcke JA: Computed tomography of the normal and pathologic muscular system. *Radiology* 137:439–444, 1980

115. Turner ML, Mulhern CB, Dalinka MK: Lesions of the sacrum: Differential diagnosis and radiological evaluation. *JAMA* 245:275–277, 1981

116. Villafana T, Lee SH, Lapayowker MS: A device to indicate anatomical level in computed tomography. *J Comput Assist Tomogr* 2:368–371, 1978

117. Vujic I, Stanley J, Tyminski LJ: Computed tomography of suspected caval thrombosis secondary to proximal extension of phlebitis from the leg. *Radiology* 140:437–441, 1981

118. Vukanovic S, Hauser H, Wettstein P: CT localization of myonecrosis for surgical decompression. *AJR* 135:1298–1299, 1980

119. Weinberger G, Levinsohn EM: Computed tomography in the evaluation of sarcomatous tumors of the thigh. *AJR* 130:115–118, 1978

120. Weiner DS, Cook AJ: Practical considerations in the use of computed tomography in the measurement of femoral anteversion. *Isr J Med Sci* 16:288–294, 1980

121. Weiner DS, Cook AJ, Hoyt WA, Oravec CE: Computed tomography in the measurement of femoral anteversion. *Orthopedics* 1:299–306, 1978

122. Weis L, Heelan RT, Watson RC: Computed tomography of orthopedic tumors of the pelvis and lower extremities. *Clin Orthop* 130:254–259, 1978

123. Weissberger MA, Zamenhof RG, Aronow S, Neer RM: Computed tomography scanning for the measurement of bone mineral in the human spine. *J Comput Assist Tomogr* 2:253–262, 1978

124. Welch DM, Gilula LA: Pseudotumor of the femur from post-traumatic false aneurysm. *AJR* 128:510–512, 1977

125. Wilson JS, Korobkin M, Genant HK, Bovill EG: Computed tomography of musculoskeletal disorders. *AJR* 131:55–61, 1978

126. Wittenberg J, Fineberg HV, Ferrucci JT, Simeone JF, Mueller PR, van Sonnenberg E, Kirkpatrick RH: Clinical efficacy of computed body tomography. II. *AJR* 134:1111–1120, 1980

127. Wright CH, Thomas ML, Young AE: Computed tomography in the evaluation of a femoral aneurysm. *Radiology* 138:404, 1981

Chapter 18

Pediatric Applications

Marilyn J. Siegel

Pediatric diseases are frequently different in type and presentation from those in the adult. But, as in the older population, valuable diagnostic information can be gained from CT scanning of the body and CT is being accepted as an important method for the diagnosis of extracranial disease in children (2,8–12,16–21, 29,30,44–46,48–52,84).

The advantages of CT compared to conventional radiography—its ability to distinguish small tissue density differences, as well as to provide three-dimensional, cross-sectional delineation of anatomic relationships unobscured by overlying structures—are as applicable to the pediatric as to the adult population. But extracranial CT in children has unique problems not present in adults. Most important of these is the relative paucity of perivisceral fat, making delineation of organs and structures more difficult in pediatric patients. Furthermore, small children frequently are unable to cooperate and sedation may be needed. The radiation doses in children from CT are different from those in adults (20,73). The skin dose and organ dose in the directly irradiated area as well as the exposure of organs outside the area examined are higher in children because of their smaller body diameter. However, the absorbed energy is lower in children than in adults because of their smaller volume (73). Newer generation CT scanners, especially, have reduced the radiation dose while improving image quality (19).

TECHNIQUE

Special Preparation for Pediatric Patients

Sedation

Children under the age of 4 years often require sedation, usually secobarbital (Seconal®) 5 mg/kg up to a maximum dose of 100 mg. The injection is given intramuscularly approximately 20 to 30 min before the procedure.

Immobilization

Immobilization on commercially available troughs specially designed to hold young infants is required occasionally. In older infants, a light sandbag on the extremities can be used for restraint. Children 4 years of age or older generally will cooperate after verbal reassurance and explanation.

Intravenous Contrast Administration

Scanning after intravenous administration of iodinated contrast media is helpful in confirming a lesion thought to be of vascular origin or closely related to vascular structures, in addition to improving differentiation of normal from pathologic parenchyma, especially in the liver and kidneys. With proper coordination, abdominal CT scans can be obtained within 1 to 2 hr following conventional urography, so that in many patients no additional contrast medium needs to be administered.

Bowel Opacification

For most examinations of the abdomen, opacification of the small and large bowel with contrast material (Gastrografin® or E-Z Cat®) given orally or through a nasogastric tube is necessary (63). If the contrast agent is given the evening before the examination and 15 to 30 min prior to scanning, the small and large bowel usually are fairly well opacified, and opacification of the large bowel with a contrast agent administered via enema is generally obviated (Fig. 1). Intramuscular sedation can be given approximately 5 to 10 min after oral contrast medium has been given. With this approach, we have had no problems with aspiration.

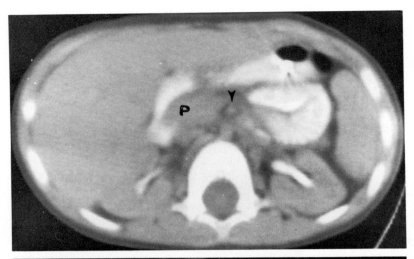

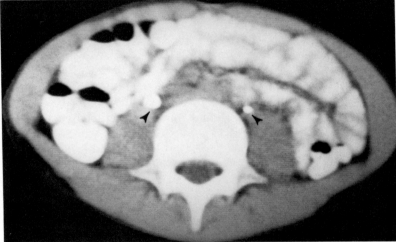

FIG. 1. Normal CT scans after intravenous contrast medium administration. **Above:** Upper abdomen in a 2-year-old boy. The pancreatic head (P) is well profiled by oral contrast in the surrounding antrum of the stomach and the duodenal loop. A small amount of fat surrounds the superior mesenteric artery (arrowhead). **Below:** Lower abdomen in a 7-year-old boy. Abundant oral contrast is used to fill both the large and small bowel completely, and thereby exclude a retroperitoneal or mesenteric mass. The opacified ureters (arrowheads) are well seen, although precise delineation of the aorta and inferior vena cava is difficult.

Imaging Techniques

For optimal examination of children, rapid scanners are necessary because patient motion can cause significant degradation of the CT image. The slice thickness and interval vary with the age of the patient, the area of interest, and the clinical indication for the examination. Generally, in chest and abdominal examinations in older children, 1-cm collimated sections at 1- or 2-cm intervals are obtained from the thoracic inlet to the subdiaphragmatic region and from the xyphoid to the symphysis pubis, respectively. Decreased collimation (2 to 5 mm) and scanning intervals (5 mm to 1 cm) are reserved for areas of maximum interest, detailed examinations such as evaluation of pulmonary nodules or the adrenal, and in the very small child. If the patient is cooperative, sections are obtained with breath holding at full inspiration. Computed tomography sections are obtained at resting lung volume if the patient is sedated.

CHEST

Mediastinum

As in adults, CT is able to identify some normal mediastinal structures not seen on conventional chest radiographs, but the lack of fat in the mediastinum frequently precludes the identification of each separate vessel. In the pediatric population, the normal thymus will be seen in virtually every patient (6) (Fig. 2). On occasion, differentiation of a mediastinal mass from the normal thymus can be difficult. Additionally, absolute distinction between a normal but prominent thymus from a pathologically enlarged organ may not be possible.

Indications for CT of the mediastinum include: (a) characterization of mediastinal widening or a mass of uncertain etiology suspected or clearly detected on chest radiography, (b) determination of the extent of a proven mediastinal tumor associated with an abnormal radiograph, and (c) evaluation of a mediastinum that is

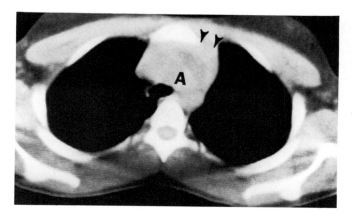

FIG. 2. Normal thymus in a 3-year-old girl. A normal left lobe of the thymus (arrowheads) is seen separated by fat from the aortic arch (A). At a lower level, the right lobe of the thymus was well seen.

normal by plain chest radiography in a patient with an underlying disease or radiographic signs that may be associated with a mediastinal mass. In these clinical settings, additional diagnostic information beyond that provided by the conventional chest radiograph is frequently provided (79).

Mediastinal Mass of Undetermined Etiology on Chest Radiograph

An abnormal mediastinum in infants and children is often due to a mass lesion, most commonly a neurogenic tumor, teratoma, lymphoma, or a cyst of foregut origin (15,39,66,76). Computed tomography can differentiate between lesions composed predominantly of fat, water, or soft tissue, and sometimes provides a more definitive diagnosis (7). Lesions that can present with attenuation values near water include pericardial cyst and duplication cysts of foregut origin. Pericardial effusions also can be documented by CT (Fig. 3). Rarely, bronchogenic cysts can have a density equal to that of soft tissue because their contents are quite viscous and not simple serous fluid. Vascular causes of mediastinal widening, such as an aortic aneurysm or a congenital anomaly of the thoracic vascular system, usually can be identified confidently following intravenous administration of contrast agent immediately prior to scanning (4) (Fig. 4).

When a mass has an attenuation value of soft tissue, the CT scan findings may be of value in predicting whether mediastinoscopy, thoracotomy, or other biopsy procedures such as bone marrow aspiration would be best to yield a diagnosis (Fig. 5). In the evaluation of posterior mediastinal masses, CT, in conjunction with metrizamide myelography, can depict intraspinal tumor extension (67,68).

Malignant Mediastinal Neoplasms and Abnormal Chest Radiograph

Lymphoma is the commonest malignant mediastinal tumor in childhood. Computed tomography may contribute diagnostic information by demonstrating more extensive disease than expected from plain chest radiography. This information is helpful as a base line for follow-up examinations but appears to have little beneficial effect on altering radiation or chemotherapy at the time of diagnosis in the patient with a known radiographic abnormality. In some patients, CT can be helpful in separating a mediastinal process from disease in the adjacent pulmonary parenchyma or pleura.

Underlying Disease and Normal Chest Radiograph

Computed tomography is useful to demonstrate thymic size and shape in patients with myasthenia gravis (5,79). This type of investigation is rewarding, particularly in children with myasthenia gravis and a normal or suspicious chest radiograph. Delineation of a focal thymic mass can prompt surgery, whereas demonstration of a normal size thymus, in conjunction with the knowledge that thymomas are rare in juvenile myasthenia gravis, can lead to medical management. Symmetric enlargement of the thymus suggests hyperplasia rather than thymoma (5) (Fig. 6). Whether removal of hyperplastic tissue is beneficial remains controversial.

Enlarged lymph nodes in the paratracheal region, due to lymphoma, metastatic carcinoma, or infectious disease, may be recognized and prompt mediastinoscopy or thoracotomy. Additionally, the intrapericardial portions of the great vessels are well delineated and congenital anomalies such as corrected transposition or absence of a pulmonary artery can be diagnosed in a noninvasive fashion (4).

Lungs

Computed tomography is a valuable technique in searching for pulmonary metastases in patients with known malignancies with a high propensity for lung dissemination, such as Wilms' tumor, osteogenic sarcoma, and rhabdomyosarcoma. Demonstration of a pulmonary nodule(s) in such a patient, as well as additional nodules in the patient with an apparent solitary metastasis for whom surgery is planned, may be critical to treatment planning. In the first instance, such detection may lead to additional treatment (surgery, chemotherapy, or radiation), whereas in the latter setting, demonstration of several metastatic nodules may negate surgical plans. Although a com-

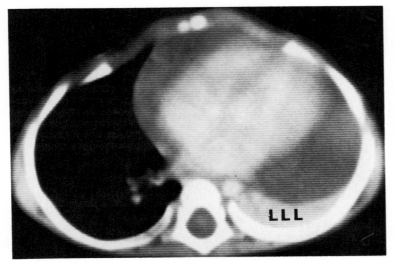

FIG. 3. Pericardial effusion. An 18-month-old girl with recurrent pericardial effusions studied to exclude a pericardial tumor. A large pericardial effusion with a low attenuation value is confirmed by CT. A collapsed left lower lobe (LLL) is seen posteriorly.

prehensive study of CT and conventional tomography in children is not yet available, our experience supports the contentions of others that CT is able to demonstrate a greater number of metastases, especially those located peripherally (pleural or subpleural) (72). Confusion with benign granulomas does not appear to be a clinically significant problem in children; almost all noncalcified nodules depicted by CT are due to metastases rather than granulomatous disease (44,45).

Chronic or recurrent segmental or subsegmental pneumonitis in children, especially at a lung base, is a finding suggestive of sequestration. Although demonstration of an anomalous vessel occasionally may be achieved by plain chest radiography or conventional tomography, CT appears more sensitive in iden-

tifying such a vessel (34) (Fig. 7), and may obviate aortography.

ABDOMEN

The appearance of the abdomen on CT examinations is comparable in adults and children except for the limitations imposed by the small size of the structures being examined and the relative paucity of perivisceral fat.

Four major categories of inquiry usually prompt CT examination of the abdomen: (a) determination of site of origin, extent, or character of an abdominal mass; (b) determination of the extent of a proven lymphoma;

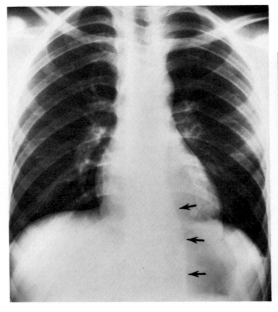
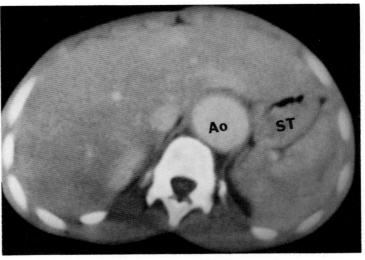

FIG. 4. Aortic aneurysm in a 12-year-old boy. **Left:** Posteroanterior chest radiograph reveals a left paraspinal mass (arrows). **Right:** Postcontrast CT demonstrates aneurysmal dilatation of the abdominal aorta (Ao) displacing the stomach (ST) laterally.

5a

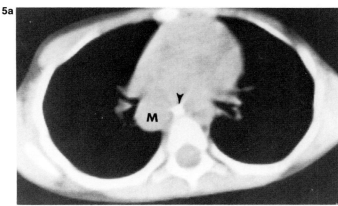

FIG. 5. Neuroblastoma in a 4-year-old girl. **a:** CT scan at the level of the left atrium shows a right paraspinal mass (M). A nasogastric tube (arrowhead) is in place. **b and c:** Sections through the lower chest and upper abdomen, respectively, show tumor extension (arrowheads) across the midline and beneath the diaphragmatic crura into the retroperitoneum. The posterior location of the tumor suggested a neuroblastoma, confirmed by bone marrow aspiration.

5b,c

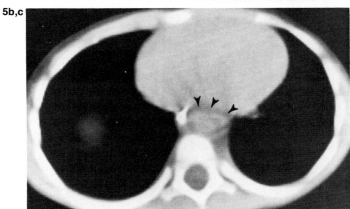
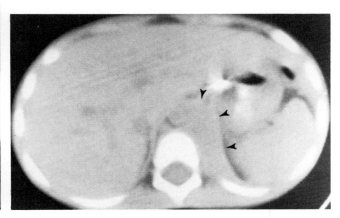

(c) determination of the existence of a suspected abscess; and (d) evaluation of extent of injury from blunt abdominal trauma. Less often, CT is used to evaluate parenchymal disease of the pancreas, liver, and kidney, as well as abnormalities of the major abdominal vessels.

Abdominal Masses

Abdominal masses in the pediatric population are primarily of retroperitoneal origin, with the kidney being the source in more than half of the cases (35,40). With increasing age, the percentage of malignant neoplasms increases while there is a decrease in benign cystic masses (42). Computed tomography can provide important diagnostic information, particularly in the older infant and child, regarding the site and extent of a mass, as well as the presence or absence of metastatic disease (16,51).

Renal Masses

Hydronephrotic and multicystic dysplastic kidneys are the cause of most abdominal masses in the neonate, although any form of renal cystic disease may present as nephromegaly and be misdiagnosed as a solid tumor (53,56,75). Although CT can delineate these

conditions (Fig. 8), it is usually unnecessary if the diagnosis can be established with urography or ultrasonography (US) (43,52,65,81). If the axis of the kidney is displaced or the etiology or level of obstruction is uncertain, such as with a horseshoe kidney or retrocaval ureter, CT may be of value in excluding a mass lesion as the cause.

Wilms' tumor is the most common primary malignant renal tumor of childhood. On CT, a Wilms' tumor usually appears as a large, spherical, and, at least partially, intrarenal mass usually with a central density lower than that of normal renal parenchyma. The peripheral area of the neoplasm usually approximates the density of the normal kidney and generally can be enhanced by the use of iodinated contrast media, although not to the same degree as the functioning normal renal parenchyma (Fig. 9). Differentiation of a Wilms' tumor from an extrarenal neuroblastoma should be possible in almost all cases. Renal vein thrombosis or tumor extension, which occurs in 4 to 10% of the cases, may be demonstrated after iodinated intravenous contrast (Fig. 10). The thrombus may be seen as a low-density intraluminal defect or suggested by renal vein or inferior vena caval enlargement (46,80). Additionally, CT may identify small exophytic tumors arising in the renal cortex and expanding outward anteriorly or posteriorly that cannot be seen on plain radiographs or

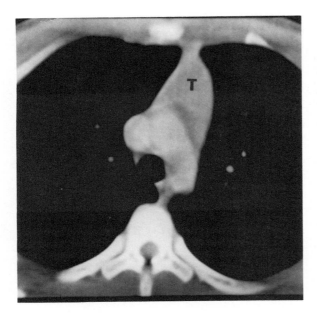

FIG. 6. Thymic hyperplasia in a 17-year-old boy with myasthenia gravis and a normal chest radiograph. The thymus (T), especially the left lobe, is too large for the patient's age. Normal mediastinal fat separates the thymus from the aorta.

urography. Otherwise occult calcifications also may be depicted. Following nephrectomy, CT can be used to detect local recurrence in the renal fossa. If the tumor is initially nonresectable or bilateral, CT may be valuable in assessing the response to radiation or chemotherapy.

In children with tuberous sclerosis, urography may suggest polycystic disease, angiomyolipoma, or a combination of both (88). Distinction with CT usually is possible in the older child based on differences in the attenuation value of cystic and lipomatous tissue (32,82) (Fig. 11).

Focal inflammatory masses may occur in the kidney and represent either an abscess or acute focal bacterial nephritis. The former often has a thick rim and a nonenhancing low-density center on CT. In contradistinction, acute focal nephritis appears as a focal area(s) of diminished density without a well-defined wall. After intravenous contrast medium administration, inhomogeneous enhancement is seen in the involved area (54). In most instances, the relative decreased density is only apparent after contrast medium administration.

Adrenal Masses

Neuroblastoma is the commonest malignant tumor in children under the age of 4 years; more than half originate in the abdomen, with two-thirds of these arising in the adrenal gland. The diagnosis can be rendered confidently with CT even when the lesion is relatively small and escapes detection on urography (78). The tumor is recognized as an irregular pararenal soft-tissue mass. Even on precontrast scans, the mass usually has a density lower than that of surrounding soft tissues; intravenous contrast medium administration accentuates this difference. Calcifications within the tumor, which may be coarse, irregular, or assume a ring-appearance (Fig. 12), can be observed in almost 80% of neuroblastomas by CT, whereas plain radiographs identify calcification only in approximately 50% of patients (16). Computed tomography usually provides information about the extent of tumor, including relationships to the great vessels, liver involvement, and intraspinal extension, which may require metrizamide CT myelography for complete assessment (20,51). Prevertebral extension across the midline is common. The interface of tumor

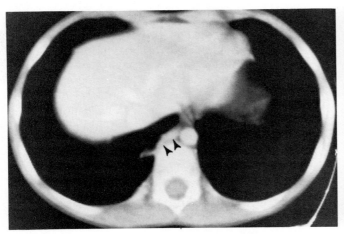

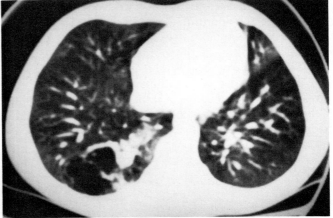

FIG. 7. Pulmonary sequestration in a 6-year-old boy with chronic right lower lobe consolidation on chest radiographs. **Left:** CT scan through the lower thorax after the administration of intravenous contrast medium shows an anomalous vessel (arrowheads) extending to the right lower lobe. **Right:** CT scan 2 cm cephalad viewed at lung window settings identifies the anomalous vessel coursing anterior to cystic changes and infiltrate in the right lower lobe.

8a,b

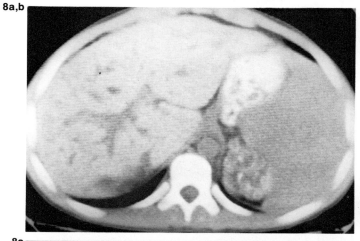

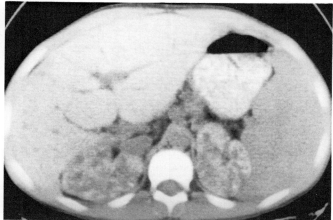

8c

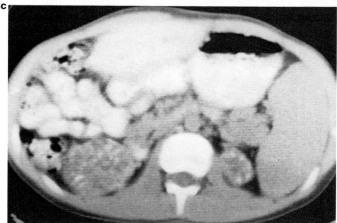

FIG. 8. Polycystic kidney disease in a 13-year-old boy with congenital hepatic fibrosis. **a:** The liver is abnormally increased in density, accentuating the portal venous structures. Splenomegaly is present. **b and c:** Lower levels through the kidneys show multiple small renal cysts, some of which have areas of high attenuation, believed to represent inspissated mucoid material.

with normal renal tissue is usually well defined and absence of a cleavage plane suggests renal parenchymal invasion by tumor. Computed tomography is also useful in the follow-up of patients with neuroblastomas (27).

Hepatic Tumors

Primary hepatic tumors are the third most frequent solid abdominal mass in children, following Wilms' tumor and neuroblastoma. The majority of malignant

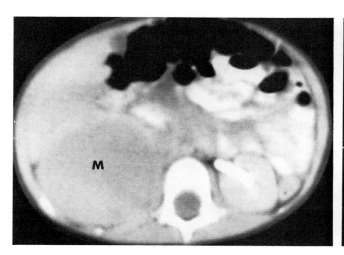

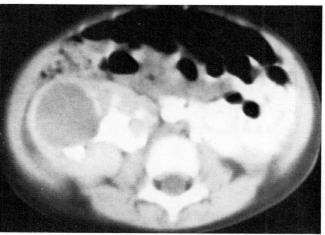

FIG. 9. Wilms' tumor in a 2-year-old girl with a palpable abdominal mass. **Left:** Postcontrast enhanced CT scan reveals a large low density mass (M) in the area of the upper pole of the right kidney. The mass, which is somewhat lower in attenuation value than the liver, has a higher density rim. **Right:** Three cm inferiorly the mass is shown to be intrarenal distorting the calyces. The density of the mass is substantially less than the enhanced renal parenchyma.

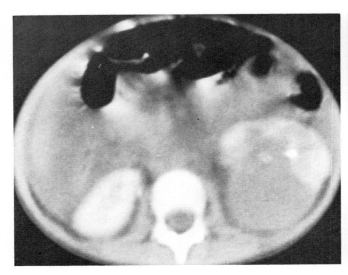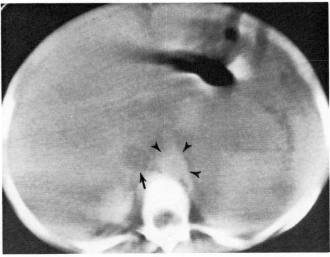

FIG. 10. Wilms' tumor in an 18-month-old girl. **Left:** CT scan through the kidneys 2 hr after an intravenous urogram demonstrates a large, round, low-density intrarenal mass that distorts and displaces the calyces. The interface with the enhanced renal parenchyma is indistinct. **Right:** At a higher level, the inferior vena cava (arrow) is noted to be of lower density than the aorta (arrowheads). A Wilms' tumor with renal vein and inferior vena caval extension was confirmed at autopsy.

tumors are hepatoblastoma or hepatocellular carcinoma, whereas vascular tumors, particularly hemangioendotheliomas or hemangiomas, are the commonest benign tumors of the liver. Computed tomography can document the presence of hepatic cysts or abscesses (Fig. 13). In general, most lesions detected by CT are of lower density than normal hepatic parenchyma. The density difference between normal tissue and some lesions can be great, as is the case with benign cysts, or minimal, as occurs with some primary hepatic tumors. The use of iodinated intravenous contrast enhancement may result in the lesions becoming relatively less, equal to, or more dense than the normal hepatic tissue (10,48). Often the CT features of a mass allow it to be characterized with more certainty, such as in the case of a cavernous hemangioma (3). With most hepatic neoplasms, however, a definitive histologic diagnosis is provided by biopsy and not by CT.

Imaging Methods (Clinical Application of Comparative Imaging)

In the evaluation of abdominal masses, it is difficult to make a dogmatic statement as to which imaging procedure should be used first or is superior because there are no large series comparing various diagnostic studies in children. Therefore, the choice of examination for a given institution strongly depends on the available equipment and expertise as well as the relative advantages and disadvantages of each imaging method. An overview of the productivity of the various diagnostic techniques is presented below.

Plain film radiography and excretory urography have been the mainstay of the investigation of suspected abdominal masses in infants and children for years. The plain abdominal radiograph is simple, readily available, inexpensive, and can serve to confirm the presence, size, and position of a mass. Although such information may be helpful in planning other investigative procedures, the plain radiograph usually is not diagnostic. Excretory urography with total-body opacification traditionally has provided the most useful and direct information about intraabdominal masses, the reason being that most masses are renal or pararenal in origin. However, urography at times not

FIG. 11. Angiomyolipomas in an 8-year-old retarded boy with tuberous sclerosis. CT scan after intravenous contrast medium administration shows bilateral renal enlargement, distortion of the collecting system, and multiple small renal masses of low attenuation values approaching fat density, consistent with angiomyolipomatosis.

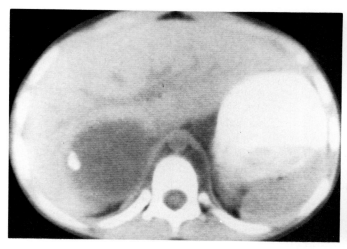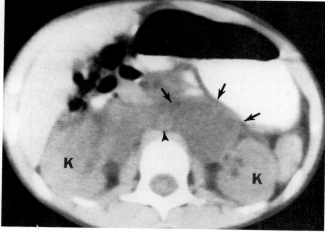

FIG. 12. Neuroblastoma in a 4-year-old girl with a palpable mass. **Left:** CT scan through the upper abdomen demonstrates a low density mass with calcification in the right side of the abdomen behind the liver. Neoplasm is also present in the retrocrural area. **Right:** At a lower level, the mass (arrows) is shown to extend across the midline in the retroperitoneum and surround the aorta (arrowhead). Both kidneys (K) are displaced laterally.

only fails to detect disease, but also may underestimate its extent (75). Additionally, contrast medium excretion by the neonatal kidney is poor and adequate delineation of the kidney often cannot be achieved.

For the most part, radionuclide scanning has its greatest application in the evaluation of masses situated in the right or left upper quadrants (liver, gallbladder, spleen). Dynamic as well as static studies can be obtained and this may be valuable in the evaluation of the vascularity of certain hepatic tumors. However, the anatomic delineation by radionuclide imaging is not as clear as with other imaging methods and the techniques are very organ specific.

Basically, ultrasound (US) and CT are procedures that provide similar information (17). Both give excellent cross-sectional anatomy and usually provide more

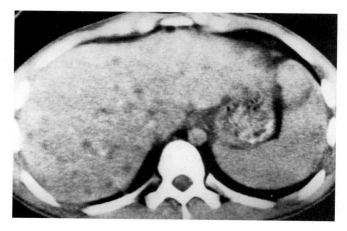

FIG. 13. Liver abscesses in a 16-year-old boy with leukemia and fever. Multiple low density lesions, consistent with abscesses, are seen throughout the liver. Repeat CT examination 1 month later following appropriate antibiotic therapy showed marked decrease in the size of the lesions.

detailed information than the aforementioned radiologic techniques (28,78). Computed tomography has an added advantage of being able to detect small density differences that are not visible on conventional radiography (calcium and fat). Furthermore, our experience, as well as that of others (11,12), suggests that CT is superior to US in detecting tumor extent and relationships to surrounding structures. In addition, gas-filled viscera, normally found in younger children, create more artifacts on US than CT. However, CT is not without certain drawbacks. Sedation is often required for CT; it involves ionizing radiation, and infants and young children frequently have little perivisceral fat, making anatomic delineation difficult in many cases.

Because of these limitations, US usually is considered the screening technique of choice or the examination to follow excretory urography in the evaluation of a pediatric abdominal mass (81). If US cannot yield adequate information or if it suggests a malignant mass, CT generally should be considered, particularly in the latter instances to delineate better the tumor extent.

Lymphoma

Although CT commonly demonstrates normal size lymph nodes in the retroperitoneum and pelvis in the adult, these are rarely recognized in children. However, lymphoma and metastatic disease of any etiology may produce sufficient lymph node enlargement to be demonstrable on CT. The appearance of such adenopathy varies from individually enlarged lymph nodes to a large homogeneous mass obscuring normal structures (51,83). In addition, CT may demonstrate the presence of extranodal disease (e.g., liver, spleen, kidney) within the abdomen. As in the adult, CT cannot differentiate normal lymph nodes from nodes that are of normal size but replaced with tumor. In addition, it is impossible to distinguish mild enlargement of lymph nodes due to inflammatory conditions from enlargement due to neoplastic involvement.

Clearly, CT is the initial radiologic procedure of choice in evaluating the abdomen in patients with lymphoma, especially since masses in childhood lymphoma can appear in the mesentery and range in size from small to bulky (Fig. 14). Ultrasound will not reliably detect the smaller mesenteric masses, and the lymphangiogram studies only a limited nodal area.

Abdominal Abscess

The CT appearance of an abscess most commonly consists of a relatively low-density mass, with or without a rim that often enhances after the administration of intravenous contrast medium. The internal contents of the mass may contain only fluid or be mixed with gas. The size and shape is affected by location, since abscesses usually are confined to various fascial or intraperitoneal compartments, expanding the spaces and displacing contiguous structures. Needle placement for drainage as well as for diagnosis can be directed by CT.

Gallium imaging, US, and CT are all accurate methods for confirming the presence of intraabdominal abscesses in adults (13,23,36,47,50,86). In children who are not acutely ill and have a fever of unknown origin without localizing signs or symptoms, use of gallium 67-citrate or ^{111}In WBC scanning is recommended as the primary screening test because of its ease of performance and its ability to offer a view of the entire body in a single image. Generally, if the scan is normal, no further evaluation is needed. If the ra-

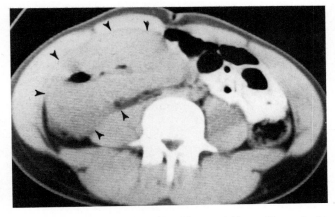

FIG. 14. Burkitt's lymphoma in a 12-year-old boy with a palpable right lower quadrant mass. A soft tissue mass (arrowheads) extends from the anterior abdominal wall to the retroperitoneum. The large mass surrounds the cecum and displaces contrast-medium-filled small bowel to the left.

dionuclide scan is abnormal, CT or US is required for documentation and to determine the full extent of the lesion. Conversely, a patient with localizing signs of disease usually is best studied initially with CT or US. If the patient is acutely ill without localizing signs, and an abdominal abscess is clinically suspected, CT or US also is the procedure of choice, particularly in view of the fact that imaging with gallium requires a delay of 24 hr or more. Although experience in children is limited, a previous report has suggested that CT is the most accurate method for diagnosing abdominal abscesses (51).

The choice of examination between CT and US depends on the individual clinical situation. A US examination is often hampered by a large amount of bowel gas; it also can be suboptimal in the immediate postoperative period because of difficulty in imaging the area directly beneath the surgical wound. Moreover, the left subphrenic area and the lesser sac may be difficult to evaluate by sonography because of the gas-filled stomach. This is especially true in patients with prior splenectomy. Since these areas are readily studied by CT examination, CT is our preferred method. The right subphrenic and subhepatic areas are at least as well studied by US as by CT, and US is the initial procedure of choice. Computed tomography is considered the method of choice when a retroperitoneal abscess is suspected (41).

Blunt Abdominal Trauma

Computed tomographic imaging provides a radiologic display of the entire abdomen following nonpenetrating injuries, and can document parenchymal injury to the liver, spleen, pancreas, and kidney, as well as the presence of a subcapsular hematoma, and intraperitoneal or retroperitoneal hemorrhage (Fig. 15). Fractures and lacerations often appear on CT as irregular, wedge-shaped abnormal densities within or surrounding an organ. Fresh hemorrhages have a density greater than surrounding tissues, whereas chronic hematomas are lower in attenuation value. Subcapsular hematomas usually are lenticular or oval in configuration and flatten or indent the lateral margin of the organ.

In renal trauma, CT is not only more accurate than excretory urography in demonstrating the extent of injury (9,16), but it also supplies information about injuries to other organs. An advantage compared to US is that it demonstrates function as well as anatomy. No transducer contact is necessary and the ileus, which is often associated with trauma, is not a deterrent to CT. Computed tomography is superior to radionuclide scanning in assessing anatomic detail and is not organ specific.

Radionuclide imaging, because of its ease of per-

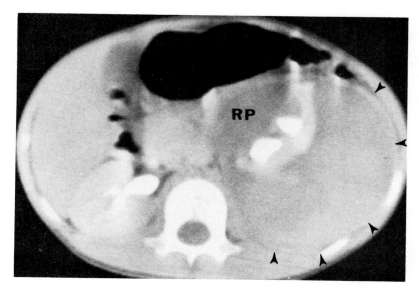

FIG. 15. Renal laceration and perirenal hematoma in an 8-year-old boy following abdominal trauma. A CT scan after contrast medium administration reveals a low density fluid collection (arrowheads) posterolateral to the markedly displaced left kidney. Also noted are dilated contrast-medium-filled renal calyces and a dilated renal pelvis (RP). The CT diagnosis of a perirenal hematoma/urinoma and ureteropelvic junction obstruction was confirmed at surgery.

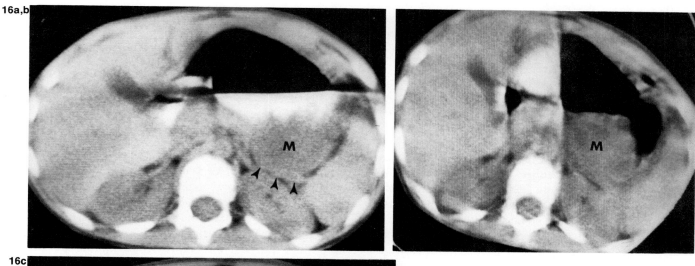

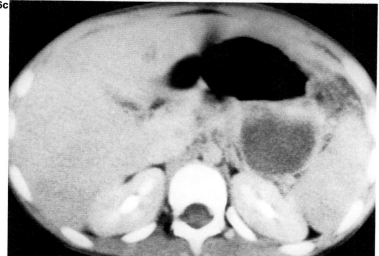

FIG. 16. Extrapancreatic fluid collection in a 7-year-old boy with pleural effusions and elevated serum amylase. **a:** Conventional supine CT scan shows a mass (M) with a low density center occupying the lesser sac anterior to the pancreatic tail (arrowheads). **b:** Scan obtained with the patient in a right lateral decubitus position confirms the presence of a mass (M). **c:** A repeat scan in the supine position after intravenous injection of iodinated contrast medium clearly defines a low density lesion with a thick enhancing wall.

17a,b

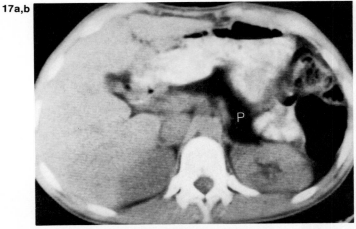
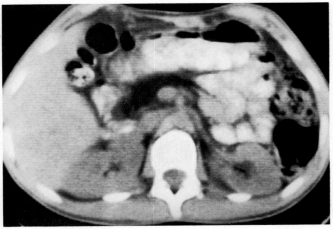

17c

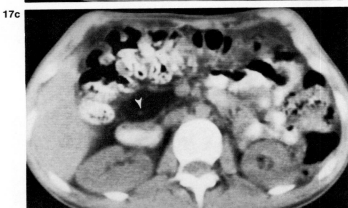

FIG. 17. Fatty pancreas in an 18-year-old girl with cystic fibrosis. Serial CT scans show the pancreas to be completely replaced by fatty tissue. **a:** Body and tail of pancreas (P). **b:** Head and neck of pancreas. **c:** Head and uncinate process of pancreas with visible duct (arrowhead).

formance and its ability to assess function (59), may be the screening procedure of choice when only hepatic or splenic injury is suspected. When a hematoma is suggested, US or CT can provide more precise definition of the extent of injury (61).

Experience with the utility of CT in managing children with blunt abdominal trauma is still evolving. Clearly, CT can be of value by providing accurate information about the presence and degree of injury. More appropriate decisions about surgical or conservative management can be reached. In almost all circumstances, angiography, which previously might have been required for diagnosis, can be obviated.

Pancreatic Disorders

Acute pancreatitis is rare in children but can follow trauma or chemotherapy. On CT, pancreatitis usually appears as diffuse enlargement of the gland with a lower density than normal. This decreased attenuation presumably represents edema and/or necrosis. Frequently, the normal fat planes surrounding the pancreas are obliterated. Pancreatic and extrapancreatic fluid collections are usually well imaged with

CT and displayed as well-defined masses of near water density. The configuration is variable and the collections may be unilocular or multilocular. Commonest sites include the anterior pararenal space, lesser sac (Fig. 16), and the mesenteric root.

In children, recurrent pancreatitis usually is due to hereditary familial pancreatitis. The pancreas and ducts are of normal size but multiple parenchymal calcifications can be identified by CT. Chronic pancreatitis may result from cystic fibrosis; parenchymal calcification as well as total replacement of the gland by fat may be observed (26) (Fig. 17).

In general, US and CT are competitive methods in evaluating pancreatic disease. In patients with good clinical evidence supporting the diagnosis of uncomplicated acute pancreatitis, neither imaging method is necessary. Diagnostic evaluation is reserved for patients with suspected complications. Ultrasound is preferred as the screening examination because it does not require ionizing radiation. In cases where US is suboptimal because of bowel gas, CT may be used to provide valuable information. Computed tomography is considered the method of choice for displaying calcification in suspected hereditary pancreatitis when plain abdominal radiographs are negative or equivocal.

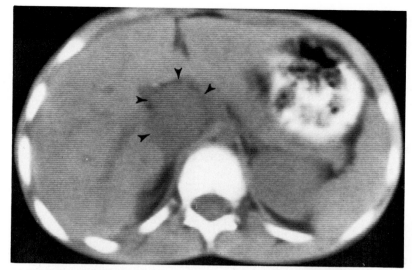

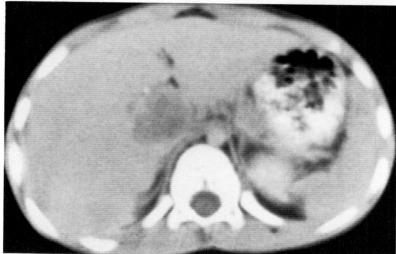

FIG. 18. Porta hepatis metastasis in a 10-year-old boy with previously treated abdominal carcinoma. **Above:** CT scan demonstrates a large low density mass (arrowheads) within the caudate lobe and porta hepatis containing a small area of calcification anteriorly. **Below:** A scan at a slightly higher level after intravenous contrast medium administration shows the tumor tissue enhances less than the normal hepatic parenchyma.

Diseases of the Liver

Diagnosis of certain parenchymal liver disorders can be made with CT because of its ability to measure tissue densities. Fatty infiltration, often associated with severe malnutrition and cystic fibrosis in children, is clearly recognizable by its diminished density (26,74). Attenuation values higher than normal can occur with hemochromatosis and glycogen storage disease (57,70).

In jaundiced patients, US is the preliminary procedure of choice to detect intrahepatic ductal dilatation associated with obstruction as well as a choledochal cyst (33). This can be supplemented by radionuclide studies utilizing the newer hepatobiliary imaging agents (60,64). Although the ability of CT to document the presence of dilated bile ducts is well known, CT should be reserved for cases in which the level or cause of obstruction cannot be determined by other radiologic methods. Choledochal cysts may be depicted by CT (1) as well as mass lesions in the porta hepatis that might result in obstruction of the biliary tree (Fig. 18).

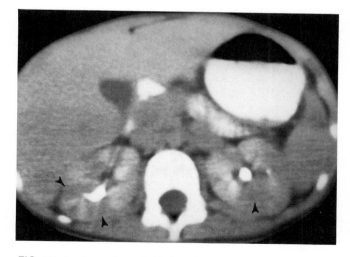

FIG. 19. Acute pyelonephritis in a 6-year-old boy. CT scan after iodinated intravenous contrast medium administration demonstrates multiple wedge-shaped low density areas (arrowheads) within the renal parenchyma, compatible with an acute inflammatory process. These lesions were not evident on urography or ultrasonography. A follow-up urogram 6 weeks after antibiotic therapy showed some bilateral renal atrophy.

Renal Parenchymal Disease

Most renal calcifications in children are associated with obstruction and infection and less frequently are due to metabolic disorders. In rare instances, CT may be of value in detecting lithiasis or nephrocalcinosis before it appears on conventional radiographs (58,62).

Acute pyelonephritis can present as uniform enlargement of the kidney. On postcontrast CT scans, single or multiple areas of lower density, presumably related to inflammatory hypovascularity or microabscesses, are seen frequently (38) (Fig. 19). A CT diagnosis of chronic pyelonephritis is based on recognition of a small kidney with an irregular contour and a blunted calyceal system; unilateral renal hypoplasia, in contradistinction, is associated with a small smooth kidney that usually lies close to the spine.

Excretory urography certainly remains the initial screening procedure for most patients with suspected renal disease because it is easy to perform, relatively inexpensive, and better displays the collecting system. Ultrasound is preferable in patients with allergy to urographic contrast medium or compromised renal function. Computed tomography may be a valuable ancillary examination in patients with acute pyelonephritis and suspected perinephric extension because it provides a better topographic display of the kidney and its adjacent structures than US.

Vascular Structures

Aneurysms are rare in children and occur most frequently in association with Marfan's syndrome, collagen diseases, sepsis, or trauma. Any severe illness associated with intense dehydration may be complicated by thrombosis, particularly of the renal veins. Computed tomography can diagnose anomalies of the abdominal aorta, vena cava, or other vascular structures (14,22,25,69). Frequently, this has been an unexpected discovery in patients studied for other clinical concerns.

Ultrasonography is the preferred examination for confirming a suspected aneurysm because it has the advantage of easily being able to determine the dimensions and the effective lumen of the aorta in longitudinal and transverse sections. However, if the abdomen is obscured by bowel gas, CT can provide the necessary information.

PELVIS

Computed tomography is well suited for evaluating pelvic pathology because most lateral pelvic structures are bilaterally symmetric and, even in very young children, respiratory motion does not interfere with the quality of the scan. Indications for pelvic CT in children include evaluating the character and extent of benign and malignant pelvic masses for treatment planning and follow-up management, and localizing nonpalpable undescended testes.

Benign Pelvic Disorders

A variety of lesions, including presacral and ovarian teratomas, and those due to an infectious, inflammatory, or traumatic nature, can be evaluated. The usefulness of CT in benign diseases is most often related to definitive characterization of a lesion based on the ability to distinguish different tissue densities rather than establishment of the extent of disease (Fig. 20). Teratomas can be confirmed by identification of fatty tissue, calcification, or associated bony anomalies (Fig. 21). Acute hematomas are recognized by their relatively high attenuation value in comparison to other parenchymal organs. Precise identification of other soft tissue masses usually requires further diagnostic evaluation, especially tissue sampling.

Malignant Neoplasms

Rhabdomyosarcoma (sarcoma botryoides) is the commonest primary malignant pelvic tumor in children, frequently involving the vagina and bladder in girls and the prostate, bladder, and urethra in boys. The testis and ovary also may be involved with primary neoplasms. With malignant pelvic neoplasms, CT is most valuable in delineating the extent of tumor as well as its relationships to surrounding structures (24,29). Metastases to pelvic lymph nodes can be detected if the nodes are enlarged. Subtle bony destruction also can be diagnosed.

Impalpable Testes

Cryptorchidism is important because of the increased risk of infertility should the testis remain undescended and because of the increased incidence of malignancy, particularly with an intraabdominal testis. Computed tomography can preoperatively localize the undescended testis and indicate its position, thereby expediting surgical management (55,87).

Clinical Application

When a pelvic mass is detected on physical examination or another radiologic study (e.g., excretory urogram, barium enema), further characterization of the mass and a suggestion of its etiology are possible with both US and CT. Ultrasound should be used in the initial evaluation of most suspected gynecologic masses because it does not require ionizing radiation. How-

20a,b

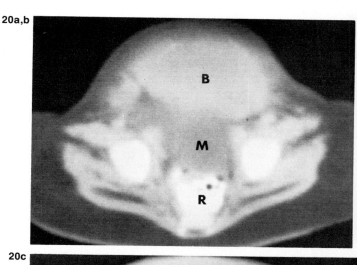

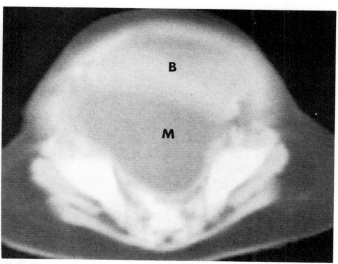

20c

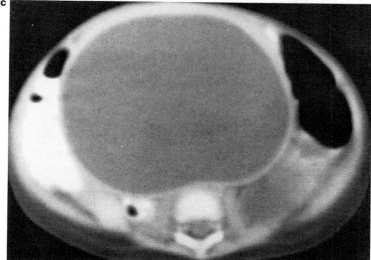

FIG. 20. Hydrocolpos in a 3-month-old girl presenting with an abdominal mass. **a and b:** CT scans through the lower and upper pelvis show a water density mass (M) interposed between the contrast-medium-filled bladder (B) and rectum (R). **c:** At a higher level, the mass almost completely occupies the abdomen. At surgery, a fluid filled vagina was drained and an imperforate vaginal membrane excised.

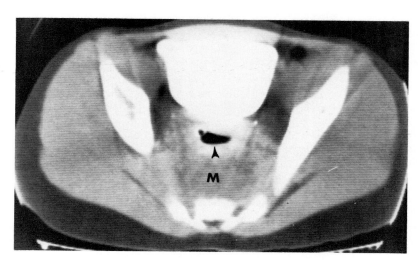

FIG. 21. Malignant presacral teratoma in a 12-year-old girl with chronic constipation. A low density soft tissue mass (M) displaces the rectum (arrowhead) anteriorly. The tumor extends into the pelvo-rectal and presacral fat.

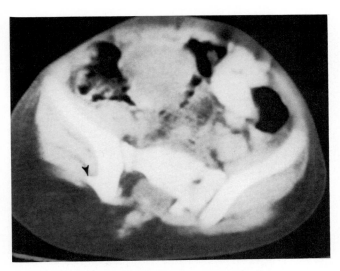

FIG. 22. Congenital iliac anomaly and buttock lipoma in a 3-year-old with a large right buttock mass since birth. Plain radiographs showed a hypoplastic right sacrum and a bony protuberance arising from the right ilium. Pelvic CT shows a lipomatous mass in the area of the right gluteal muscle as well as the extra bony density (arrowhead) arising from the ilium. The sacrum posteriorly is underdeveloped and the spinal contents are contiguous with the fatty tissue, suggesting a lipomeningocele, confirmed at surgery.

ever, US is often suboptimal in the posterior pelvic compartment and the presacral space; CT is useful in these areas in confirming the presence of a suspected pelvic mass and in detecting possible bony involvement. When a pelvic malignancy has been diagnosed, CT is preferable to detect the extent of pelvic invasion prior to surgery, chemotherapy, or radiation therapy (77).

MUSCULOSKELETAL SYSTEM

Computed tomography has several important clinical applications in the evaluation of musculoskeletal disorders. Computed tomography is indicated in patients in whom delineation of soft tissue involvement is important and in the evaluation of abnormalities of complex bony structures (pelvis and spine).

Osseous Tumors

Routine radiographs are comparable or superior to CT in providing a specific diagnosis. When the lesion appears benign but large or appears malignant on plain radiographs, CT is superior in determining the full extent of soft tissue involvement, including information about adjacent blood vessels (8). Such information can often affect the surgical or nonsurgical management of the patient and can be helpful in designing radiation ports (31).

Soft Tissue Tumors

Although CT generally is unable to suggest a specific histologic diagnosis unless the lesions contain predominantly fatty components, it is useful and accurate in delineating the anatomy prior to surgical extirpation (24,85) (Fig. 22). This is especially true around the pelvis and upper thigh. In the more distal extremities, where a paucity of fat and readily recognizable tissue planes exist, US is a superior method for delineating tumor extent.

Osteomyelitis

Computed tomography can display clearly the medullary portion of bone. Normally the marrow cavity of a long bone has a density equal to that of fat; when infected, the density increases to near that of water. In patients in whom the diagnosis of osteomyelitis is uncertain, CT may be helpful by showing this increased density in the abnormal extremity compared to the normal side (49). Such an appearance, however, is not specific for osteomyelitis but also can be observed in neoplasms, storage diseases, trauma, and primary bone marrow disorders.

Pelvis and Spine

The axial skeleton and pelvis frequently are difficult to evaluate with plain radiographs because of the superimposition of bony parts (Fig. 23). Computed tomography is especially useful in symptomatic patients with trauma and equivocal or normal routine radiographs (71). Other special indications in infants

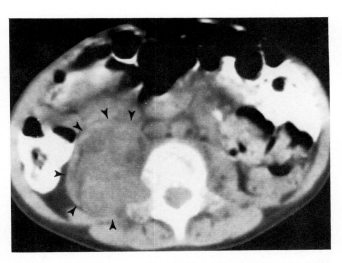

FIG. 23. Ewing's sarcoma in a 7-year-old boy with a 1-year history of back pain. Spine radiographs suggested expansion of the right transverse process of L_3. A CT scan shows a large paraspinal soft tissue mass (arrowheads) with destruction of the adjacent L_3 vertebral body.

and children include evaluation of the dislocated hip in plaster cast and the angle of anteversion of the hip (37).

REFERENCES

1. Araki T, Itai Y, Tasaka A: CT of choledochal cyst. *AJR* 135:729–734, 1980
2. Arger PH, Mulhern CB, Littman PS, Meadows AT, Coleman BG, Jarrett PT: Management of solid tumors in children: Contribution of computed tomography. *AJR* 137:251–255, 1981
3. Barnett PH, Zerhouni EA, White RI, Siegelman SS: Computed tomography in the diagnosis of cavernous hemangiomas of the liver. *AJR* 134:439–447, 1980
4. Baron RL, Gutierrez FR, Sagel SS, Levitt RG, McKnight RC: CT of anomalies of the mediastinal vessels. *AJR* 135:571–576, 1981
5. Baron RL, Lee JKT, Sagel SS, Levitt RG: Computed tomography of the abnormal thymus. *Radiology* 142:127–134, 1982
6. Baron RL, Lee JKT, Sagel SS, Peterson RR: Computed tomography of the normal thymus. *Radiology* 142:121–125, 1982
7. Baron RL, Levitt RG, Sagel SS, Stanley RJ: Computed tomography in the evaluation of mediastinal widening. *Radiology* 138:107–113, 1981
8. Berger PE, Kuhn JP: Computed tomography of tumors of the musculoskeletal system in children: Clinical applications. *Radiology* 127:171–175, 1978
9. Berger PE, Kuhn JP: CT of blunt abdominal trauma in childhood. *AJR* 136:105–110, 1981
10. Berger PE, Kuhn JP: Computed tomography of the hepatobiliary system in infancy and childhood. *Radiol Clin North Am* 19:431–444, 1981
11. Berger PE, Kuhn JP, Munschauer RW: Computed tomography and ultrasound in the diagnosis and management of neuroblastoma. *Radiology* 128:663–667, 1978
12. Berger PE, Munschauer RW, Kuhn JP: Computed tomography and ultrasound of renal and perirenal diseases in infants and children: Relationship to excretory urography in renal cystic disease, trauma and neoplasm. *Pediatr Radiol* 9:91–99, 1980
13. Biello DR, Levitt RG, Melson GL: The roles of gallium-67 scintigraphy, ultrasonography and computed tomography in the detection of abdominal abscesses. *Semin Nucl Med* 9:58–65, 1979
14. Boldt DW, Reilly BJ: Computed tomography of abdominal mass lesions in children. *Radiology* 124:371–378, 1977
15. Bower RJ, Kiesewetter WB: Mediastinal masses in infants and children. *Arch Surg* 112:1003–1009, 1977
16. Brasch RC: Computed tomography in the evaluation of pediatric genitourinary disease. *Urol Clin North Am* 7:223–230, 1980
17. Brasch RC, Abols IB, Gooding CA, Filly RA: Abdominal disease in children: A comparison of computed tomography and ultrasound. *AJR* 134:153–158, 1980
18. Brasch RC, Boyd DP, Gooding CA: Computed tomographic scanning in children: Comparison of radiation dose and resolving power of commercial CT scanners. *AJR* 131:95–102, 1978
19. Brasch RC, Cann CE: Computed tomographic scanning in children. II. An updated comparison of radiation dose and resolving power of commercial scanners. *AJR* 138:127–133, 1982
20. Brasch RC, Gooding CA: Extracranial computerized tomography in children: Initial clinical experiences and radiation dose considerations. *Prog Pediatr Radiol* 7:100–131, 1980
21. Brasch RC, Korobkin M, Gooding CA: Computed body tomography in children: Evaluation of 45 patients. *AJR* 131:121–125, 1978
22. Buschi AJ, Harrison RB, Brenbridge AN, Williamson BR, Gentry RR, Cole R: Distended left renal vein: CT/sonographic normal variant. *AJR* 135:339–342, 1980
23. Callen PW: Computed tomographic evaluation of abdominal and pelvic abscesses. *Radiology* 131:171–175, 1979
24. Carter BL, Kahn PC, Wolpert SM, Hammerschlag SB, Schwartz AM, Scott RM: Unusual pelvic masses: A comparison of computed tomographic scanning and ultrasonography. *Radiology* 121:383–390, 1976
25. Coleman CC, Saxena KM, Johnson KW: Renal vein thrombosis in a child with the nephrotic syndrome: CT diagnosis. *AJR* 135:1285–1286, 1980
26. Cunningham DG, Churchill RJ, Reynes CJ: Computed tomography in the evaluation of liver disease in cystic fibrosis patients. *J Comput Assist Tomogr* 4:151–154, 1980
27. Damgaard-Pedersen K: Neuroblastoma follow-up by computed tomography. *J Comput Assist Tomogr* 3:274–275, 1979
28. Damgaard-Pedersen K: CT and IVU in the diagnosis of Wilms' tumor. A comparative study. *Pediatr Radiol* 9:207–211, 1980
29. Damgaard-Pedersen K, Edeling CJ, Hertz H: CT whole body scanning and scintigraphy in children with malignant tumors. *Pediatr Radiol* 8:103–107, 1979
30. Damgaard-Pedersen K, Jensen J, Hertz H: CT whole body scanning in pediatric radiology. *Pediatr Radiol* 6:222–229, 1978
31. deSantos LA, Bernardino ME, Murray JA: Computed tomography in the evaluation of osteosarcoma: Experience with 25 cases. *AJR* 132:535–540, 1979
32. Frija J, Lardé D, Belloir C, Botto H, Martin N, Vasile N: Computed tomography diagnosis of renal angiomyolipoma. *J Comput Assist Tomogr* 4:843–846, 1980
33. Gates GF, Sinatra FR, Thomas DW: Cholestatic syndromes in infancy and childhood. *AJR* 134:1141–1148, 1980
34. Goodwin JD, Webb WR: Dynamic computed tomography in the evaluation of vascular lung lesions. *Radiology* 138:629–635, 1981
35. Griscom NT: The roentgenology of neonatal abdominal masses. *Am J Roentgenol Radium Ther Nucl Med* 93:447–463, 1965
36. Haaga JR, George C, Weinstein AJ, Cooperman AM: New interventional techniques in the diagnosis and management of inflammatory disease within the abdomen. *Radiol Clin North Am* 17:485–513, 1979
37. Hernandez RJ, Tachdjian MO, Poznanski AK, Dias LS: CT determination of femoral torsion. *AJR* 137:97–101, 1981
38. Hoffman EP, Mindelzun RE, Anderson RU: Computed tomography in acute pyelonephritis associated with diabetes. *Radiology* 135:691–695, 1980
39. Hope JW, Borns PH, Koop CE: Radiologic diagnosis of mediastinal masses in infants and children. *Radiol Clin North Am* 1:17–50, 1963
40. Hope JW, Koop CE: Abdominal tumors in infants and children. *Med Radiogr Photogr* 38:1–51, 1962
41. Jeffrey RB, Callen PW, Federle MP: Computed tomography of psoas abscesses. *J Comput Assist Tomogr* 4:639–641, 1980
42. Kasper TE, Osborne RW Jr, Semerdjian HS, Miller HC: Urologic abdominal masses in infants and children. *J Urol* 116:629–633, 1976
43. Kelsey JA, Bowie JD: Grey-scale ultrasonography in the diagnosis of polycystic kidney disease. *Radiology* 122:791–795, 1977
44. Kirks DR, Korobkin M: Computed tomography for chest examinations in children. *Pediatr Ann* 9:192–199, 1980
45. Kirks DR, Korobkin M: Chest computed tomography in infants and children: An analysis of 50 patients. *Pediatr Radiol* 10:75–82, 1980
46. Kirks DR, Ponzi JW, Korobkin M: Computed tomographic diagnosis of calcified inferior vena cava thrombus in a child with Wilms' tumor. *Pediatr Radiol* 10:110–112, 1980
47. Knochel JW, Koehler RP, Lee TG, Welch DM: Diagnosis of abdominal abscesses with computed tomography, ultrasound, and 111In leukocyte scans. *Radiology* 137:425–432, 1980
48. Korobkin M, Kirks DR, Sullivan DC, Mills SR, Bowie JD: Computed tomography of primary liver tumors in children. *Radiology* 139:431–435, 1981
49. Kuhn JP, Berger PE: Computed tomographic diagnosis of osteomyelitis. *Radiology* 130:503–506, 1979
50. Kuhn JP, Berger PE: Computed tomographic diagnosis of abdominal abscesses in children. *Ann Radiol (Paris)* 23:153–158, 1980
51. Kuhn JP, Berger PE: Computed tomographic imaging of abdominal abnormalities in infancy and childhood. *Pediatr Ann* 9:200–209, 1980
52. Kuhn JP, Berger PE: Computed tomography of the kidney in infancy and childhood. *Radiol Clin North Am* 19:445–461, 1981

53. Lebowitz RL, Griscom NT: Neonatal hydronephrosis: 146 cases. *Radiol Clin North Am* 15:49–59, 1977

54. Lee JKT, McClennan BL, Melson GL, Stanley RJ: Acute focal bacterial nephritis: Emphasis on grey scale ultrasonography and computed tomography. *AJR* 135:87–92, 1980

55. Lee JKT, McClennan BL, Stanley RJ, Sagel SS: Utility of computed tomography in the localization of the undescended testis. *Radiology* 135:121–125, 1980

56. Leonidas JC, Carter BL, Leape LL, Ramenofsky ML, Schwartz AM: Computed tomography in diagnosis of abdominal masses in infancy and childhood: Comparison with excretory urography. *Arch Dis Child* 53:120–125, 1978

57. Long JA Jr, Doppmann JL, Nienhus AW, Mills SR: Computed tomographic analysis of Beta-thalassemic syndrome with hemochromatosis: Pathologic findings with clinical and laboratory correlations. *J Comput Assist Tomogr* 4:159–165, 1980

58. Luers PR, Lester PD, Siegler RL: CT demonstration of cortical nephrocalcinosis in congenital oxalosis. *Pediatr Radiol* 10:116–118, 1980

59. Lutzker L, Koenigsberg M, Meng CH, Freeman LM: The role of radionuclide imaging in spleen trauma. *Radiology* 110:419–425, 1974

60. Majd M, Reba RC, Altman RP: Hepatobiliary scintigraphy with 99mTcPIPIDA in the evaluation of neonatal jaundice. *Pediatrics* 67:140–145, 1981

61. Mall JC, Kaiser JA: CT diagnosis of splenic laceration. *AJR* 134:265–269, 1980

62. Manz F, Jaschke W, vanKaick G, Waldherr R, Willich E: Nephrocalcinosis in radiographs: Computed tomography, sonography and histology. *Pediatr Radiol* 9:19–26, 1980

63. Megibow AJ, Bosniak MA: Dilute barium as a contrast agent for abdominal CT. *AJR* 134:1273–1274, 1980

64. Miller JH, Sinatra FR, Thomas DW: Biliary excretion disorders in infants: evaluation using 99mTcPIPIDA. *AJR* 135:47–52, 1980

65. Rabinowitz R, Segal AJ, Rao HKM, Pathak A: Computed tomography in diagnosis of infantile polycystic kidney disease. *J Urol* 120:616–617, 1978

66. Ravitch MM, Sabiston DC: Mediastinal infections, cysts and tumors. In: *Pediatric Surgery,* ed. by MM Ravitch, KJ Welch, CD Benson, E Aberdeen, JG Randolph, Chicago, Year Book Medical Publishers, 1979, pp 499–512.

67. Resjo IM, Harwood-Nash DC, Fitz CR, Chuang S: Normal cord in infants and children examined with computed tomographic metrizamide myelography. *Radiology* 130:691–696, 1979

68. Resjo IM, Harwood-Nash DC, Fitz CR, Chuang S: CT metrizamide myelography for intraspinal and paraspinal neoplasms in infants and children. *AJR* 132:367–372, 1979

69. Royal SA, Callen PW: CT evaluation of anomalies of the inferior vena cava and left renal vein. *AJR* 132:759–763, 1979

70. Royal SA, Goldberg HI, Thaler MM: *Evaluation of Cryptogenic Hepatomegaly by Computed Tomography.* Presented at the 22nd Annual Meeting of the Society of Pediatric Radiologists, Toronto, 1979

71. Sauser DA, Billimoria PE, Rouse GA, Mudge K: CT evaluation of hip trauma. *AJR* 135:269–274, 1980

72. Schaner EG, Chang AE, Doppman JL, Conkle DM, Flye MW, Rosenberg SA: Comparison of computed and conventional whole lung tomography in detecting pulmonary nodules: A prospective radiologic-pathologic study. *AJR* 131:51–54, 1978

73. Schmidt T, Stieve FE: Radiation exposure of infants and children in computed tomography. *Ann Radiol* 23:143–149, 1980

74. Scott WW Jr, Sanders RC, Siegelman SS: Irregular fatty infiltration of the liver: Diagnostic dilemmas. *AJR* 135:67–71, 1980

75. Shackelford GD, McAlister WH: Errors in the diagnosis of Wilms' tumor. *CRC Crit Rev Radiol Sci* 3:171–196, 1972

76. Shackelford GD, McAlister WH: Mediastinal teratoma confused with loculated pleural fluid. *Pediatr Radiol* 5:118–119, 1976

77. Siegel MJ, Glasier CM, Sagel SS: Computed tomography of pelvic disorders in children. *AJR* 137:1139–1143, 1981

78. Siegel MJ, Sagel SS: Computed tomography as a supplement to urography in the evaluation of suspected neuroblastoma. *Radiology* 142:435–438, 1982

79. Siegel MJ, Sagel SS, Reed K: The value of computed tomography in the diagnosis and management of pediatric mediastinal abnormalities. *Radiology* 142:149–155, 1982

80. Slovis TL, Cushing, B, Reilly BJ, Farooki ZQ, Philippart AI, Berdon WE, Baker DH, Reed JO: Wilms' tumor to the heart: Clinical and radiographic evaluation. *AJR* 131:263–266, 1978

81. Slovis TL, Perlmutter AD: Recent advances in pediatric urological ultrasound. *J Urol* 123:613–620, 1980

82. Totty WA, McClennan BL, Melson GL, Patel R: Relative value of computed tomography and ultrasonography in the assessment of renal angiomyolipoma. *J Comput Assist Tomogr* 5:173–178, 1981

83. Tschappeler H: Computed tomography (CT) and lymphoma in children. *Ann Radiol* 23:87–91, 1980

84. Vinocur CD, Dinn WM, Dudgeon DL: Computed tomographic scanning in children. *J Pediatr Surg* 12:847–856, 1977

85. Wilson JS, Korobkin M, Genant HK, Bovill EG: Computed tomography of musculoskeletal disorders. *AJR* 131:55–61, 1978

86. Wolverson MK, Jagannadharao B, Sundaram M, Joyce PF, Riaz MA, Shields JB: CT as a primary diagnostic method in evaluating intraabdominal abscess. *AJR* 133:1089–1095, 1979

87. Wolverson MK, Jagannadharao B, Sundaram, M, Riaz MA, Nalesnik WJ, Houttuin E: CT in localization of impalpable cryptorchid testes. *AJR* 134:725–729, 1980

88. Wright FW, Ledingham JGG, Dunnill MS, Grieve NWT: Polycystic kidneys, renal hamartomas, their variants and complications. *Clin Radiol* 25:27–43, 1974

Chapter 19

Comparative Imaging

G. Leland Melson, Daniel R. Biello, and Joseph K. T. Lee

Just as computed tomography (CT) has rapidly developed and has become established as a major imaging technique, important advancements have also occurred in ultrasonography (US) and radionuclide imaging (RI). The availability of these three imaging methods has resulted in many interesting and perplexing problems for clinicians, radiologists, and health care administrators and planners. Questions that must be faced almost daily include: which imaging method should be utilized in a given clinical situation? If more than one technique is to be employed, what is the optimum sequence? Which is the most ''cost effective''? In many instances definitive answers to these questions are not known or are still evolving. A discussion of the accuracy of CT in evaluating each anatomical area has been incorporated into the appropriate chapters elsewhere in this textbook. The major objectives of this chapter will be: (a) to compare and contrast the physical principles on which CT, US, and RI are based and which in many situations result in complementary information being provided by these competing modalities; (b) to compare the relative advantages and disadvantages of each method; and (c) to examine those factors that make it difficult to achieve categorical conclusions regarding the relative accuracy of these techniques.

PHYSICAL BASES FOR CT, US, AND RI IMAGING

A detailed discussion of the physical principles and instrumentation of CT is found elsewhere in this text (Chapter 1). For purposes of comparison the basic characteristics of the interrogating energy and the physical properties of matter that are responsible for image production in CT, US, and RI are shown in Table 1.

Electromagnetic, ionizing radiation is employed by both CT and RI. X-rays, usually in the 120 kVp energy range, are utilized in CT whereas gamma rays in the 80 to 360 keV range form the basis of the most widely used nuclear medicine studies. In comparison, US employs high frequency (2.25–10 MHz), nonionizing mechanical waves that require a molecular medium for propagation. The energy that is processed to produce an image is transmitted in the case of CT, reflected in US, and emitted in RI. Although preliminary work in US transmission scanning incorporating reconstruction techniques has been reported and transmission scans were formerly performed in nuclear medicine, neither of these methods is currently employed clinically.

Both CT and US images represent tomographic sections of the body. The slice thickness in CT may be varied by collimation and is relatively uniform in thickness throughout a given section. In US the thickness of the image ''slice'' varies with the distance of the tissue from the transducer and the focal characteristics of the transducer, being relatively thicker in the near and far fields of the image and thinner within the focal zone of the transducer (11).

Images in all three methods represent the spatial distribution of certain physical and physiological properties of the area studied. The characteristics of matter that are responsible for image production, however, are quite different for the three techniques. CT images depict the X-ray attenuating properties of the area examined. For the energy range utilized in clinical scanning, X-ray attenuation is determined by the physical density, the effective atomic number, and the electron density (15).

The physical properties determining the reflection of US waves vary with the relative size of the reflecting surface and the wave length (λ) of the interrogating beam. If the reflecting surface is larger than λ (specular reflector), the proportion of energy reflected is related to the difference in acoustic impedance (Z) between the two media separated by the interface and is dependent on the angle of incidence of the beam, but is independent of the frequency of the beam. Specular reflectors are responsible for the sonographic demonstration of borders of organs, blood vessels, and a va-

TABLE 1. *Physical bases for imaging with CT, US, and RI*

Bases	CT	US	RI
Type of interrogating energy	Electromagnetic ionizing	Mechanical nonionizing	Electromagnetic ionizing
Energy producing image	Transmitted	Reflected	Emitted

Physical properties of matter depicted by image	Effective atomic number
	Electron density
	Physical density
		Acoustic impedance
		  Physical density
		  Speed of propagation of sound
		Bulk modulus of elasticity
		Size of reflectors
			Varied physical and physiological
			  Active transport
			  Capillary blockade
			  Cell sequestration
			  Compartmental localization
			  Diffusion
			  Phagocytosis

riety of other structures. Acoustic impedance, in turn, is the product of the physical density of the medium (ρ) and the velocity of US propagation within that medium (C)(9). In equation form these relationships are expressed as:

$$Z = \rho C$$

and

$$\% \text{ reflected} = \left| \frac{Z_2 - Z_1}{Z_2 + Z_1} \right|^2 \times 100$$

where: Z, acoustic impedance; C, velocity of US propagation; ρ, physical density of the medium; Z_1, acoustic impedance of medium 1; Z_2, acoustic impedance of medium 2.

When the reflector is smaller than λ (diffuse reflector), the factors governing reflection of the sonic beam are more complex. Diffuse reflections are independent of beam angulation and vary with both the frequency of US and the diameter of the reflector (8). Such reflections are responsible for the patterns of "tissue texture." In most clinical situations the proportion of incident sound reflected by diffuse reflectors correlates well with the bulk modulus of elasticity of the tissue interrogated (5).

Radionuclide images represent the spatial distribution of an administered radiopharmaceutical within an area of interest. In the visualization of organs two general types of images may be obtained (14). In one the administered radiopharmaceutical localizes in the area of abnormality, resulting in a region of increased uptake or "hot" area, such as in bone scanning or ^{67}Ga citrate scanning for abscess or neoplasm. In the second type, labeled compound localizes in normal tissues with abnormalities represented as areas of decreased or absent activity ("cold" areas). Examples of studies of the second type are lung scanning using labeled particles and liver scanning using a sulfur colloid preparation. Generally, the most sensitive studies result from uptake of the radiopharmaceutical by areas

of abnormality. Mechanisms of radiopharmaceutical localization include compartmental localization, simple or exchange diffusion, active transport, phagocytosis, cell sequestration, and capillary blockade (14).

It might be expected that the differing physical and physiological properties on which these three imaging techniques are based would in some instances result in the generation of complementary or supplementary information or provide a clear advantage to one method in a given situation. Indeed, this has proven to be true in both *in vitro* and *in vivo* studies. The US and CT appearance of various fluids has been studied using a phantom composed of material having US and CT characteristics of liver tissue (6). For selected fluids,

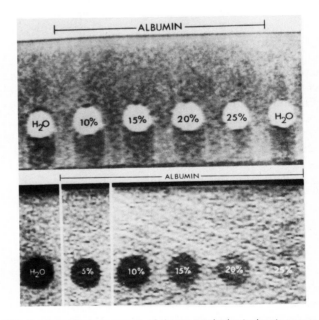

FIG. 1. **Top.** Ultrasonogram of tissue-equivalent phantom containing from left to right: water, albumin solutions of concentrations 10, 15, 20, and 25% by weight, and water. **Bottom:** CT scan of the phantom containing from left to right: water, albumin solutions of concentrations 5, 10, 15, 20, and 25% by weight. All fluids exhibit classic US criteria for fluid. Most of the fluids are well differentiated from the phantom by CT, but the 25% of albumin solution is poorly detected. (From Filly et al., ref. 6, with permission.)

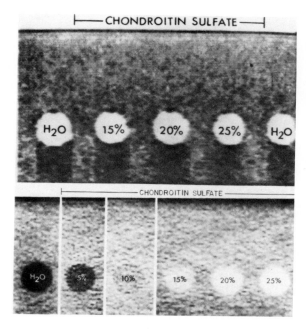

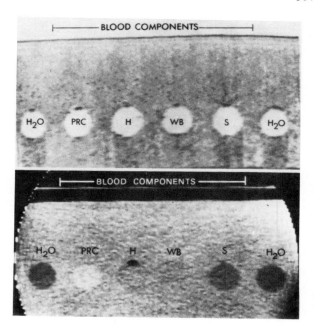

FIG. 2. Top: Ultrasonogram of tissue-equivalent phantom containing from left to right: water, chondroitin sulfate solutions of concentrations 15, 20, and 25% by weight, and water. **Bottom:** CT scan of the phantom containing from left to right: water, condroitin sulfate solutions of concentrations 5, 10, 15, 20, and 25% by weight. By US all fluids demonstrate classic criteria for fluid. Water and 5% chondroitin sulfate are clearly detected by CT but 10% condroitin sulfate is poorly separated from the phantom by CT. The 15, 20, and 25% condroitin sulfate solutions are more dense than the phantom. (From Filly et al., ref. 6, with permission.)

FIG. 3. Ultrasound **(top)** and CT **(bottom)** scans of phantom containing from left to right: water, packed red cells (PRC), hemolysate (H), whole blood (WB), serum (S), and water. All fluids are anechoic, but packed red cells show no acoustic enhancement and the hemolysate exhibits more acoustic enhancement than whole blood. Whole blood and hemolysate are nearly indistinguishable from the phantom by CT whereas packed red cells are denser than the phantom. (From Filly et al., ref. 6, with permission.)

measurements of CT number, ultrasound absorption, and viscosity were also obtained. All fluids, including blood and blood products and concentrated solutions of albumin and chondroitin sulfate, were anechoic and exhibited acoustic enhancement on US scans, and could therefore be easily differentiated from the phantom itself (Figs. 1–3). Fluids having CT numbers much lower than the phantom were readily detected by CT whereas those having CT numbers similar to the phantom (whole and hemolyzed blood, 25% albumin, and 10% chondroitin sulfate) were either poorly detected or undetectable. Concentrated solutions of chondroitin sulfate and packed red cells appeared more dense than the phantom (Figs. 2 and 3).

These theoretical considerations and *in vitro* observations explain findings encountered in clinical practice in which CT and US clearly may provide complementary information concerning the nature of fluids and the differentiation between solid tissue and fluid. For example, septations in ovarian or renal cysts may be clearly demonstrated on US scans but not shown by CT (Fig. 4). In these instances the difference in acoustic impedance between the thin but solid septations and the surrounding cyst fluid results in a strong, specular reflection on US scanning whereas the small

difference in X-ray attenuation by these two components of the lesion is not sufficiently great to resolve the thin septations from the adjacent fluid by CT.

Differentiation of high-density bloody fluid from adjacent solid tissue may not be possible on noncontrast enhanced CT scans although the distinction can be clearly shown on US (Fig. 5). In contradistinction, CT may differentiate bloody ascites from urine because the former has a higher attenuation value whereas US will display both types of fluid as being anechoic (Fig. 5). Although freshly clotted blood usually has a higher density on CT than flowing blood, CT may be unable to differentiate old clotted blood from a seroma, since both have low attenuation values (Fig. 6). On sonography, freshly clotted blood is anechoic or has low echogenicity whereas organized hematomas are echogenic (Fig. 6) and true seromas are sonolucent.

Low-density solid lesions such as metastases may occasionally be confused with cysts or abscesses on CT but their solid nature is more clearly shown by US (Fig. 7). On the other hand, CT is clearly superior to US for distinguishing small collections of air from small calcifications, both of which are highly echogenic and may cause acoustic shadowing but have highly characteristic CT numbers. For the same rea-

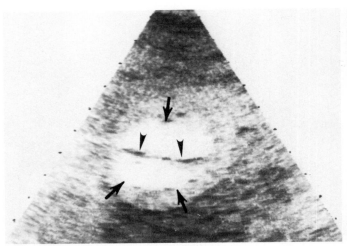

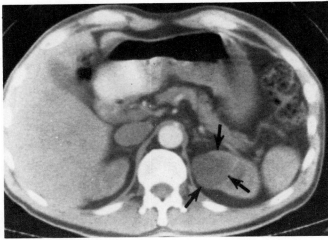

FIG. 4. Septated renal cyst. **Left:** Transverse real-time mechanical sector US demonstrates a sharply marginated sonolucent mass (arrows) surrounded by renal cortex. An echogenic septation, subsequently proven by cyst aspiration and cystogram, extends through the central portion of the cyst (arrowheads). **Right:** Contrast-enhanced CT scan shows a left upper pole smoothly marginated water density mass (arrows) but no septation. The septation is well demonstrated by US due to the difference in acoustic impedance between the cyst fluid and the septation. Because the septation and cyst fluid cause essentially identical X-ray attenuation, they are not separated by CT.

5a

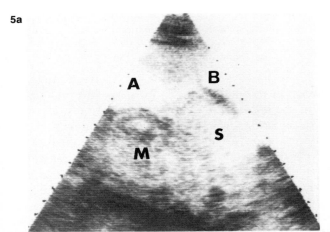

FIG. 5. Ovarian carcinoma with hemorrhagic ascites. **a:** Transverse real-time mechanical sector sonogram shows an inhomogeneous solid mass in the right pelvis (M) deviating the sigmoid colon (S) laterally. Ascites (A) is present anterior to the mass and lateral to the bladder (B). **b:** CT scan of the pelvis demonstrates the solid pelvic mass (M) to be essentially the same density as the bloody ascites (A). S, sigmoid colon. **c:** CT scan 2 cm caudal to **b** shows urine within the bladder (B) to be lower in density than the bloody ascites (A). S, sigmoid colon. US clearly separated the solid pelvic mass from ascites, but was unable to distinguish between urine and bloody ascites.

5b,c

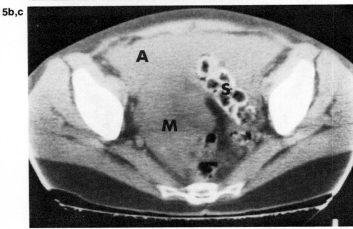

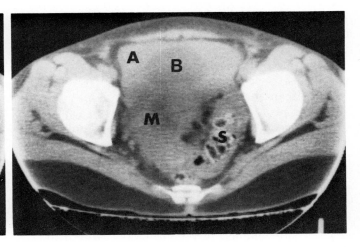

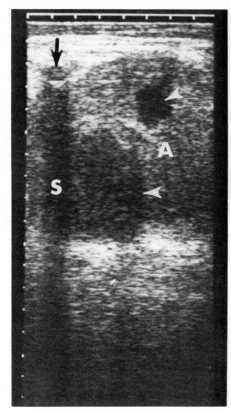
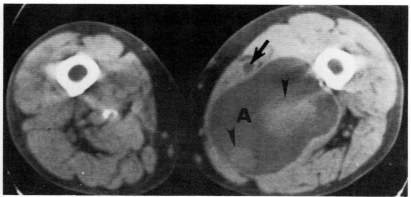

FIG. 6. Large clot-filled pseudoaneurysm in the left thigh following femoral popliteal arterial bypass graft surgery. **Left:** Transverse US obtained with linear array real-time scanner demonstrates the pseudoaneurysm (A) to be filled primarily by material of medium echogenicity. There are a few irregular, relatively hypoechoic zones (arrowheads). The synthetic arterial graft (arrow) casts an acoustic shadow (S). **Above:** CT scan shows the pseudoaneurysm (A) to consist largely of near-water density material with scattered zones of near soft tissue density (arrowheads). Arrow, arterial graft. The low density material could have been either an old blood clot or a seroma but the US characteristics are typical of clotted blood. The zones that are hypoechoic on US and higher density on CT are due to more recent hemorrhage.

son, CT may unequivocally distinguish fat from other echodense solid tissue.

RELATIVE ADVANTAGES AND DISADVANTAGES OF IMAGING TECHNIQUES

In addition to their ability to image different properties of tissues, CT, US, and RI have inherent characteristics that confer relative advantages or disadvantages to each in given situations (Table 2). Ultrasound is the least invasive of the three techniques since, at the present time, no adverse biological effects from US at the power level and frequency used in clinical scanning have been documented in intact mammals. Longitudinal studies of infants and children subjected to US scanning *in vitro* are in progress and a variety of *in vitro* assessments of the adverse effects of US on organisms or subcellular structures have been reported (3). A careful assessment of all of these studies will be necessary before it is definitely established that US as utilized in clinical scanning had no deleterious effects. Radionuclide imaging subjects the patient to variable, but generally small amounts of radiation. The distribution of this exposure varies throughout the body with the "target organ," i.e., the organ concentrating the radiopharmaceutical, receiving the highest dose, which may range from 1 to 4 rad. In patients who

undergo CT without the administration of intravenous iodinated contrast medium, the only invasive feature of the study is a low dose of radiation that varies somewhat depending on the scanner employed and the number of scans obtained but generally is comparable to that from established radiographic studies of the abdomen such as an excretory urogram or barium enema. If intravenous contrast medium is used, the risks of adverse reaction to this material are added to the procedure.

Computed tomography is by far the most expensive of the three methods, with state-of-the-art scanners now costing well over $1,000,000. In contrast, the cost of US scanners has remained relatively stable for the past several years or actually decreased. Most static B-mode and real-time scanners currently cost $50,000 to $70,000. Some technically advanced but "stripped down" real-time instruments now sell for under $25,000, and are easily afforded by smaller hospitals and even physicians' offices. Standard and large field of view gamma cameras with advanced electronics are priced in the $100,000 to $175,000 range.

Current US and RI equipment is highly reliable, whereas most CT scanners are subject to small-to-moderate amounts of downtime related chiefly to computer and mechanical malfunction.

Image and examination quality in CT and RI have a low degree of dependence on the skill of the tech-

7a,b

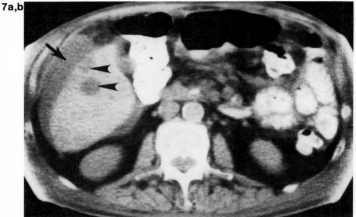
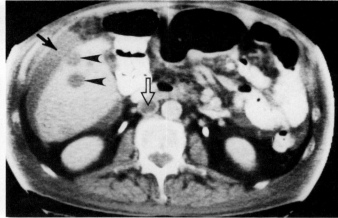

7c

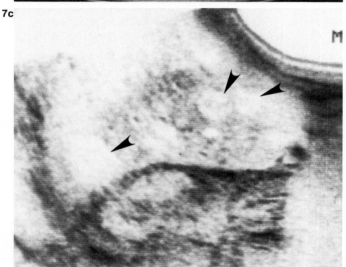

FIG. 7. Low-density hepatic metastases from carcinoma of the pancreas. **a:** Precontrast CT scan shows round well-circumscribed lesions (arrowheads) within the liver that are the same density as ascitic fluid (arrow). **b:** Postcontrast CT scan demonstrates that the lesions (arrowheads) fail to enhance and that a thrombus is present in the inferior vena cava (open arrow). **c:** Parasagittal US of the liver shows multiple hypoechoic areas (arrowheads), some of which are indistinctly marginated, without acoustic enhancement or refraction shadows. The CT characteristics suggest that the hepatic lesions are possibly benign cysts, but the US features establish that they are solid.

nologist operating the equipment. Despite considerable improvement in US instrumentation, the technique remains highly dependent on the skill of the operator. Clinician acceptance, i.e., the ability of clinicians to appreciate imaging findings and to understand their significance, is highest for CT, in which images "look just like a section through a cadaver." Nuclear medicine studies are moderately well accepted by most clinicians, but fewer feel comfortable with sonograms.

Spatial resolution in CT has progressively improved and now is approximately 1 to 2 mm for most scanners and less than 1 mm for high-contrast objects. The major determinant of spatial resolution in US is the transducer. Axial resolution is dependent on frequency and pulse length whereas lateral resolution is determined by beam focusing. State-of-the-art articulated arm and real-time scanners achieve in clinical scanning conditions an axial resolution of approximately 1 to 2 mm and lateral resolution of 2 to 3 mm. Superficial parts, high-resolution scanners employing 7.5 to 10 MHz transducers may have both axial and lateral resolutions of approximately 1 mm. In RI, res-

olution is dependent on the instrument and collimation used, but generally is approximately 2 to 3 cm in most examinations. High-resolution collimators may achieve spatial resolution of 0.5 to 1.0 cm. For all three techniques, spatial resolution is related to the contrast range present in the image. The greater the difference in contrast between the object resolved and its surroundings, the smaller the spatial resolution that may be attained. For example, minimally dilated bile ducts or small metastases may be resolved by CT only after administration of intravenous contrast medium that increases the contrast difference between these alterations and surrounding normal liver.

In CT, spatial resolution is uniform throughout the entire image, whereas in US and RI maximal resolution is achieved only within the focal zone of the transducer or collimator. More uniform resolution is accomplished by dynamic focusing of electronically phased array US transducers, but such instruments have thus far gained widespread acceptance only in echocardiography. Also, CT images display information about the entire portion of the body contained within the plane of the image, whereas most high-

TABLE 2. Relative advantages and disadvantages of CT, US, and RI

Characteristic	CT	US	RI
Invasiveness	Noninvasive to mildly invasive	Noninvasive	Noninvasive
Adverse biological effects	Minimal	None	Minimal
Cost	High	Lowest	Low
Reliability	Moderate	High	High
Operator dependence	Low	High	Low
Clinician acceptance	High	Fair	Good
Resolution	1−2 mm	Variable: optimally 1 mm axial 2 mm lateral	2−3 cm
Field of high resolution	Entire image	Limited	Limited
Area of interest	Limited	Limited	Limited in some, entire body in others
Dependence of image on perivisceral fat	Moderate	Non−minimal	None
Image degradation by:			
Patient motion	Min−moderate	Least	Minimal
Bone	None	Marked	Minimal
Gas	None	Marked	None
Obesity	None	Min−moderate	None
Multiplane capability	With special programs	Easily accomplished	With special instrumentation
Portability	Fixed	Portable	Portable units available
Ability to evaluate function	Min−moderate blood flow and renal function only	Minimal: displays motion	Highest
Obstetrical applications	Not used	Very useful	Rarely used
Neurological applications	Most valuable	Useful only in neonates and infants	Moderately useful
Cardiac applications	Low	High	High
Direction of interventional procedures	High	High	None

resolution sonograms consist of a sector or limited single pass scan through the area of interest and RI represents only the organ system(s) within which the radiopharmaceutical is localized. Thus, CT is the technique most likely to result in appreciation of significant findings outside a predetermined area of interest. Furthermore, CT permanently records all information in the plane imaged, thereby facilitating retrospective review.

Both US and CT are directed to an area of interest; the entire body is not imaged. In patients with fever or suspected bone pathology, but having no localizing symptoms, whole body RI may detect an area of abnormality that may be further characterized by CT or US (Fig. 8).

The quality of CT images, particularly in the mediastinum and retroperitoneum, is partially dependent on the amount of perivisceral fat that outlines the margins of the soft tissue density structures. On the other hand, the borders of structures in US are provided by specular reflectors and are much less dependent on the presence of surrounding tissue of different echogenicity. In some patients having a paucity of fat, US may provide clearer delineation of structures than the latest CT scanners (Fig. 9). Radionuclide imaging is relatively unaffected by this factor other than the increased narrow angle scatter in obese patients.

Patient body habitus and condition generally have greater effect on image quality in US than in CT or RI. Obesity, large amounts of bowel gas, and bone are impediments to obtaining high-quality US scans that are not likely to be overcome in the near future. Sector real-time instruments have greatly reduced the problem of obtaining an adequate "window" for scanning. Patient motion significantly degraded CT images on early scanners but is a minor problem in most cases for "fast" scanners. Ultrasonography has always been relatively less limited by patient motion than CT and real-time scanners have maintained this advantage. Radionuclide imaging is affected by patient motion but compensatory data manipulations are available.

In the ease with which images can be obtained in multiple planes, US has a clear advantage, particularly when real-time scanners are used. Parasagittal, coronal or oblique sections having equal information content may be rapidly obtained simply by reorienting the plane of the transducer. Images in these planes may be very helpful in defining anatomical relationships and the precise origin and position of pathological processes, particularly with respect to the diaphragm (Fig. 10). Although such images may also be produced by many CT scanners, the process normally involves reconstruction from information originally obtained in transverse planes of section. In many instances for optimal results the original imaging planes must be more closely spaced than normally obtained for a

8a

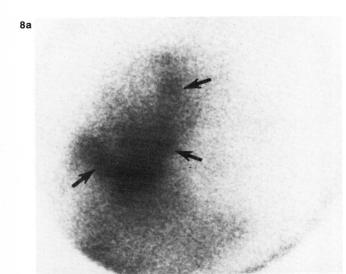

8b,c

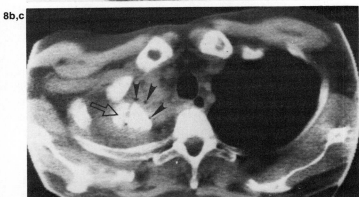
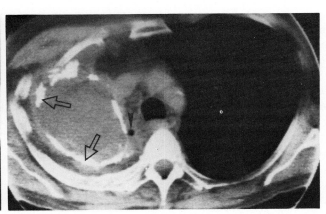

FIG. 8. Thoracic abscess in a patient with fever of unknown origin 16 years following a pneumonectomy for bronchogenic carcinoma. **a:** ⁶⁷Ga citrate scan of the thorax and upper abdomen demonstrates increased uptake in the right hemithorax (arrows). **b,c:** CT scans show peripheral calcification (open arrows) and a few gas bubbles (arrowheads) compatible with an abscess or bronchopulmonary fistula. Placement of a chest tube resulted in drainage of more than 500 ml of pus. In this patient having no localizing symptoms and a normal CT scan of the abdomen 2 weeks previously, RI localized an unsuspected area of pathology.

9a,b

9c,d

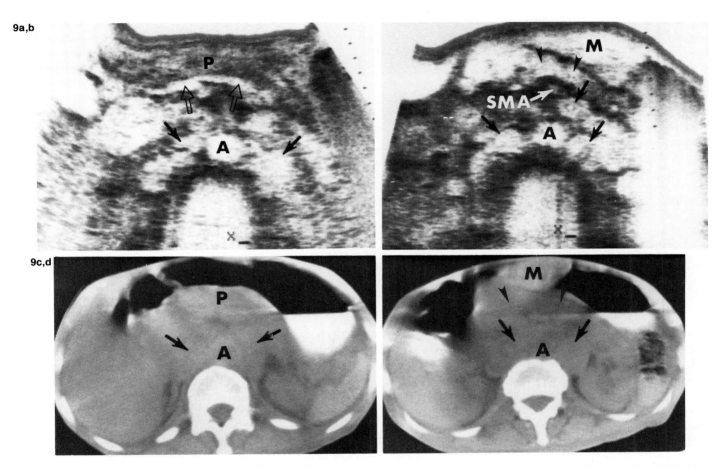

FIG. 9. Elderly cachectic man with palpable abdominal mass due to lymphoma. **a:** Limited transverse sonogram demonstrates the normal pancreas (P) anterior to the splenic vein (open arrows). Multiple lobulated masses of low-to-medium echogenicity (arrows) surrounding the aorta (A) are enlarged lymph nodes. **b:** Limited transverse sonogram at the level of palpable mass (M) shows this mass to involve the anterior abdominal wall. The mass is similar in echogenicity to enlarged retroperitoneal (arrows) and mesenteric lymph nodes (arrowheads). SMA, superior mesenteric artery; A, aorta. **c:** CT scan at the same level as **a**. The pancreas (P) and a mantle of soft tissue density, characteristic of prevertebral lymphadenopathy (arrows), surrounding the aorta (A) are shown. The enlarged lymph nodes are essentially the same density as the aorta and pancreas and are poorly delineated from these structures. **d:** CT scan at the same level as **b** demonstrates the palpable mass (M) and enlarged mesenteric (arrowheads) and retroperitoneal lymph nodes (arrows). A, aorta. In this patient having a paucity of body fat, the lobulated nature of the matted lymph nodes involved with lymphoma and the distinction between lymphomatous tissue and the pancreas and aorta are much more clearly demonstrated by US than by CT.

10a,b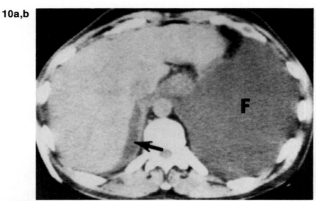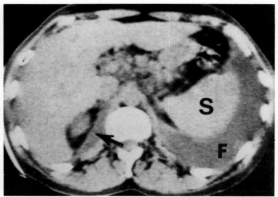

10c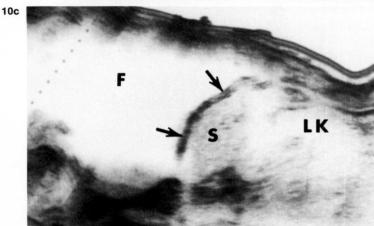

FIG. 10. Large left pleural effusion in a patient with pancreatitis. **a:** CT scan of upper abdomen shows a large fluid collection in the left upper quadrant (F). A small right pleural effusion (arrow) is present. **b:** CT scan 2 cm caudal to **a** reveals the fluid collection (F) to be posterolateral to the spleen (S). Arrow, right pleural effusion. **c:** Coronal sonogram with the patient in the right lateral decubitus position shows the fluid (F) all to be above the diaphragm (arrows). No subdiaphragmatic fluid is present. S, spleen; LK, left kidney. The CT study was originally interpreted as showing the fluid collection to be beneath the diaphragm, most likely a pancreatic pseudocyst. The US scan clearly established that the fluid was a large pleural effusion.

study consisting only of transverse sections, resulting in higher radiation exposure to the patient. Image degradation may result from registration errors related to patient motion or respiration. Direct coronal CT of the abdomen and pelvis using specially designed positioning devices can provide useful, high-quality images (16). However, this technique may not be possible in uncooperative or very ill patients.

Portability of real-time scanners has made US the method of choice for examining and directing invasive procedures on critically ill patients in intensive care units who are dependent on multiple life support systems. Portable gamma cameras are also available but are more cumbersome than US. However, bedside RI evaluation of lung, renal, and cardiac function is readily performed in critically ill patients. Some CT scanners are suitable for mobile installations in vehicles for movement among institutions, but it is unlikely that this technique will become truly portable.

Radionuclide imaging, particularly with computer processing of data, has much greater ability to assess organ function than US or CT at the present time (Fig. 11). Qualitative evaluation of blood flow within the kidney and other organs and some parameters of cardiac function may be accomplished by dynamic CT following intravenous injection of iodinated contrast

materials. Quantitation of flow is possible by analysis of the appearance time and density of contrast within a vessel or organ under research conditions, but has not become as generally applicable, or as sophisticated, as the RI determination of thyroid function, pulmonary ventilation and perfusion, myocardial perfusion, or cardiac and renal function. Ultrasonographic assessment of physiology is at present limited to qualitative evaluation of motion, except for echocardiography in which quantitative determinations of wall and valve motion, aortic valve area, and left and right ventricular function have been reported. Doppler US has potential for providing considerable information regarding blood flow in the heart and vessels but current applications are limited to the peripheral vessels.

Because of several of the previously discussed characteristics, these three major imaging techniques have differing ranges of applicability. Computed tomography has had perhaps its greatest impact in evaluating the cranial contents, where, except in infants and neonates, US is severely limited by bone. Likewise, virtually total reflection of sound by the air-containing lung and, to a lesser degree, by ribs renders US of limited utility in assessing the thorax other than for localizing pleural effusions and cardiac evaluation. On the other hand, the lack of known adverse biological effects,

11a

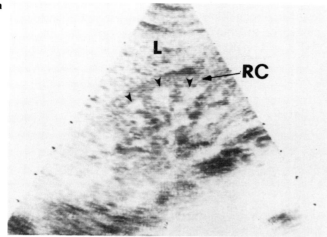

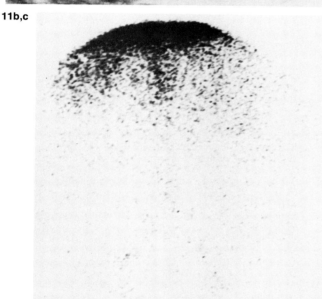

11b,c

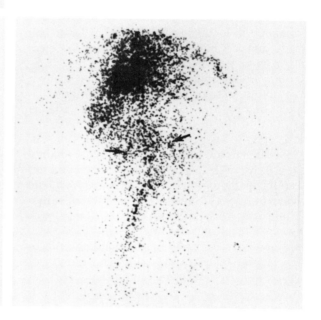

FIG. 11. Acute renal cortical necrosis in a 4-year-old girl. **a:** Oblique parasagittal real-time sonogram shows the renal cortex (RC) to be more echogenic than the liver (L) and clearly separated from the relatively sonolucent renal pyramids (arrowheads). **b:** ^{99m}Tc glucoheptonate flow study performed the same day as the sonogram, at a time when the patient was anuric, shows no blood flow to the kidneys. **c:** Repeat RI study done after 2 weeks of hemodialysis when the serum creatinine clearance was approximately 5 ml/min demonstrates some blood flow to the kidneys (arrows).

ease of assessing motion, and portability make US the ideal method for evaluating obstetric and pediatric patients.

Both CT and US may be used to direct interventional procedures, such as percutaneous biopsies, percutaneous nephrostomies, and abscess drainage. Computed tomography has the distinct advantage of providing direct confirmation of the position of the needle tip, wherever it might be, including within bone. Its demonstration is unaffected by interposed bowel gas or bone. Some real-time US scanners also permit confirmation of needle position and may be used intraoperatively. Generally, we have found that many procedures may be more quickly and easily accomplished and more readily coupled with fluoroscopic evaluation using US guidance than with CT without the necessity of localizing needle position. This is especially true when the needle needs to be inserted into a cystic space or a large mass.

COMPARATIVE ACCURACY OF CT, US, AND RI

Experience in many centers has established that CT, US, and RI are highly accurate in diagnosing a wide spectrum of pathological processes. The results of studies that have assessed the accuracy of these techniques have been incorporated into the appropriate chapters. At the present time, several factors make definitive conclusions concerning the absolute diagnostic accuracy and most appropriate utilization of these techniques difficult to achieve.

First, there have been relatively few centers in which technical expertise, technology, and interpreter experience and interest are equally highly developed for all methods. Radionuclide imaging was well established prior to the emergence of US and CT. In most academic centers in which either US or CT became especially well developed early in their evolution, development of the other method generally lagged significantly. More recently an increasing number of institutions have achieved parity among all techniques.

Second, relatively few well-designed and conducted prospective studies utilizing sophisticated statistical analysis to assess all imaging modalities have been published. Major sources of initial enthusiasm for the accuracy of a technique, not borne out by subsequent experience, are failure to include an adequate proportion of patients without disease and interpreter bias based on the knowledge of previously conducted tests (13). Recently reported, well-designed prospective studies found that CT was superior to US for the evaluation of the adrenal (1) and pancreas (7) and to US and RI for detecting hepatic metastases from breast or colon cancer (2), but all three methods were equally valuable in localizing the source of fever (12) and that CT and US had equal sensitivities for diagnosing obstructive jaundice (4).

Third, rapid advancement of technology has made it difficult to obtain state-of-the-art studies on large patient populations before "significant" improvements in one or more of the imaging technologies make the conclusions open to question. "Fast" 3rd and 4th generation CT scanners are generally felt to have distinct advantages over their predecessors. Improved instrumentation, including digital signal processing, the use of higher frequency transducers, and the development of improved real-time scanners, together with new knowledge regarding the interaction of US with matter and carefully designed and conducted clinical studies have contributed to the continued growth of sonography. Improved instrumentation, but particularly new radiopharmaceuticals, offers unlimited potential for new applications in RI.

Finally, as previously discussed, each method demonstrates different properties of tissue and in many situations provides complementary or supplementary information. All of these factors will likely make necessary ongoing re-evaluation of the accuracy and most appropriate utilization of these valuable methods.

In conclusion, no single imaging method has proven superior to the other two in all patients and in all clinical situations. Whether one method is selected over another depends not only on the strengths and weaknesses of that technique, but also on machine availability and relative expertise existing in each institution.

REFERENCES

1. Abrams HL, Siegelman SS, Adams DF, Sanders R, Finberg HJ, Hessel SV, McNeil BJ: Computed tomography versus ultrasound of the adrenal gland: A prospective study. *Radiology* 143:121–128, 1982
2. Alderson PO, Adams DF, McNeil BJ, Sanders R, Siegelman SS, Finberg H, Hessel SJ, Abrams HL: A prospective study of computed tomography, ultrasound and nuclear imaging of the liver in patients with breast or colon cancer. *J Nucl Med* 22:35, 1981
3. Baker ML, Dalrymple GV: Biological effects of ultrasound: A review. *Radiology* 126:479–483, 1978
4. Baron RL, Stanley RJ, Lee JKT, Koehler RE, Melson GL, Balfe DM, Weyman PJ: Prospective comparison of the evaluation of biliary obstruction with CT and US. *Radiology (in press)* 1982
5. Chivers RC: Phase and amplitude fluctuations in the propagation of acoustic waves in lossless inhomogeneous continua with velocity, density and bulk modulus variations. *Ultrasound Med Biol* 4:353–361, 1978
6. Filly RA, Sommer FG, Minton MJ: Characterization of biological fluids by ultrasound and computed tomography. *Radiology* 134:167–171, 1980
7. Hessel SJ, Siegelman SS, McNeil BJ, Sanders R, Adams DF, Alderson PO, Finberg HJ, Abrams HL: A prospective evaluation of computed tomography and ultrasound of the pancreas. *Radiology* 143:129–133, 1982
8. Hill CR: Ultrasonic attenuation and scattering by tissues. In: *Handbook of Clinical Ultrasound*, ed. by deVlieger, M et al., New York, John Wiley and Sons, 1978, pp 91–98
9. Kremkau FW: *Diagnostic Ultrasound—Physical Principles and Exercises*, New York, Grune and Stratton, 1981, p 24
10. Kremkau FW: *Diagnostic Ultrasound—Physical Principles and Exercises*, New York, Grune and Stratton, 1981, pp 29–32
11. Kremkau FW: *Diagnostic Ultrasound—Physical Principles and Exercises*, New York, Grune and Stratton, 1981, pp 54–71
12. McNeil BJ, Sanders RC, Alderson PO, Hessel SJ, Finberg HJ, Siegelman SS, Adams DF, Abrams HJ: Prospective study of computed tomography, ultrasound and gallium imaging in patients with fever. *Radiology* 139:647–653, 1981
13. Ransohoff DF, Feinstein AR: Problems of spectrum and bias in evaluating the efficacy of diagnostic tests. *N Engl J Med* 299:926–930, 1978
14. Subramanian G, Rhodes BA, Cooper JF, Sodd VF: *Radiopharmaceuticals*, New York, The Society of Nuclear Medicine, Inc., 1975
15. Ter-Pogossian MM: *The Physical Aspects of Diagnostic Radiology*, New York, Hoeber Medical Division, Harper and Row, Publishers, 1967, pp 64–95
16. van Waes PFGM, Zonneveld FW: Direct coronal body computed tomography. *J Comput Assist Tomogr* 6:58–66, 1982

Chapter 20

Radiation Oncology

Miljenko V. Pilepich, Satish C. Prasad, and Todd H. Wasserman

Computed tomography has profoundly affected the management of a large proportion of cancer patients, including those treated with radiotherapy. The optimal applications of CT within the diversity of tumor sites and stages are emerging but are far from being completely defined.

The strategy of the diagnostic work-up and treatment of cancer grows increasingly complex. Following the initial *diagnosis,* an accurate *staging* (definition of tumor extent) is required for most malignancies before a rational application of surgical, radiotherapeutic, and chemotherapeutic *treatment* can be planned. Of obvious importance is lifelong *follow-up* for evaluation of the results of treatment and early detection of possible recurrences and complications of treatment. Computed tomography can play an important role in each of these four steps: diagnosis, staging, treatment, and follow-up.

A large percentage of cancer patients with localized or local-regional disease receive radiotherapy (either alone or in combination with other therapeutic modalities) with curative intent. Success of such treatment will depend, among other factors, on the radiotherapist's ability to deliver an adequate dose to the tumor in its entirety while preserving the normal structures. There are several steps involved in achieving this rather complex goal. These steps include: (a) accurate localization of tumor volume and surrounding normal structures; (b) prescription of a dose to be delivered to tumor volume(s) and the definition of limiting doses to normal tissues; (c) accurate computation of dose distribution within the treatment volume of the patient, and (d) precise delivery of radiation dose over the entire course of treatment.

COMPUTED TOMOGRAPHY AND DETERMINATION OF TREATMENT VOLUME

The accurate localization of normal structures and tumor and their three-dimensional representation has long been a weak link in radiation treatment planning.

Moreover, accurate computation of absorbed dose distribution within a patient requires a precise knowledge of the patient's surface contour and radiation absorption properties of internal tissues. Computed tomography has become a useful tool in radiotherapy planning by providing the above information with a precision that was not possible in the past.

Before making a rational decision on the choice of equipment, beam quality, position and shape of ports, use of accessories, doses, and fractionation pattern, the radiation therapist needs to define: (a) clinically and radiographically *detectable tumor volume;* (b) *volume at risk for subclinical (microscopic) involvement,* although clinically and radiographically free of disease (in some instances, this volume of tissue will be defined by anatomical boundries such as bony structures, fascias, organ capsules, and serosal surfaces); (c) *location of the critical normal structures* that are dose-limiting (e.g., spinal cord, bowel, kidney, lung); and (d) *treatment volume* and the doses to be delivered within the volume. These terms are defined in some detail in Figs. 1–3.

The cross-sectional CT scan images delineating body contour, tumor, and internal structures are well suited for immediate application in radiotherapy (2,3,10,14,18,19,22,27,32,33,40,43,46,49,50).

The important considerations to be reviewed during interpretation of the CT scans for radiotherapy by the diagnostic radiologist are: (a) anatomical and quantitative definition of tumor extent; (b) relationship of tumor mass to bone structures as well as to key organs (i.e., heart, liver, kidney, spinal cord); and (c) identification of tumor in distant anatomical compartments (e.g., mediastinum versus hilum, mesenteric versus retroperitoneal). It is very important that the tumor extent be defined quantitatively in centimeters and in all directions, as well as relative to key organs within the anatomical region. It also may be useful to represent tumor extent in relation to vertebral body position. It is helpful if the tumor mass can be somewhat defined on a supine conventional or computed (digital) radiograph. It is also important to identify

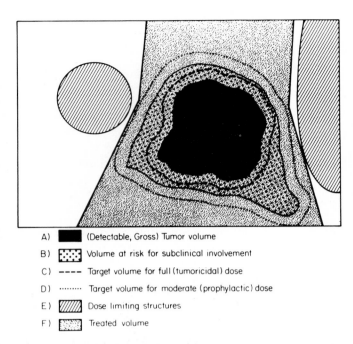

A) ■ (Detectable, Gross) Tumor volume

B) ▨ Volume at risk for subclinical involvement

C) ---- Target volume for full (tumoricidal) dose

D) ········ Target volume for moderate (prophylactic) dose

E) ▨ Dose limiting structures

F) ▨ Treated volume

FIG. 1. Schematic description of the frequently used terminology in radiotherapy treatment planning. **A:** *Gross tumor volume* implies the radiographically and clinically detectable tumor. **B:** *Volume at risk for subclinical involvement* is the volume of tissue in which the tumor is not clinically and radiographically detectable, but is at high risk for microscopic involvement. In defining this volume, the radiotherapist uses the known characteristics of the primary tumor, such as tendency to lymphatic spread, or permeation of tissues, as judged by the degree of histological differentiation. **C:** *Target volume,* which needs *to receive high tumoricidal doses* to eradicate a tumor, is somewhat larger than the gross tumor volume. A safety margin has been added around the tumor to provide for the daily variation in positioning of the patient and the treatment beams. **D:** *Target volume* that needs *to be treated to lower (prophylactic) doses* includes the volume at risk for subclinical involvement with a safety margin to provide for variations in the positioning of the patient and the treatment beam. In most tumors, the prophylactic doses range between 4,000 and 5,500 rad. **E:** *Dose-limiting structures* are an important consideration in the treatment planning. The spinal cord is an example, the dose to which is limited to 4,500 rad in 4 to 5 weeks. If a large area of the lung is to be treated, the dose is usually limited to 2,000 rad or less in 2 weeks or longer. The kidneys and the liver are also dose-limiting structures. The usually accepted level of tolerance for the kidneys, if the whole of the kidney parenchyma is to be treated, is 2,000 rad in 2 weeks or longer. For the liver, the accepted tolerance limit is 3,000 rad in 3 weeks. **F:** *Treated volume* is comprised of all tissues that get irradiated, including those that happen to be in the passage of the beam only incidentally.

separately other tumor masses that may exist in distinct anatomical compartments. Examples would be to separate mediastinal from hilar lymph node disease, and mesenteric from retroperitoneal lymph node disease.

There have been several attempts to quantitate the impact of CT on radiotherapy treatment planning. Munzenrider et al. (33) analyzed retrospectively one of the first sizable groups of patients for whom CT information had been systematically utilized in treatment planning. In their experience, CT data were con-

sidered essential for therapeutic decision-making in 55% of patients studied and prompted a change in treatment volume in 45% of cases.

Goitein et al. (18) reported the results of a prospective study designed to assess the value of CT in radiotherapy treatment planning for 77 patients. Conventional studies were performed first and computer-generated treatment plans were drawn up. Subsequently, CT scans were used to delineate the location of the tumor and adjacent normal tissues and the treatment plans were altered when necessary. In 32 patients (42%), techniques were changed because of inadequate tumor coverage. Considerations of normal tissue coverage were the only reason for field changes in 4 patients. In 36 patients (47%), radiotherapy plans were changed as a result of the CT examination.

The available literature indicates that, depending on tumor type, CT information has prompted changes in treatment planning in 34 to 61% of studied cases (8,14,18,19,33,36). Although there is no doubt that CT has a major influence on radiotherapy planning, the degree to which these CT-induced modifications alter the clinical course (tumor control and treatment-related morbidity) remains to be quantitated through a controlled study. Yet the CT scan has had an almost universal acceptance and utilization as a novel and noninvasive approach to definition of internal structures. The design of a prospective controlled study of the impact of CT on therapeutic results would be greatly hampered because of this.

TECHNICAL CONSIDERATIONS

Certain technical problems associated with whole body scanners must be eliminated before CT scans can be used in treatment planning. For example, most scanner couches that support the patient are concave. The radiotherapy treatment machine couches are generally flat. The difference in couch design causes the patient's body contour and location of internal organs to be different during treatment compared to that during scanning. Also, a few of the older scanners employ bolus material around patients to obtain good quality images. The weight of the bolus distorts the patient's surface contour and the internal anatomy. In general, the setup of a patient during CT should be identical to that used during radiation treatment. If a patient is to be treated in a position other than supine, the CT scan should also be done in that position. This was not always possible because the scanning aperture size on some early generation scanners was small (40 cm for an EMI 5005 scanner). In addition, the small diameter of the image reconstruction size results in edge cutoff of the patient's contour in many anatomical regions. This limitation poses a problem in treatment

2a,b

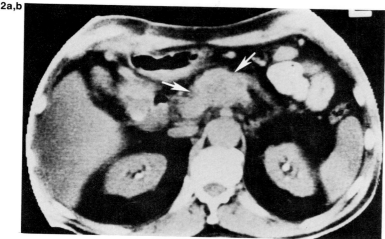

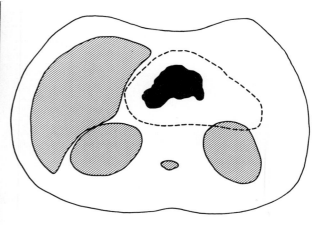

2c

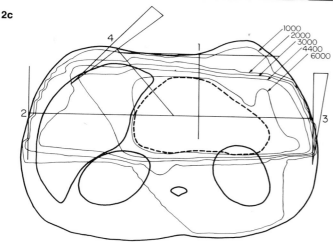

1000
2000
3000
4400
6000

FIG. 2. Seventy-one-year-old man with carcinoma of the pancreas. **a:** The scan delineates the tumor (arrows) in the body of the pancreas. At this level, the tail of the pancreas and the major part of the head of the pancreas are not visualized. **b:** The volume to receive the full tumoricidal doses has been delineated on the basis of several slices. Provision is made for inclusion of the tail. The dose-limiting structures are the spinal cord, kidneys, and liver. The delineation of the kidneys and the liver does not correspond exactly to Fig. 2a since other representative cuts above the slice shown in Fig. 2a are taken into account. **c:** Treatment plan delineating four-field arrangement. Fields 3 and 4 are wedged. The vicinity of the tumor volume to critical structures (spinal cord, kidneys, and liver) makes irradiation of the pancreas a particularly difficult one. In this case, the tumor with generous margins receives a dose of approximately 6,000 rad. The major portion of the renal parenchyma remains outside the 2,000 rad isodose. A large portion of the hepatic parenchyma receives 3,000 rad or less. *Isodose lines in this and subsequent figures refer to lines delineating areas within a treatment plan receiving the same dose.*

planning because lateral radiation beams are often employed for treatment. If it can be anticipated that the scan will be used for radiotherapy treatment planning, an appropriate number of full contour scans should be obtained above, through, and below the tumor bearing areas. To utilize the CT scan for planning, one must properly register CT slices with respect to appropriate landmarks on a patient's skin surface or on computed or conventional radiographic film. The use of radiopaque marks on key external surfaces is often helpful.

Most existing radiation therapy centers have dedicated treatment planning computers that use patient contour and internal structure information obtained from means other than CT scans. These data are usually entered into the computer by means of light pen or tracing devices. Optically or photographically enlarged CT images also can be entered into a treatment planning computer. Although this procedure can be used without any modification of existing treatment planning computers, the matrix of CT data should be transferred to the treatment planning computer di-

rectly via a magnetic tape or a floppy disk for the sake of efficiency and accuracy of dose computation.

Based on our experience and that of others (11,17, 24,42), the design features of a CT scanner that will be useful in radiation therapy are as follows: (a) large scanner aperture (60 cm or more); (b) flat couch surface; (c) capability of producing anteroposterior and lateral digital radiographs to reference scan slices; (d) scanning without bolus material; (e) availability of patient immobilization devices and alignment lasers; (f) good spatial and contrast resolution; (g) fast scan time and capability of producing a large number of slices within a reasonable time period; (h) sagittal and coronal reconstruction capability; and (i) data storage and transfer capability for treatment planning.

Most of the problems discussed above have been eliminated in the newer generation CT scanners. These scanners have larger aperture size (60 cm for EMI 7070 scanner) and do not require bolus material. A larger reconstruction field of view (50 cm for the EMI 7070 scanner) capability is available and may be used to obtain images containing the full contour of a patient.

3a,b

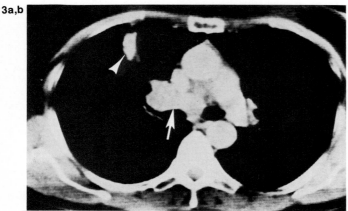

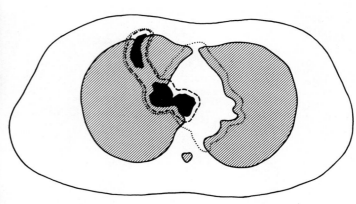

3c

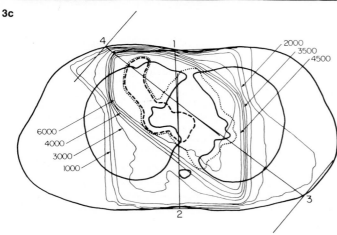

FIG. 3. Sixty-three-year-old woman with carcinoma of the lung. **a:** Primary tumor (arrowhead) is a relatively small lesion located anteriorly adjacent to the chest wall and most likely invading the chest wall. The hilum and the adjacent mediastinum are involved (arrow). **b:** Blackened area is grossly detectable tumor. The areas to receive full tumoricidal doses (in this case 6,000 rad), and the area to receive prophylactic doses (in this case 4,500 rad), are delineated. The shaded areas represent the dose-limiting structures, which are, in this case, the lungs and the spinal cord. **c:** Treatment plan that utilizes a complex set of four beams. Beams 1 and 2 are AP and PA; 3 and 4 are oblique opposed beams. A combination of 18 and 4 MV X-ray beams is used. A substantial portion of the lung parenchyma at the treated level is included in the treated volume. Even at this level, a substantial portion of the lung receives less than 2,000 rad. It should be stressed that in this patient, the bases of the lung need not be included in the treatment volume; the total volume of irradiated lung is, therefore, not excessive.

The location of CT slices can be registered with respect to a digital radiograph obtained on the scanner. The concave couch on a CT scanner can be made flat by means of a hard foam or wooden insert.

Table 1 lists technical factors to be considered when obtaining CT images for radiotherapy treatment planning. Most of these suggestions will help ensure that the CT scan conforms to the patient position parameters that will be used during radiotherapy. Therefore, prior to CT it is essential that the radiation therapist informs the diagnostic radiologist about the planned treatment position to be used. It is important that the CT study fully defines the extreme dimensions of the tumor, with at least several levels of normal anatomy above and below the gross disease.

Table 2 lists the parameters of radiotherapy treatment that can be determined by CT scan information. Some of these measurements can be determined accurately only by modern CT scan information and were not used prior to the advent of CT. These data provide not only for better tumor localization but also for better and truer physical representation of the effects of the radiation.

Radiation therapists often use a *simulator*, a ma-

chine that mimics the physical parameters of a radiation therapy machine, but is capable of producing X-rays of diagnostic energies only. The simulator is designed to test the options that may be available for treatment of a patient, to test the ability of a patient to maintain a reproducible position, and to provide clear X-ray images of the paths of the photon beam. A number of commercial prototype units that integrate the CT scanner directly into the simulator currently are being developed. Most of these have a computer interface that allows for on-line treatment planning and

TABLE 1. *Technical considerations in CT scans for radiotherapy*

Use flat couch surface, not concave one.
Scan patients in reproducible treatment position: supine, prone, lateral.
Scan patient with arms and legs in intended treatment position.
Represent position of scan slices on an AP computed or conventional radiograph.
Show entire patient contour on scan.
Avoid bolus material or use thin sheet of bolus only so as not to distort the body contour by external weight.
Use sufficient number of scan slices to define tumor's extent in all directions.

TABLE 2. *Parameters of radiotherapy treatment that can be determined by CT scan information*

Patient diameters—cross-sectional dimensions
Field size
Depth for dose specification
  From skin (depth dose)
  From skin to axis (distance for isocentric treatment)
Depth from surface of dose-limiting organs or structures
Portal or field angles for oblique and rotational fields
Absorption data (tissue density)
Isodose distribution

control of the simulator to show the dose delivery capability of such treatment planning.

COMPUTED TOMOGRAPHY AND DOSE COMPUTATION

At the present time, most radiotherapy treatments are delivered by Cobalt-60 gamma rays or high energy (megavoltage) X-rays produced by linear accelerators and betatrons. Electron beams produced by linear accelerators and betatrons are also gaining wider acceptance. In addition, a few specialized radiotherapy research centers are using charged particles such as protons, pions, and heavy ions (41).

In radiotherapy, an accurate delivery of radiation dose to many anatomical sites within a patient is complicated by the presence of dose-perturbing inhomogeneities such as bone and lung tissue. To take into account the effects of dose-perturbing tissues, the location and absorption properties of these inhomogeneities must be known. For beam modalities used in radiotherapy, the absorption properties of tissues are determined primarily by the electron density (electron per cc) or the physical density (grams per cc) of the tissue. Some of the most useful information obtained from CT scans is the linear attenuation coefficients of tissues for diagnostic X-ray energies. Several investigators (9,20,21,34,35,39) have shown how these CT numbers, which are relative linear attenuation coefficients at diagnostic energies, can be related to electron or physical density of the tissue. This has generated considerable interest in the development of treatment planning programs that utilize CT scan data. Several commercial companies have developed CT-based treatment planning computers where two-dimensional dose distributions are overlayed on CT scans. For the purposes of dose computation, the CT scan data are transferred to the treatment planning computer via floppy disk or magnetic tape. The CT number of each pixel is converted to electron density by an experimentally determined (computer-stored) curve correlating CT numbers with electron density. Absorbed dose is computed in two dimensions where the difference in electron density of an individual pixel element relative to water is taken into account (34,39). For photon beam dose calculations,

the inhomogeneity corrections are significant in the lung tissue (3,39,40,47). Inhomogeneity correction is particularly important for charged particle dose calculations because the infinite range of charged particles in tissue makes it critical that the location of tumor, tissue inhomogeneities, and their electron densities are accurately known. The application of CT scan in treatment planning with charged particle beams has been reported by several authors (9,16,20,27).

CT IN THE MANAGEMENT OF SELECTED TUMORS

Bronchogenic Carcinoma

Although the majority of intrapulmonary lesions can be easily identified by conventional radiographs, CT has proven invaluable in the definition of tumor extent. It is particularly useful in the evaluation of the involvement of mediastinal lymph nodes and direct extension of the tumor to mediastinal structures and the chest wall. Invasion of any of these structures is usually considered a contraindication for surgical resection; therefore, this information is important in the selection of patients for radiotherapy. Documentation of the presence of gross tumor in the mediastinal lymph nodes or the chest wall indicates a need to increase the dose and the field size substantially in these areas.

An example of the use of CT in treatment planning in carcinoma of the lung is shown in Fig. 3. Because patients breathe freely during radiation treatment, it is best to obtain the CT images in resting mid-expiration. In most instances, treatment is given with the arms positioned along the chest rather than raised above the head. Obtaining the CT images with arms in the same position prevents from distortion of the patient contour and shifting of the internal structures. Also, window level should be taken into account while determining the size of the lung lesion (25).

Carcinoma of the Bladder

Determination of the depth of penetration of the primary tumor through the bladder wall is essential in staging and choice of therapy for bladder carcinoma. The customary clinical staging procedures are cystoscopy, transurethral resection of the tumor, and bimanual examination under anesthesia. Clinical staging differs from pathological staging in a large percentage of cases. In most instances, the error is due to clinical understaging, which occurs in approximately one-third of the cases (52). Since patients with deeply invasive tumors usually receive preoperative radiotherapy, identification of these patients prior to exploration-resection (cystectomy) is essential. Several reports indicate a high degree of correlation between CT staging and pathological staging in deeply invasive tumors (23,54); however, CT is not useful in assessing the depth of penetration in more superficial tumors. Although CT can show grossly enlarged lymph node metastases, it will not indicate spread within normal-sized lymph nodes, resulting in understaging.

Computed tomography has also been shown to be useful in the optimization of radiotherapy treatment planning primarily by providing better definition of position and topographic relationship of the bladder. In the series of Schlager et al. (45), CT information caused revisions in 29% of treatment plans.

A potentially promising area of CT application in the radiotherapy of bladder cancer is the evaluation of tumor response following preoperative irradiation. In patients whose tumors regress significantly following a course of preoperative radiotherapy to moderate doses, cystectomy may be avoided if additional radiotherapy to full tumoricidal doses is given (53). Results of a study reported by Veenema et al. (51) support this approach.

Carcinoma of the Prostate

Radiotherapy is playing an increasingly important role in the curative management of carcinoma of the prostate. With the exception of early stage B (B₁), which is usually treated with radical prostatectomy, most potentially curable patients are treated with definitive radiotherapy. The selection of treatment modality (surgery versus radiotherapy) and determination of the radiotherapy fields and doses are usually based on clinical staging. Clinical staging is largely dependent on the findings of rectal examination; tumor extent is often underestimated.

The value of CT in the definition of local and regional spread of prostatic carcinoma has been studied but remains unresolved (48). Since most patients with more advanced tumors do not undergo exploration and prostatectomy, which would confirm or disprove the CT findings, it is difficult to compile a substantial number of cases with CT and surgical-pathological correlation. The value of CT in the optimization of treatment planning, on the other hand, has been well documented (28,36,37). The target volume, which is to receive high tumoricidal doses and should include primary tumor and its extension into the periprostatic tissue, is difficult to define with conventional radiographic techniques, which fail to demonstrate lateral extent of the tumor and position and shape of the seminal vesicles, a frequent site of involvement.

In a series of 82 patients treated with curative intent

at the Mallinckrodt Institute of Radiology (MIR) with external beam radiotherapy (37), 7% of treatment plans done without CT information were found inadequate in stage B and early stage C carcinoma of the prostate. Fifty-three percent (17 of 32) of patients with (clinically) involved seminal vesicles would not have had adequate treatment of the entire tumor volume without the CT information. Similar findings have been reported by Lee et al. (28) and Asbell et al. (2).

A promising area for application of CT is the localization of radioactive implant sources in patients with carcinoma of the prostate treated with an implant (13).

Testicular Tumors

Management of testicular tumors depends to a great extent on the accurate assessment of the retroperitoneal lymph nodes. Status of the periaortic and renal hilum lymph nodes in seminoma determines the extent of the radiation fields and the total dose. In testicular carcinomas, the nodal status determines the need for lymphadenectomy, radiotherapy, and chemotherapy. Although lymphangiography is superior to CT in detecting minor deposits that do not cause enlargement of the lymph nodes, CT can assess the areas not visualized on lymphangiography, primarily those in the renal hilum and above the L₂ level (29).

It is usually agreed that patients with questionable or negative CT should also have a lymphangiogram directed primarily at the evaluation of intranodal architecture.

In terms of treatment planning, CT is particularly useful in patients with large retroperitoneal masses requiring an enlargement of the routine radiotherapy fields and an increase in doses. Massively involved lymph nodes frequently are not demonstrated with lymphangiography due to total replacement of the nodal tissue.

Lymphomas

Evaluation of intra-abdominal lymphatics is essential for adequate management of Hodgkin's disease and non-Hodgkin's lymphomas. The status of the retroperitoneal and mesenteric lymph nodes, among other factors, determines not only the need for irradiation, the extent of the abdominal fields, and the doses of irradiation, but also the need for chemotherapy.

Hodgkin's disease is characterized by orderly progression along the axial lymphatics. Periaortic lymph nodes are much more likely to be involved than celiac and mesenteric lymph nodes. The customary staging policies at most institutions include lymphangiogram and laparotomy in most lesser stage clinical presentations.

Non-Hodgkin's lymphomas tend to involve multiple intra-abdominal sites and produce bulky enlargement of the celiac and mesenteric lymph nodes and also those in the splenic and hepatic hilum. Staging laparotomy is not a customary procedure in non-Hodgkin's lymphomas.

Major advantages of CT relative to lymphangiography and exploratory laparotomy are the simplicity and noninvasiveness of the procedure and its ability to assess nodes not ordinarily seen on a lymphangiogram (mesenteric, retrocrural, celiac, splenic, and hepatic hilar nodes). A major disadvantage of CT versus lymphangiography is its inability to detect abnormalities in intranodal architecture. Computed tomography can detect nodal involvement only if the nodes are enlarged; CT is unable to identify a replaced but normal-sized lymph node as abnormal. However, in most cases of nodal involvement with lymphoma, in comparison to carcinoma, the nodes are enlarged enough to be detectable with CT.

Several reports attest to a high degree of correlation between findings obtained by CT, lymphangiography, and laparotomy (1,5–7,12,30,31,44,55).

It appears reasonable to use abdominal CT as the primary staging method in non-Hodgkin's lymphomas. Its use in Hodgkin's disease varies considerably from institution to institution and depends largely on the institutional policies regarding laparotomy. At MIR, CT is used as one of the first steps in the workup of patients with Hodgkin's disease, lymphangiography being reserved for cases with negative or equivocal CT.

Chest CT can be of considerable usefulness in optimization of treatment planning in a subgroup of patients with Hodgkin's disease and non-Hodgkin's lymphomas who present with sizable mediastinal masses spreading along or invading the chest wall. This type of involvement is frequently not detected by conventional radiographic means and may be an important cause of treatment failure (38).

Examples of the use of CT in treatment planning optimization in lymphomas are illustrated in Figs. 4 and 5.

4a,b

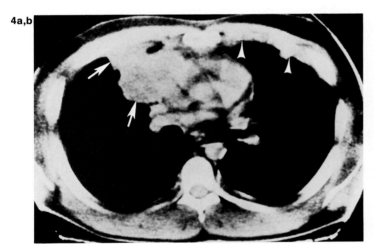

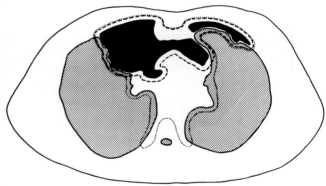

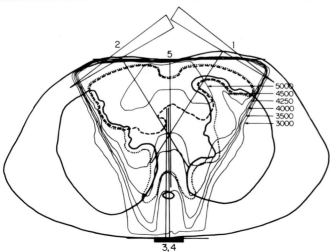

FIG. 4. Twenty-year-old man with locally advanced, poorly differentiated lymphocytic lymphoma. **a:** A large tumor mass (arrows) involves the right chest wall and mediastinum. In addition, considerable extension across the midline to involve the left anterior pleura and chest wall (arrowheads) is present. **b:** To the area containing the gross tumor, 4,400 rad is to be given. The prophylactic dose is 4,000 rad. **c:** Five beams have been utilized. Beams 1 and 2 are oblique-wedged 4 MV X-ray beams. Beams 3, 4, and 5 are parallel opposed. A block is added posteriorly to reduce the spinal cord dose. The spinal cord dose, according to the plan, is limited to 3,500 rad.

Sarcomas

Soft tissue malignancies show certain characteristics that make them a particularly promising area for application of CT. These tumors are generally bulky at the time of diagnosis and frequently can be separated easily from the surrounding tissues. The attenuation values of these malignancies are usually lower than surrounding normal tissues. This phenomenon is most prominent in well-differentiated liposarcomas (Fig. 6) where the attenuation value approaches that of normal fat (−50 to −90 Hounsfield units).

Sarcomas permeate the surrounding tissues far beyond the grossly detectable tumor. The natural barriers to tumor spread are fasciae and aponeurotic membranes surrounding the muscle groups and forming the anatomic compartments. Recognition of the compartmental type of tumor spread forms the basis for the treatment of sarcomas that, under optimal circumstances, should be directed not only toward the gross tumor but toward the whole compartment within which the tumor arises. This therapeutic principle applies to both surgery and radiotherapy.

It has been shown that radiotherapy can consistently control subclinical (microscopic) extensions of sar-

comas. Surgical removal of the gross tumor preceded or followed by adjuvant radiotherapy directed to the sites of potential spread, yields high control rates without the mutilation associated with radical surgery, such as amputation.

Radiotherapy of soft tissue sarcomas (either adjuvant or definitive) poses a challenge to the radiation oncologist. The volumes that need to be treated are generally quite large and the doses required for tumor control are substantial. Highly sophisticated treatment techniques are needed to achieve adequate dose distribution and maximal preservation of normal tissues. It has been shown that a "strip" of normal tissues needs to be preserved when an extremity is irradiated in order to spare lymphatic channels and prevent crippling extremity edema. Adequate coverage of all areas at risk along with maximal preservation of normal tissues is frequently a formidable task in patients with soft tissue sarcomas. Computed tomography has proven invaluable in treatment planning for this group of patients. The compartments are easily identified and the positioning of the beam and the choice of the spared tissue are greatly facilitated (Figs. 6 and 7). In patients to be treated postoperatively, CT images should ideally be obtained prior to surgical resection. In addition,

5a,b

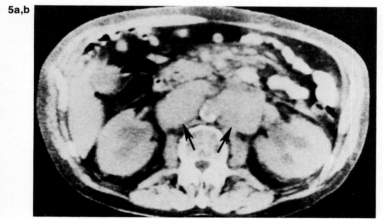

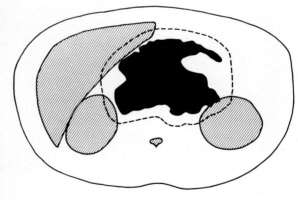

5c

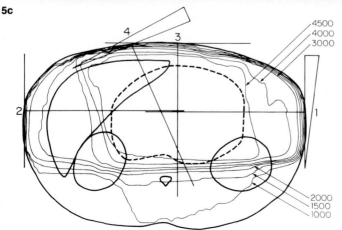

FIG. 5. Sixty-six-year-old man with poorly differentiated nodular lymphocytic lymphoma presenting with massive retroperitoneal and mesenteric lymphadenopathy. Patient is to be treated with a combination of radiotherapy and chemotherapy. **a:** The retroperitoneal (periaortic and pericaval) lymphadenopathy (arrows) and mesenteric lymphadenopathy are shown. Bilateral moderate degree hydronephrosis is caused by encasement of ureters at a lower level. **b:** The delineated volume is to receive 4,500 rad. Slices above the level shown in Fig. 5a have been utilized to delineate the liver. **c:** Treatment plan using four 18 MV X-ray beam setup. A large percentage of kidney parenchyma is in the treatment volume. A reduction of target volume during the treatment course is indicated and is often facilitated by the prompt shrinkage of tumor in patients with lymphoma.

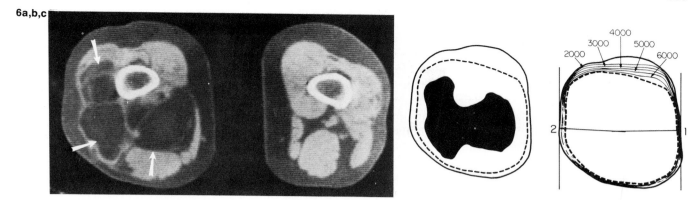

FIG. 6. Sixty-two-year-old woman with myxo-liposarcoma of the thigh. **a:** Tumor (arrows) is of strikingly low density and clearly delineated in relation to the muscular groups involved. **b:** The delineated volume is to receive 6,000 rad. The patient will be treated with a combination of surgery and radiotherapy. **c:** A simple setup of two parallel-opposed 4 MV beams is used. Computed tomography has proven essential in choosing the site of the spared strip of tissue and its width. Due to the extent of the tumor, width of the preserved tissue is minimal.

CT is invaluable in the follow-up of patients with deep-seated lesions in whom early detection of recurrences may be lifesaving, with the application of further therapy. Recent studies (4) suggest that ultrasound also may play a role in defining the limits of these tumors, especially in areas where there is little or no perimuscular fat.

Future Applications of CT in Radiotherapy

At the present time, most radiotherapy treatment plans consist of two-dimensional dose calculations in transverse planes of a patient. For photon beams, improved geometrical description of anatomy and a knowledge of tissue density from CT scans have re-

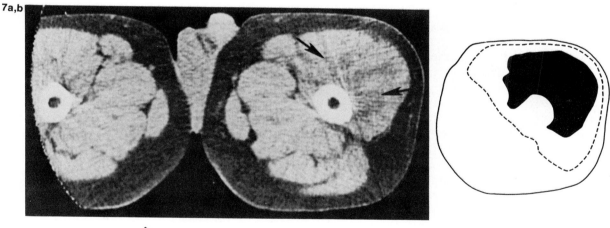

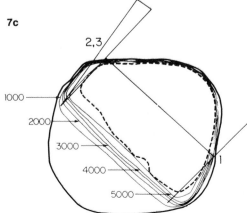

FIG. 7. Thirty-seven-year-old man with malignant fibrohistiocytoma of the antero-lateral compartment of the left thigh. Patient is to be treated with a course of preoperative radiotherapy, chemotherapy, and limited resection. **a:** The tumor (arrows) is confined to the antero-lateral muscle group. It extends to the femur but does not appear to invade other compartments of the thigh. **b:** The delineated area is to receive approximately 5,000 rad. **c:** Parallel-opposed beams, one of which is wedged, are utilized, preserving postero-medial portion of the extremity to prevent lymphatic obstruction. Computed tomography imaging is essential in choosing the angle of the beams and the width of the preserved strip of normal tissues.

sulted in only a modest improvement over the accuracy of dose computation on existing treatment planning computers that take into account the effect of inhomogeneities only in the plane of calculation (15,39). The present computational methods, which are two-dimensional, ignore the dose-perturbing influences of inhomogeneities in planes other than the plane of the dose calculation. Therefore, one of the major limitations of current radiotherapy planning is that the absorbed doses are generally computed in a single plane through the central axis of the radiation beam rather than in the three-dimensional volume actually treated. Attempts are being made to develop three-dimensional computational methods that utilize electron density information over the entire irradiated volume of a patient (26,47). Computed tomography scans with contiguous slices over the treated volume will be required to obtain electron density information within the patient; thus, CT scanners will be essential for *three-dimensional treatment planning* and optimization of dose distribution in the treated volume. An important issue that requires future investigation is the method of presenting computed doses to the clinician in a manner that will allow visualization of the predicted three-dimensional dose distribution. The human brain is limited in its ability to conceptualize such three-dimensional information displayed on two-dimensional screens. Coronal and sagittal reconstructed CT images will play an important role in displaying these dose distributions.

One can anticipate that, in the future, CT capability might be integrated into radiotherapy machines directly and that this capability would provide for more *dynamic treatment*. By dynamic it is meant that the radiation treatment would automatically, on a real-time basis, adjust for physiological manifestations or changes that may occur in the tumor mass configuration as a direct result of previous radiation treatments. This form of dynamic radiotherapy would be highly promising in providing for more selective treatment of tumor while sparing normal tissues.

REFERENCES

1. Alcorn FS, Mategrano VC, Petasnick JP, Clark JW: Contributions of computed topography in the staging and management of malignant lymphoma. *Radiology* 125:717–723, 1977
2. Asbell SO, Schlager BA, Baker AS: Revision of treatment planning for carcinoma of the prostate. *Int J Radiat Oncol Biol Phys* 6:861–865, 1980
3. Battista JJ, Rider WD, VanDyk J: Computed tomography for radiotherapy planning. *Int J Radiat Oncol Biol Phys* 6:99–107, 1980
4. Bernardino ME, Jing B-S, Thomas JL, Lindell MM, Zornoza J: The extremity soft-tissue lesion: A comparative study of ultrasound, computed tomography and xeroradiography. *Radiology* 139:53–59, 1981
5. Best JJK, Blackledge G, Forbes WStC, Todd IDH, Eddleston B, Crowther D, Isherwood I: Computed tomography of abdomen in staging and clinical management of lymphoma. *Br Med J* 2:1675–1677, 1978
6. Blackledge G, Best JJK, Crowther D, Isherwood I: Computed tomography in the staging of patients with Hodgkin's disease: A report on 136 patients. *Clin Radiol* 31:143–147, 1980
7. Breiman RS, Castellino RA, Harell GS, Marshall WH, Glatstein E, Kaplan HS: CT-pathologic correlations in Hodgkin's disease and non-Hodgkin's lymphoma. *Radiology* 126:159–166, 1978
8. Brizel HE, Livingston PA, Grayson EV: Radiotherapeutic applications of pelvic computed tomography. *J Comput Assist Tomogr* 3:453–466, 1979
9. Chen GTY, Singh RP, Castro JR, Lyman JT, Quivey JM: Treatment planning for heavy ion radiotherapy. *Int J Radiat Oncol Biol Phys* 5:1809–1819, 1979
10. Chernak ES, Rodriquez-Antunez A, Jelden GL, Dhaliwal RS, Lavik PS: The use of computed tomography for radiation therapy treatment planning. *Radiology* 117:613–614, 1975
11. deWinter J: Computed tomography and the radiotherapist. In: *Medical Imaging,* ed. by L Kreel and RE Steiner, Chicago, Year Book Medical Publishing, 1979, pp 168–177
12. Earl HM, Sutcliffe SBJ, Kelsey Fry I, Tucker AK, Young J, Husband J, Wrigley PFM, Malpas JS: Computerised tomographic abdominal scanning in Hodgkin's disease. *Clin Radiol* 31:149–153, 1980
13. Elkon D, Kim JA, Constable WC: Anatomic localization of radioactive gold seeds of the prostate by computer-aided tomography. *Comput Tomogr* 5:89–93, 1981
14. Emami B, Melo A, Cater BL, Muzenrider JE, Piro AJ: Value of computed tomography in radiotherapy of lung cancer. *Am J Roentgenol* 131:63–67, 1978
15. Geise RA, McCullough EC: The use of CT scanners in megavoltage photon-beam therapy planning. *Radiology* 124:133–141, 1977
16. Goitein M: Compensation for inhomogeneities in charged particle radiotherapy using computed tomography. *Int J Radiat Oncol Biol Phys* 4:499–508, 1978
17. Goitein M: Computed tomography in planning radiation therapy. *Int J Radiat Oncol Biol Phys* 5:445–447, 1979
18. Goitein M, Wittenberg J, Mendiondo M, Doucette J, Friedberg C, Ferucci J, Gunderson L, Linggood R, Shipley WU, Fineberg HV: The value of CT scanning in radiation therapy treatment planning: A prospective study. *Int J Radiat Oncol Biol Phys* 5:1787–1798, 1979
19. Hobday P, Hodson NJ, Husband J, Parker RP, MacDonald JS: Computed tomography applied to radiotherapy treatment planning: Techniques and results. *Radiology* 133:477–482, 1979
20. Hogstrom KR, Smith AR, Simon SL, Somers JW, Lane RG, Rosen II, Kelsey CA, VonEssen CF, Kligerman MM, Berardo PA, Zink SM: Static pion beam treatment planning of deep seated tumors using computerized tomographic scans. *Int J Radiat Oncol Biol Phys* 5:875–886, 1979
21. Isherwood I, Pullan BR, Rutherford RA, Strang FA: Electron density and atomic number determination by computed tomography. Part I: Methods and limitation. Part II: A study of colloid cysts. *Br J Radiol* 50:613–619, 1977
22. Jelden GL, Chernak ES, Rodriquez-Antunez A, Haaga JR, Lavik PS, Dhaliwal RS: Further progress in CT scanning and computerized radiation therapy treatment planning. *Am J Roentgenol* 127:179–185, 1976
23. Kellett MJ, Oliver RTD, Husband JE, Fry IK: Computed tomography as an adjunct to bimanual examination for staging bladder tumors. *Br J Urol* 52:101–106, 1980
24. Kelsey CA, Berardo PA, Smith AR, Kilgerman MM: CT scanner selection and specification for radiation therapy. *Med Phys* 7:555–558, 1980
25. Koehler PR, Anderson RE, Baxter B: The effect of computed tomography view controls on anatomical measurements. *Radiology* 130:189–194, 1979
26. Larson KB, Prasad SC: Absorbed-dose computations for inhomogeneous media in radiation-treatment planning using differential scatter-air ratios. In: *Proceedings of the Second Annual Symposium on Computer Application in Medical Care,* Long Beach, California, IEEE Computer Society, 1978, pp 93–99
27. Laughlin JS, Chu F, Simpson LD: Radiation treatment planning. *Cancer* 39:719–728, 1977

28. Lee D-J, Leibel S, Shiels R, Sanders R, Siegelman S, Order S: The value of ultrasonic imaging and CT scanning in planning the radiotherapy for prostatic carcinoma. *Cancer* 45:724–727, 1980

29. Lee JKT, McClennan BL, Stanley RJ, Sagel SS: Computed tomography in the staging of testicular neoplasms. *Radiology* 130:387–390, 1979

30. Lee JKT, Stanley RJ, Sagel SS, Levitt RG: Accuracy of computed tomography in detecting intraabdominal and pelvic adenopathy in lymphoma. *Am J Roentgenol* 131:311–315, 1978

31. Marshall WH Jr, Breiman RS, Harell GS, Glatstein E, Kaplan HS: Computed tomography of abdominal paraaortic lymph node disease: Preliminary observations with a 6 second scanner. *Am J Roentgenol* 128:759–764, 1977

32. McCullough EC: Potential of CT in radiation therapy treatment planning. *Radiology* 129:765–768, 1978

33. Munzenrider JE, Pilepich M, Rene-Ferrero JB, Tchakarova I, Carter BL: Use of body scanner in radiotherapy treatment planning. *Cancer* 40:170–179, 1977

34. Parker RP, Hobday PA, Cassell KJ: The direct use of CT numbers in radiotherapy dosage calculation for inhomogeneous media. *Phys Med Biol* 24:802–809, 1979

35. Phelps ME, Gado MH, Hoffman EJ: Correlation of effective atomic number and electron density with attenuation coefficients measured with polychromatic x-rays. *Radiology* 117:585–588, 1975

36. Pilepich MV, Perez CA, Prasad S: Computed tomography in definitive radiotherapy of prostatic carcinoma. *Int J Radiat Oncol Biol Phys* 6:923–926, 1980

37. Pilepich MV, Prasad SC, Perez CA: Computed tomography in definitive radiotherapy of prostatic carcinoma. Part 2: Definition of target volume. *Int J Radiat Oncol Biol Phys* 8:235–240, 1982

38. Pilepich MV, Rene JB, Munzenrider JE, Carter BL: Contribution of computed tomography to the treatment of lymphomas. *Am J Roentgenol* 131:69–73, 1978

39. Prasad SC, Glasgow GP, Purdy JA: Dosimetric evaluation of a computed tomography treatment system. *Radiology* 130:777–781, 1979

40. Prasad SC, Pilepich MV, Perez CA: Contribution of CT to quantitative radiation therapy planning. *Am J Roentgenol* 136:123–128, 1981

41. Proceedings of the Symposium on Particles and Radiation Therapy, Second International Conference. *Int J Radiat Oncol Biol Phys* 3:1977

42. Purdy JA, Prasad SC: Computed tomography applied to radiation therapy treatment planning. In: *Medical Physics of CT and Ultrasound: Tissue Imaging and Characteristics,* Medical Physics Monograph No. 6, ed. by GD Fullerton and JA Zagzebski, New York, American Institute of Physics, pp 221–250, 1980

43. Ragan DP, Perez CA: Efficacy of CT-assisted two-dimensional treatment planning: Analysis of 45 patients. *Am J Roentgenol* 131:75–79, 1978

44. Redman HC, Glatstein E, Castellino RA, Federal WA: Computed tomography as an adjunct in the staging of Hodgkin's disease and non-Hodgkin's lymphoma. *Radiology* 124:381–385, 1977

45. Schlager B, Asbell SO, Baker AS, Sklaroff DM, Seydel HG, Ostrum BJ: The use of computerized tomography scanning in treatment planning for bladder carcinoma. *Int J Radiat Oncol Biol Phys* 5:99–103, 1979

46. Seydel HG, Kutcher GJ, Steiner RM, Mohiuddin M, Goldberg B: Computed tomography in planning radiation therapy for bronchogenic carcinoma. *Int J Radiat Oncol Biol Phys* 6:601–606, 1980

47. Sontag MR, Cunningham JR: Clinical applications of a CT based treatment planning system. *Comput Tomogr* 2:117–130, 1978

48. Stanley RJ, Sagel SS, Fair WR: Computed tomography of the genitourinary tract. *J Urol* 119:780–782, 1978

49. Sternick ES, Lane FW, Curran B: Comparison of computed tomography and conventional tranverse axial tomography in radiotherapy treatment planning. *Radiology* 124:835–836, 1977

50. Stewart JR, Hicks JA, Boone ML, Simpson LD: Computed tomography in radiation therapy. *Int J Radiat Oncol Biol Phys* 4:313–324, 1978

51. Veenema RJ, Harisiadis L, Chang C, Puchner P, Romas N, Wechsler M, Guttman R: Bladder carcinoma: Preliminary external radiotherapy used as a means for selecting complete treatment. In: *Progress in Cancer Research and Therapy. Volume 18: Carcinoma of the Bladder,* ed. by JG Connolly, New York, Raven Press, 1981, pp 183–191

52. Whitmore WF: Bladder cancer. *Cancer* 28:170–177, 1978

53. Wizenberg MJ: Invasive bladder cancer: Definitive irradiation and salvage cystectomy. *Semin Oncol* 6:229–235, 1979

54. Yu WS, Sagerman RH, King GA, Chung CT, Yu YW: The value of computed tomography in the management of bladder cancer. *Int J Radiat Oncol Biol Phys* 5:135–142, 1979

55. Zelch MG, Haaga JR: Clinical comparison of computed tomography and lymphangiography for detection of retroperitoneal lymphadenopathy. *Radiol Clin North Am* 17:157–168, 1979

Chapter 21

The Economics and Politics of Computed Tomography

Ronald G. Evens and R. Gilbert Jost

Computed tomography (CT) was more than a new diagnostic technique for medicine; it had significant political and economical ramifications. Within a year after its introduction in 1973, this invention was known worldwide and became a major topic of discussion in the houses of congress, state legislatures, and at cocktail parties. Widespread acclaim for CT was constrained because CT became a symbol of extravagance to individuals concerned with mounting health care costs. Most of these critics had no immediate responsibility for the ill. The early years of CT (1973–1978) created as many enemies as friends because of the social and political concerns about medical costs.

Nearly everyone would agree that medical care in the United States had dramatically improved since World War II in almost every aspect. A series of major technological developments during the 1940s, 1950s, and 1960s, having an impact on every medical specialty, had resulted in dramatically improved care for American citizens. This was an era of antibiotics, modern anesthetics, open heart surgery, cobalt and linear accelerator radiation therapy, specialty medicine and substantive advances in our understanding of biology and pathophysiology. These medical advances became available to larger segments of the population as health care was "a right, not a privilege." Medical schools were scientifically based, the National Institutes of Health routinely obtained increased funding, and the modern hospital-based medical complex became a visible part of the landscape in most cities. Physicians, with the support of the biomedical sciences and hospitals, became more effective and more powerful.

At the same time, the cost of medical care was receiving increasing attention due to a combination of factors. Improved care and its accessibility made the total cost go up; patients became increasingly knowledgeable about health and demanded the best in care; insurance and other third-party programs became increasingly available through employers and government; and, most importantly, medical care became a political issue. A series of congressional actions resulted in programs to provide medical care for various segments of the population that were not covered by personal or employer-supported insurance programs. These included Title V (Maternal and Child Health), Title XVII (Medicare), and Title XIX (Medicaid). During the 1970s it was recognized by taxpayers, legislatures, and corporations that health care costs were rising faster than other segments of the economy and it was easy to predict that health care would soon consume as much as 10% of our gross national productivity. A political and societal change in philosophy occurred during the 1970s, with an increasing demand from politicians, big business, and the public to reduce or at least control costs.

HEALTH CARE PLANNING IN THE UNITED STATES

A system of health planning was first required by congressional legislation in 1966 (Public Law 89–749), which funded the development of local comprehensive health planning councils and established a Certificate of Need (CON) review process for new health care proposals. There were several objectives for local planning councils, including data gathering, long-range planning, and the approval or disapproval of capital expenditure projects in each geographic region. In general, the local planning councils did little planning and their primary role became the review and comment on specific projects.

The federal initiative for health planning was strengthened in 1972 when Section 1122 was added to the Social Security Act under Public Law 92–603. Section 1122 required prior approval by both local and state planning agencies for any capital expenditures exceeding $100,000 or for any significant change in clinical services if reimbursement was sought from federal funds through Medicare, Medicaid, Maternal and Child Health Legislation, or federal employee insurance programs. Section 1122 gave "teeth" to the planning process since denial of reimbursement was a major problem to most health care institutions. The responsibility for long-range planning and data collection in each local and state planning agency continued.

No one was particularly happy with the directives of Section 1122. Medical providers found them restrictive, highly bureaucratic, and inconsistent. Planning agencies were hampered by a lack of data, and had difficulty in developing long-range plans. These agencies commonly stimulated considerable controversy when reviewing individual projects—particularly when a project was turned down. Congress was dissatisfied with progress toward goals in cost containment and improving the accessibility of medical care.

Further revision of planning activities was legislated by Congress in the National Health Planning and Resource Development Act of 1974 (Public Law 93–641). This law mandated extensive changes in the health planning system that included changing the geography of local planning areas, and adding consumer representation to planning agencies (now called Health Systems Agencies or HSAs) and their state counterpart. State planning agencies were required to develop a health systems plan to control costs and improve accessibility of care by defining criteria and standards for specific health service needs. To aid the HSAs in developing these plans, the secretary of the Department of Health, Education, and Welfare (HEW), which in 1981, was renamed the Department of Health and Human Services, was directed to develop a set of national goals "expressed where practicable in quantitative terms" (15) to guide the more than 200 local HSAs in their planning.

The secretary of HEW did not actively pursue the development of such "guidelines" until 1977 when then Secretary Califano saw the use of national guidelines as a mechanism to control health care costs, particularly to reduce the perceived inefficiency of hospitals (described by the secretary as "fat") and the growth of costly technologies.

On September 23, 1977, HEW published a set of guidelines and standards related to 11 specific areas. Of the 11, 3 specifically related to radiology—cardiac catheterization, megavoltage radiation therapy, and CT scanners. The guidelines stimulated a wave of protest as more than 50,000 individual comments were received by HEW. Most concerns were expressed on specific standards, including the impact of the guidelines on rural hospitals and teaching facilities, and the loss of local control or responsibility for health planning. This protest resulted in revised guidelines,

published on January 20, 1978. The guidelines were considered reasonable by most radiologists, with the exception of those for CT.

CT BECOMES THE SYMBOL OF "TECHNOLOGY RUN WILD"

The introduction of CT in 1973 was greeted by radiologists and other physicians as a great advance that would revolutionize medical diagnosis and, perhaps, therapy (5,14). To those concerned with the cost of medical care and to critics of the expanding role of technology, CT was another dangerous force with which to reckon (8). During the early years, when CT was limited to examinations of the head, these concerns were not widespread, but in 1975, the British firm of EMI announced an 18-sec scanner capable of examining the entire body. Soon other companies had similar scanners and total body CT became practical with an associated dramatic increase in the desire of all radiologists and hospitals (and many ambulatory facilities) to provide CT services.

Computed tomography became *the* example for politicians and planners to symbolize the "inappropriate" use of medical technology with its ultimate associated increase in cost. Computed tomography was in many respects a nearly perfect scapegoat—it was expensive, of great interest to physicians, could easily be shown in a photograph, and even had an eponym, CAT. It seemed that everyone from local planners to Secretary Califano to the President of the United States began to use the phrase "CAT scanner" and described the dangers of "CAT fever" (34).

It was initially difficult to debate the opponents of CT effectively because few data were available on economics, utilization, and medical efficacy of CT—particularly for the body. Supportive documentation had not been published because of the limited time that prototype units had been in clinical use; yet most radiologists and other physicians were convinced of the importance of CT not only for the head, but for the body as well. Although politicians and planners made CT a scapegoat because of its high cost, this approach clearly was a serious mistake as CT has proven to be a major revolution in diagnostic imaging, so beneficial, in fact, that it could not be stopped by legislation and guidelines.

ECONOMICS AND UTILIZATION OF CT

Realizing the need for data on CT economic utilization, a study was begun to obtain data from multiple CT users in the United States (19). With the cooperation of all known CT equipment manufacturers, a list of all operating CT installations as of January 1976 was compiled. Information was obtained from 98 to 140 operating installations. At that time, the overwhelming experience was with head CT units and the first understanding of the equipment's utilization, efficiency, and cost was limited to neuroradiology activity. The CT units were operated an average 64 hr a week and examined 50 to 55 patients per week. Even at this early stage, radiologists were responsible for the performance and interpretation of CT scans (92 of 98 facilities) and most equipment (90%) was installed in association with a hospital. Scheduling delays were lengthy, averaging 1.6 days for inpatients and 11.5 days for outpatients. An economic break-even point analysis (13) was performed using data on equipment cost and its method of depreciation, equipment maintenance, space remodeling and upkeep, personnel, and the cost of iodinated contrast material and other supplies. The "typical" unit had an annual technical cost of $325,000 to $371,000, depending on patient volume. Data on charges indicated the net technical revenue was $138 per patient as compared to a net technical cost of $130 per patient. It was emphasized that this study obtained data on CT installations in order to satisfy interests and concerns about this new imaging method's use, but that most CT installations were not independent activities and needed to be considered as an integral part of a diagnostic radiology department or office.

This project in 1976 became the first in a series of publications because of the continued need to justify the cost and utilization of CT to its opponents. A study in early 1978 (21) of the first CT installations capable of obtaining images with "breath holding" (18 sec or less scanning time) demonstrated different results. Even though 60% of studies were for evaluation of the head, fewer patients were studied per week (33) on these early multipurpose scanners, and the units were operating at a significant financial loss.

A follow-up study (22,23) in November 1978 summarized information obtained from 134 installations (70 head only and 64 body and head units). At that time, dedicated head CT units were examining an average of 63 patients per week with an annual technical cost of $383,000, and each installation was generating excess revenues over expenses (a profit) of approximately $123,000 per year. Body CT scanners were examining 34 patients per week, consisting of 55% head studies, at an average annual technical cost of $384,000. Each body unit was operating at an average economic loss of $77,000 per year. Most importantly, 73% of the head units were meeting the national guidelines of 1978, whereas only 17% of body CT scanners were meeting this level of activity.

The guidelines published by the Health Resource Administration for CT scanners were simple, yet deadly:

1. A computed tomographic scanner (head and body) should operate at a minimum of 2,500 medically necessary patient procedures per year, for the second year of its operation and thereafter.

2. There should be no additional scanners approved in a geographic region unless each existing scanner in the health service area is performing at a rate greater than 2,500 medically necessary patient procedures per year.

3. There should not be additional scanners approved unless the operators of the proposed equipment set in place data collection and utilization review systems.

The guidelines went on to define a "patient procedure" to include all diagnostic studies performed on the same visit, in the same area of anatomy, and with the same diagnostic interest—a definition specifically developed to count a patient examination with and without intravenous contrast material as a single procedure. The standard also stated that this level of activity should be possible in a 50- to 55-hr week, with a head to body ratio of 60/40, but no basis for possible adjustments were given. Data from our surveys demonstrated that 2,500 patient procedures per year was an impossible goal for most installations with body CT scanners of the technology available in 1978. Yet, the second guideline permitted *no* additional scanners within an HSA area unless *all* other scanners were performing more than 2,500 procedures per year. This essentially established a moratorium on the further purchase of CT scanners in most geographic regions.

Economic data on CT scanners was important for other reasons in addition to demonstrating the moratorium effect of the national guidelines.

1. They were the first economic studies of a radiologic procedure or installation from national data that documented economic and utilization adjustments with time, experience, and improved technology (Table 1).

2. This approach demonstrated a model for analyzing costs based on standard utilization and expense data and suggested a method for establishing charges that would allow coverage of these costs.

3. The data and reports emphasized the critical importance of patient volume with most radiology procedures, where the vast majority of costs are fixed (unrelated to examination activity) and only a small portion of costs are variable (related to examination activity) (21). When most costs are fixed, patient volume is a critical component in evaluating the charge necessary to break-even since total costs vary little with examination volume while the cost per patient changes dramatically (Table 2).

Other investigators reported on the cost of CT in their own departments, including studies on the effect

TABLE 1. *CT economic and utilization data from national surveys of experienced radiology facilities*

	Jan. 1976 (Head CT)	May 1977 (Body)	Nov. 1978 (Head)	Nov. 1978 (Body)
No. installations reporting	98	74	70	64
Operating hours/week	64	52	59	52
Patients/week	55	32	63	34
Percent head/body	100/0	60/40	100/0	55/45
Typical total charge ($)	258	286	247	273
Annual technical cost ($)	345,000	373,000	388,000	384,000
Annual technical profit (loss) ($)	22,880	(72,000)	123,000	(77,000)

of CT in reducing other examinations or procedures. Wortzman et al. (39) described cost effectiveness in Canada; Turcke and Gilmore (35) reported a marked reduction in radionuclide brain imaging after CT was initiated in adjacent community hospitals in a small metropolitan area (Medford, Oregon); Whalen (37) reported a 30% reduction in lymphangiography, 50% in abdominal aortograms, 30% in other arteriographic procedures, 25% in retrograde pyelograms, and 35% in intravenous cholangiography after the initiation of CT and ultrasound use.

These authors were developing an analysis of CT cost. At the same time, and most importantly, an evaluation of the benefits of CT to patients (efficacy) was in progress.

EFFICACY STUDIES AND CT

While opponents were criticizing the lack of efficacy data in 1976–1978 (1), multiple studies were in progress from several medical centers and results were beginning to be reported. These reports in the first year or two of head and body CT experience were necessarily limited to clinical descriptions and impact on diagnosis. Studies soon followed describing and documenting the impact of CT on treatment, clinical decision making, other diagnostic procedures, and, subsequently, on mortality and morbidity.

Ambrose et al. (4) noted a dramatic fall in the number of brain scans, arteriography, and air studies and a significant fall in exploratory surgery after the intro-

duction of CT, but without a real change in mortality in patients after head injuries. Several authors (2,10,20) compared head CT to radionuclide brain scanning as a primary or screening test and showed CT to be slightly more accurate but providing substantially more diagnostic data. Fineberg et al. (25), reporting on patients from the Massachusetts General Hospital, demonstrated a marked decrease in the perceived need by clinicians for brain scans, angiograms, and pneumoencephalograms after CT. In the Fineberg series, therapy was altered in 19% of those examined, including the abandonment of certain proposed treatments deemed worthless after CT findings. Larson et al. (30) showed a marked reduction in normal arteriograms following CT. The same group (28,29) found no change in the length of hospital stay or treatment plans in patients with cerebrovascular disease but a reduction in the time to diagnosis, with alteration of the therapeutic approach, in patients with suspected hydrocephalus and with brain tumors.

Efficacy studies of body CT began in 1978 and soon demonstrated improvement in diagnosis, reduction in the cost of work-up, and alterations in treatment plans, but without definite evidence for a reduction of morbidity and mortality. Robbins et al. (33) found 16% of CT examinations in the chest and abdomen produced clinically important information that was otherwise not available, which altered patient diagnosis, prognosis, and therapy. Wittenberg et al. (38) performed studies in 184 selected patients demonstrating that CT improved diagnostic understanding in 41%, reassured physicians about planned therapy in 43%, and changed therapy in 17%. Weyman et al. (36) compared CT and arteriography in patients with renal cell carcinoma, demonstrating that arteriography can be obviated in most patients. In summary, data from multiple institutions, essentially all favorable, were being reported on the benefit to patients and overall efficacy of CT in both the head and extracranial portions of the body.

Several authors recommended more extensive efficacy studies (1,12,24) and indicated the need for multi-institutional approaches. One such study on head CT (6) was funded by the National Cancer

TABLE 2. *Effect of patient volume on CT technical costs*

	Patients/weeks			
	25	30	40	50
Fixed costs	$217,183	217,183	217,183	217,183
Variable costs	22,230	26,676	35,568	44,460
Indirect costs	119,770	121,930	126,376	130,822
Total costs	359,183	365,789	379,127	392,465
Cost/patient	276	234	182	151

Reprinted from Evens and Jost (21).

Institute and data were obtained from five university centers. This study began in 1974 and collected data for several years (during the critical time of controversy), but was not reported until July 1980, when it was of little use. Efficacy studies with new technology are critically important but multi-institutional projects were not timely and the responsibility for efficacy data rested primarily with the medical institutions who had early access to the equipment.

CT IS NATIONALLY ACCEPTED

For the United States, 1976 was a good year (our bicentennial celebration), but a bad year for CT. Computed tomography was "CAT" scanning, and a major challenge to medical cost control. Local HSAs became battlegrounds with physicians and radiologists (and sometimes patients) against planners and politicians. Meaney (32), Cloe (11), and Evens (15) advised radiologists and others to cooperate with planning agencies and provide data to evaluate CT effectively, without emotion. Economic and efficacy data (as described above) were being reported.

Important institutions and societies, often coordinated by the American College of Radiology, were particularly effective in the formulation and publication of statements dealing with efficacy. In April 1977, radiologists from five institutions (the Cleveland Clinic Foundation, Mallinckrodt Institute of Radiology at Washington University, Mayo Clinic, New York Hospital-Cornell Medical Center, and the University of California at San Francisco) jointly stated their opinion that body CT was a clinically important and efficacious radiologic procedure (18). The Society of Computed Body Tomography soon reported on a list of indications for CT that they deemed appropriate based on their members' evaluation (3), experience, and published sources.

In 1979, the increasing amount of data demonstrating the efficacy of CT and the increasing number of patients who benefited from its use began to sway the opinions of the public and the planners. Economic data from several sources were utilized in a study by Arthur D. Little, Inc. (26), which predicted that CT would not increase the cost of diagnostic procedures because of a reduction in other medical tests. This view was further documented (16) with an economic report, using data from the economic studies of Evens and Jost with an analysis of operational CT units in 1980, showing that improved diagnostic information was provided at essentially no cost to the medical public. This study emphasized that CT equipment must be readily available to patients to prevent the use of less effective diagnostic procedures and associated hospital patient days. The pendulum for CT swung further with a report by Maloney and

Rogers (31), emphasizing that expensive new technologies (CT) do not actually cost that much, but "little ticket" (i.e., less expensive but high volume) technologies result in very high cost.

Further studies confirmed the economic and medical necessity for CT in contemporary medical care. Computed tomography sharing had not been effective for patient care (9) in municipal health care facilities (i.e., city and state hospitals) that relied on other institutions for CT due to difficulties in patient scheduling and patient transportation, often because the patients were too ill to be moved. Dr. David Banta, a member of the Office of Technology Assessment (OTA) of Congress, published an article entitled "Computed Tomography: Cost Containment Misdirected" (7), reporting major problems in health care due to lack of CT facilities to major segments of United States citizens.

A major milestone for CT came with the dramatic announcement that the 1979 Nobel Prize in Medicine was awarded to Hounsfield and Cormack for their pioneering efforts in the development of CT. Computed tomography is now well accepted as an important diagnostic radiologic procedure. A Consensus Conference at the National Institutes of Health in late 1981 has reported on the major advances of head CT and encouraged its use in neurologic studies. It will indicate that it is not available in appropriate locations and will recommend that *more* CT is needed for effective medical care in the United States.

THE FUTURE FOR RADIOLOGY AND NEW MEDICAL TECHNOLOGY

The notoriety of CT was in large measure unrelated to its medical use. Computed tomography was developed by Godfrey Hounsfield and the EMI Corporation at an inopportune time—a period of history with increasing concerns about medical costs and the impact of new technology. Computed tomography was the first example of new technology in our specialty subjected to critical scrutiny and rigorous assessment of its medical and economic efficacy. Fortunately, for radiology, the early claims for its applications and value (18) have been substantiated.

The specialty of radiology is a relatively small component of medical care. Less than 4% of physicians are radiologists, and less than 10% of the total medical cost in the United States relates to radiology. Yet radiology is a highly visible aspect of medical care (more than one of every two citizens in the United States has a radiograph each year) and future developments seem likely to be associated with new "inventions" with a high price tag (17). Radiologists should assume that future concerns about costs will often be focused toward our speciality.

Radiologists have learned a lot from this experience with CT that should certainly prove additionally useful in the future. The primary goal for most radiologists should continue to be the evaluation of medical efficacy (both diagnostic and therapeutic) with new techniques for patient care. Computed tomography demonstrated the need to develop economic data (cost, resources required, and appropriate revenues) in a timely fashion to answer questions about costs, benefits, and the allocation of new technology for the benefit of patients.

The next several decades will be a time of exciting developments in technology, constant demands for health care to all citizens, and relatively limited resources. The United States has not yet decided on an appropriate allocation of the gross national product to health needs. Is 8, 10, 15, or 20% enough? The specialty of radiology is an easy focus for debate. New technology in radiology is expensive and easy to question—note a recent article (27) where a discussion on the use of information theory in clinical medicine used eight clinical examples with seven from the specialty of radiology because data were available for evaluation.

Our specialty has learned that new improvements are highly likely to be costly, will require important economic and personnel commitments, and will quickly become a public and political focus. Economic evaluation of emerging technology should be started at the same time as medical studies in order to achieve public acceptance, a lesson learned from CT experience.

REFERENCES

1. Abrams HL, McNeil BJ: Computed tomography: Cost and efficacy implications. AJR 131:81–87, 1978
2. Alderson PO, Mikhael M, Coleman R, Gado M: Optimal utilization of computerized cranial tomography and radionuclide brain imaging. Neurology 26:803–807, 1976
3. Alfidi RJ, Evens RG, Glenn W, et al. (Society for Computed Body Tomography): Special report: New indications for computed body tomography. AJR 133:115–119, 1979
4. Ambrose J, Gooding, MR, Uttley D: EMI scan in the management of head injuries. Lancet 1:847–848, 1976
5. Baker HL Jr: Computed tomography and neuroradiology: A fortunate primary union. AJR 127:101–110, 1976
6. Baker HL, Houser OW, Campbell JK: National Cancer Institute Study: Evaluation of computed tomography in the diagnosis of intracranial neoplasms. I. Overall results. Radiology 136:91–96, 1980
7. Banta D: Computed tomography: Cost containment misdirected. Am J Public Health 70:215–216, 1980
8. Bogue T, Wolfe SM: CAT Scanners: Is Fancier Technology Worth a Billion Dollars of Health Consumer Money? Washington, DC, Health Resource Group, 1976
9. Brust JMC, Dickinson PCT, Healton EB: Failure of CT sharing in a large municipal hospital. N Engl J Med 304:1388–1393, 1981
10. Clifford JR, Connolly ES, Vorhees RM: Comparison of radionuclide scans with computer assisted tomography in diagnosis of intracranial disease. Neurology 26:1119–1123, 1976
11. Cloe LE: Health planning for computed tomography: Perspectives and problems AJR 128:187–190, 1976
12. Creditor MC, Garrett JB: The information base for diffusion of technology: Computed tomography scanning. N Engl J Med 297:49–52, 1977
13. Evens RG: Cost accounting in radiology and nuclear medicine. CRC Crit Rev Clin Radiol Nucl Med 6:67–80, 1975
14. Evens RG: New frontier for radiology: Computed tomography. AJR 126:1117–1129, 1976
15. Evens RG: National guidelines and standards for health planning: Their relation to radiology. AJR 131:1101–1104, 1978
16. Evens RG: The economics of computed tomography: Comparison with other health care costs. Radiology 136:509–510, 1980
17. Evens RG: Economic implications of a new technology installation: A CT model. AJR 136:673–677, 1981
18. Evens RG, Alfidi RJ, Haaga JR, et al.: Body computed tomography: A clinically important and efficacious radiologic procedure. Radiology 123:239–240, 1977
19. Evens RG, Jost RG: Economic analysis of computed tomography units. AJR 127:191–198, 1976
20. Evens RG, Jost RG: The clinical efficacy and cost analysis of cranial computed tomography and the radionuclide brain scan. Semin Nucl Med 7:129–136, 1977
21. Evens RG, Jost RG: Economic analysis of body computed tomography units including data on utilization. Radiology 127:151–157, 1978
22. Evens RG, Jost RG: Utilization of head computed tomography units in installations with greater than two-and-a-half years' experience. Radiology 131:691–693, 1979
23. Evens RG, Jost RG: Utilization of body computed tomography units in installations with greater than one-and-a-half years' experience. Radiology 131:695–698, 1979
24. Fineberg HV: Editorial: Evaluation of computed tomography: Achievement and challenge. AJR 131:1–4, 1978
25. Fineberg HV, Bauman R, Sosman M: Computerized cranial tomography: Effect on diagnostic and therapeutic plans. JAMA 238:224–227, 1977
26. Gempel PA, Harris GH, Evens RG: Comparative Cost Analysis: Computed Tomography Versus Alternative Diagnostic Procedures, 1977–1980. Cambridge, Massachusetts, Arthur D. Little, Inc., 1977
27. Harris JM: The hazards of bedside Bays. JAMA 246:2602–2605, 1981
28. Larson EB, Omenn GS, Loop JW: Computed tomography in patients with cerebrovascular disease: Impact of new technology on patient care. AJR 131:35–40, 1978
29. Larson EB, Omenn GS, Magno J: Impact of computed tomography on the care of patients with suspected hydrocephalus. AJR 131:41–44, 1978
30. Larson EB, Omenn GS, Margolis MT, Loop JW: Impact of computed tomography on utilization of cerebral angiograms. AJR 129:1–3, 1977
31. Maloney TW, Rogers DE: Medical technology: A different view of the contentious debate over costs. N Engl J Med 301:1413–1419, 1979
32. Meaney TF: CT and the planners. AJR 126:1095–1097, 1976
33. Robbins AH, Pugatch RD, Gerzof SG, Faling LJ, Johnson WC, Sewell DH: Observations on the medical efficacy of computed tomography of the chest and abdomen. AJR 131:15–19, 1978
34. Shapiro SH, Wyman SM: CAT fever. N Engl J Med 294:954–956, 1976
35. Turcke DA, Gilmore GT: Computed tomography's impact on nuclear medicine service in two community hospitals. Appl Radiol 6:149–151, 1977
36. Weyman PJ, McClennan BL, Stanley RJ, Levitt RG, Sagel SS: Comparison of computed tomography and angiography in the evaluation of renal cell carcinoma. Radiology 137:417–424, 1980
37. Whalen JP: Radiology of the abdomen: Impact of new imaging methods. AJR 133:587–618, 1979
38. Wittenberg J, Fineberg HV, Black EB, Kirkpatrick RH, Schaffer DL, Ikeda MK, Ferrucci JT Jr: Clinical efficacy of computed body tomography. AJR 131:5–14, 1978
39. Wortzman G, Holgate RC, Morgan PP: Cranial computed tomography: An evaluation of cost effectiveness. Radiology 117:75–77, 1975

Subject Index

Subject Index

A

Abdomen, 131–165
  abscess in childhood, 528
  acetabular roof in, 154–159
  aortic-caval bifurcation in, 151–152, 154
  gallbladder in, 140–142
  gastroesophageal junction in, 131–134, 136, 312–313
  mesentery in, 149–151
  pancreatic head in, 142–145
  in pediatric patients, 522–532
  pelvic inlet in, 152–154
  porta hepatis in, 137–140
  renal hilus in, 145–149
  splenic hilus in, 134–137
  symphysis pubis in, 159–164
  trauma in childhood, 528–530
  tumors in childhood, 523–526
Abdominal wall, 287–289
  abscess in, 288, 289
  hematoma in, 288, 289
  hernias in, 287–288
  inflammation in, 288
  metastases to, 289, 290, 291
  neoplasms in, 288–289
  normal anatomy of, 287
Abdominoperineal resection, pelvic anatomy after, 409–411
Abscess
  abdominal, in childhood, 528
  of abdominal wall, 288, 289
  adrenal, 390
  appendiceal, 293, 295
  Brodie's, 503
  drainage of, percutaneous, 31–34, 297
    catheters in, 31–32
    complications of, 34
    imaging guidance in, 31
    indications for, 31
    results of, 34
    technique of, 32–33
  iliopsoas, 298
  intraperitoneal, 292–299
  of kidney, 367
    in childhood, 524
    perirenal, 368, 372
  of liver, 185–186
    in childhood, 526, 527

  of lung, 118, 119, 120
  mesenteric, 293
  pancreatic, 229–233, 234
  paraspinal, 91
  pelvic, 294
  pericolonic, 337
  presacral, 402
  of psoas muscle, 284, 294
  of spleen, 252
  subhepatic, 294, 297
  subphrenic, 292
  thoracic, 544
  tubo-ovarian, 404, 405
Accuracy of imaging methods, 547–548
Acetabular fractures, 489, 492
Acetabular roof, 154–159
  female, 158–159
  male, 154–158
Adenocarcinoma, *see* Carcinoma
Adenoma
  adrenal
    Cushing's syndrome in, 383, 384, 385, 391
    nonfunctioning, 381, 387–388
  of liver, 179, 180
  of pancreas
    macrocystic, 224, 225
    microcystic, 225, 226
Adrenal glands, 135, 140, 379–392
  abscess of, 390
  adenoma of
    Cushing's syndrome in, 383, 384, 385, 391
    nonfunctioning, 381, 387–388
  in aldosteronism, 380, 383, 385
  in bronchogenic carcinoma, 112–113
  calcifications in, 389, 390
  carcinoma of, 385–386, 388
  in Cushing's syndrome, 383, 384–385, 391
  cysts of, 385, 388, 389
  hematoma in, 390
  hemorrhage in, 389–390
  in histoplasmosis, 389
  hyperplasia of, 383, 384
  metastases to, 383, 388
  myelolipoma of, 388–389
  normal anatomy of, 379, 380, 381
  pheochromocytoma of, 386–387
  pseudotumors of, 380–382

Adrenal glands *(contd.)*
  scintigraphy of, 391
  sonogrpahy of, 391
  techniques for CT studies of, 23
  tumors of, 385–388
    in childhood, 524–525
    nonfunctioning, 387
  venous sampling of, 391–392
Afferent loop syndrome, 329–330, 332
Alcoholic liver disease, 187
Aldosteronism, primary, 380, 383, 385
Aldosteronomas, 385
Alimentary tract, 307–339
  colon, 330–339
  duodenum and small intestine, 322–330
  esophagus, 307–312
  stomach, 312–322
Amebic abscess of liver, 185
Aneurysm
  aortic, 80, 82, 83, 257–261
    in childhood, 522
    dissecting, 81–82, 83, 84, 258
    leakage from, 258, 260
    mycotic, 258
  in childhood, 532
Aneurysmal bone cyst, 459, 473
Angiography
  adrenal, 391
  computed tomography, *see* Dynamic scanning
Angiomyolipomas, of kidney, 350, 359–360, 362
  in childhood, 524, 526
Aorta, 257–261
  aneurysms of, 80, 82, 83, 257–261
    in childhood, 522
    leakage from, 258, 260
    mycotic, 258
  ascending, 55
  atherosclerosis of, 257, 259
  bifurcation of, 151, 154
  circumaortic left renal vein, 263
  dissection of, 81–82, 83, 84, 258
  grafts of, infected, 259, 261
  normal anatomy of, 257
  periaortic lymph nodes, 267–280
  pseudoaneurysm of, 258, 260, 269
  retroaortic left renal vein, 264, 265
  tortuous, 80
  in transposition of great vessels, 85
Aortic arch, 58
  right, 73, 84
Aortopulmonary window, 59, 60
  lymphadenopathy in, 92
Apparatus for CT, 2–4
Appendiceal abscess, 293, 295
Arteriovenous fistula, postliver biopsy, 189, 192
Arteriovenous malformations, renal, 360, 362
Arthritis of hip, 495, 497
Artifacts, 5
  from barium retention, 17
  in liver studies, 172

photopenia, 10
  in superior vena cava, 71
Aryepiglottic fold, 40
Arytenoid cartilages, 42
Ascites
  hemorrhagic, in ovarian carcinoma, 540
  malignant, 291, 302
  pancreatic, 227
  in pouch of Douglas, 292
Atelectasis, round, 115, 118
Atherosclerosis of aorta, 257, 259
Artria, cardia, 62
Atrophy
  of pancreas
    in carcinoma, 216, 219
    in chronic pancreatitis, 234
  of psoas muscle, 284
Attenuation values, 13
Axial resolution in CT, 542
Azygoesophageal recess, 61
Azygous vein, 56, 58, 63, 68, 134, 136
  continuation of vena cava, 89, 262–263, 264

B

Beam hardening, 5
Biliary tract, 167–209
  in Caroli's disease, 206–207
  common bile duct, 139, 142, 214, 217, 322
    cyst of, 204–206
    stones in, 200, 201
  cystic duct, 139, 141
  cysts of , 204–206
  dilatation of ducts, 195–196, 197
  diseases of, 193–207
  hepatic ducts, 138, 139, 141
  normal anatomy of, 167–172
  obstruction of, 193–202
    common bile duct in, 195, 196, 198, 200
    hepatic duct in, 197, 202
    in hepatoma, 174
    in lymphoma, 196, 199
    stones in, 199, 200, 201
  size criteria for ducts, 195
  techniques for CT studies, 193
Biopsy, CT-guided, 21–31
  complications of, 30
  contraindications to, 31
  imaging methods in, 25–27
  indications for, 27
  localization aids in, 30
  musculoskeletal, 509–512, 513, 514, 515
  needles for, 24–25, 27
  results of, 25
  technique of, 27–30
  triangulation method in, 30
Bladder, 154
  carcinoma of, 394–397
    radiotherapy of, CT application in, 553–554

recurrent, 409
    transitional cell, 394, 395
  compression from pelvic lymph nodes, 401
  cystectomy of, pelvic anatomy after, 405–409
  cystitis of, 394
Bone cyst, aneurysmal, 459, 473
Bone tumors, 455–473
  benign, 457–459
  in childhood, 534
  chondroma, 463
  chondrosarcoma, 457, 458, 463, 482, 486
  enchondroma, 461
  evaluation of extent of, 456, 457, 459
  Ewing's sarcoma, 471, 534
  lymphoma, 465, 468
  myeloma, 466, 469
  osteoid osteoma, 459
  osteochondroma, 457
  osteosarcoma, 458, 464–465, 466, 467
  plasmacytoma, 466, 469, 472
Brachiocephalic artery, 57
  tortuous, 78
Brachiocephalic vein, 57, 58
Breast carcinoma, 128
  metastasis of
    to colon, 336
    to liver, 175
    to mesentery, 305
    to stomach, 320
    to thoracic wall, 126
  recurrent, 125
Brodie's abscess, 503
Bronchi, 57, 65
  right upper lobe, 59
Bronchiectasis, 104, 107
Bronchogenic carcinoma, see Lungs, carcinoma of
Bronchogenic cysts, 73
  in childhood, 521
Bronchopleural fistula, empyema with, 117
Bullae in lungs, 103, 106, 107
Burkitt's lymphoma, 528

C

Calcifications
  in adrenal glands, 389, 390
  in hepatoma, 174
  in herniated nucleus pulposus, 420–421, 422
  pancreatic ductal, in chronic pancreatitis, 235
  pericardial, 126
  in renal masses, 368–370
  in solitary pulmonary nodule, 99, 100
  in spleen, 251
  in uterine myoma, 402
Calculi
  bile duct, 200, 201, 202
  gallstones, 199, 200, 202–204
  renal
    radiolucent, 374
    staghorn, 368, 369
    urate, 357
Calf muscles, 475
Carcinoid tumors of duodenum, 325
Carcinoma
  adrenal, 385–386, 388
  of bladder, 394–397
    radiotherapy of, CT application in, 553–554
    recurrent, 409
    transitional cell, 394, 395
  bronchogenic, see Lungs, carcinoma of
  of cecum, 332
  of cervix uteri, 397–399
    recurrent, 399
  of colon, 230, 330–336, 337
    metastasis to adrenals, 388
    recurrent, 333, 334, 336
  of duodenum, 324
  of esophagus, 309–311, 312
    metastasis to adrenals, 388
  of gallbladder, 204, 205
  of hepatic flexure of colon, 335
  hepatocellular, 172–173
    in childhood, 526
  of kidney, see Kidney, carcinoma of
  of larynx, 43–52
  of ovary, 400–401; see also Ovary, carcinoma of
  of pancreas, 215–221, 222, 223; see also Pancreas, carcinoma of
  of prostate, 396, 397
    metastatic, 269
    radiotherapy of, CT application in, 553
    recurrent, 398
  of rectum, 332, 333, 335
    recurrent, 334, 409, 411
  of splenic flexure of colon, 335
  of stomach, 314, 315, 316
    recurrent, 320
  of uterus, 399–400
Cardioesophageal junction, adenocarcinoma of, 315
Caroli's disease, 206–207
Catheters, for percutaneous abscess drainage, 31–32
Cauda equina
  compression of, 418
  in degenerative spinal stenosis, 428, 429
  in meningioma, 437
Cecum, carcinoma of, 332
Celiac axis, 141
Celiac ganglia, 143, 147
Cerebrospinal fluid, intraperitoneal collection of, 296
Cervical spine injury, 441–443, 444
Cervix uteri, carcinoma of, 397–399
  recurrent, 399
Chest wall masses, 124, 125, 126–128
Childhood conditions, see Pediatric patients
Cholangiocarcinoma, 196, 202
Cholangitis, sclerosing, 194
Choledocholithiasis, 200, 201
Cholelithiasis, 199, 200, 202–204
Chondroma, 463

Chondrosarcoma, 457, 458, 463, 482, 486
Circumflex arteries, femoral, 164
Cirrhosis of liver, 186–189
    caudate lobe in, 189, 191, 197
Colitis
    Crohn's, 337, 338
    cystica profunda, 337, 338
    pseudomembranous, 337
Collimation, 10
    thin collimatedscans
        of liver, 172
        of pulmonary nodule, 99, 100
Colon, 330–339
    abdominoperineal resection of, 409–411
    abscesses of, 337
    anatomic variations in, 330
    ascending, 330
        normal variant of, 297
    carcinoma of, 230, 330–336, 337
        metastasis to adrenals, 388
        recurrent, 333, 334, 336
    descending, 330
    diverticulitis of, 337
    hepatic flexure of, 141, 143, 144, 330
        carcinoma of, 335
    inflammatory disease of, 336–337
    ischemia of, 339
    lipomas of, 336
    lymphoma of, 336
    metastases to, 336
    mucin-producing tumors of, metastatic, 176, 177
    normal anatomy of, 330
    obstruction of, 337–338
    in pancreatitis, 228
    radiation damage to, 338–339
    sigmoid, 153
    splenic flexure of, carcinoma of, 335
    transverse, 141, 145, 146, 289, 290, 330
    tumors of, 330–336
    wall thickness of, 330
Comparative imaging, 537–548
    advantages and disadvantages of techniques in, 541–547
    in childhood, 526–527
    physical bases for methods in, 1–2, 537–541
Components of CT system, 3
Computed radiograph, 11
Contrast enhancement, 16–21
Contrast media
    EOE–13, 21, 191, 244
    intravenous, 17–21
        agents in, 20–21
        bolus technique for, 18, 19
        in dynamic scanning, 20
        indications for, 17
        infusion of, 18, 19
        in kidney studies, 341–343
        in mediastinal studies, 68–70
        in pediatric applications, 519
        techniques in administration of, 17–20
    oral, 16–17

Contrast resolution, 6, 9
Coronal scans
    direct
        of kidney, 348
        of pelvis, 13, 393
    reformated, 5, 11–13
        of kidney, 348
        of mediastinum, 71
Costovertebral joints, 502
Cricoid cartilage, 41
Crohn's disease
    of colon, 337, 338
    of ileum, 326
Cryptorchidism, 404–405, 407, 532
    pelvic studies in, 23
Cushing's syndrome, 384–385
    adrenal cortical adenoma in, 383, 384, 385, 391
Cyst
    adrenal, 385, 388, 389
    of biliary tree, 204–206
    of bone, aneurysmal, 459, 473
    bronchogenic, 73
        in childhood, 521
    choledochal, 204–206
    of kidney, 346–352
    of liver, 183–185
    of mediastinum, 71–74
    mesenteric, 306
    neurenteric, 434
    of ovary, 402, 403
    pericardial, 72
    of spleen, 252–253
Cystadenocarcinoma of ovary, 404
Cystadenoma of ovary, 403, 404
Cystectomy, pelvic anatomy after, 405–409
Cystic tumors of pancreas, 221–225, 237
Cystitis, 394

D

Degenerative disease of lumbar spine, 415–430
Densitometry of bone, 512–515
Dermoid cysts of ovary, 403
Desmoid tumors
    of abdominal wall, 289
    mesenteric, 299
Dialysis patients, cystic renal disease in, 350
Diaphragmatic crura, 63, 68, 131, 132, 148
Diastematomyelia, 445, 447, 449
Direct coronary scans
    of kidney, 348
    of pelvis, 13, 393
Disc, intervertebral, 416, 417
    herniated, 418–426, see also Herniated intervertebral disc
Discitis, tuberculous, 504
Diverticulitis of colon, 337
Diverticulosis of sigmoid colon, 337
Diverticulum
    duodenal, 322, 323

gastric, 313, 314
  Zenker's, 76
Dose of radiation, 7
Douglas pouch, 290
  ascites in, 292
Drainage of abscesses, percutaneous, 31–34, 297
Dromedary hump in kidney, 346
Dual energy scanning, 9
Ductus deferens, 158, 159
Duodenitis, radiation, 326
Duodeno-jejunal flexure, 136
Duodenum, 144, 322–330
  adenocarcinoma of, 324
  in afferent loop syndrome, 329–330, 332
  anatomic variations in, 322
  carcinoid tumors of, 325
  diverticulum of, 322, 323
  hematoma of, 328, 329
  inflammatory disease of, 325–327
  leiomyoma of, 325
  leiomyosarcoma of, 324–325
  lipoma of, 325
  lymphoma of, 324, 325
  malrotation of, 322, 323
  metases to, 325
  normal anatomy of, 322–324
  obstruction of, 329–330
  trauma of, 329
  wall thickness of, 323
Dural sac, 416, 419
  deformity of, 419–420
Dynamic scanning, 11, 20
  of liver, 182
  mediastinal, 68
Dysraphism, spinal, 445

E

Echinococcal disease of liver, 186, 187
Economic utilization of CT, 562–564
Efficacy of CT, 564–565
Effusions
  in knee joint, 478
  pericardial, 121, 122, 123–124
    in childhood, 522
  pleural, 110, 117
    in pancreatitis, 546
Emboli, tumor, in mesentery, 303
Empyema, 119
  bronchopleural fistula with, 117
  epidural, 440
Endometrium, adenocarcinoma of, 399
Enteritis, radiation, 326
EOE-13, use of, 21, 191, 244
Epidural fat, 416, 419
  displacement of, 419
  in empyema, 440
Epigastric vessels, 153, 157
Epiglottis, 40

Esophagogastric junction, 131–134, 136, 312–313
  carcinoma of, 311
Esophagus, 57, 59, 307–312
  carcinoma of, 309–311, 312
    metastasis to adrenals, 388
  cervical, 307, 308
  duplication cyst of, 311
  gastroesophageal junction, 131–134, 136, 312–313
  inflammatory disease of, 311
  leiomyomas of, 311, 312
  normal anatomy of, 307–309
  thoracic, 307, 308
  varices of, 89, 190, 311–312
Ethiodized oil emulsion, 21, 191, 244
Ewing's sarcoma, 471
  in childhood, 534

F

Falciform ligament, 136, 138
Fat collections
  extrapleural, 111, 114
  mediastinal, 55, 71, 73
    paraspinal, 88
    retrocrural, 87
  perinephric, 147
Fat, epidural, 416, 419
  displacement of, 419
  in empyema, 440
Fat pad, pericardial, 72
Fatty infiltration
  of liver, 187–188
    in childhood, 531
  of pancreas, 213, 215, 234, 238
Fatty replacement of kidney, 368, 369
Fibrolipoma of spine, 433
Fibroma of kidney, 360, 362
Fibrosarcoma of soft tissue, 479, 480, 481
Fibrosis, retroperitoneal, 269, 270, 280
Field of view, 11
Fistula
  arteriovenous
    postliver biopsy, 189, 192
    renal, 360, 362
  bronchopleural, empyema with, 117
Foot vein infusions, and laminar flow phenomenon in inferior vena
    cava, 266, 267, 356
Foreign bodies in hip, 496
Fractures, see Trauma

G

Gallbladder, 140–142, 169, 170
  anomalous position of, 143
  carcinoma of, 204, 205
  diseases of, 202–204
Gallstones, 199, 200, 202–204

Gantries, 2
  tilt of, 11
Gastric lymph nodes, left
  in duodenal carcinoma, 324
  in esophageal carcinoma, 309
Gastrinoma, 224
Gastritis, hypertrophic, 322
Gastroesophageal junction, 131–134, 136, 312–313
  carcinoma of, 311
Gastrohepatic ligament, 133, 136
Gastrointestinal tract, see Alimentary tract
Gastrosplenic ligament, 133
Gerota's fascia, 147, 148
  in perirenal abscess, 372
  in renal cell carcinoma, 354
Glomerulonephritis, chronic, 373, 374
Goiters, thoracic, 74, 75, 76
Gonadal vessels, 150, 152
  enlargement of 261, 262, 270

H

Heart, 62
Hemangioma of liver, cavernous, 181, 182, 183, 184
Hematoma
  in abdominal wall, 288, 289
  adrenal, 390
  in duodenum, 328, 329
  hepatic, 189, 192
  in mesentery, 306
  perirenal, 372
    in childhood, 528, 529
  in psoas muscle, 284
  in soft tissue, 481, 483
    in childhood, 532
  splenic, 252, 253
Hemiazygous vein, 63, 68, 134, 136
Hemochromatosis, liver in, 188, 189
Hemorrhage
  adrenal, 389–390
  intestinal, 326
  perirenal, 372
    in childhood, 528, 529
  retroperitoneal, 280
  soft tissue, 480–481
    in childhood, 532
Hepatic arteries, 139, 170–171
  variations in 140, 141
Hepatic ducts, 138, 139, 141
Hepatic flexure of colon, 141, 143, 144, 330
  carcinoma of, 335
Hepatic veins, 169–170, 261
Hepatoblastoma, in childhood, 526
Hepatoma, 172–173, 178
  biliary obstruction in, 174
  calcifications in, 174
  portal vein in, 172

Hernia
  abdominal, 330
  femoral, 288
  hiatus, 308, 309
  inguinal, 287–288
  Spigelian, 287
  ventral, in abdominal wall, 287, 288
Herniated intervertebral disc, 418–426
  calcification of, 420–421, 422
  differential diagnosis of, 421–423
  dural sac deformity in, 419–420, 421, 424
  gas associated with, 421, 423
  myelography compared to CT in, 423–426
  nerve root sheath compression in, 420, 422
  pathogenesis of, 418
  posterior border deformity in, 419, 420, 423
  recurrent, 426
  and soft tissue density in extradural space, 419, 422
  vacuum phenomenon in, 421
High resolution scans, 3
Hip, 474, 486–489
  in adults, 490–491
  avascular necrosis of femoral head, 497
  in childhood, 488
  foreign bodies in, 496
  fracture of, 489, 492, 493, 494, 504
  osteoarthritis of, 495, 497
Histoplasmosis, adrenal glands in, 389
Hodgkin's disease
  kidney in, 359
  lymph nodes in, 271, 272–274
  spleen in, 250
  radiotherapy of, CT application in, 554–556
  thymus in, 94, 95
Horseshoe kidney, 344, 346
Hounsfield unit or number, 4, 5
Hydatid disease
  of kidney, 370
  of liver, 186, 187
Hydrocolpos, in childhood, 532
Hydromyelia, 434
Hydronephrosis, 372–373
Hyoid bone, 39
Hyperplasia
  adrenal, 383, 384
  of liver, focal nodular, 179–181
  of thymus, 93, 94, 95, 524
Hypertension, pulmonary arterial, 86

I

Ileocecal valve, lipoma of, 336, 337
Ileocolic intussusception, 329, 330, 338
Ileum, Crohn's disease of, 326
Iliac arteries, 153, 155, 156, 158
Iliac muscle, 155

Iliac veins, 153
  left external, enlarged, 394
Ilipsoas muscle, 155, 158, 283
  abscess of, 298
Ilium, 154
Image characteristics, 4–5
Image manipulation, 13–15
Infarction
  of kidney, 343, 345
  splenic, 254
Inguinal canal, 405, 406
  normal anatomy of, 158
Innominate artery, tortuous, 78
Intervals between scans, 10
Intervertebral disc, 416, 417
  herniated, 418–426; see also Herniated intervertebral disc
Intestines
  large, 330–339
  small, 322–330
Intussusception
  entero-enteric, 331
  ileocolic, 329, 330, 338
Iodinated intravenous contrast agents, 17–21
Ischemia
  colonic, 339 .
  renal, 373, 374
Islet cell tumors of pancreas, 221, 224

J

Jaundice, techniques in, 22
Jejunum
  in Whipple's disease, 326, 327
  in Zollinger-Ellison syndrome, 321, 326
Jugular veins, 43

K

Kidney, 341–375
  abscesses of, 367
    in childhood, 524
    perirenal, 368, 372
  acute focal bacterial nephritis of, 366
    in childhood, 524
  anatomic variations in, 344–345
  angiomyolipomas of, 350, 359–360, 362
    in childhood, 524, 526
  arteriovenous malformations of, 360, 362
  calcified masses in, 368–370
    cysts, 369
    indeterminate mass, 369, 370
    renal cell carcinoma, 369
    transitional cell carcinoma, 359
  calculi in
    radiolucent, 374
    staghorn, 368, 369
    urate, 357

carcinoma of
  adenocarcinoma, 352, 357
  adrenal metastasis of, 383
  hepatic metastasis of, 355
  hyperdense, 353
  inferior vena cava in, 355, 356
  laminar flow phenomenon in, 356
  lymph node metastases in, 354, 355
  nutcracker phenomenon in, 356
  recurrent, 357
  renal vein invasion in, 354, 356
  spinal metastasis of, 415
  transitional cell, 357–359, 360, 361
  tumor thrombus in, 355, 356
changes after nephrectomy, 345, 348
congenital anomalies of, 344–345
contrast media for, 341–343
  rapid bolus injection of, 342
  infusion of, 342
cystic disease of, 346–352
  in dialysis patients, 350
  hyperdense, 348, 350
  multicystic dysplastic, 352
  multilocular cystic nephroma, 352
  peripelvic/parapelvic, 349, 350
  polycystic disease, 349–350, 351, 525
  septated cyst, 540
  simple cysts, 346–349, 350
  in tuberous sclerosis, 350, 352
  in Von Hippel–Lindau disease, 350, 352
dromedary hump in, 346
duplex, 344, 347
evaluation of masses in, 342, 345–346
failure of, 372–373
fascia of, 147, 148, 149
fatty replacement of, 368, 369
fibroma of, 360, 362
filling defect in pelvis, 374–375
glomerulonephritis of, chronic, 373, 374
hematoma of, 371, 372, 374
hilus of, 145–149
horsehoe, 344, 346
hydatid disease of, 370
hydronephrosis of, 372–373
indeterminate masses in, 363–366
  calcified, 369, 370
indications for CT of, 342
infarction of, 343, 345
inflammatory masses in, 366–368
ischemia of, 373, 374
lymphoma of, 359, 361
nephrogram of, 343
  patchy, 343
  persistent, 372–373
normal anatomy of, 341, 343, 344
parenchymal disease in childhood, 532
perirenal and pararenal spaces, 149
  in pancreatic pseudocyst, 370, 371

Kidney (contd.)
  polycystic disease
    in adults, 349–350, 351
    in childhood, 525
  pyelogram of, 343
  pyelonephritis of
    acute, in childhood, 531, 532
    chronic atrophic, 373
    emphysematous, 367
    xanthogranulomatous, 366–368
  renal sinus lipomatosis, 345, 348
  splenomegaly affecting, 344, 347
  techniques for CT studies of, 22
  transplants of, 375
  trauma of, 371, 372, 373–374
    in childhood, 528, 529
  tumors of, 352–363
    in childhood, 523–524, 525, 526
    Wilms' tumor, 523–524, 525, 526
Kilovoltage, 9
Knee
  effusions in, 478
  muscles and tendons of, 474–475

L

Laminar flow phenomenon, in inferior vena cava, 266, 267, 356
Larynx, 37–53
  anatomic variations in, 41
  anterior commissure of, 42
  aryepiglottic fold in, 40
  arytenoid cartilages in, 42
  carcinoma of, 43–52
    in anterior commissure, 49
    applications of CT in, 51–52
    in aryepiglottic fold, 50
    cartilaginous invasion of, 46–48
    epiglottic, 44
    laryngography compared to CT in, 51
    limitations of CT in, 49–51
    in pyriform sinus, 47
    supraglottic, 44, 45, 50, 51
    transglottic, 45
    in vocal cords, 46, 48, 49
  cricoid cartilage in, 41
  epiglottis in, 40
  hyoid bone in, 39
  normal anatomy of, 37–43
  paralaryngeal space, 43
  posterior commissure of, 42
  pyriform sinus in, 40
  techniques for CT studies of, 25, 26, 37
  thyroid cartilages in, 40–41
  trauma of, 52–53
    in cricoid lamina, 52
    occult fracture in, 46, 48
    in thyroid lamina, 52

  vascular structures of, 43
  vestibule of, 43
  vocal cords in, 42–43
Leg muscles, 474–475
Leiomyoma
  of duodenum, 325
  of esophagus, 311, 312
Leiomyosarcoma
  of duodenum, 324–325
  retroperitoneal, 281, 282
  of stomach, 316, 318, 319
Leukemia, skeletal system in, 465, 467
Ligamentum teres, 138, 140
  fissure for, 139, 140, 168
Ligamentum venosum, fissure for, 136, 137
Lipoma
  of chest wall, 127
  of duodenum, 325
  of ileocecal valve, 336, 337
  mediastinal, 73, 76, 77
  mesenteric, 305, 306
  retroperitoneal, 281
  of soft tissue, 478, 480
Lipomatosis, renal sinus, 345, 348
Liposarcoma
  retroperitoneal, 281
  of soft tissue, 478–479, 480
Liver, 167–209
  abscess of, 185–186
    in childhood, 526, 527
  adenoma of, 179, 180
  arteries of, 138–139, 170–171
  caudate lobe of, 138, 169
    in cirrhosis, 189, 191, 197
  childhood diseases of, 531
  cirrhosis of, 186–187, 188–189
    caudate lobe in, 189, 191, 197
  cysts of, 183–185
  diffuse disease of, 186–189
  fatty infiltration of, 187–188
    in childhood, 531
  focal nodular hyperplasia of, 179–181
  hemangioma of, cavernous, 181, 182, 183, 184
  hematoma in, 189, 192
  in hemochromatosis, 188, 189
  hydatid disease of, 186, 187
  metastases to, 173–178, 179, 542
  normal anatomy of, 167–172
  parenchyma of, 171
    diseases of, 172–193
  postbiopsy arteriovenous fistula, 189, 192
  radiation injury to, 190–191
  regenerating nodules in, 189
  in renal cell carcinoma, 355, 356
  techniques for CT studies of, 22, 167
    in jaundiced patients, 22
  trauma of, 189–190
  tumors of, 172–183
    benign, 178–183

in childhood, 525–526
  malignant, 172–173
  volume measurement of, 192–193
venous systems of, 169–170
volume measurement of, 192–193
Lumbar nerve plexus, 151
Lumbar spine, degenerative disease of, 415–430
Lumbar vessels, 151, 152
Lungs, 57, 65, 99–114
  abscess of, 118, 119, 120
  atelectasis of, round, 115, 118
  blood flow in, 66
  in bronchiectasis, 104, 107
  bullae in, 103, 106, 107
  carcinoma of, 86, 104, 105, 106, 107–114, 120
    adrenals in, 112–113
    chest wall invasion of, 109
    hepatic metastasis of, 178
    hilar lymph node involvement in, 111
    in left hilum, 87
    mediastinal lymph nodes in, 109, 110, 113
    mediastinal vessels in, 108
    radiotherapy of, CT application in, 553
    in right hilum, 86
    spinal metastasis of, 435
  density affected by diseases, 106
  hilum of, 88
    enlarged, 86
    lymph node involvement in bronchogenic carcinoma, 111
    normal anatomy of, 57, 85
  interlobar fissures in, 66
  metastases to
    in childhood, 521–522
    occult, 101, 102–106
  nodules detected in, 102–106
  occult processes in, 106–107
  parenchymal disease differentiated from pleural disease,
      119–121
  in pediatric patients, 521–522
  pneumothorax space in, 111
  postpneumonectomy space in, 119, 120, 121–122
  in radiation fibrosis, paramediastinal, 104, 107
  sequestration in childhood, 522, 524
  solitary nodule in, 99–102
    calcified, 99, 100
    partial volume effect in, 99, 100
    thin collimated scan of, 99, 100
  techniques for CT studies of, 24
Lymph nodes
  in aortopulmonary window, 92
  celiac, in esophageal carcinoma, 309
  gastric, left
    in duodenal carcinoma, 324
    in esophageal carcinoma, 309
  iliac, in bladder cancer, 395
  mediastinal, 56–57, 63, 68, 77
    in bronchogenic carcinoma, 109, 110, 113
    calcified, 64
    enlargement of, 69, 79, 80

in esophageal carcinoma, 309
    retrocrural adenopathy of, 88
  pelvic, 161, 393
    in bladder cancer, 395
    bladder compression from, 401
    in prostatic cancer, 397
  periaortic and pericaval, 150–151, 153, 267–280
  pericardial, 72
    adenopathy of, 80
  retrocrural
    adenopathy of, 88
    in esophageal carcinoma, 309
  retroperitoneal, 267–280; see also Retroperitoneum,
      lymph nodes of
Lymphangiography
  in lymphomas, 270–275
  in testicular tumors, 278
Lymphomas
  abdominal, 545
  abdominal wall in, 290
  biliary obstruction in, 196, 199
  Burkitt's, 528
  in childhood, 527–528
  of colon, 336
  of duodenum, 324, 325
  gastric, 272, 314, 317, 318
  hepatic, 178, 272
  Hodgkin's, see Hodgkin's disease
  mediastinal, 78
    in childhood, 521
  mesentery in, 304
  musculoskeletal, 465, 468
  pancreas in, 225, 226
  peritoneum in, 304
  psoas muscle in, 284
  radiotherapy of, CT application in, 554–556
  renal, 272, 359, 361
  retroperitoneal lymph nodes in, 270–275
  spleen in, 250–251, 272

M

Machine variables, 9–13
Macrodystrophia lipomatosa, 479
Mediastinum, 55–96
  cystic lesions of, 71–74
  fat collections in, 55, 71, 73
  lymph nodes of, see Lymph nodes, mediastinal
  masses in, 71–76
  occult disease detection in, 90–96
  paraspinal line widening in, 87, 88–90, 91
  parathyroid adenoma, 95–96
  in pediatric patients, 520–521
  techniques for CT studies of, 23, 24, 68–71
  thymus in, 90–95
  vasculature of, 55–56
    congenital anomalies of, 82–86
  widening of, 69, 76–88

Melanoma, metastatic, 176, 438
Meningioma, 435, 437
Mesenteric artery
    inferior, 150, 151
    superior, 144, 149
Mesenteric vein
    in colonic ischemia, 339
    superior, 144, 149, 151, 214, 217
Mesenteritis, retractile, 306
Mesentery, 149–151, 289
    cysts of, 306
    desmoid tumor of, 299
    hematomas in, 306
    lipoma of, 305, 306
    in lymphomas, 304
Mesothelioma
    peritoneal, 300
    pleural, malignant, 116, 119
Metrizamide, in spinal examinations, 430, 431, 432, 433, 434,
436, 438, 439, 440, 447, 448, 450
Milliamperage, 9–10
Morrison's pouch, 141, 144
    ascending colon in, 297
Musculoskeletal system, 453–515
    aneurysmal bone cyst, 459, 473
    biopsy of, CT-guided, 509–512, 513, 514, 515
    childhood disorders of, 534–535
    dystrophies of, 475
    fibrous dysplasia of bone, 460
    hip, 474, 486–489
    in leukemia, 465, 467
    metastases to, 466, 470, 511, 512
    osteodensitometry of, 512–515
    Paget's disease, 508–509
    pelvis, 484–487
    psuedotumors, 468, 473, 474
    ribs, 494, 502
    sacroiliac joint, 486, 487
    shoulder girdle, 489, 498
    skeletal neoplasms, 455–473; see also Bone tumors
    soft tissue diseases and masses, 473–483; see also Soft tissue
    sternum and sternoclavicular joint, 493–494, 499
    technique for CT studies of, 454–455
    trauma of, 502–508
Myasthenia gravis, in childhood, 521
Myelography
    in degenerative spinal stenosis, 430
    in disc herniation diagnosis, 423–426
Myelolipoma of adrenals, 388–389
Myeloma, bone lesions in, 466, 469

N

Needle biopsy, CT-guided, 21–31
    needles in, 24–25
Nephritis, acute focal bacterial, 366
    in childhood, 524

Nephrograms, 343
    patchy, 343
    persistent, 372–373
Nephroma, multilocular cystic, 352
Neuroblastoma
    in childhood, 523, 524–525, 527
    in spinal canal, 439
Neurofibromatosis
    bone changes in, 468
    pseudotumor of, 474
Nucleus pulposus herniation, 418–426; see also Herniated
        intervertebral disc

O

Obstruction
    of biliary tract, 193–202
    of colon, 337–338
    of small bowel, 329–330
Oil emulsion, ethiodized, 21, 191, 244
Omentum, 289
    metastases to abdominal wall, 289, 290, 291, 400
Osteoarthritis of hip, 495, 497
Osteochondroma, 457, 459, 461, 462
Osteodensitometry, 512–515
Osteoma, osteoid, 459
Osteomyelitis, 502, 503, 504
    in childhood, 534
Osteosarcoma, 458, 464–465
    after Paget's disease, 509, 510
    central, 464, 465
    parosteal, 464, 466, 467
Ovary
    carcinoma of, 400–401
        abdominal wall metastasis of, 290, 291, 400
        duodenal metastasis of, 325
        hemorrhagic ascites with, 540
        hepatic and splenic metastasis of, 177
        peritoneal metastasis of, 300, 303
    cyst of, 402, 403
    cystadenocarcinoma of, 404
        metastatic, 176
    cystadenoma of, 403, 404
    dermoids of, 403
    in Stein-Leventhal syndrome, 160, 403
    tubo-ovarian abscess, 404, 405

P

Paget's disease of bone, 508–509
    transformation to osteosarcoma, 509, 510
Pancreas, 135, 213–240
    abscess in, 229–233, 234
    adenoma of
        macrocystic, 224, 225
        microcystic, 225, 226

atrophy of
  in carcinoma, 216, 219
  in chronic pancreatitis, 234
body of, 213, 214
carcinoma of, 215–221, 222, 223
  accuracy of CT in, 238
  ampullary, 220
  atrophy in, 216, 219
  biliary obstruction in, 195, 198, 199, 200
  in body, 219
  common bile duct dilatation in, 216, 220
  in head, 216, 219, 220
  hepatic metastasis of, 176, 542
  pancreatic duct dilatation in, 216, 220
  peripancreatic fat planes in, 217, 222
  in uncinate process, 216, 219, 221
  vascular encasement in, 220, 222, 223
childhood disorders of, 530
clinical applications of CT in, 238–240
cystic tumors of, 221–225, 237
extrapancreatic fluid collections, 227, 229, 232
fatty infiltration of, 213, 215, 234, 238
fluid collections in, 227, 229, 231
  in childhood, 530
focal mass in, 220, 234
  problems in CT diagnosis of, 239
head of, 142–145, 213, 214
  vascular anatomy of, 148
islet cell tumors of, 221, 224
in lymphomas, 225, 226
neck of, 214
normal anatomy of, 213–215
phlegmon in, 229, 231, 232
pseudocyst of, 216, 221, 225, 231
  in chronic pancreatitis, 235–237
  pararenal space in, 370, 371
  spleen in, 252
pseydotumors of, 215, 218, 219
retention cysts of, 237
tail of, 213, 214, 217
techniques for CT studies of, 22
  in jaundiced patient, 22
trauma of, 237
tumors of, 215–221
uncinate process of, 146, 147, 214, 218
  neoplasms of, 216, 219, 221
Pancreatic duct, 147, 171, 214
dilatation of, 196, 213
  in carcinoma of pancreas, 220
  in chronic pancreatitis, 234–235
Pancreatitis
acute, 225–234
  accuracy of CT in, 238
  anterior pararenal space in, 227, 231, 232, 233
  in childhood, 530
  focal mass in, 220
  lesser sac in, 227, 232, 233
chronic, 194, 234–237

  accuracy of CT in, 238
  focal mass in, 220, 234
colon in, 334
focal, 225, 228
henorrhagic, 234
pleural effusion in, 546
stomach in, 320
traumatic, 237
Pancreatography, endoscopic retrograde, 239
Parathyroid gland, 95–96
Partial volume effect, 5, 15, 99, 100, 171
Patient variables, 15
Pediatric patients, 519–535
abdomen in, 522–532
  abscess of, 528
  trauma of, 528–530
adrenal masses in, 524–525
aneurysms in, 532
bronchogenic cyst in, 521
chest in, 520–522
comparative imaging in, 526–527
extrapancreatic fluid collections in, 529, 530
hip in, normal, 488
liver disease in, 531
liver tumors in, 525–526
lungs in, 521–522
  sequestration of, 522, 524
lymphomas in, 527–528
mediastinum in, 520–521
musculoskeletal disorders in, 534–535
myasthenia gravis in, 521
neuroblastoma in, 523, 524–525, 527
osteoomyelitis in, 534
pancreatic disorders in, 530
pelvic pathology in, 532–534
renal masses in, 523–524
renal parenchymal disease in, 532
techinques for CT studies of, 519–520
thymus in, 521
  hyperplasia of, 521
tuberous sclerosis in, 524, 526
Pelvic lymph nodes, 161, 393
in bladder cancer, 395
bladder compression from, 401
in prostatic cancer, 397
Pelvis, 393–411
bladder tumors, 394–397
childhood pathology of, 532–534
fractures of, 489, 492, 493, 504, 505, 506
inlet of, 152–154
female, 153–154
male, 152–153
osseous anatomy of, 484, 485
ovarian tumors, 400–404
postoperative assessment of, 405–411
  after abdominoperineal resection, 409–411
  after cystectomy, 405–409
presacral masses, 401–402

Pelvis *(contd.)*
  prostatic cancer, 396, 397
  soft tissue anatomy of, 484–487
  techniques for CT studies of, 21, 23
    in undescended testicle, 23
  trauma in childhood, 534
  tubo-ovarian abscess, 404
  undescended testis, 404–405, 407, 532
  uterine tumors, 399–400, 402
    cervical, 397–399
Performance of CT devices, 6–7
Pericardial effusions, 121, 122, 123–124
  in childhood, 522
Pericardial fat pad, 72
Pericardial lymph nodes, 72
  adenopathy of, 80
Pericarditis, constrictive, 90, 125
Pericardium, 62, 122–126
  congenital absence of, 122–123
  cyst of, 72
  metastases to, 126
  thickening of, 124–126
Perineum, 164–165
  female, 164–165
  male, 163, 164
Peritoneal cavity, 289–306
  abscess in, 292, 299
  cerebrospinal fluid in, 296
  folds connecting structures in, 289, 291
  intraperitoneal fluid, 290–291
  in lymphomas, 304
  metastases to, 299–303
    direct spread of, 301–302
    embolic, 303
    intraperitoneal seeding of, 302, 303
    lymphatic dissemination of, 302–303
  necrotic neoplasms in, 293, 295, 296
  normal anatomy of, 289–292
  pseudomyxoma peritonei, 301, 302
  tumors of, 299
Peritoneal space
  at gallbladder fossa, 144
  at gastroesophageal junction, 133
  at porta hepatis, 138
  at splenic hilus, 136
Phantoms, imaging of, 538–539
Pheochromocytoma, 386–387
Phlegmon, pancreatic, 229, 231, 232
Photopenia artifact, 10
Physical basis for computed tomography, 1–2, 537–541
Pixels, 4
  determination of size, 11
Plasmacytoma, bone lesions in, 466, 469, 472
Pleura, 114–122
  confirmation of disease in, 117–119
  effusions in, 110, 117
    in pancreatitis, 546
  lesions differentiated from parenchymal lung disease, 119–121
  in mesothelioma, malignant, 116, 119

  plaques in, 114, 117–118
  in round atelectasis, 115, 118
Pneumonitis, in childhood, 522
Pneumothorax, 111
Porta hepatis, 137–140
  metastasis, in childhood, 531
Portable units for imaging, 546
Portal vein, 138, 143, 169–170, 214
  in colonic ischemia, 339
  in hepatoma, 172
  thrombosis by tumor, 175
Positioning of patient, 15
Presacral masses, 401–402
  teratoma in childhood, 532, 533
Proctitis, 337
  radiation, 338
Prostate, 162
  carcinoma of, 396, 397
    metastatic, 269
    radiotherapy of, CT application in, 553
    recurrent, 398
Pseudoaneurysm
  after femoral popliteal bypass graft, 541
  of aorta, 258, 260, 269
Pseudocyst of pancreas, 216, 221, 225, 231
  in chronic pancreatitis, 235–237
  pararenal space in, 370, 371
  spleen in, 252
Pseudomyxoma peritonei, 301, 302
Pseudotumor
  abdominal or pelvic, 16
  adrenal, 380–382
  of pancreas, 215, 218, 219
  of skeleton, 468, 473, 474
  splenic, 380, 382
  of stomach, 313, 382
Psoas muscles, 149–150, 153, 155, 283–285, 474
  abscess of, 284, 294
  atrophy of, 284
  hematoma in, 284
  in lymphomas, 284
  minor, 148, 150, 283
Pulmonary arteries, 55, 57, 60, 61, 70
  dilatation of, 81
    in hypertension, 86
  right, 85
    measurement of diameter, 88
  in transposition of great vessels, 85
Pulmonary outflow tract, dilatation of, 81
Pulmonary veins, 57
  inferior, 62
  superior, 59, 85
Pyelograms, 343
Pyelonephritis
  acute, in childhood, 531, 532
  chronic atrophic, 373
  emphysematous, 367
  xanthogranulomatous, 366–368
Pyonephrosis, 372

Pyopneumothorax, compared to lung abscess, 119–120
Pyriform sinus, 40
Pyriformis muscles, 153, 156, 158

R

Radiation dose, 7
 determining factors in, 10–11
Radiation exposure, 7
Radiation injury
 of colon, 338–339
 duodenitis in, 326
 of liver, 190–191
 paramediastinal fibrosis in, 104, 107
 proctitis in, 338
Radiograph, computed, 11
Radionuclide imaging
 accuracy of, 547–548
 adrenal, 391
 advantages and disadvantages of, 541–547
 physical basis for, 537–541
 portable units for, 546
Radiotherapy and CT applications, 549–558
 in bladder carcinoma, 553–554
 in bronchogenic carcinoma, 553
 dose computation in, 553
 dose-limiting structures in, 550, 551
 inhomogeneity corrections in, 553
 parameters determined by CT information, 553
 in prostatic cancer, 554
 target volume in, 550
 technical considerations in, 550–553
 treatment planning in, 549–550, 552, 556
 treatment volume in, 549–550, 552, 556
 and tumor extent related to tumor mass, 549–550
Rectum
 abdominoperineal resection of, 409–411
 carcinoma of, 332, 333, 335
  recurrent, 334, 409, 411
Reformated sagittal or coronal images, 5, 11–13
 of kidney, 348
 of mediastinum, 71
Reidel's lobe, 167
Renal arteries, 145, 341, 343
Renal veins, 145, 261, 341, 343
 invasion by renal cell carcinoma, 354, 356
 left
  circumaortic, 263
  retroaortic, 264
  thrombosis of, 267
Resolution
 in comparative imaging, 542
 contrast, 6, 9
 spatial, 6, 9, 542
 temporal, 6–7
Retrocrural lymph nodes
 adenopathy of, 88
 in esophageal carcinoma, 309

Retrocrural space, 134, 135
Retroperitoneum, 257–285
 abdominal aorta, 257–261
 fibrosis of, 269, 270, 280
 hemorrhage in, 280
 leiomyosarcoma of, 281, 282
 lipoma of, 281
 liposarcoma of, 281
 lymph nodes of, 267–280
  fibrolipomatous changes in, 268
  in lymphomas, 270–275, 305
  in metastatic disease, 269
  in renal cell carcinoma, 354, 355–356
  in testicular tumors, 275–279
  in Whipple's disease, 270
 normal anatomy of, 258
 psoas muscles, 283–285
 sarcoma of, 281, 282
 techniques for CT studies of, 21
 tumors of, 280–283
 vena cava, inferior, 261–267
Ribs, 494, 502
Rotate-rotate configuration, 2, 3
Rotate stationary detector array, 2, 3
Round ligament of uterus, 159, 160

S

Sacroiliac joint, 486, 487
Sacroiliitis, 486, 488
Sagittal image
 direct
  of kidney, 348
  of pelvis, 13, 393
 reformated, 5, 11-13
  of kidney, 348
  of mediastinum, 71
Saphenous vein, greater, 164
Sarcoma
 chondrosarcoma, 457, 458, 463, 482, 486
 Ewing's, 471
  in childhood, 534
 fibrosarcoma, 479, 480, 481
 liposarcoma, 478–479, 480
 osteosarcoma, 458, 464–465, 466, 467
 radiotherapy of, CT application in, 556–557
 retroperitoneal, 281, 282
 soft tissue, 481
 of spleen, 251, 252
Schwannoma, soft tissue, 479, 481
Sciatic nerve, 164
Sclerosis, tuberous
 in childhood, 524, 526
 kidney in, 350, 352
Seminal vesicles, 157, 159
Seminomas, 275
Seroma, poltsplenectomy, 296
Shoulder girdle, 489, 498

Size determinations, for objects on display, 14–15
Skeletal tumors, 455–473; *see also* Bone tumors
Soft tissue
  fibrosarcoma of, 479, 480, 481
  hematoma in, 481, 483
  hemorrhage into, 480–481
  lipoma of, 478, 480
  liposarcoma of, 478–479, 480
  normal anatomy of, 473–475, 476–477
  sarcoma of, 481
  schwannoma of, 479, 481
  tumors of, 478–480
    in childhood, 534
Sonography; *see* Ultrasonography
Spatial resolution in CT, 6, 9, 542
Speed of scanning, 10
Spermatic cords, 161, 162, 405, 406
Spinal cord, tethered, 445, 448, 449
Spine, 415–449
  congenital anomalies of, 445–450
  diastematomyelia of, 445, 447, 449
  discitis, tuberculous, 504
  dural sac, 416, 419
    deformity of, 419–420
  dysraphism of, 445
  epidural empyema of, 440
  epidural fat, 416, 419
    displacement of, 419
    in empyema, 440
  fibrolipoma of, 433
  hydromyelia of, 434
  hypertrophic neuritis of, 435, 438
  intervertebral disc, 416, 417
    herniation of, 418–426; *see also* Herniated intervertebral disc
  intervertebral foramen, 416
  lumbar degenerative disease, 415–430
  meningioma of, 435, 437
  metastasis to, 422, 425, 435, 438, 439
  nerve root sheath in, 418
    compression and displacement of, 420
    conjoined anomaly of, 422–423, 425
    in degeneration of posterior articular joints, 426–427
    neurofibroma of, 425
  neurenteric cyst of, 434
  neuroblastoma of, 439
  normal anatomy of, 415–518, 419
  paraspinal muscles, 475
  posterior articular joints of, 416
    degeneration of, 426–427
  spondylolisthesis of, 429
  stenosis of
    central, 428
    degenerative, 428–430
    foraminal, 430
    idiopathic developmental, 427–428
    lateral, 428–430
  superior articular processes of, 418
  syringomyelia of, 434, 435, 449–450

  trauma of, 436–444
    cervical, 441–443, 444
    in childhood, 534
    fractures, 440, 441, 442, 443, 444, 445, 446, 447
    gunshot injury, 447
    thoracolumbar, 443–445
  tumors of, 430–436
    extradural, 436
    extramedullary, intradural, 435–436
    intramedullary, 433–435
Spleen, 243–255
  abscess of, 252
  acessory, 248
  anatomic variations in, 245–248
  calcified granulomata in, 251–252
  cysts of, 252–253
  displacement of
    affecting stomach, 321
    postoperative, 246, 247
  enlargement of, 248–249, 250
    renal displacement in, 344, 347
  hematoma of, 252, 253
  hilus of, 134–137, 243
  infarction of, 254
  inflammatory disease of, 251–252
  in lymphomas, 250–251
  metastases to, 177, 251
  normal anatomy of, 243–244
  parenchyma of, 244
  polysplenia, 248
  pseudotumors of, 380, 382
  sarcoma of, 251, 252
  techniques for CT studies of, 22
  trauma of, 253–254
  volume measurements of, 249
  wandering, 246–248
Splenic artery, 135, 243, 244
Splenic flexure of colon, carcinoma of, 335
Splenic vein, 135, 213–214, 216, 243, 244
Splenomegaly, 248–249, 250
  renal displacement in, 344, 347
Spondylitis, ankylosing
  of costovertebral joints, 502
  of hip, 497
  sacroiliac, 487, 488
Spondylolisthesis, 429
Stein-Leventhal syndrome, 160, 403
Sternum and sternoclavicular joint, 57, 493–494, 499
  infections of, 494, 501
  trauma of, 494, 500
  tumors of, 494, 501
Stomach, 312–322
  carcinoma of, 314, 315, 316
    recurrent, 320
  diverticulum of, 313, 314
  esophagogastric junction, 131–134, 136, 312–313
  hypertrophic gastritis of, 322
  inflamatory disease of, 318–322

leiomyosarcoma of, 316, 318, 319
lymphoma of, 314, 317, 318
metastases to, 320
normal anatomy of, 312–313
pseudotumor of, 313, 382
splenic displacement affecting, 321
wall thickness of, 312
in Zollinger-Ellison syndrome, 318, 321
Subclavian artery, aberrant, 84
Symphysis pubis, 159–164
female, 162, 164
male, 159–164
Syringomyelia, 434, 435, 449–450

T

Techniques for various regions, 21–24, 25
Temporal resolution, 6–7
Teratoma
mediastinal, 74
presacral, in childhood, 532, 533
Testis
tumors of
nodal metastasis of, 275–279
radiotherapy of, CT application in, 554
undescended, 404–405, 407, 532
pelvic studies in, 23
Thigh muscles, 474, 475
Thin collimated scan
of liver, 172
of pulmonary nodule, 99, 100
Thoracic duct, 63, 68
Thoracolumbar spine injuries, 443–445
Thorax, 55–96; see also Mediastinum
abscess in, 544
indication for CT of, 71–96
normal anatomy of, 55–68
in pediatric patients, 520–522
Thrombosis
of inferior vena cava, 266–267
tumoral
mesentery, 303
portal vein, 175
in renal cell carcinoma, 355, 356
Thymoma, 92, 93
Thymus, 59, 66, 67, 68, 90–95
in Hodgkin's disease, 94, 95
hyperplasia of, 93, 94, 95, 524
in pediatric patients, 521
teratoma of, 74
Thyroid cartilages, 40–41
Thyroid gland, 56
mediastinal, 74
Tibia, fracture of, incomplete union of, 507
Trachea, 56
Transplanted kidney, 375
Transposition of great vessels, 85

Trauma
abdominal, in childhood, 528–530
of duodenum, 329
of hip, 489, 492, 493, 494
of kidney, 371, 372, 373–374
in childhood, 528, 529
of larynx, 52–53
of liver, 189–190
skeletal, 502–508
of spine, 436–444
of spleen, 253–254
of sternoclavicular joint, 494, 500
Tuberous sclerosis
in childhood, 524, 526
kidney in, 350, 352
Tubo–ovarian abscess, 404, 405
Tumors; see also Carcinoma and other specific tumors
abdominal, in childhood, 523–526
of abdominal wall, 288–289
adrenal, 385–388
in childhood, 524–525
of bladder, 394–397
breast carcinoma, 125, 126, 128
bronchogenic carcinoma, 86, 104, 105, 106, 107–114
chest wall masses, 124, 125, 126–128
cholangiocarcinoma, 196, 202
of colon, 330–336
of duodenum, 324–325
of esophagus, 309–311
extent of, related to tumor mass, 549–550
of kidney, 352–363
in childhood, 523–524, 525, 526
of liver, 172–183
in childhood, 525–526
mesothelioma
peritoneal, 330
pleural, malignant, 116, 119
of pancreas, 215–221
pericardial, 126
of peritoneum, 299
radiotherapy of, see Radiotherapy and CT applications
retroperitoneal, 280–283
skeletal, 455–473
of soft tissue, 478–480
in childhood, 534
of spine, 430–436
of sternoclavicular joint, 494, 501
of stomach, 313–318
thrombosis in; see Thrombosis, tumoral
of thymus, 92, 93, 94, 95

U

Ultrasonography
accuracy of, 547–548
adrenal, 391
advantages and disadvantages of, 541–547

Ultrasonography *(contd.)*
  physical basis for, 537–541
  portable units for, 546
Umbilical artery, 158
Unbilical vein, 138
Uncinate process of pancreas, 214, 218
  neoplasms of, 216, 219, 221
Ureter
  circumcaval, 265–266
  periureteral vessels, 153
Urinoma, 372, 374
Uterus, 158, 160
  carcinoma of, 399–400
  cervical carcinoma, 397–399
    recurrent, 399
  leiomyosarcoma metastasis to mesentery, 303
  myoma of, calcified, 402

V

Vagina, 164
Varices, esophageal, 89, 190, 311–312
Vas deferens, 158, 159
Vater papilla, 144
Vena cava
  inferior, 62, 261–67
    anatomic variations in, 261–266
    azygous continuation of, 89, 262–263, 264
    bifurcation of, 151, 154
    circumcaval ureter, 265–266
    duplication of, 264–265, 266
    laminar flow phenomenon in, 266, 267, 356
    normal anatomy of, 261

pericaval lymph nodes, 267–280
    pseudothrombus in, 266, 267
    in renal cell carcinoma, 355, 356
    thrombosis of, 266–267
    transposition of, 264, 265
  superior, 56, 70
    artifact in, 71
Venous sampling, adrenal, 391–392
Ventricles, cardiac, 62
  interventricular septum, 62
Vertebrae; *see* Spine
Vocal cords
  false, 43
  true, 42–43
Von-Hippel–Lindau disease, kidney in, 350, 352
Voxel, 5

W

Whipple's disease, 326, 327
  retroperitoneal lymph nodes in, 270
Wilms' tumor, 523–524, 525, 526
Window level, 5, 13–14
Window width, 5, 13–14
Winslow foramen, 138

Z

Zenker's diverticulum, 76
Zollinger-Ellison syndrome, 225
  jejunum in, 321, 326
  stomach in, 318, 321